Self-Assessment and Review of MICROBIOLOGY AND IMMUNOLOGY

Self-Assessment and Review of MICROBIOLOGY AND IMMUNOLOGY

14th Edition

Rachna Chaurasia MD (Radiodiagnosis)
Professor
MLB Medical College, Jhansi, India
(Ex-Registrar, Indraprastha Apollo Hospital, New Delhi)

Anshul Jain MD (Anaesthesia)
Professor
MLB Medical College, Jhansi, India
(Ex-Senior Resident, Anaesthesiology, AIIMS, New Delhi)

Edited by
Suman P Singh MBBS MD (Microbiology)
Professor
Department of Microbiology, Pramukhswami Medical College and
HM Patel Centre for Medical Care and Education,
Karamsad, Anand, Gujarat, India

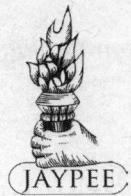

JAYPEE BROTHERS MEDICAL PUBLISHERS
The Health Sciences Publisher
New Delhi | London | Panama

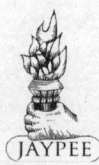
Jaypee Brothers Medical Publishers (P) Ltd

Headquarters
Jaypee Brothers Medical Publishers (P) Ltd
4838/24, Ansari Road, Daryaganj
New Delhi 110 002, India
Phone: +91-11-43574357
Fax: +91-11-43574314
Email: jaypee@jaypeebrothers.com

Overseas Offices

J.P. Medical Ltd
83, Victoria Street, London
SW1H 0HW (UK)
Phone: +44 20 3170 8910
Fax: +44 (0)20 3008 6180
E-mail: info@jpmedpub.com

Jaypee-Highlights Medical Publishers Inc
City of Knowledge, Bld. 235, 2nd Floor, Clayton
Panama City, Panama
Phone: +1 507-301-0496
Fax: +1 507-301-0499
E-mail: cservice@jphmedical.com

Jaypee Brothers Medical Publishers (P) Ltd
Bhotahity, Kathmandu, Nepal
Phone: +977-9741283608
E-mail: kathmandu@jaypeebrothers.com

Website: www.jaypeebrothers.com
Website: www.jaypeedigital.com

© 2019, Jaypee Brothers Medical Publishers

The views and opinions expressed in this book are solely those of the original contributor(s)/author(s) and do not necessarily represent those of editor(s) of the book.

All rights reserved. No part of this publication may be reproduced, stored or transmitted in any form or by any means, electronic, mechanical, photocopying, recording or otherwise, without the prior permission in writing of the publishers.

All brand names and product names used in this book are trade names, service marks, trademarks or registered trademarks of their respective owners. The publisher is not associated with any product or vendor mentioned in this book.

Medical knowledge and practice change constantly. This book is designed to provide accurate, authoritative information about the subject matter in question. However, readers are advised to check the most current information available on procedures included and check information from the manufacturer of each product to be administered, to verify the recommended dose, formula, method and duration of administration, adverse effects and contraindications. It is the responsibility of the practitioner to take all appropriate safety precautions. Neither the publisher nor the author(s)/editor(s) assume any liability for any injury and/ or damage to persons or property arising from or related to use of material in this book.

This book is sold on the understanding that the publisher is not engaged in providing professional medical services. If such advice or services are required, the services of a competent medical professional should be sought.

Every effort has been made where necessary to contact holders of copyright to obtain permission to reproduce copyright material. If any have been inadvertently overlooked, the publisher will be pleased to make the necessary arrangements at the first opportunity. The **CD/DVD-ROM** (if any) provided in the sealed envelope with this book is complimentary and free of cost. **Not meant for sale.**

Inquiries for bulk sales may be solicited at: jaypee@jaypeebrothers.com

Self-Assessment and Review of Microbiology and Immunology

Tenth Edition: 2015
Eleventh Edition: 2016
Twelfth Edition: 2017
Thirteenth Edition: 2018
Fourteenth Edition: **2019**

ISBN: 978-93-5270-933-5

Printed at: Rajkamal Electric Press, Plot No. 2, Phase-IV, Kundli, Haryana.

> **Dedicated to**
>
> *Our family members, teachers
> and above all God
> who created us*

Preface

"First of all we want to thank all of the readers for their immense support—the key of success."

The overwhelming success of the previous edition has encouraged us to carry this 14th edition a step ahead to revise and update the book, so as to match the pace of present PGMEE requirement of this difficult subject.

PGMEE is a battlefield in which everyone fights for success but only few succeed because only a few know the correct use of

weapon of "Knowledge, hard work and guidance".

So, guys learn the golden words:

"You cannot cross the sea merely by standing and staring at the water, you need to take the plunge"

Why this book is different?
- This book provides important points of each topic in continuous manner not in parts as given in previous guides.
- This book consists of theory of each topic followed by its questions so theory portion helps you to solve new questions.
- This pattern of book allows you to revise whole infectious diseases very clearly and quickly.
- This book provides sufficient matter which can be revised without any problem.

Always keep one thing in your mind:

There's one thing, we cannot recycle and that's wasted time, so guys !

"Schedule a daily time for relaxing, reflecting, planning and brainstorming."

Rachna Chaurasia
Anshul Jain

Acknowledgements

"To Bhagwan Mahavir and Ganesha whose blessing made our goal possible"

We are extremely grateful and obliged to :
Prof KK Gupta (Professor Endocrinology, Director General Medical Education, Uttar Pradesh
Prof Sadhna Kaushik (Principal, MLB Medical College, Jhansi)
Prof Ganesh Kumar (Principal BRD Medical College Gorakhpur)
Prof NS Sengar (Professor, Nephrology, MLB Medical College, Jhansi)
Prof Anjan Tirika (Professor, Anaesthesiology, AIIMS New Delhi)
Prof Poonam Malhotra (Professor, Cardiac Anaesthesiology, AIIMS New Delhi)
Prof GK Aneja (Principal SN Medical College Agra)
Dr Chhavi (Additional Professor, Anaesthesia, AIIMS New Delhi)
We would always remain obliged to our lifelong teachers:
Dr BC Tiwari
Dr Atish Sharma and Mr Amod Yadav
We are extremely thankful to Mr Rajesh Kardam for his suggestions and encouragement.
We would be extremely thankful to Dr Vikas Chaurasia and Dr Gaurav Tiwari whose inspiration makes the task possible.
We are highly grateful to Dr Suman Singh for reviewing and updating the text.
We extend our sincere thanks and gratitude to our beloved family members for their encouragement and useful suggestions:

Father	:	Dr PC Chaurasia
Mother	:	Mrs Shakuntla Chaurasia
Uncle and Aunty	:	Mr Subhash Chandra Chaurasia and Mrs Rashmi Chaurasia
Brother and Bhabhi	:	Dr Vikas Chaurasia and Dr Mrs Anahita Chaurasia
		Mr Vishal Chaurasia and Mrs Kavita Chaurasia
Nephew and Niece	:	Priyanshu, Aashi and Paras

— **Rachna Chaurasia**

Father	:	Dr DB Jain
Mother	:	Mrs Saroj Jain
Sisters	:	Ayusha Jain and Ankita Jain
Brother	:	Mr Kapil Jain

— **Anshul Jain**

And above all to our little Riya and Ansh whose innocence empowers us in every moment

We offer cordial thanks to our colleagues for their support:
Dr Naveen Yadav, Fellow Anaesthesia, SGH Australia
Dr Dushyant Agarwal, Associate Professor Anatomy, AIIMS Jodhpur
Dr Apoorva Abhinandan Mittal, Associate Prof Anaesthesia, SN Medical College, Agra
Dr Deepak Singhal, Max Hospital, New Delhi
Dr Hazari M Shukla, Fortis Hospital, Delhi
Dr Mayank singh, Associate Professor, Pathology, MLB Medical College Jhansi
Dr Om Shankar Chaurasia, Associate Professor Pediatrics, MLB Medical college Jhansi
Dr Sachin Maheshwari
Dr Dushyant Agarwal
Dr Monika Agarwal

Dr Nidhi Singh
Dr Neha
Dr Anil Kumar Suryavanshi
Dr Preeti MD SPM

We cannot forget to acknowledge:
Mr Bishan Lal (Librarian, MLB Medical College, Jhansi) and All Staff.
Mr CP Lavania (Librarian, SN Medical College, Agra) and All Staff.

We would also like to acknowledge:
Mr Sandeep Tiwari
Mr Adeep Tiwari
Mr CP Lamba

We would also like to thank Mr Jitendar P Vij (Group Chairman), Mr Ankit Vij (Managing Director), Ms Chetna Malhotra Vohra (Associate Director—Content Strategy), Ms Payal Bharti (Senior Manager—Professional Publishing), and the complete production team of Jaypee Brothers Medical Publishers (P) Ltd, New Delhi, India.

Last but not least, most important we gratefully acknowledge all readers, who will act as a guide to improve and upgrade the content of this book.

From the Publisher's Desk
We request all the readers to provide us their valuable suggestions/errors (if any)
at: jppgmee@gmail.com
so as to help us in further improvement of this book in the subsequent edition.

How to use this book?

Read the theory first, then do the questions. You will realize that this way of learning makes topic easy-to-understand and easy-to- grasp for long-term memory.

Try to complete each topic in one sitting.

In the last, we would like to say all the best for your PGMEE preparation and hope you will work hard with positive attitude in your mind.

Salient features of this edition

- All NEET pattern questions with full explanations.
- Reference from latest edition of Harrison, Ananthanarayan.
- Older questions have been removed so as to make it more efficient.
- New AIIMS pattern questions and Index available online on *www.accesspgmee.com* & App.

Contents

Color Plates
(Important Images, Image-based Questions and Other Informative Images) — XVII

SECTION–A: REVISION AT A GLANCE

1. Basics of Bacteriology★★★★★ — 3
2. Basics of Virology★★★★★ — 10
3. Basics of Mycology★★★★★ — 14
4. Basics of Clinical Microbiology★★★★★ — 16
5. Culture and Sterilization★★★★ — 19
6. Bacterial Genetics★★★ — 34

SECTION–B: BACTERIOLOGY

Unit–I Bacteriology

Gram-positive Cocci
7. Staphylococci★★★★ — 45
8. Streptococci★★★★★ — 57

Gram-negative Cocci
9. Neisseria★★★ — 78

Gram-positive Bacilli
10. Clostridium★★★★★ — 88
11. Corynebacterium★★★★ — 102
12. Actinomycetes and Bacillus★★★ — 113
13. Listeria Monocytogenes★★★ — 126
14. Mycobacteria★★★★ — 132

Gram-negative Bacilli
15. Enterobacteriaceae★★★★ — 153
16. Vibrio★★★★ — 175
17. Pseudomonas and Yersinia★★★★ — 188

Gram-negative Bacilli and Cocco-bacilli
18. Hemophilus, Bordetella and Brucella★★★★ — 199
19. Campylobacter and Helicobacter★★★★ — 211
20. Legionella★★★★ — 219
21. Rickettsiae and Chlamydiae★★★★★ — 225

Others
22. Spirochetes★★★★★ — 241
23. Mycoplasma★★★★ — 257

Unit-II Virology

24. DNA Virus★★★★★ — 265
25. RNA Virus★★★★★ — 289
26. Slow Virus Disease★★★ — 323
27. Hepatitis Virus★★★★★ — 328
28. HIV and Other Retrovirus★★★★ — 344

Unit-III Mycology

29. Superficial and Subcutaneous Mycosis★★★ — 369
30. Yeast and Yeast-like Fungus★★★ — 374
31. Aspergillus and Mucormycosis★★★ — 385
32. Dimorphic Fungi★★★ — 392

Unit-IV Parasitology

33. Basics of Parasitology★★★★★ — 401
34. Protozoa★★★★★ — 408
35. Helminths★★★★★ — 438

Unit-V Immunology

36. Basics of Immune System★★★★ — 465
37. Antigen and Antibody★★★★ — 487
38. Hypersensitivity★★★★ — 508

Unit-VI Miscellaneous

39. Miscellaneous★★★ — 515

SECTION–C: EMERGING DISEASES

40. Swine Flu★★★ — 539
41. Zika Virus★★★ — 541

Most Important★★★★★
Very Important★★★★
Important★★★

COLOR PLATES

Important Images

Image-based Questions with Explanations

Other Informative Images

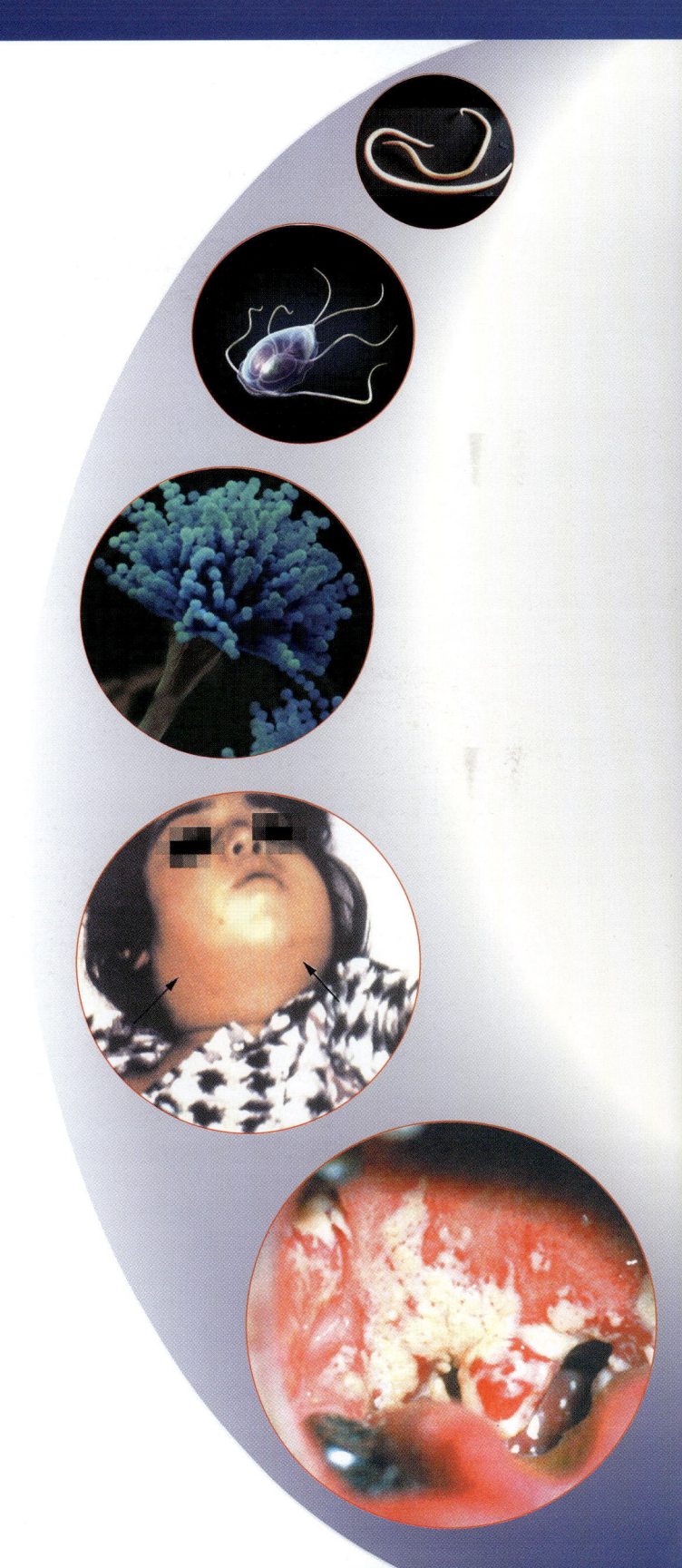

Important Images

Chapter 5 — Culture and Sterilization

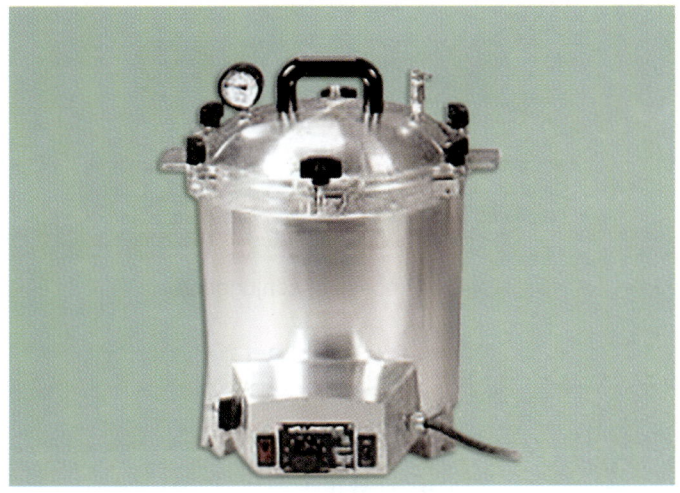

Fig. 1: Autoclave

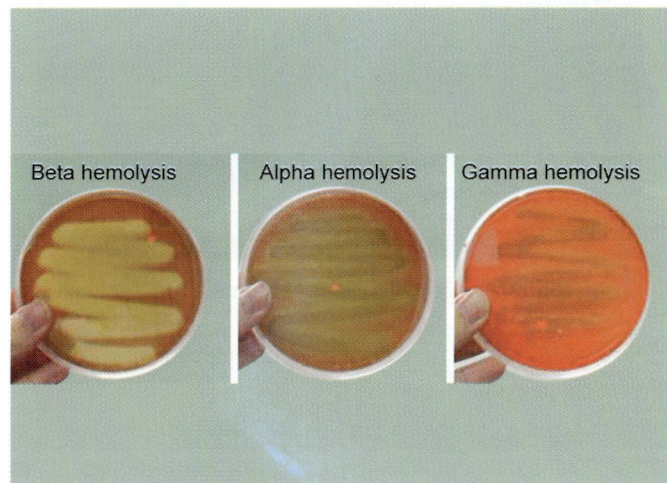

Fig. 2: Hemolysis on blood agar

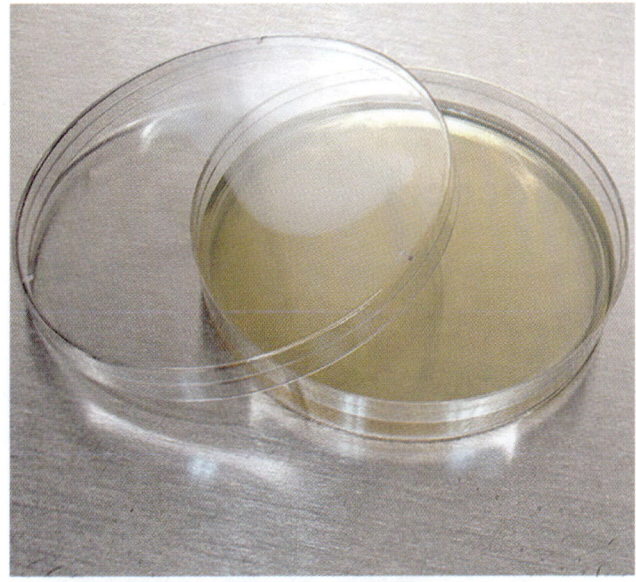

Fig. 3: Nutrient agar

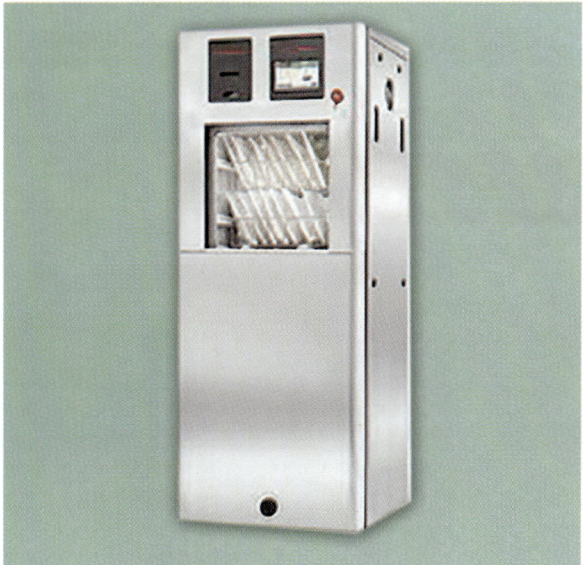

Fig. 4: Plasma sterilizer

Chapter 6 — Bacterial Genetics

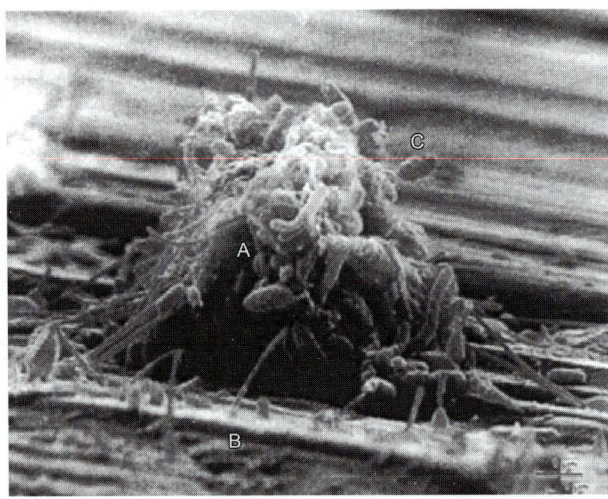

Fig. 5: Biofilm A biofilm B substratum C attached cell

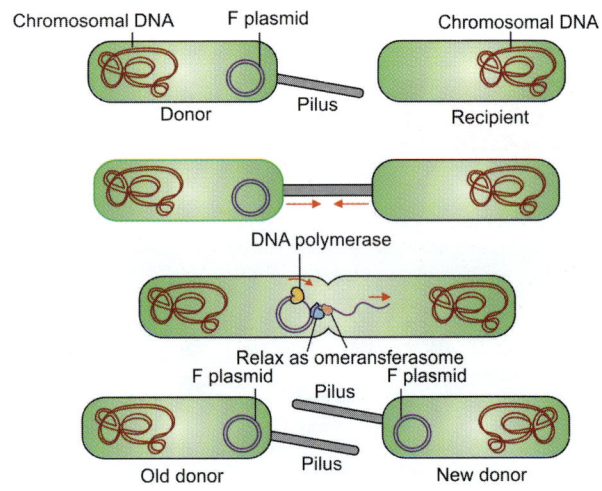

Fig. 6: Process of conjugation

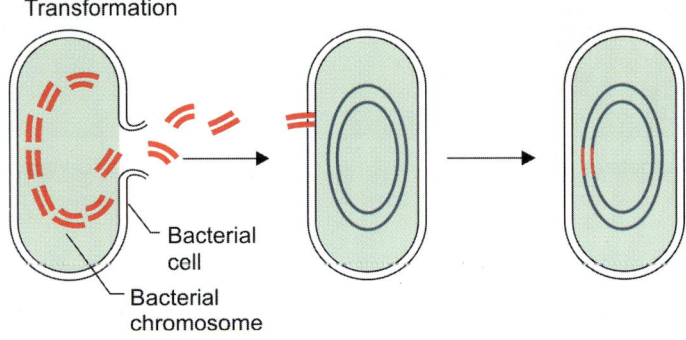

Fig. 7: Transformation

Chapter 7 — Staphylococci

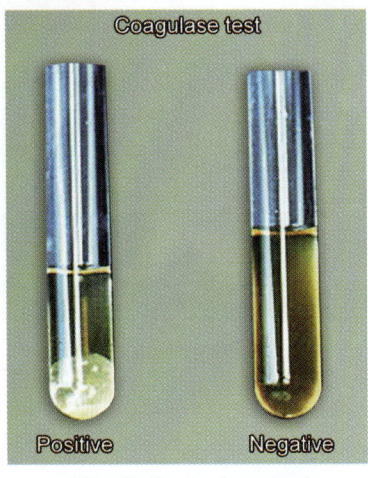

Fig. 8: Coagulase test

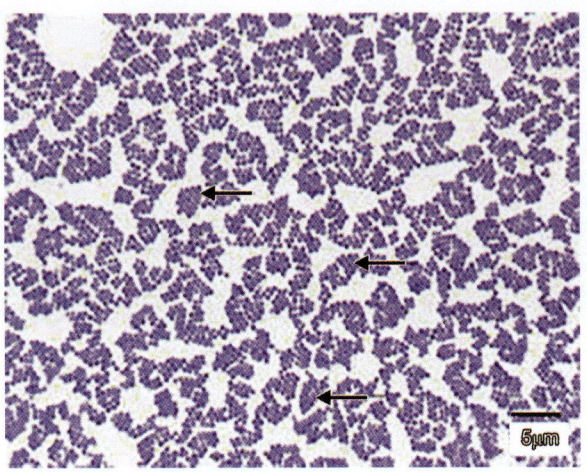

Fig. 9: Gram positive staph. aureus

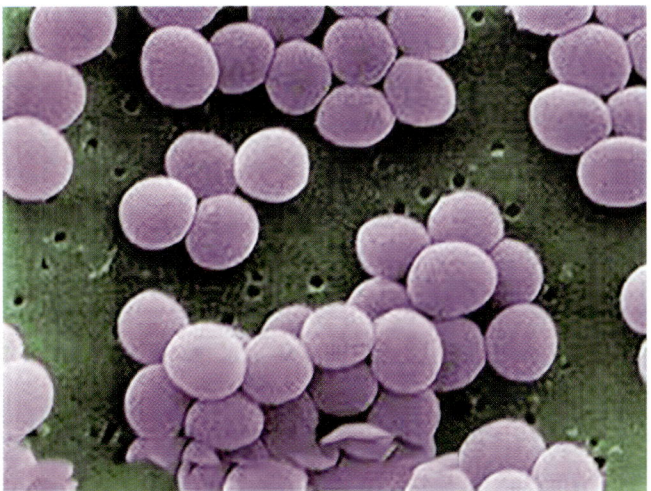

Fig. 10: Grape like pattern of staphylococci

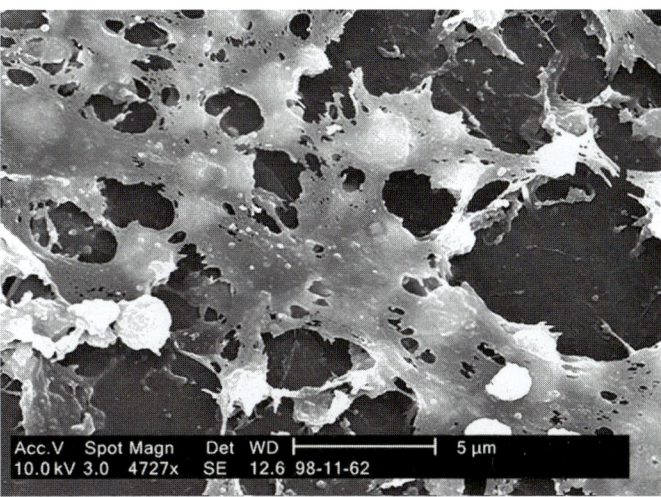

Fig. 11: Staph aureus in biofilm

Chapter 8 — Streptococci

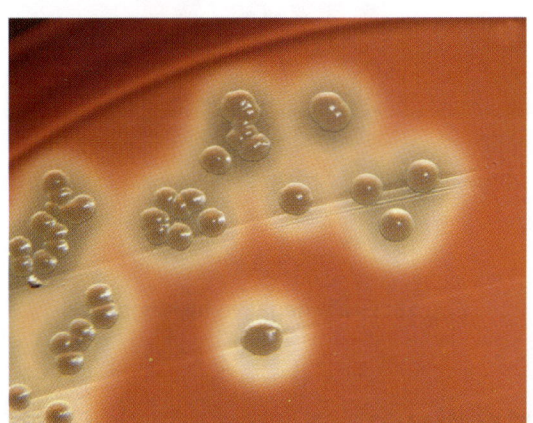

Fig. 12: Beta hemolysis of streptococci

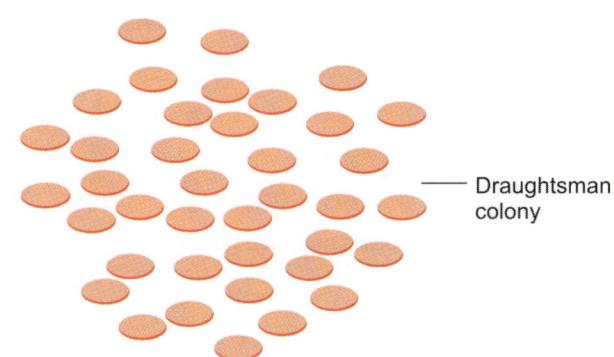

Fig. 13: Draughtsman colony of pneumococci

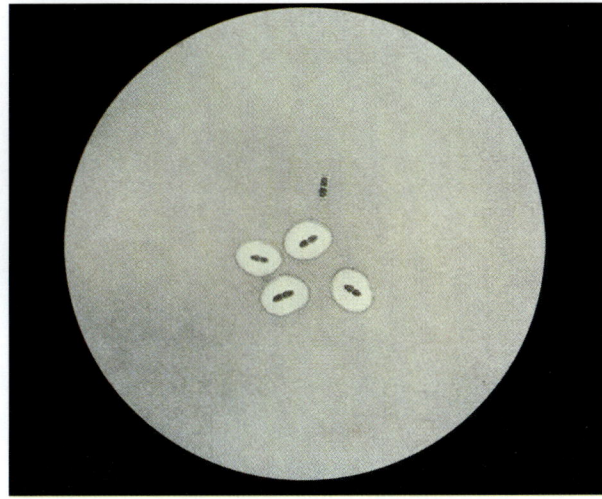

Fig. 14: Quellung test

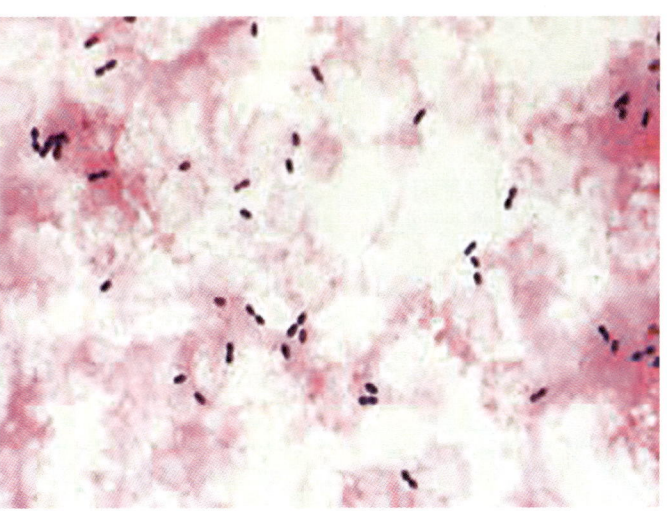

Fig. 15: Short chain of pneumococci

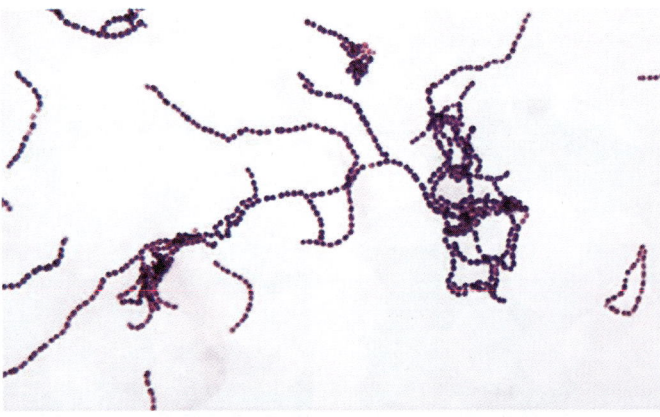

Fig. 16: Streptococci in chain

Chapter 9 — Neisseria

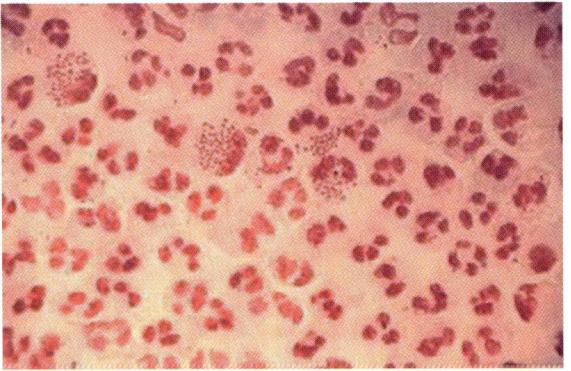

Fig. 17: Gram negative gonococci

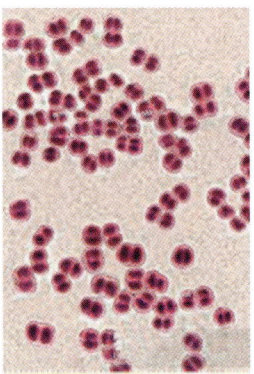

Fig. 18: Gram negative meningococci

Chapter 10 — Clostridium

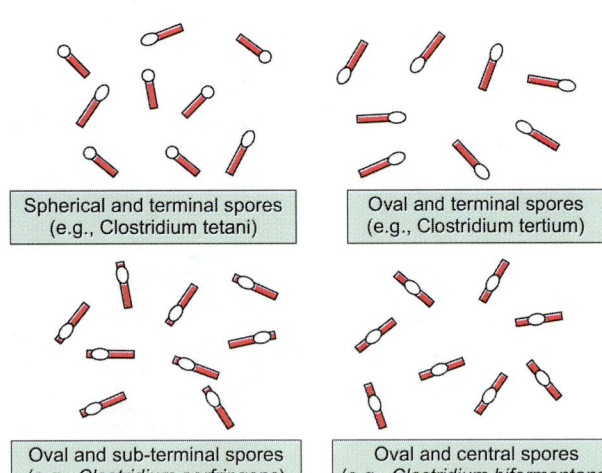

Fig. 19: Distribution of spores

- Spherical and terminal spores (e.g., Clostridium tetani)
- Oval and terminal spores (e.g., Clostridium tertium)
- Oval and sub-terminal spores (e.g., Clostridium perfringens)
- Oval and central spores (e.g., Clostridium bifermentans)

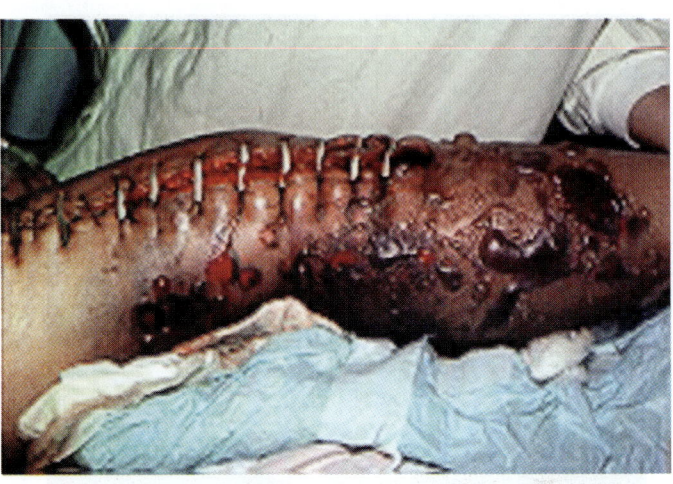

Fig. 20: Gans gangrene

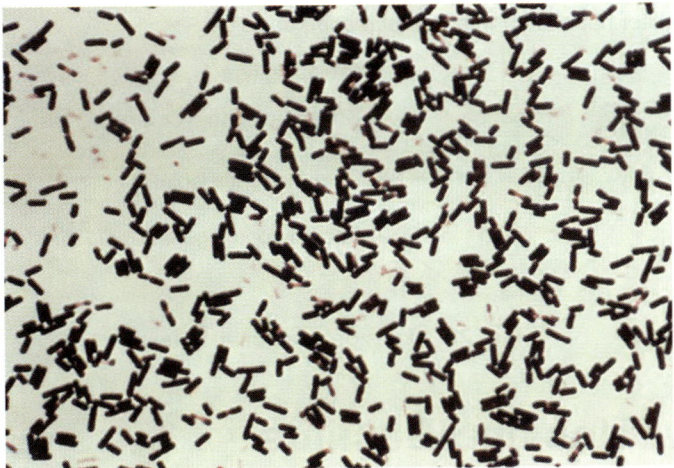

Fig. 21: Gram negative Cl. perfringens (absent spores)

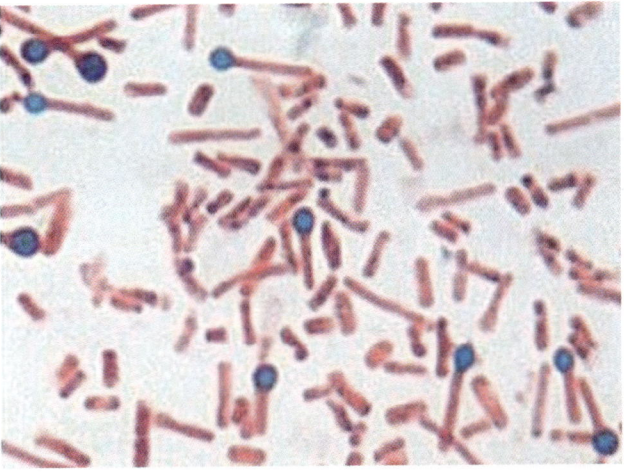

Fig. 22: Gram negative closridium (drumstick spores)

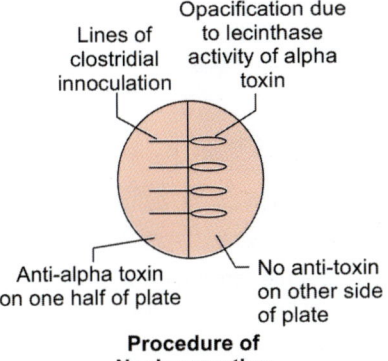
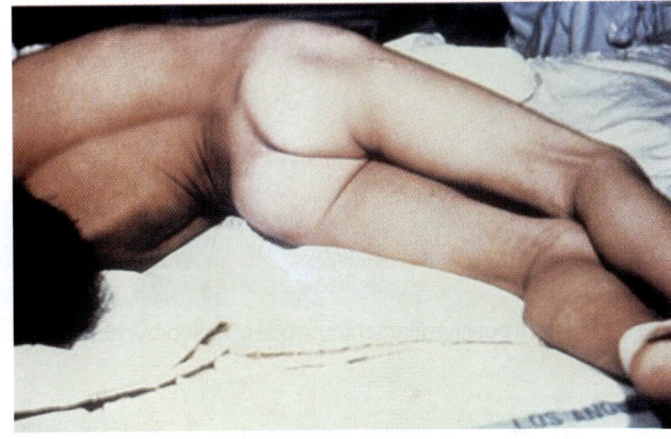

Fig. 23: Nagler's reaction

Fig. 24: Opisthotonus of tetanus

Chapter 11

Corynebacterium

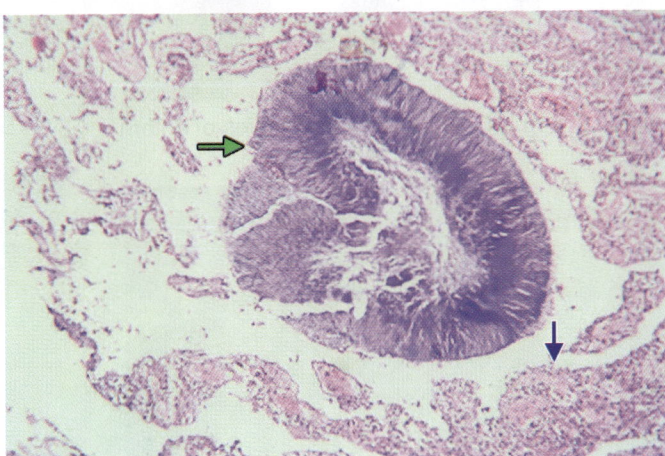

Fig. 25: Characteristic-sulfur-granule-Green-arrow-typical-of-Actinomyces-sp

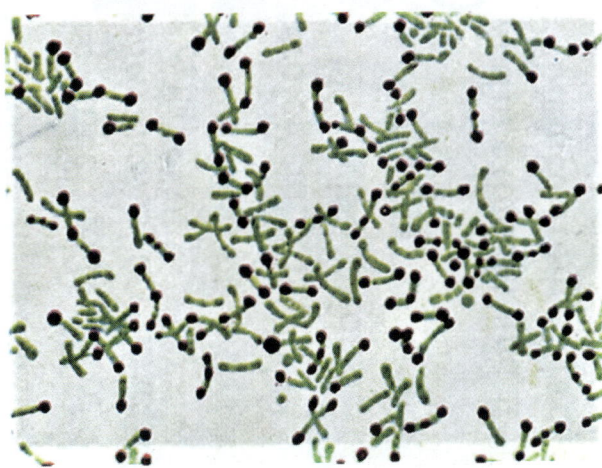

Fig. 26: Corynebacterium on Albert stain

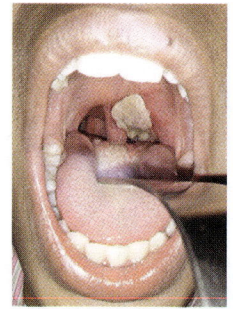

Fig. 27: Diphtheria membrane

Fig. 28: Elek's gel precipitation test

Chapter 12 — Actinomycetes and Bacillus

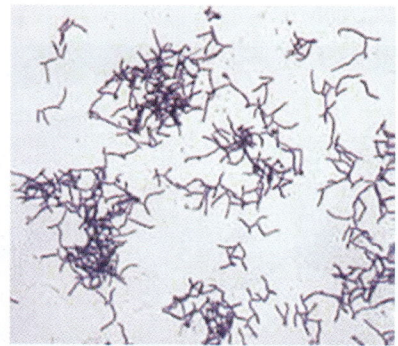

Fig. 29A: Gram positive filamentous rods of actinomycetes in pus

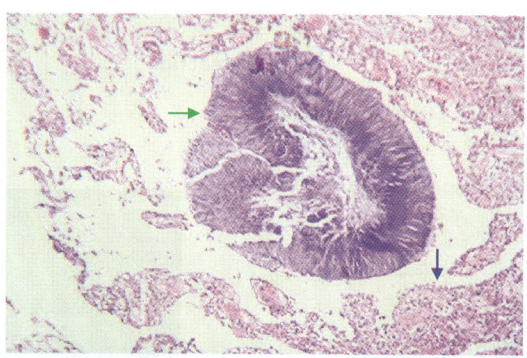

Fig. 29B: Characteristic sulfur granule (green arrow) typical of Actinomyces spp. in histological section of liver and agnio-fibroblastic growths (blue arrow)

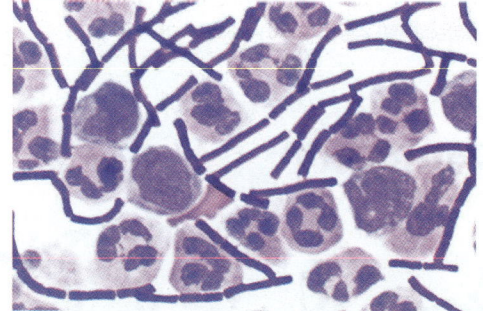

Fig. 30: Gram positive rod shaped anthrax bacilli

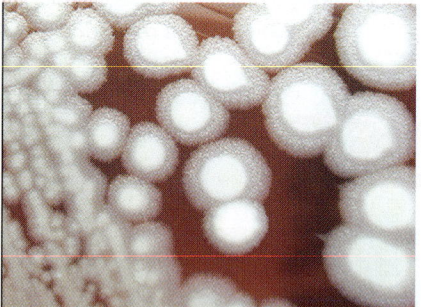

Fig. 31: Medusa head colonies of anthrax

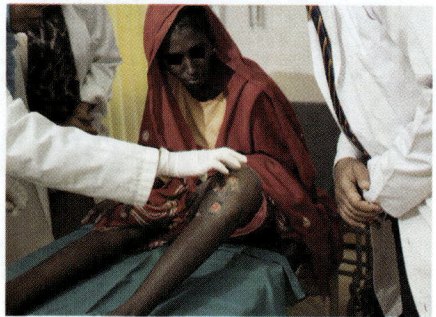

Fig. 32: Mycetoma in patient

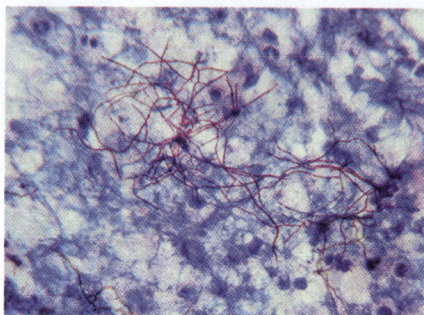

Fig. 33: Nocardia (acid fast partially branching)

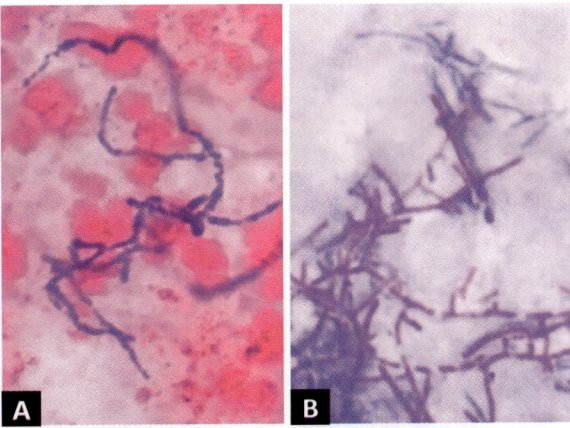

Figs. 34A and B: Nocardia sp on A. Direct Gram smear B. Modified Kinyoun acid fast stain

Chapter 13 — Listeria Monocytogenes

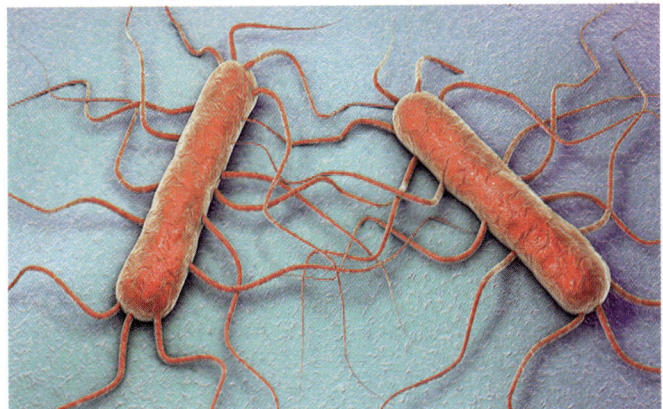

Fig. 35: Peritrichous flagella of Listeria

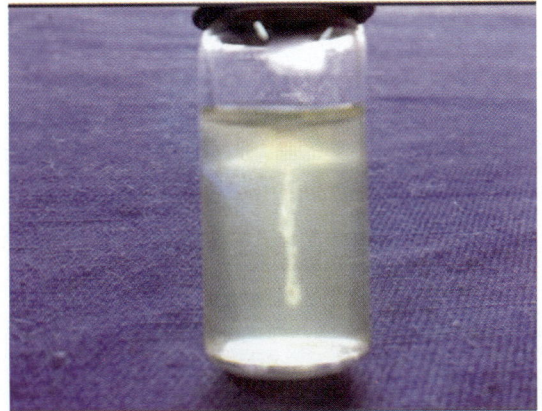

Fig. 36: Tumbling motility of Listeria (looks like umbrella)

Chapter 14 — Mycobacteria

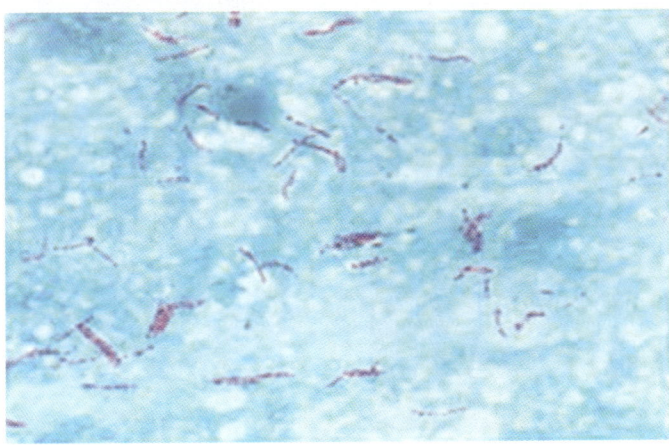

Fig. 37: AFB positive mycobacteria

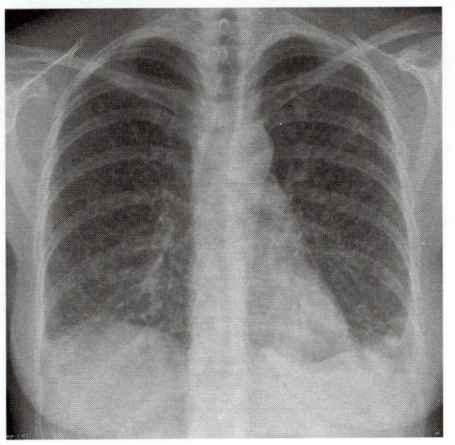

Fig. 38: Chest X-ray of miliary tuberculosis

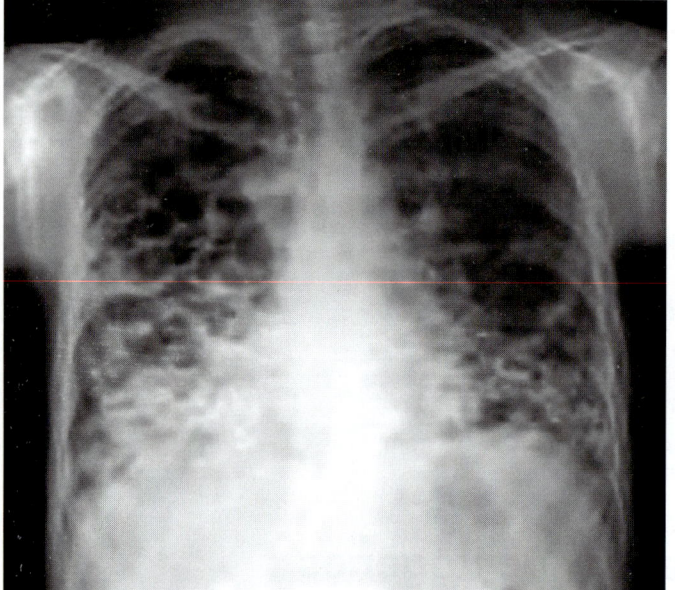

Fig. 39: Infiltration and cavitation of tuberculosis

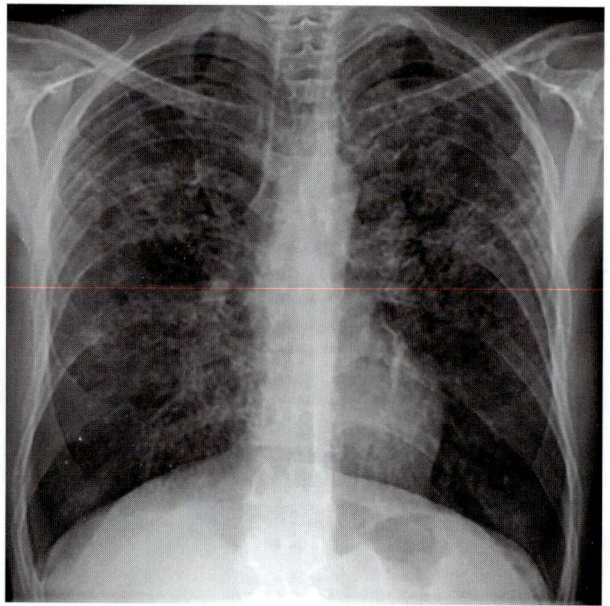

Fig. 40: Infiltration and cavitation of tuberculosis

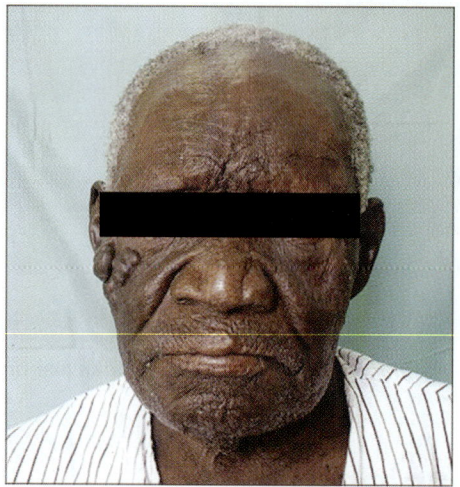

Fig. 41: Lepromatous leprosy

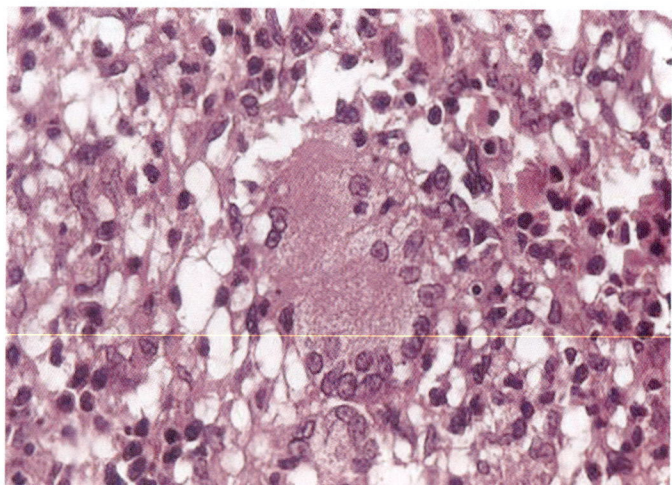

Fig. 42: Mycobacterium Laprae

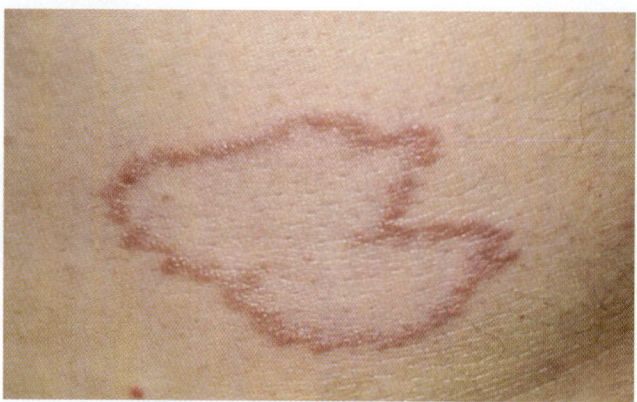

Fig. 43: Tuberculoid leprosy

Chapter 15: Enterobacteriaceae

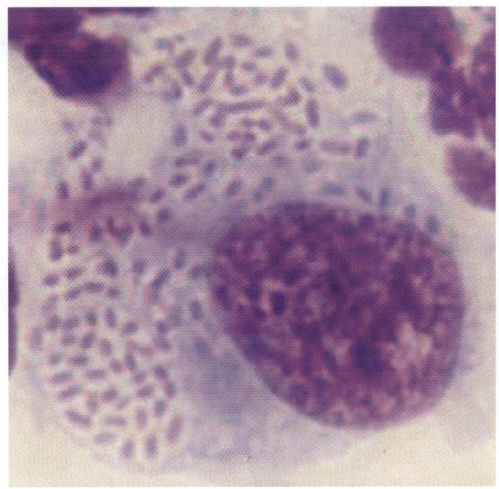

Fig. 44: Donovan bodies of klebsiella

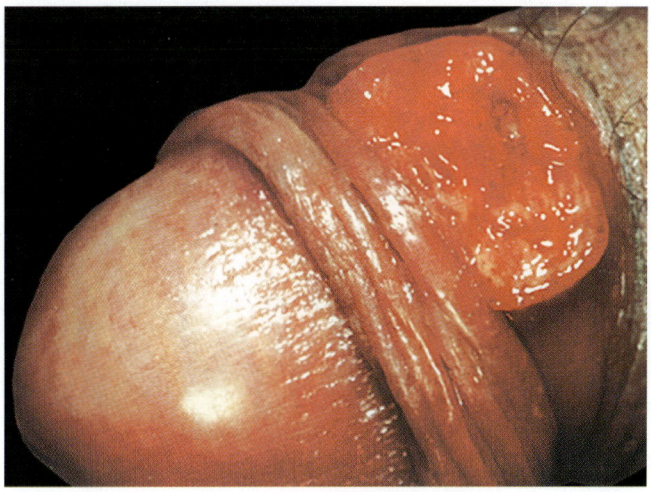

Fig. 45: Granuloma inguinale

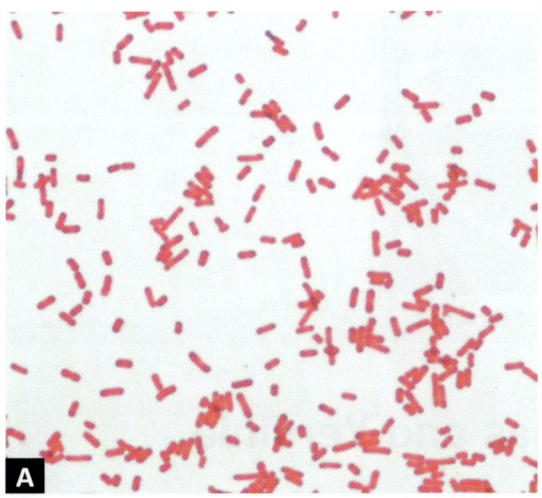

Fig. 46A and B: E coli rod on smear and its structure

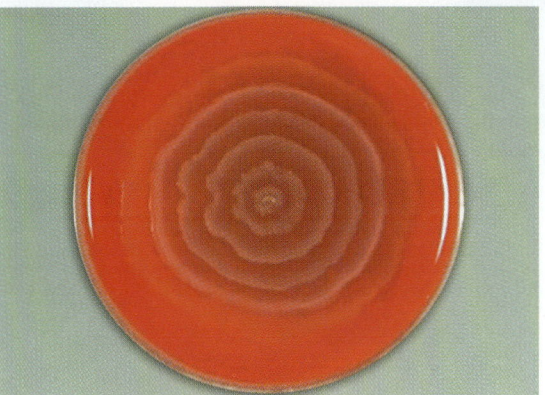

Fig. 47: Swarming growth of proteus

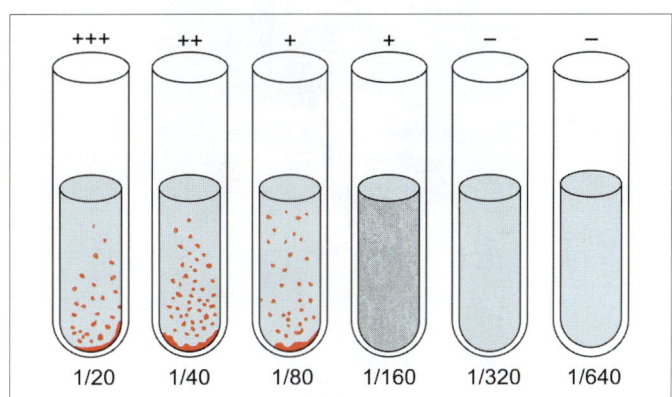

Fig. 48: Widal test

Chapter 16 — Vibrio

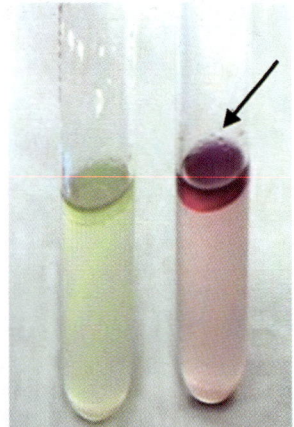

Fig. 49: Cholera red reaction

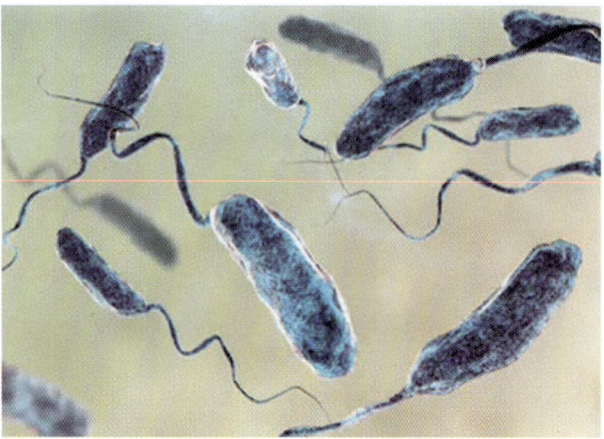

Fig. 50: Cholera vibrio

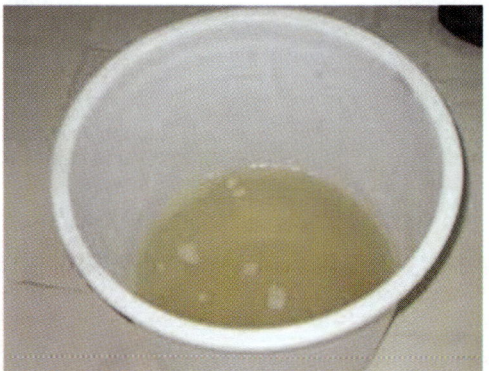

Fig. 51: Rice water stool of cholera

Chapter 17 — Pseudomonas and Yersinia

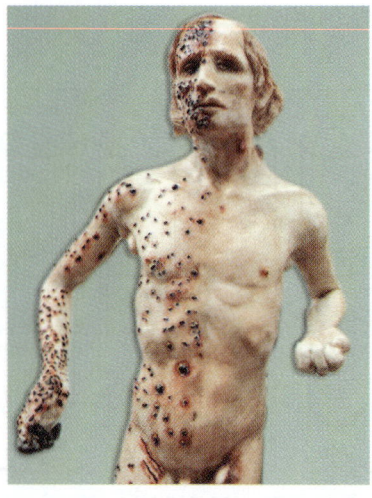

Fig. 52: Bubonic plague wax sclipture

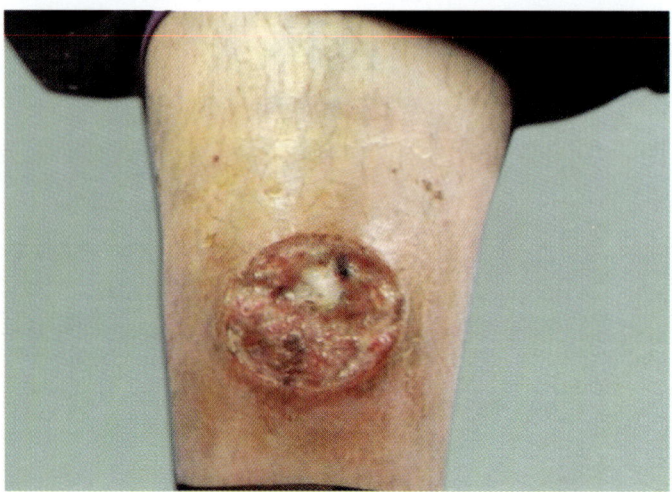

Fig. 53: Ecthyma gangrenosum

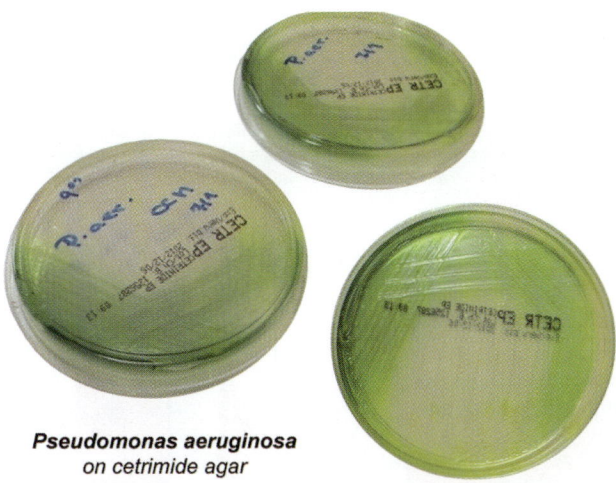

Fig. 54: Green pigment on cetrimide agar

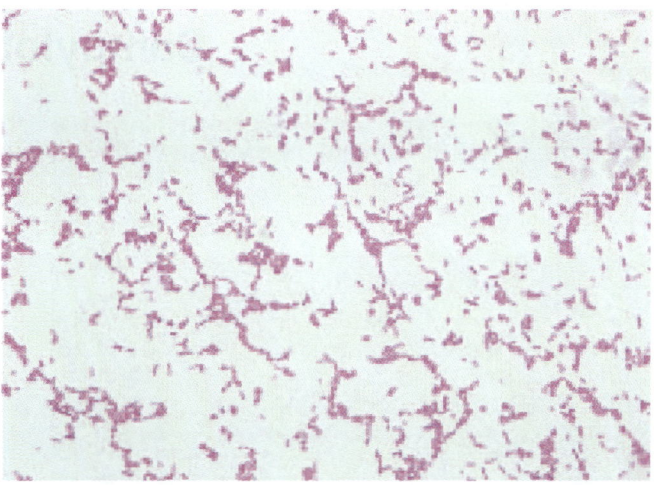

Fig. 55: Safety pin appearance of Burkholderia pseudomallei in a Gram stain

Chapter 18: Hemophilus, Bordetella and Brucella

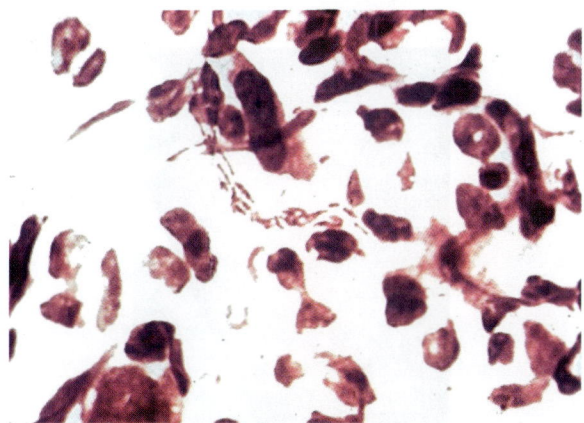

Fig. 56: Chancroid school of fish appearance

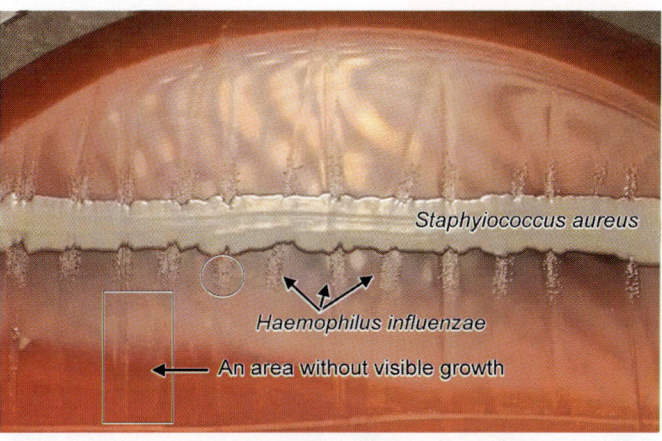

Fig. 57: H. influenzae satellitism

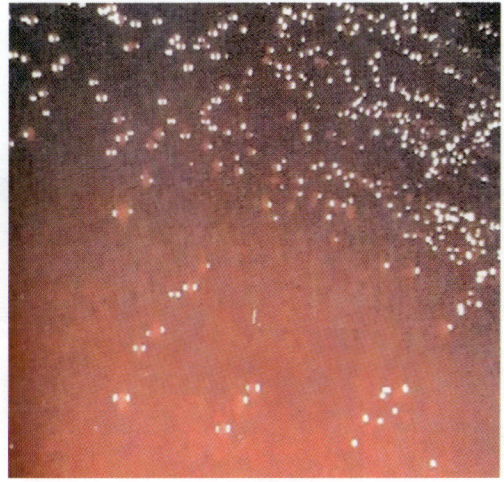

Fig. 58: Mercury drop appearance of bordetella

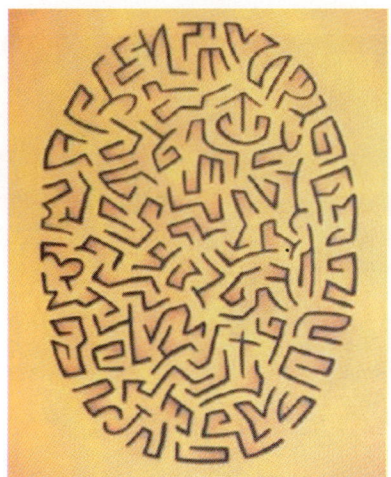

Fig. 59: Thumbprint appearance of bordetella

Chapter 19: Campylobacter and Helicobacter

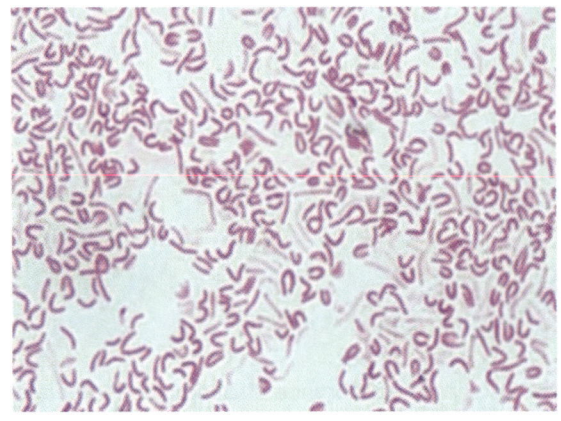

Fig. 60: S shaped U shaped helicobacter

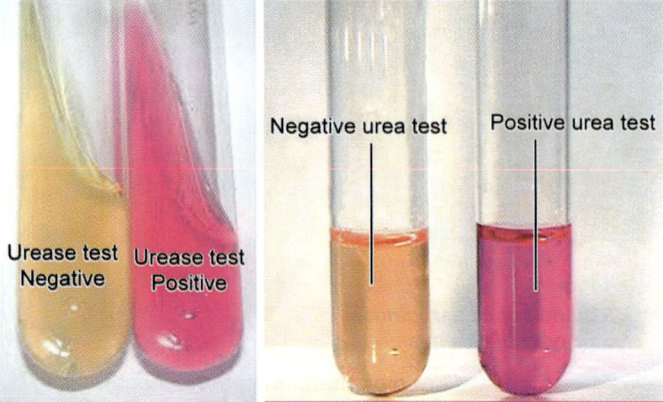

Fig. 61: Urease test

Chapter 21: Rickettsiae and Chlamydiae

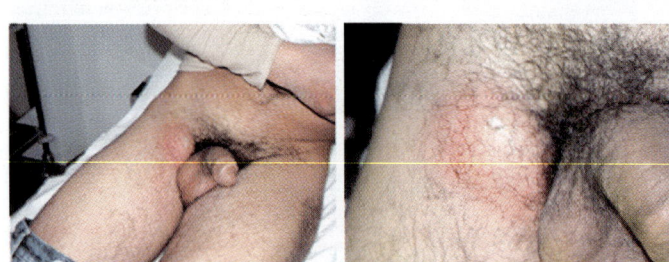

Fig. 62: Inguinal lypmhogranuloma venereum

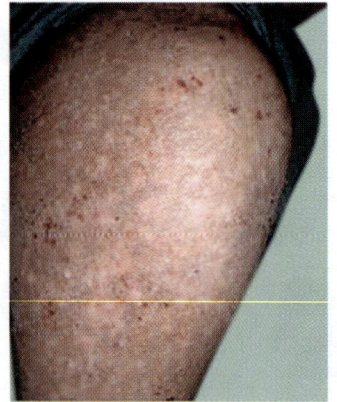

Fig. 63: Louse borne epidemic typhus

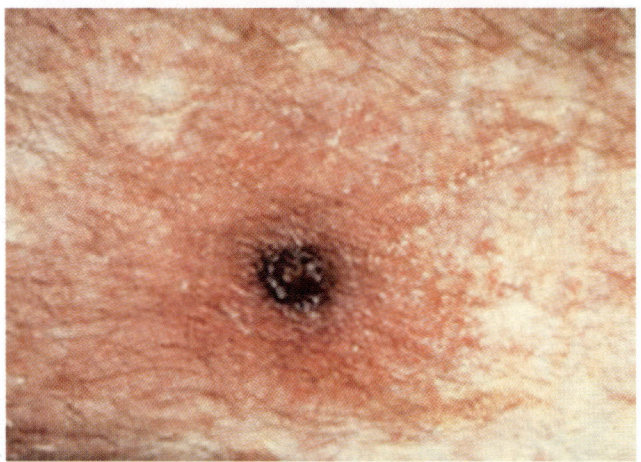

Fig. 64: Scrub-typhus-eschar

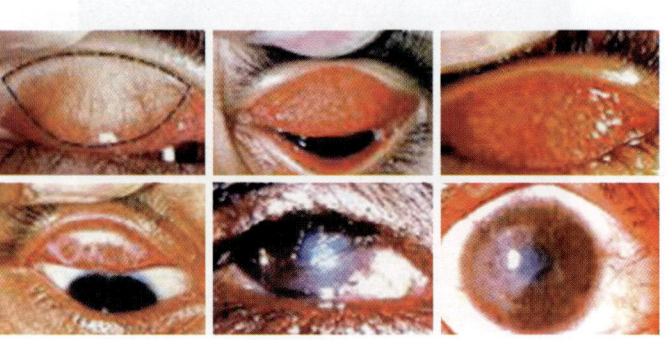

Fig. 65: Trachoma

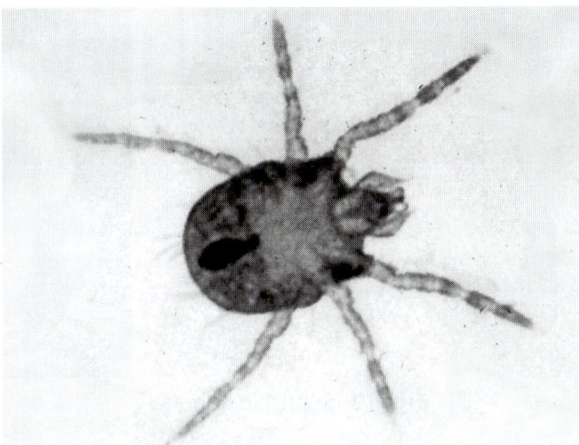

Fig. 66: Trombiculid mite

Chapter 22 — Spirochetes

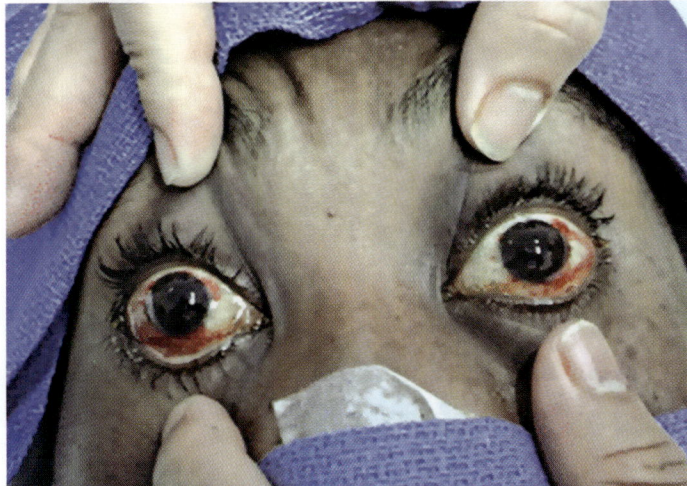
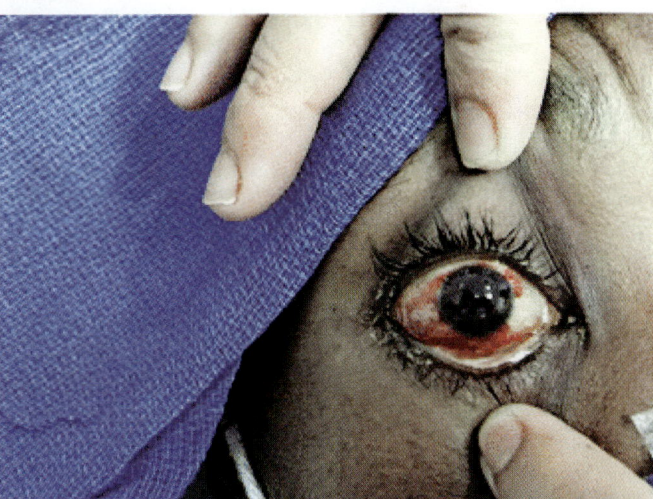

Fig. 67: Ecchymosis of leptospira

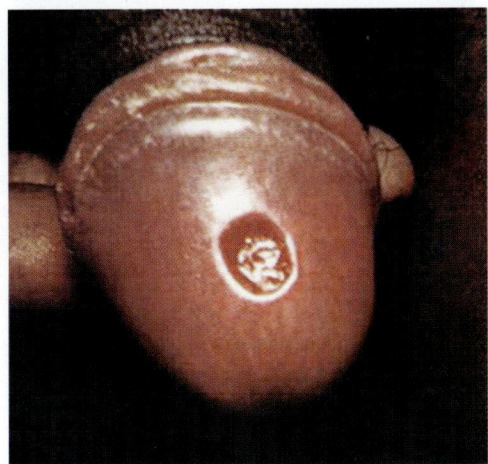

Fig. 68: Penile chancre of primary syphilis

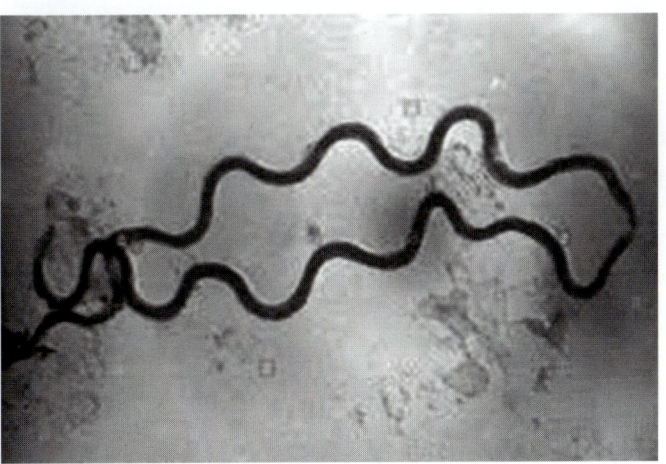

Fig. 69: Spiral shaped treponema

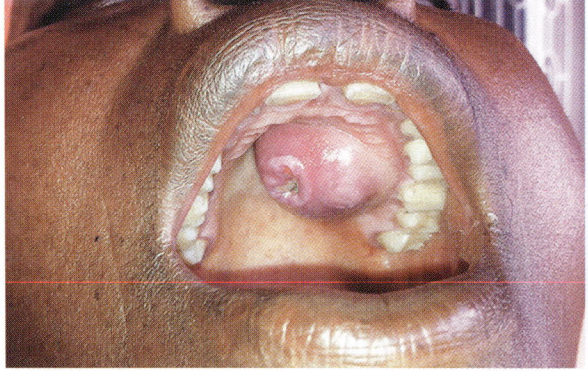
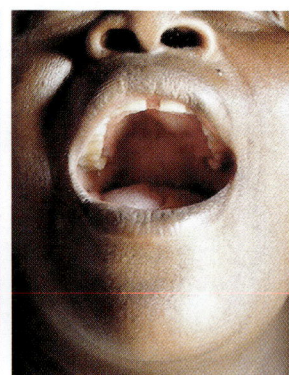

Fig. 70: Syphilitic gumma

Chapter 23 — Mycoplasma

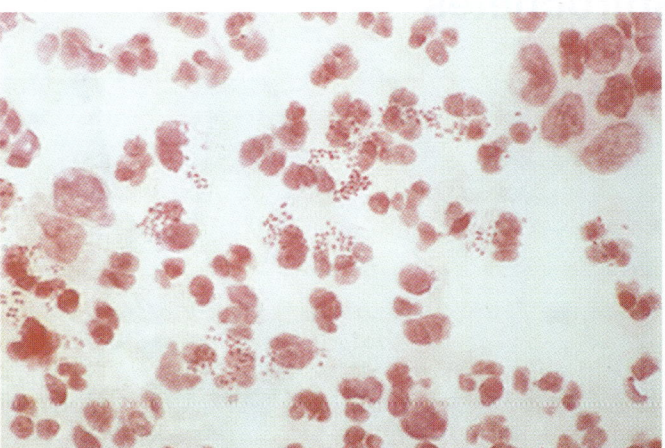

Fig. 71: Exudate smear of non gonococcal urethritis

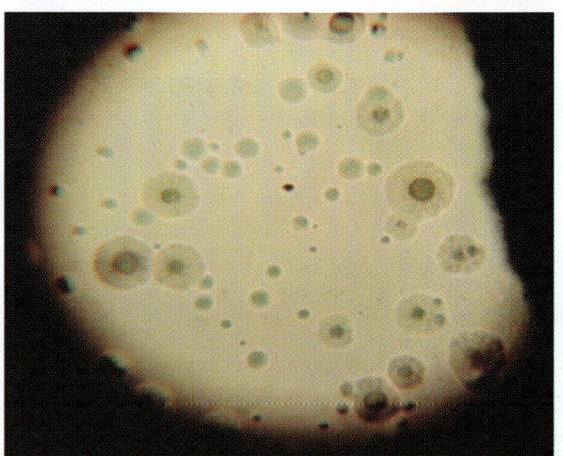

Fig. 72: Fried egg appearance of mycoplasma

Chapter 24 — DNA Virus

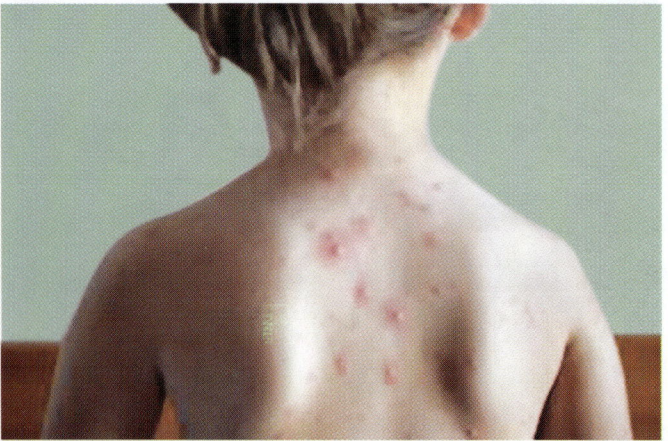

Fig. 73: Chicken pox rash

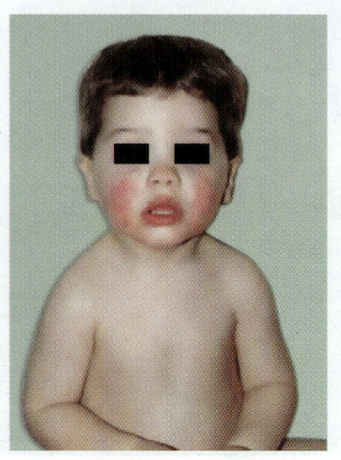

Fig. 74: Erythema infectiosum

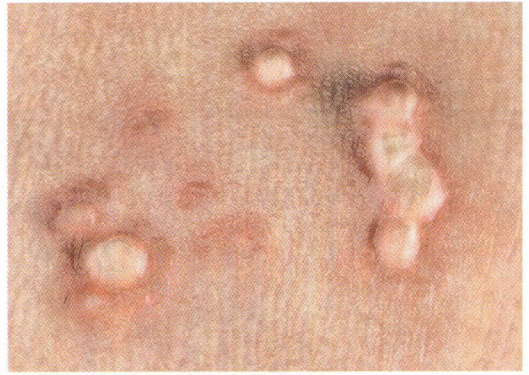

Fig. 75: HPV warts

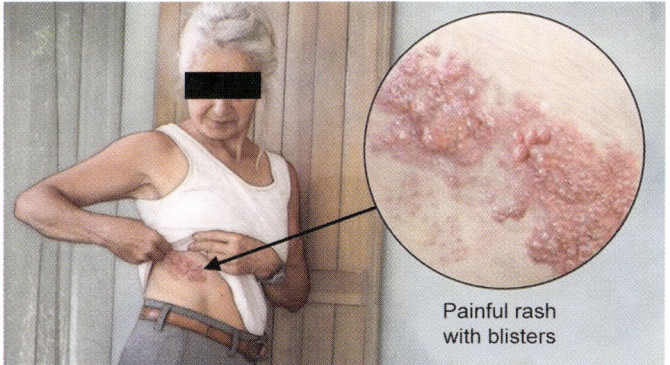

Fig. 76: Herpes Zoster

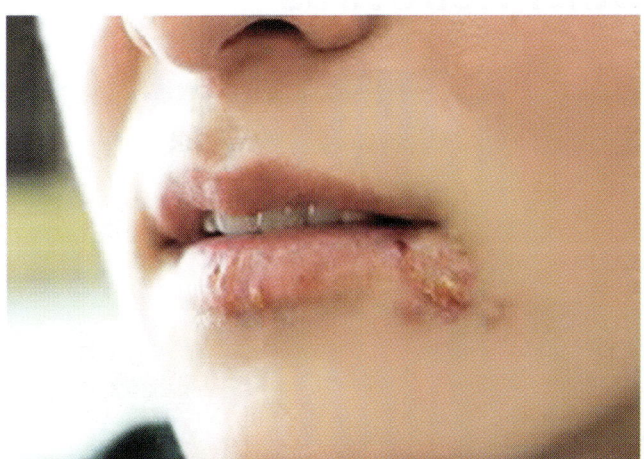

Fig. 77: HSV type 1

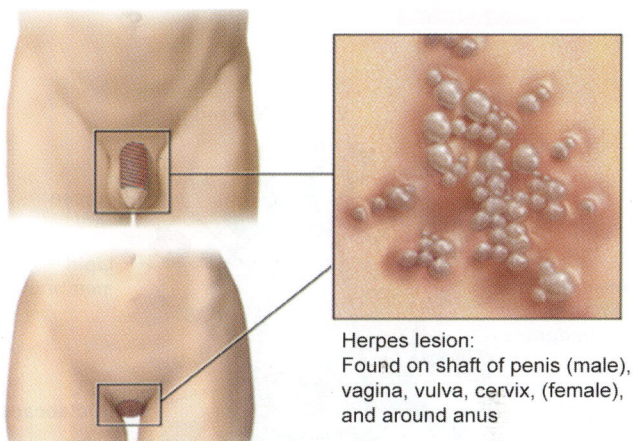

Fig. 78: HSV type 2

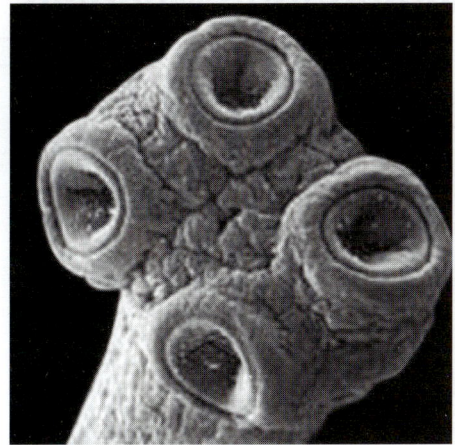

Fig. 79: Tinea saginata

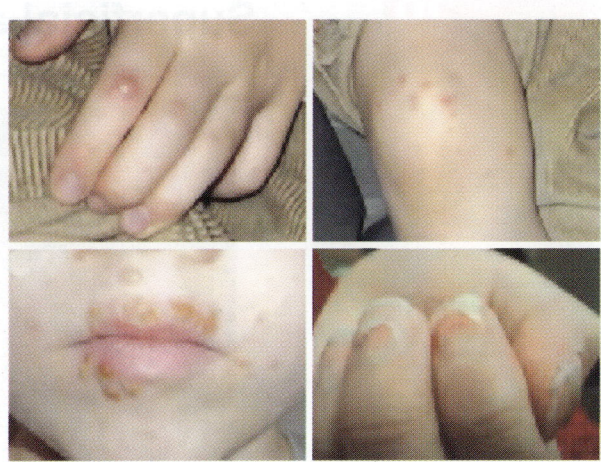

Fig. 80: Vesicular eruptions of cox sackie virus

Chapter 25 — RNA Virus

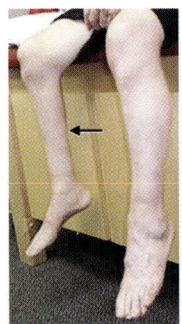

Fig. 81: Asymmetric paralysis of polio

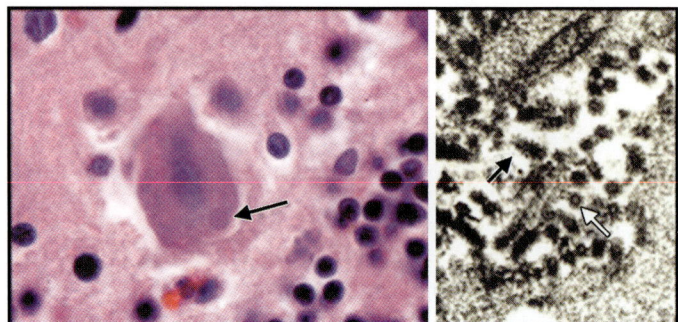

Fig. 82: Eosinophilic negri bodies

Chapter 28 — HIV and Other Retrovirus

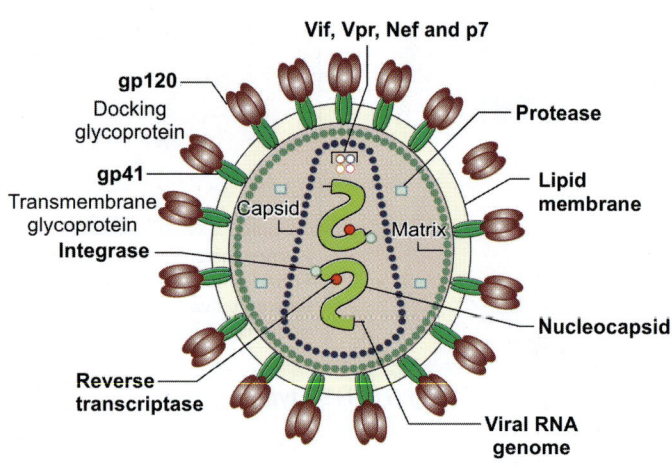

Fig. 83: HIV viriod

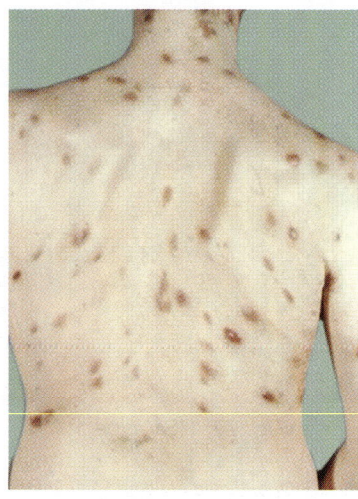

Fig. 84: Kaposi sarcoma

Chapter 29 — Superficial and Subcutaneous Mycosis

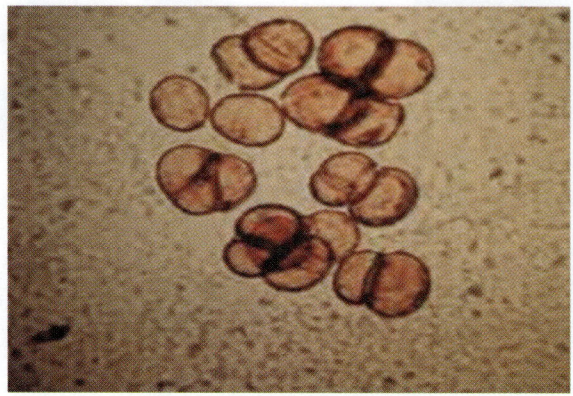

Fig. 85: Sclerotic bodies

Chapter 30: Yeast and Yeast-like Fungus

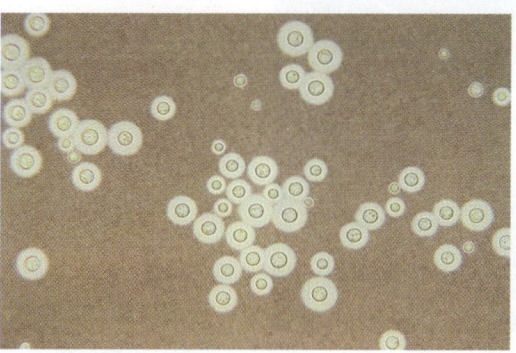

Fig. 86: India ink of cryptococcus

Chapter 31: Aspergillus and Mucormycosis

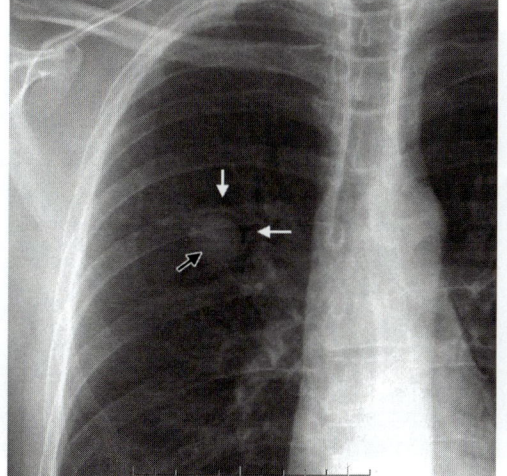

Fig. 87: Aspergilloma

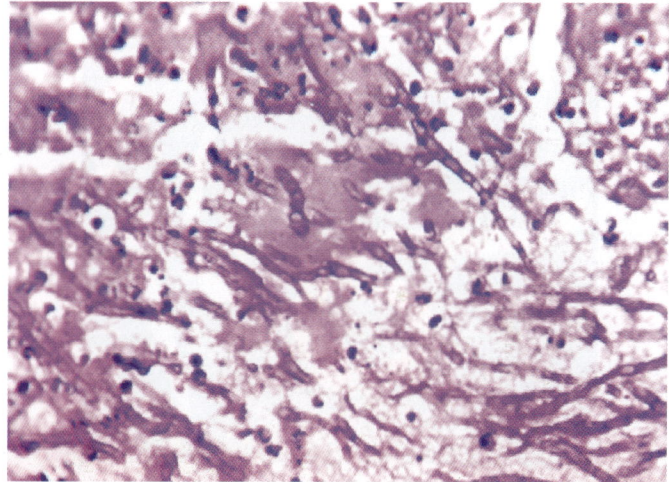

Fig. 88: Silver stain showing narrow angled septate hyphae of aspergillus

Chapter 34: Protozoa

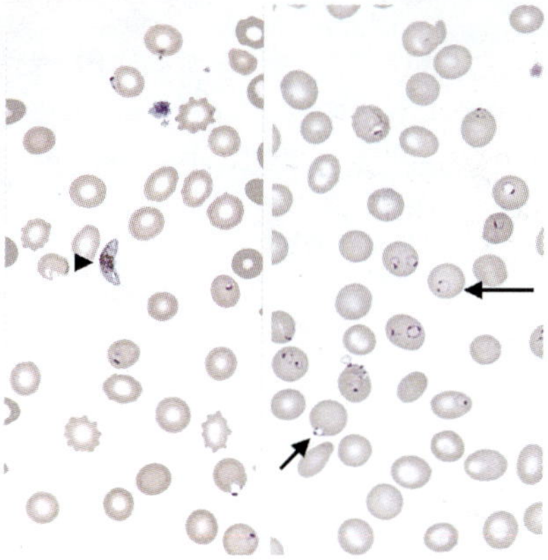

Fig. 89: Blood picture of plasmodium falciparum

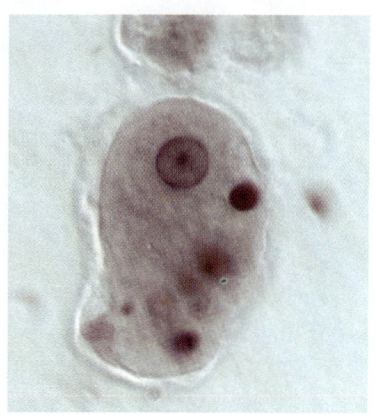

Fig. 90: Entamoeba histolytica

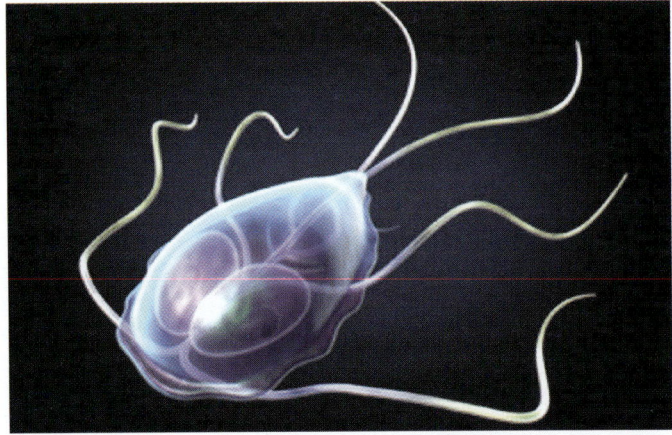
Fig. 91: Giardia lamblia

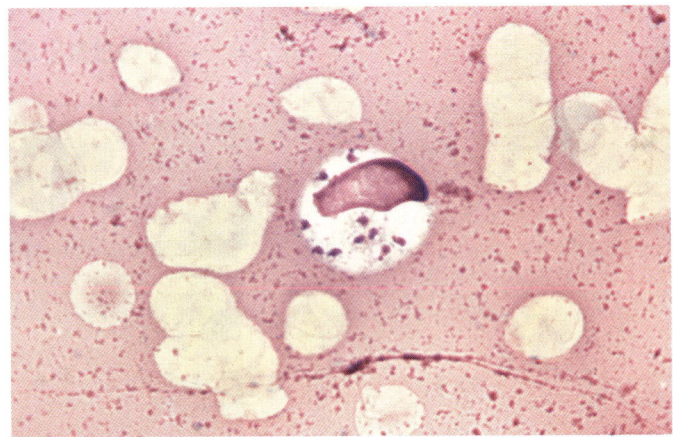
Fig. 92: Leishmania in bone marrow cell

Chapter 35

Helminths

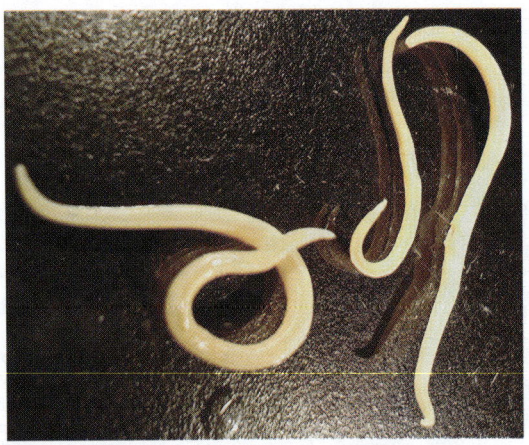
Fig. 93: Ankylostoma Duodenale

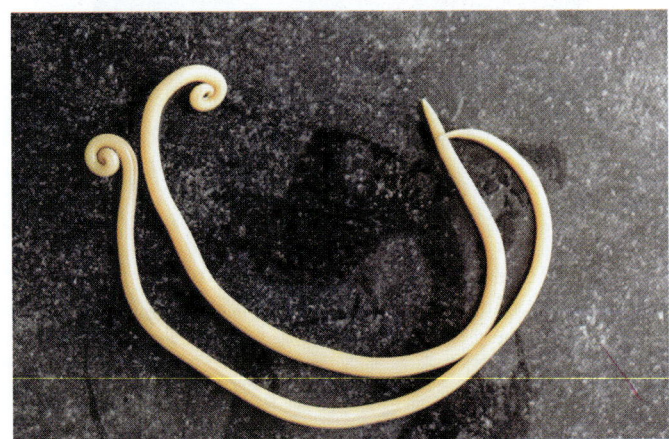
Fig. 94: Ascaris lumbricoides

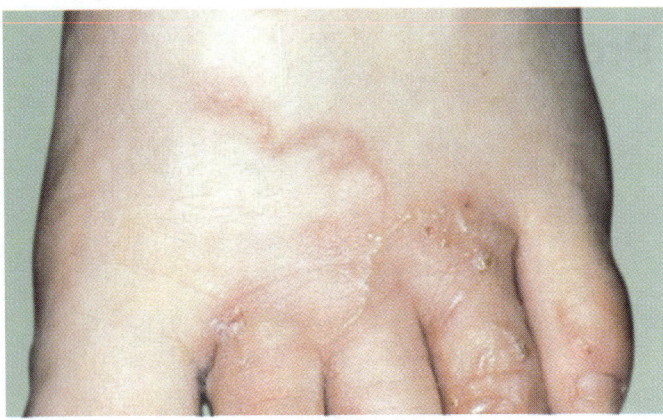
Fig. 95: Larvae Migrans

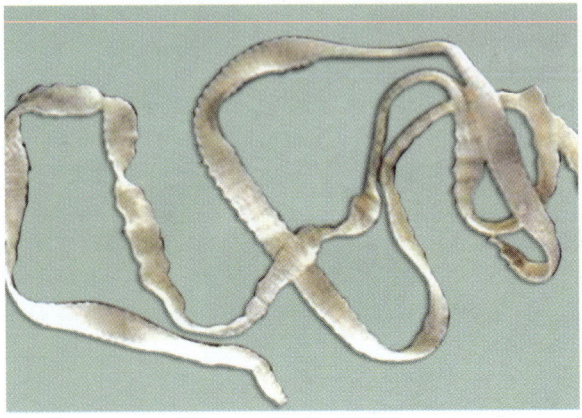
Fig. 96: Tinea solium

Image-based Questions

1. A Dutch tradesman whose hobby was to make lenses. His image is shown below. Identify the great scientist:

   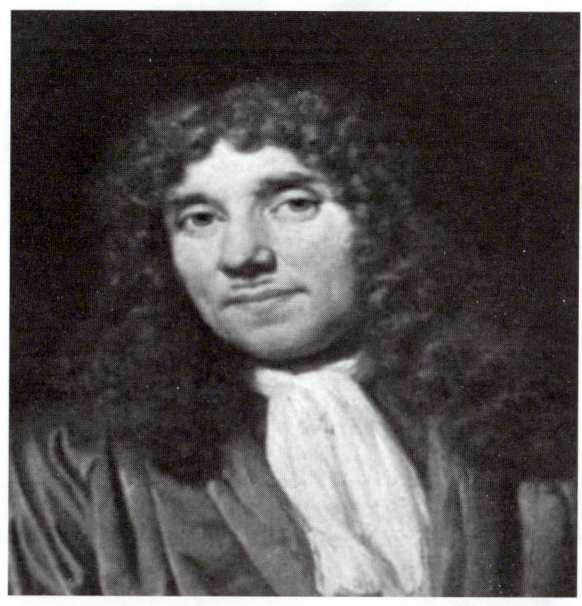

   a. Robert Koch
   b. A.V Leeuwenhoek
   c. Louis Pasteur
   d. Edward Jenner

2. Which type of bacterial morphology is shown below:

   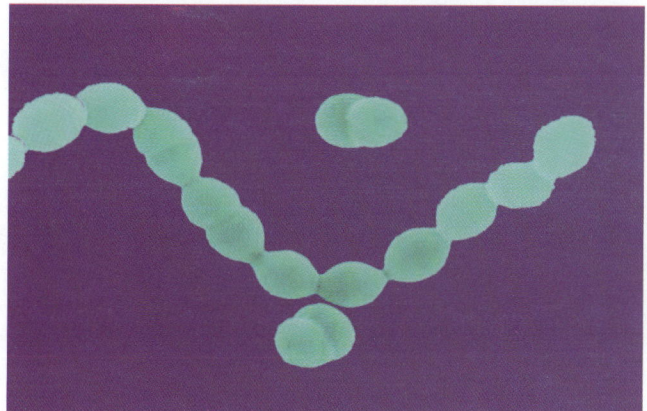

   a. Pneumococcus
   b. Streptococcus
   c. Staphylococci
   d. Meningococci

3. What type of genetic exchange is being exhibited by the *E. coli* in the picture below?

   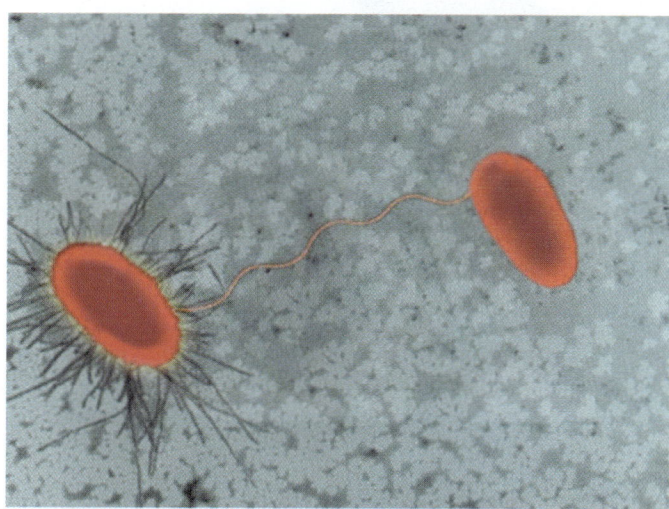

   a. Conjugation
   b. Transduction
   c. Transformation
   d. Mutation

4. What group of organisms is represented by the image below?

   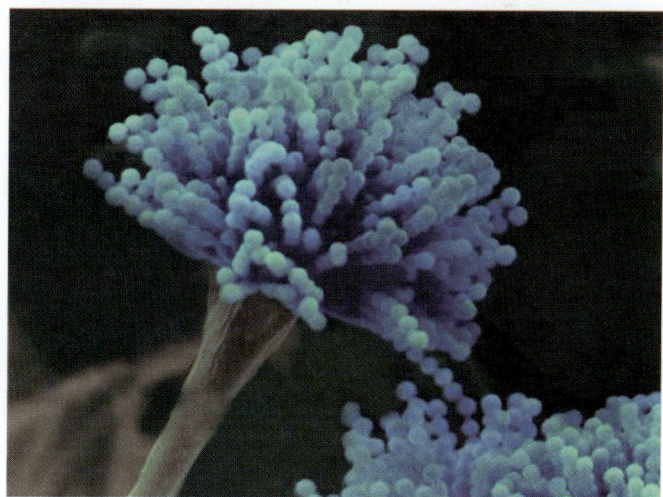

   a. Fungi
   b. Bacteria
   c. Virus
   d. Filaria

5. What flagella arrangement is exhibited in the image below?

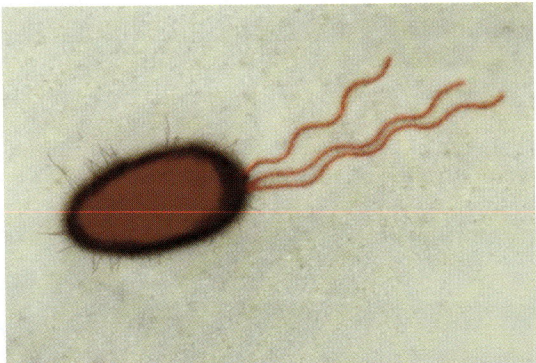

   a. Peritrichous
   b. Lophotrichous
   c. Monotrichous
   d. Amphitrichous

6. What classification group of parasite is shown in picture?

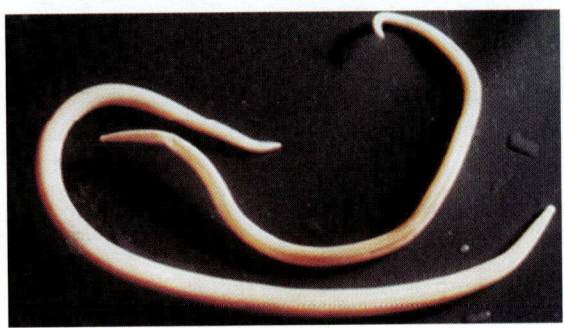

   a. Protozoa
   b. Nematoda
   c. Cestode
   d. Trematoda

7. The microorganism circled in the image below is the causative agent of a disease that is transmitted sexually. Identify the organism.

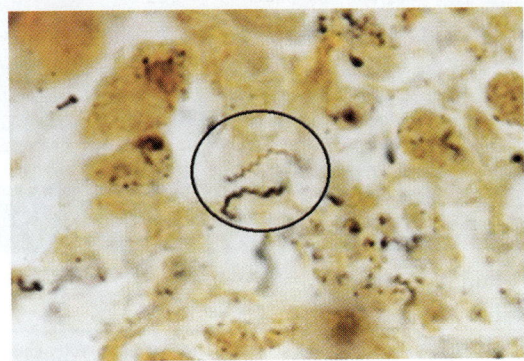

   a. Gonococci
   b. Treponema pallidum
   c. Hemophilus ducreyi
   d. Calymmobacter granulomatis

8. The symbol shown in the image below represent:

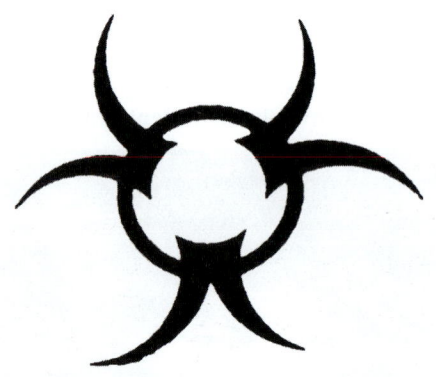

   a. Radiation hazard
   b. Cytotoxic hazards
   c. Biohazard
   d. Magnetic field inside

9. Identify the instrument:

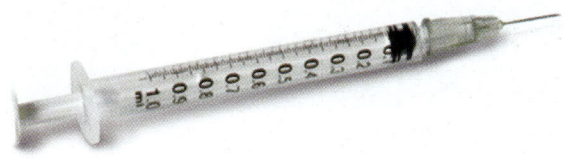

   a. Tuberculin syringe
   b. Insulin syringe
   c. 2 mL syringe
   d. Micro syringe

10. Identify the material shown below in petridish:

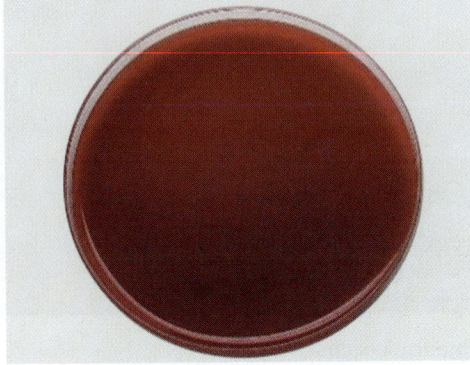

   a. Chocolate Agar
   b. Blood Agar
   c. LJ medium
   d. VP medium

Explanation

1. **Answer is (b) A.V Leeuwenhoek**

    Images of Some Famous Scientists

    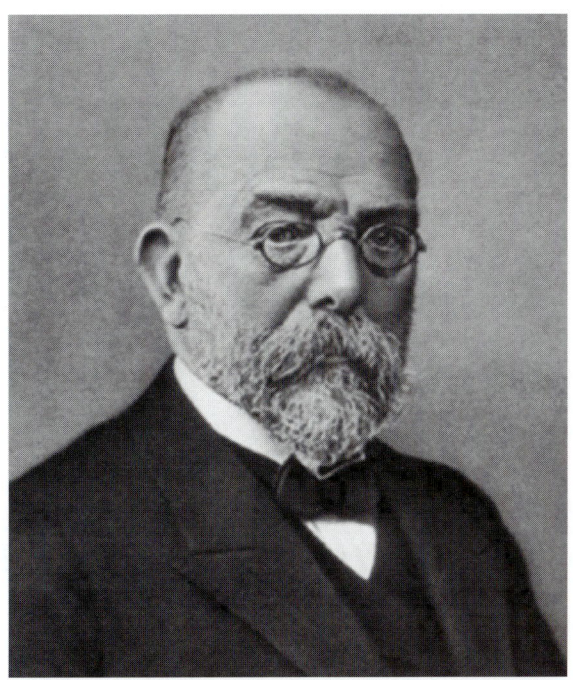
    Robert Koch

    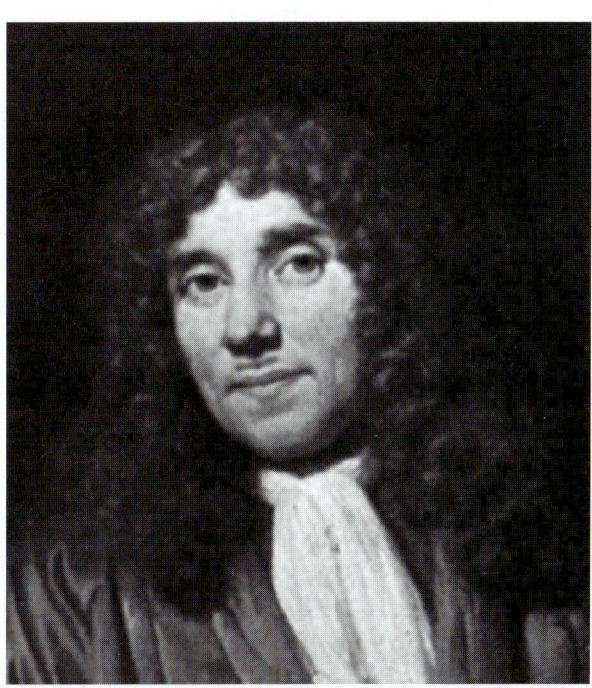
    A.V Leeuwenhoek

    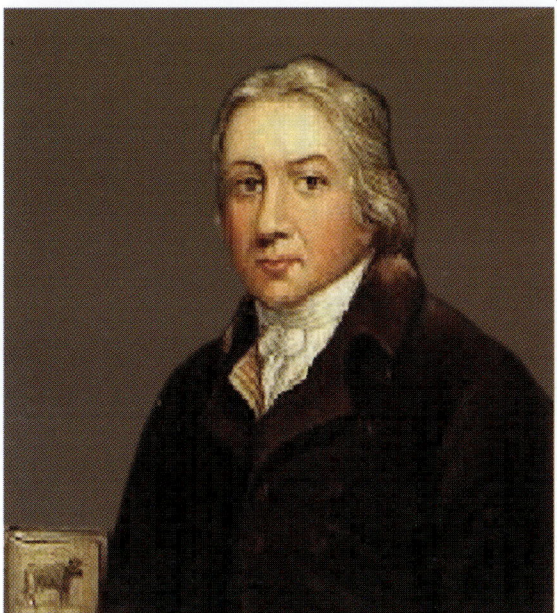
    Edward Jenner

    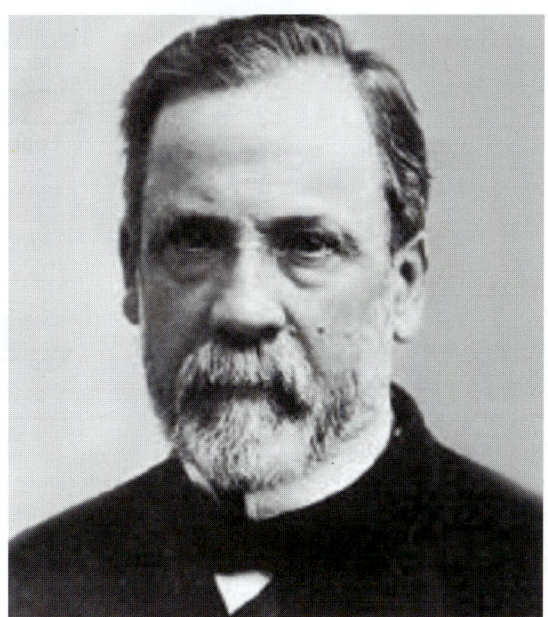
    Louis Pasteur

2. **Answer is (b) Streptococcus**

   Gram (+)ve cocci arranged in linear cluster can be none other than Streptococci. Staphylococci divide is three planes to form grape like clusters.

   Growth pattern of some important bacteria

   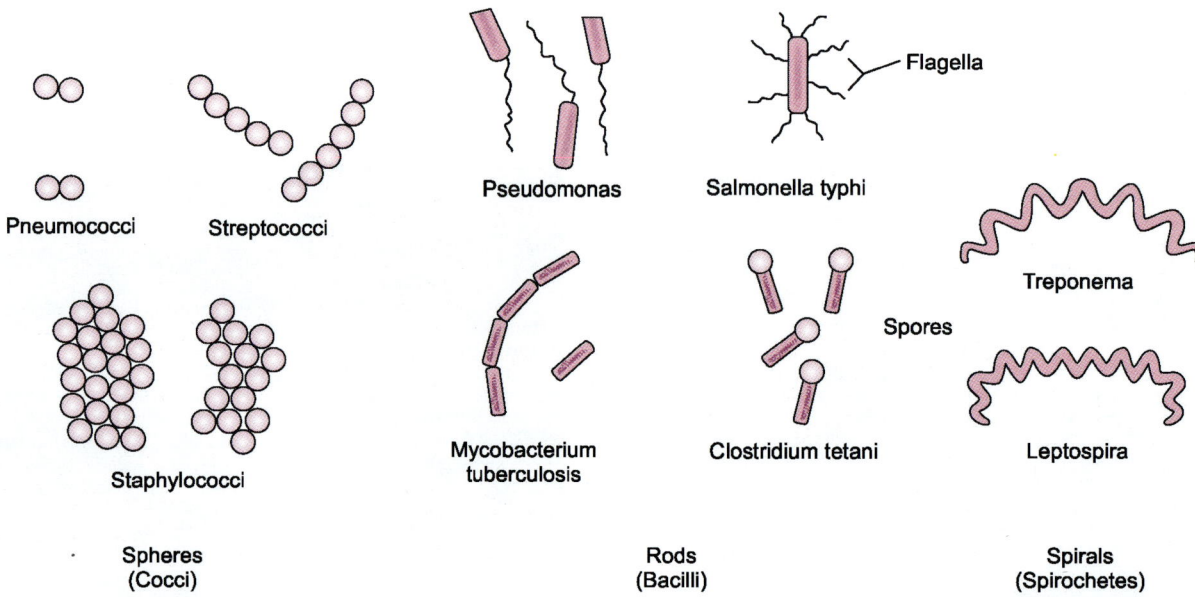

3. **Answer is (a) Conjugation**

   Here one can see the presence of sex pilli (red in image)

4. **Answer is (a) Fungi**

   Note the bluish spheres these are spores.

5. **Answer is (b) Lophotrichous**

   Types of flagella

   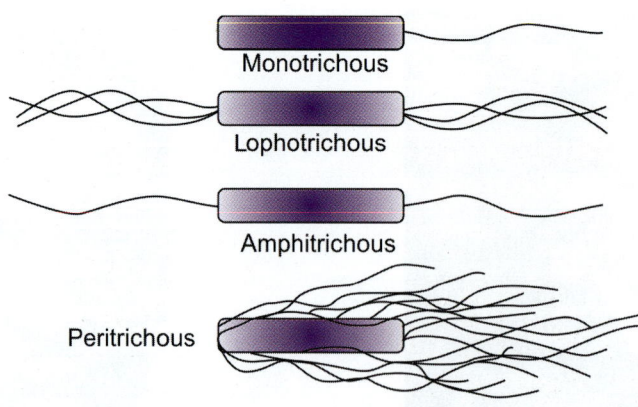

6. **Answer is (b) Nematoda**

   A parasite with long thin ungesmented tubular body can be none other than nematode. (See image below)

   Nematode (roundworms): They have long thin unsegmented tube-like bodies with anterior mouths and longitudinal digestive tracts. They have a fluid-filled internal body cavity (pseudocoelum) which acts as a hydrostatic skeleton providing rigidity (so-called *'tubes under pressure'*). Adult worms form separate sexes with well-developed reproductive systems.

   Cestodes (tapeworms): They have long flat ribbon-like bodies with a single anterior holdfast organ (scolex) and numerous segments. They do not have a gut and all nutrients are taken up through the tegument. They do not have a body cavity (acoelomate) and are flattened to facilitate perfusion to all tissues. All tapeworms are hermaphroditic and each segment contains both male and female organs.

Trematodes (flukes): They have small flat leaf-like bodies with oral and ventral suckers and a blind sac-like gut. They do not have a body cavity (acoelomate) and are dorsoventrally flattened with bilateral symmetry. Most species are hermaphroditic (individuals with male and female reproductive systems) although some blood flukes form separate male and female adults

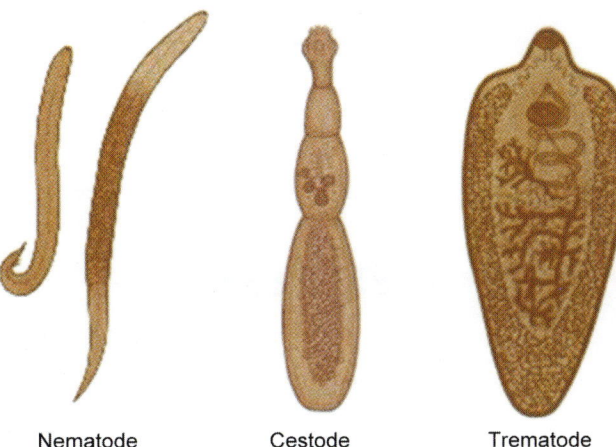

Nematode   Cestode   Trematode

7. **Answer is (b) Treponema pallidum**
   Refer answer no. 2 for image of Treponema

8. **Answer is (c) Biohazard**
   Some Important medical symbols

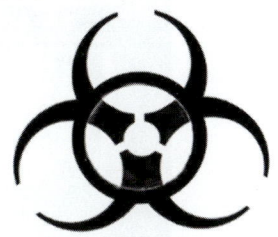

Biohazard

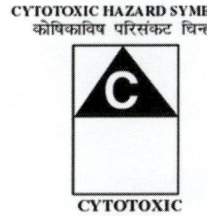

Cytotoxic Hazard

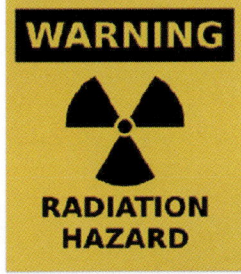

Radiation Hazard

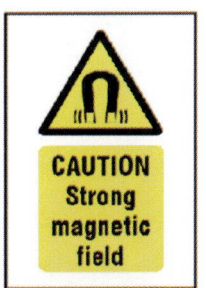

Magnetic field symbol

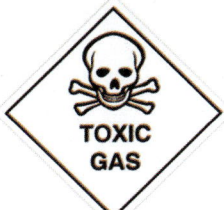

Toxic Gas

Toxic Chemicals

9. **Answer is (a) Tuberculin syringe**
   Tuberculin syringe has calibrations from 0.1 to 1.0 whereas insulin syringe has calibrations either up to 40 or up to 100 which represent 40 IU and 100 IU respectively. See figure below

   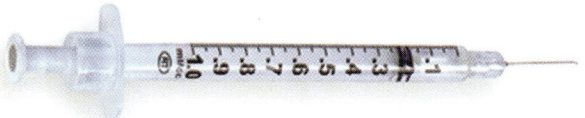
   Tuberculin syringe

   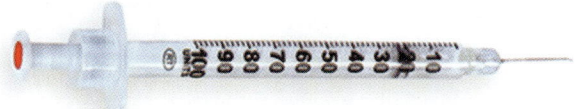
   Insulin syringe

10. **Answer is (b) Blood Agar**
    Image plates of some important culture mediums

    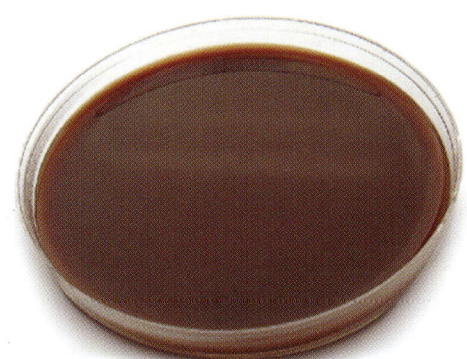
    Chocolate Agar

    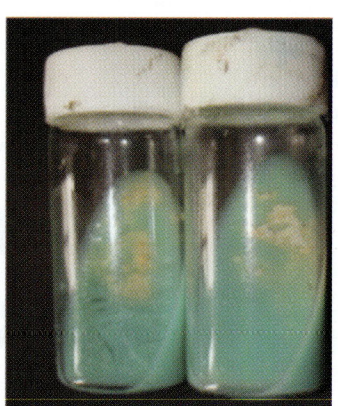
    LJ Media

Other Informative Images

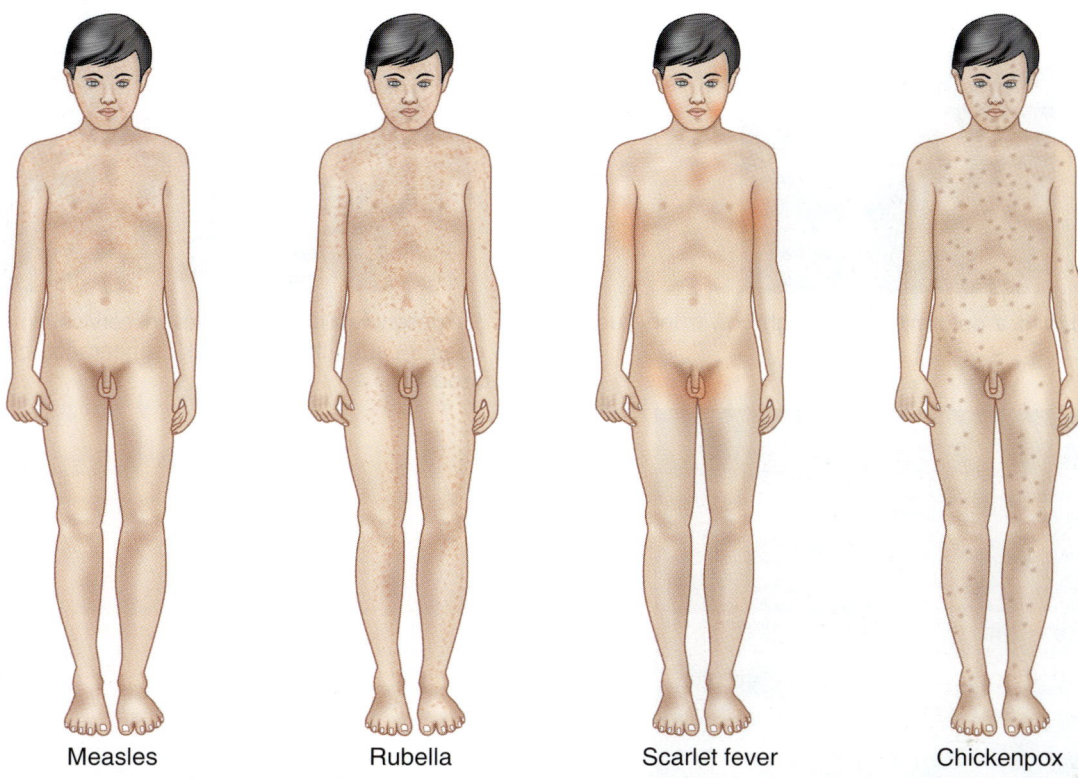

Measles Rubella Scarlet fever Chickenpox

Fig. 1: The distribution and comparison of the rash of measles, rubella, scarlet fever, and chickenpox, which can be helpful in determining the diagnosis of these childhood exanthems.

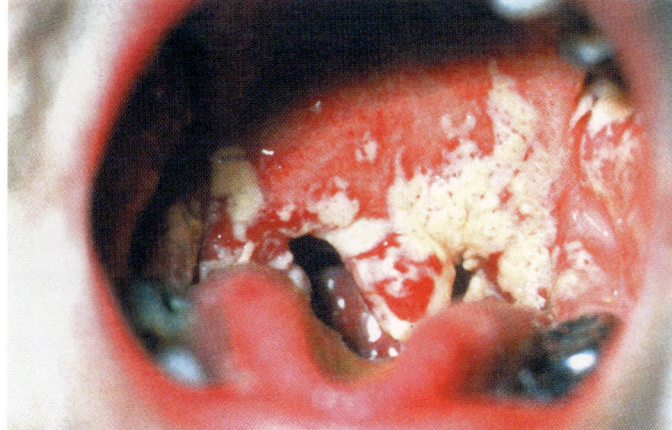

Fig. 2: A photograph of an infection of the oral cavity with thrush caused by *Candida albicans*. Note the creamy appearance of the pseudomembrane and the erythematous appearance of the mucosa.

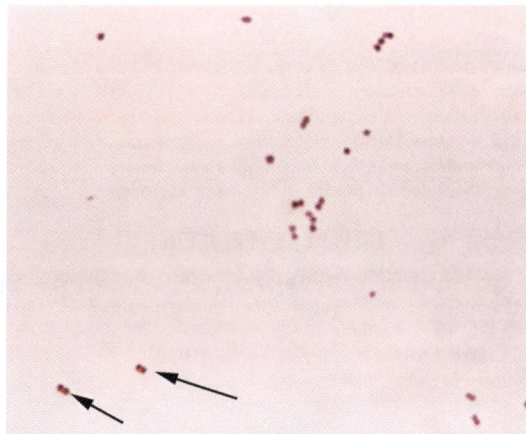

Fig. 3: Gram stain of *Neisseria meningitidis*. Notice the gram-negative diplococci (black arrows) joined together on their longer side.

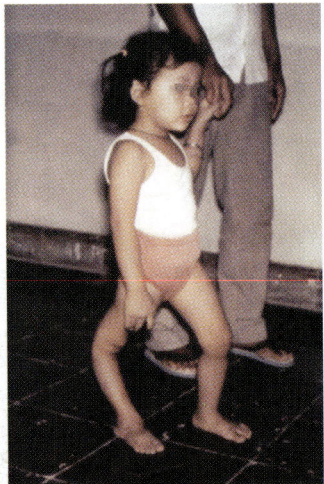

Fig. 4: A child with a deformity of the right lower leg due to poliomyelitis.

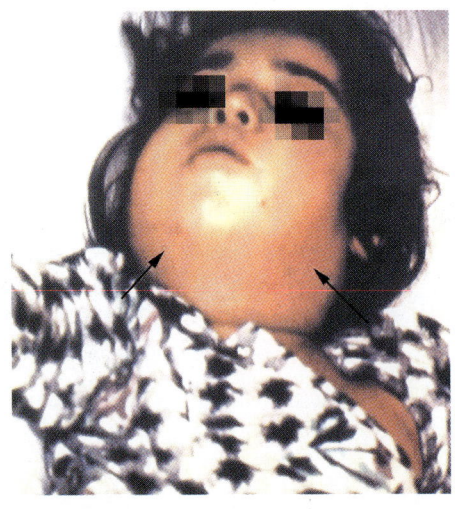

Fig. 5: A patient with diphtheria. Severe cervical lymphadenopathy and edema cause the "bull neck" appearance characteristic of this disease.

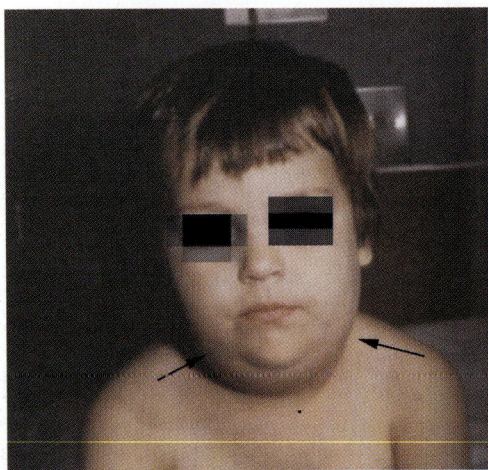

Fig. 6: A child with parotitis *(black arrows)* due to the mumps virus.

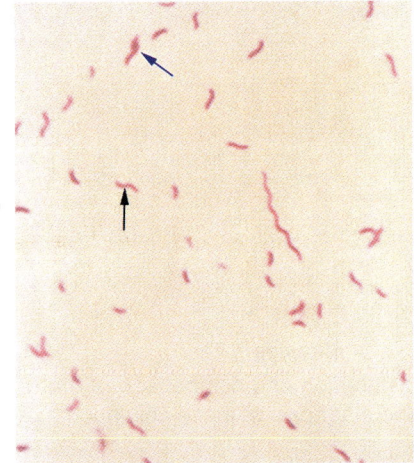

Fig. 7: A photomicrograph of *Campylobacter* demonstrating the S-shaped *(black arrow)* and gull wing-shaped *(blue arrow)*, gram-negative rod (Gram stain).

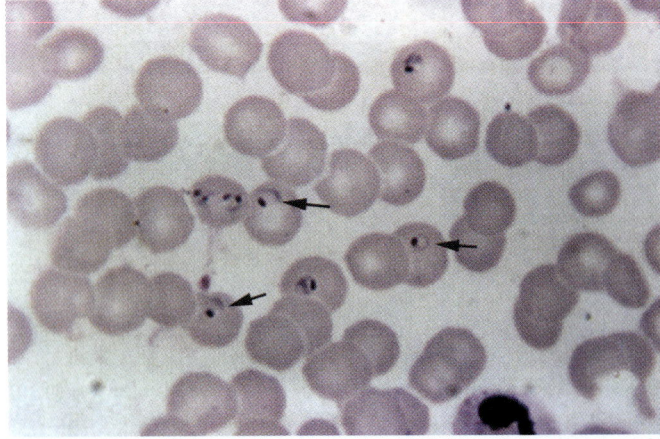

Fig. 8: A photomicrograph of a Giemsa-stained thin blood film that reveals the ring-cell stage of the Plasmodium falciparum trophozoites *(black arrows)*.

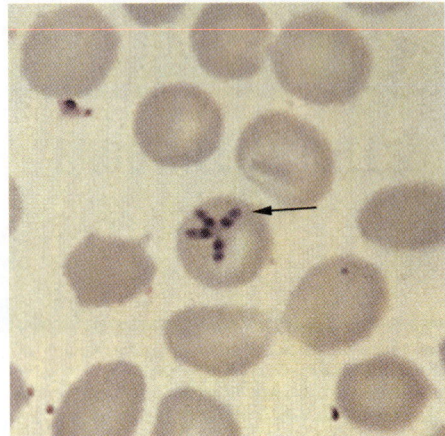

Fig. 9: A photomicrograph of a Giemsa-stained thin blood smear containing the tetrad of trophozoites showing the Maltese cross *(black arrow)*, characteristic of babesiosis.

SECTION A

Revision at a Glance

- Basics of Bacteriology
- Basics of Virology
- Basics of Mycology
- Basics of Clinical Microbiology
- Culture and Sterilization
- Bacterial Genetics

Basics of Bacteriology

CHAPTER 1

CATALASE POSITIVE BACTERIA
• *Staphylococci*
• *N. meningitidis*
• *Atypical mycobacteria*
• *Pseudomonas*
• *Coliform*
• *H. influenza*
• *H. pylori*
• *Yersinia, Pasteurella*
• *Shigella except,* • *S. dysenteriae type I*
• *L. monocytogenes*
• *Nocardia*
• *Legionella*
• *Brucella except B.neotomae, B. ovis*

HEMOLYTIC ORGANISM
• *Strep. pyogenes* - β
• *S. aureus* - β
• *Vibrio eltor*
• *Clostridium perfringes*
• *Bacillus subtilis*
• *E. coli* (pathogenic strain)
• *Mycoplasma*
• *Corynebacterium mitis*
• *Bacillus cereus*
• *L. monocytogens* - β
• *Strep. viridans*
• *Pneumococci*
• *Strep. sanguis*   α-**hemolysis**
• *Strep. mutans*
• *Enterococcus*

TRANSPORT MEDIA	ORGANISM
Pike's Media	S.pyogenes
Stuart's Media	Gonococci
Cary Blair Media	V. cholera
Sach's buffered glycerol saline	Shigella

CAPSULATED BACTERIA
• **P**neumococcus
• **B**acillus **a**nthrax
• **K**lebsiella
• **H**. influenza
• **Y**ersinia
• **B**ordetella
• N. **m**eningococci
• **Cl**. perfringes and butyricum
• **V**. parahemolyticus
Mnemonic: PAKIYB. M.C.V.

TYPES OF MOTILITY	
• Darting	– V. cholera, Campylobacter
• Tumbling	– Listeria at 20-25°C
• Stately	– Clostridia
• Cork screw	– T. pallidum
Lashing	– Borrelia
• Gliding	– Mycoplasma
• Swarming	– Proteus mirabilis, P. vulgaris,
	– Cl. tetani, Bacillus cereus

MOTILE BACTERIA

Peritrichous flagella
- All clostridia except Cl. perfringens and Cl. tetani VI
- Bacillus except B. anthrax
- Listeria monocytogens
- E. coli
- Proteus
- Salmonella except, • S. gallinarum — pullorum

Polar flagella
- Vibrio
- Pseudomonas
- H. pylori
- Campylobacter
- Spirochetes
- Legionella

ACID-FAST ORGANISM
- **N**ocardia
- **L**egionella micdadei
- **B**acterial spores
- **C**ryptococcus cyst
- **R**hodococcus
- **I**sospora
- **M**ycobacterium
- **S**permatic head

Mnemonic: **N**o **L**onger **S**eparate **B**ooking for **RIM S**im **C**ard

SHAPE OF BACTERIA

Club shape		Corynebacteria
Lanceolate (flame shaped)	💧	Pneumococi
Halfmoon (Lens)	(	Meningococci
Kidney	( )	Gonococci
Comma	〜	V. cholera, Campylobacter

PIGMENT PRODUCING BACTERIA
- Pseudomonas — Green (Ps aeroginosa)
- S. aureus — Golden yellow
  Rhodococcus — Red
- Bacteroides melanogenicus — Black
- Nocardia — Yellow to red
- Pepto and Peptostreptococcus
- Photo and Scotochromogen — Yellow orange
- Atypical mycobacteria
- Hafnia, Serratia marcescens

PLEOMORPHIC ORGANISM
- Mycoplasma
- Clostridium
- H. influenza
- V. cholera
- V. parahemolyticus
- Proteus

DEAD END INFECTION
- Leptospirosis
- Legionella
- Endemic typhus (Rickettsia typhi)
- Tetanus (Cl. tetani)
- Human rabies (Rhabdovirus)
- Japanese encephalitis
- T. solium
- Echinococcus granulosus and Trichinella spiralis

Basics of Bacteriology

AEROBIC BACTERIA
• **B**acillus anthrax I.
• **B**ordetella pertusis
• **B**rucella
• **K**lebsiella
• **L**isteria monocytogenes
• **M**ycobacteria
• **N**ocardia
• **N**eiserria
• **P**seudomonas
• **P**roteus
• **P**asteurella group except Y. pseudo TB, Y. enterocolitica
• **V**ibrio cholera
Mnemonic: B_3 KLMN$_2$ P$_3$V

ANAEROBES	
I. Cocci	
• Gram-positive	: Peptococcus, Peptostreptococcus
• Gram-negative	: Veilonella
II. Bacilli	
• Endospores forming	: Clostridia
• Nonsporing:	
Gram-positive:	– Eubacterium – Propionibacterium – Lactobacillus – Mobiluncus – Bifidobacterium – Actinomyces
Gram-negative :	– Bacteroides – Prevotella – Fusobacterium – Leptotrichia
III. Spirochetes	– Treponema – Borreli

SPORE PRODUCING BACTERIA
• **B**. anthrax and subtilis
• **S**porosarcina
• **C**lostridia
• **C**oxiella burnetti
Mnemonic: BSC Chemistry

BACTERIA IN PAIR
• Neiserria
• Branhemella (Neisseria catarrhalis) and other Neiserria
• Pneumococcus
• Klebsiella

BIPOLAR STAINING = SAFETY PIN APPEARANCE
• Hemophilus ducreyi
• Vibrio parahemolyticus
• Yersinia pestis
• Calymmatobacterium or Donovani granulomatis
• Pseudomonas mallei
• Pseudomonas pseudomallei

INTRACELLULAR BACTERIA
• Brucella and Bordetella
• Mycobacteria tuberculosis and leprae
• Legionella
• Rickettsia and Chlamydia
• Listeria monocytogenes
• Yersinia pestis
• Pneumococci
• Salmonella and Shigella
• Donovani granulomatis
• Neisseria meningococci and gonococci

CASTANEDA'S STAINS
• Rickettsiae
• Chlamydiae

GIEMSA STAIN	
• Rickettsiae	• Mycoplasma
• Chlamydiae	• Treponema pallidum
• Helicobacter pylori and Malarial parasite	

UREASE POSITIVE

- **P**roteus
- **S**. aureus
- **M**organella
- **K**lebsiella
- **N**ocardia
- **Y**ersinia pseudotuberculosis, Y. enterocolitica
- **C**ryptococcus
- **D**iphtheroids
- **M**ycobacteria except MAC
- **H**. pylori
- **Corynebacterium urealyticum**

Mnemonic: PSM Ky NaYi Cory CD Meri Hai

ORGANISM NOT GROW IN ARTIFICIAL MEDIA

- M. leprae
- Rickettsiae
- Chlamydia
- Pathogenic treponemas
- Virus
- Rhinosporidium

DESCENDING PARALYSIS

- Polio
- Tetanus
- Botulism
- Diphtheria

TOXINS INHIBITING PROTEIN SYNTHESIS

- Sh. dysenteriae I
- Diphtheria
- Pseudomonas
- Verotoxin = Shiga like toxin of *E.coli*

ACUTE PHASE REACTANT (APR)

- C - Reactive protein (CRP)
- Mannose binding protein
- Alpha-1-acid glycoprotein
- Serum amyloid P component
- ESR
- Platelets
- Ferritin
- I L-1
- TNF
- Coagulation protein
- Complement
- α1 antitrypsin
- Fibrinogen
- Haptoglobin
- Ceruloplasmin

CAUSES OF TRAVELLER'S DIARRHEA

- **Enterotoxigenic Escherichia coli (MC)**
- Enteroaggregative E. coli
- Shigella and enteroinvasive E. coli
- Salmonella
- Campylobacter jejuni
- Vibrio cholerae
- Rotavirus and Norwalk-like virus
- Entamoeba histolytica
- Giardia lamblia
- Cryptosporidium
- Cyclospora

PULMONARY INFILTRATES IN IMMUNOCOMPROMIZED PATIENTS

Infiltrate	Causative organism
Localized	Bacteria, Legionella, Mycobacteria
Nodular	Fungi (e.g., Aspergillus or Mucor), Nocardia
Diffuse	Viruses (especially CMV), Chlamydia, Pneumocystis, Toxoplasma gondii, Mycobacteria

INFECTIONS AFTER HEMATOPOIETIC STEM CELL TRANSPLANTATION

Infection site	Period after transplantation		
	Early (< 1 month)	Middle (1-4 months)	Late (> 6 months)
Disseminated	Aerobic gram-negative, gram-positive bacteria	Nocardia, Candida, Aspergillus, EBV	Streptococcus pneumoniae, Haemophilus influenzae, Neisseria meningitidis
Skin and mucous membranes	HSV	HHV-6	VZV
Lungs	Aerobic, bacteria, Candida, Aspergillus, HSV	CMV, Pneumocystis, Toxoplasma	Pneumocystis, Nocardia
Gastrointestinal tract	C. difficile	CMV	
Kidney		BK virus, adenovirus	
Brain		HHV-6, Toxoplasma	Toxoplasma, JC Virus
Bone marrow			CMV, HHV

INFECTIONS AFTER KIDNEY TRANSPLANTATION

Infection Site	Period after transplantation		
	Early (< 1 month)	Middle (1-4 months)	Late (> 6 months)
Urinary tract	Bacteria (*Escherichia coli, Klebsiella,* Enterobacteriacea, *Pseudomonas,* Enterococcus) associated with bacteremia; Candida	CMV (*fever, bone marrow suppression, hepatitis*); BK virus (*nephropathy, graft failure, vasculopathy*), JC virus.	Bacteria (late urinary tract infections usually not associated with bacteremia); BK virus (nephropathy, graft failure, generalized vasculopathy)
Lungs	Bacteria – *Legionella* in endemic settings)	CMV diffuse; pneumonitis, Legionella	Nocardia, invasive fungi
Central nervous system		*Listeria* (meningitis), Toxoplasma gondii	CMV *disease; Listeria* (meningitis), Cryptococcus (meningitis), *Nocardia*

SEXUALLY TRANSMITTED MICROORGANISMS

Bacteria	Viruses	Other
Transmitted in adults predominantly by sexual intercourse		
Neisseria gonorrhoeae Chlamydia trachomatis Treponema pallidum Calymmatobacterium granulomatis Ureaplasma urealyticum	HIV (types 1 and 2) Human T-cell lymphotropic virus type-I Herpes simplex virus type-2 Human papillomavirus Hepatitis B virus Molluscum contagiosum virus	Trichomonas vaginalis Phthirus pubis
Sexual transmission repeatedly described but not well defined or not predominant mode		
Mycoplasma hominis Mycoplasma genitalium Gardnerella vaginalis and other vaginal bacteria Group B Streptococcus Mobiluncus spp.	Cytomegalovirus Human T-cell lymphotropic virus type-2 Epstein-Barr virus Kaposi's sarcoma – associated herpesvirus	Candida albicans Sarcoptes scabiei

GASTROINTESTINAL PATHOGENS CAUSING ACUTE DIARRHEA				
Mechanism	**Location**	**Illness**	**Stool findings**	**Examples of pathogens involved**
Noninflammatory (enterotoxin)	Proximal small bowel	Watery diarrhea	No fecal leukocytes; mild or no increase in fecal lactoferrin	*Vibrio cholerae*, Enterotoxigenic, *Escherichia coli* (LT and ST), *Clostridium perfringens*, *Bacillus cereus*, *Staphylococcus aureus*, Rotavirus, Norwalk-like viruses, Enteric adenoviruses, *Giardia lamblia*, *Cryptosporidium* spp., *Microsporidia*
Inflammatory (invasion or cytotoxin)	Colon or distal small bowel	Dysentery or inflammatory diarrhea	Fecal polymorphonuclear leukocytes; substantial increase in fecal lactoferrin	*Shigella* spp., *Salmonella* spp., *Campylobacter jejuni*, Enterohemorrhagic, *E. coli*, Enteroinvasive, *E. coli*, *Yersinia enterocolitica*, *Vibrio parahaemolyticus*, *Clostridium difficile*, *Entamoeba histolytica*
Penetrating	Distal small bowel	Enteric fever	Fecal mononuclear leukocytes	*Salmonella typhi*, *Y. enterocolitica*, *Campylobacter fetus*

NORMAL BACTERIAL FLORA	
Skin	• *Staphylococcus epidermidis* • Staphylococcus aureus • Micrococcus species • Nonpathogenic *Neisseria species* • Alpha-hemolytic and nonhemolytic streptococci • Diphtheroids • Propionibacterium species • *Peptostreptococcus species* • *Candida species, Acinetobacter species*
Nasopharynx	• Diphtheroids, Nonpathogenic *Neisseria* species, α-hemolytic streptococci; • *S. epidermidis*, Nonhemolytic streptococci, Anaerobes • Yeasts, *Hemophilus* species, pneumococci, *S. aureus*, gram-negative rods, *Neisseria meningitidis*
Gastrointestinal tract and rectum	• Various *Enterobacteriaceae* **except** Salmonella, Shigella; Yersinia; Vibrio, and Campylobacter species • Enterococci • Alpha-hemolytic and nonhemolytic streptococci • *Diphtheroids* • *S. aureus* in small numbers • Yeasts in small numbers • Anaerobes in large numbers (**MC** *Bacteroides*)

Genitalia	• *Any amount of the following:*
	   – Corynebacterium species, Lactobacillus species, α-hemolytic and nonhemolytic streptococci, Nonpathogenic *Neisseria* species.
	• *The following when mixed and not predominant:*
	   – Enterococci, *Enterobacteriaceae* and other gram-negative rods, *S. epidermidis*, *Candida albicans* and other yeasts.
	   – Anaerobes especially prevotella, *Clostridium* and *Peptostreptococcus* species.

TRANSPLACENTAL INFECTION		
• Toxoplasmosis	• Rubella	• CMV (**MC**)
• HSV	• Syphilis	• Varicella ZV
• Parvo B-19	• *Plasmodium*	• *T. cruzi*
• HIV	• Coxsackie virus	• Enteroviruses
• West Nile virus	• Measles	• Hepatitis B
• HCV	• TB	• Lymphocytic choriomeningitis virus

ONCOGENIC MICROBES AND PARASITES	
Organism	Neoplasm
Human papilloma virus (papovaviridae)	Cervical, vulvar, penile cancers, squamous cell carcinoma, oropharyngeal carcinoma
HSV type 2	Cervical carcinoma, B cell lymphoma
Hepatitis B virus (Hepadnaviridae)	Hepatocellular carcinoma
Hepatitis C virus (Flaviviridae)	Hepatocellular carcinoma, Lymphoplasmacytic lymphoma
HTLV - I (Retroviridae)	Adult T-cell leukemia/lymphoma
HTLV - I (Retroviridae)	T-cell variant of hairy cell leukemia
HTLV - III (Retroviridae)	AIDS related malignancies, NHL, Kaposi sarcoma, SCC (especially of urogenital tract), Diffuse large B-cell lymphoma, Burkitt's lymphoma
Epstein-Barr Virus (Herpesviridae)	Mixed cellularity Hodgkin's, Nasopharyngeal carcinoma (anaplastic), African Burkitt's lymphoma, Post organ transplant lymphoma, Primary CNS diffuse large B-cell lymphoma, Extranodal NK/T cell lymphoma (nasal type)
H. pylori	Gastric malt lymphoma, Gastric cancer
Human Herpes virus 8	Primary effusion lymphoma, Multicentric Castleman's disease
Schistosoma hematobium	Bladder cancer (squamous cell)
Clonorchis	Cholangiocarcinoma
Opisthorchis	Cholangiocarcinoma

CHAPTER 2

Basics of Virology

DEFINITIONS

Virion	• Extracellular infectious virus particle
Capsid	• Protein coat that protects nucleic acid.
Envelope	• Lipoprotein coat which surrounds some virus particles. Lipid is of host cell origin while protein in the form of peplomers is virus coded.
Viroids	• Subviral infectious agent which is protein free and consist of low molecular weight RNA *(mostly double stranded, small RNA)*. It is resistant to heat and organic solvents but sensitive to nucleases.
Prion	• Proteinaceous infectious particles causing chronic neurological degenerative disease of human

Virus is obligate intracellular parasite, without cellular organization and contains only one type of nucleic acid either DNA or RNA but never both. So classified as:

	CAPSID	VIRION	NUCLEIC ACID	VIRUS FAMILY	MEMBERS
DNA VIRUS					
I.	Icosahedral	Naked	SS (-ve)	Parvoviridae	B-19 parvovirus
II.	Icosahedral	Naked	ds circular (±)	Papovaviridae	Papilloma virus, JC, BK virus, polyomavirus
III.	Icosahedral	Naked	ds (±)	Adenoviridae	Human adenovirus
IV.	Icosahedral	Enveloped	ds with ss (±) circular	Hepadnaviridae	HBV
V.	Icosahedral	Enveloped	ds (±)	Herpesviridae	VZ; HSV I, II; CMV; EBV
VI.	Complex	Complex coats	ds (±)	Poxviridae	Variola (small pox) Molluscum contagiosum
RNA VIRUS					
I.	Icosahedral or (cubical)	Naked	SS (+)	Picornaviridae	Polio, Coxsackie, Entero, Rhino, HAV
II.	Icosahedral	Naked	SS	Astroviridae	Human Astrovirus
III.	Icosahedral	Naked	SS (+)	Caliciviridae	HEV, Norwalk
IV.	Icosahedral	Naked	ds segmented (±)	Reoviridae	Rota, Reo, Orbivirus
V.	Icosahedral	Enveloped	SS (+)	Togaviridae	Rubella virus
VI.	Unknown or complex	Enveloped	SS (+)	Flaviviridae	HCV, HGV, Yellow fever, Dengue virus
VII.	Unknown or complex	Enveloped	SS (-) segmented	Arenaviridae (sandy appearance)	Lassa fever virus
VIII.	Unkonwn or complex	Enveloped	SS (+)	Coronaviridae	Corona virus
IX.	Unknown or complex	Enveloped	SS diploid (+)	Retroviridae	HIV 1, 2; HTLV I, II; slow virus group
X.	Helical	Enveloped	SS (-) segmented	Orthomyxoviridae	Influenza A, B, C
XI.	Helical		SS (-) segmented	Bunyaviridae	Hantavirus, Sandfly fever virus
XII.	Helical	Enveloped	SS	Bornaviridae	
XIII.	Helical	Enveloped	SS (-)	Rhabdoviridae	Rabies virus, Vesicular stomatitis virus
XIV.	Helical	Enveloped	SS (-)	Paramyxoviridae	Parainfluenza, RSV, Mumps, Rubeola, New castle virus
XV.	Helical	Enveloped	SS (-)	Filoviridae	Marburg virus, Ebola virus

> **Mnemonic:**
> - Segmented Nucleic acid
>   = **'PARBO virus'** = **P**icornaviruses, **A**rena, **R**eo, **B**unya, **O**rthomyxovirus
> - Enveloped virus are sensitive to ether, chloroform, bile salts while non-enveloped are resistant
> - All RNA virus are enveloped except **'PARC'** = **P**icorna, **A**stro, **R**eo, **C**alciviridae

- **Viruses with both DNA and RNA:** – Retrovirus
  – Lentivirus
  – HBV
- **Complex capsid:** – Pox
  – Bacteriophage
- **Shapes:**
  - *Bullet shaped* : Rabies virus
  - *Brick shaped* :– Pox virus
  - *Rod shaped* : Tobacco mosaic virus
  - *Space vehicle* : Adenovirus
- Smallest size virus : Parvovirus
- Largest size virus : Filoviridae > Pox viridae
- Virus with smallest genome: Circoviridae
- Virus with largest genome: Pandoraviruses

HEMAGGLUTINATION (HA)

- It is agglutination of erythrocytes by virus.
- It is unstable in myxovirus because *Neuraminidase (RDE- receptor destroying enzyme)* cause reversal of hemagglutination called as *Elution*. RDE also produced by cholera vibrios and many vertebrate cells.
- In other viruses HA is stable.
- In arbovirus, it is reversible by variation in pH and temperature.
- HA measures total quantity of virus.
- HA of *human* RBC is seen in - **R**eo, **I**nfluenza, **P**ara-influenza, **E**ntero and some cox and ECHO, **M**umps.
  Mnemonic: RIPE Mango
- HA also seen in measles, toga, rhino, rabies, pox, adenovirus.

POCK ASSAY

Used for quantitative infectivity assay of viruses [also done by plaque assay] since each infectious virus particle can form one pock, for example, variola, vaccinia, HSV, Pox (Monkey, Cow, Camel).

PHAGE ASSAY

- Used for titrating number of viable bacteriophage and for purification of phages.

PHAGE TYPING

- Used for typing and identification of bacteria, for example, Intraspecies typing of S. typhi (by using Vi antigen) and S. aureus; species specific bacteriophage of B. anthracis, MukerJee's phage IV for classical V. cholerae.

VIRUS MULTIPLICATION

- Critical step in viral biosynthesis is transcription of mRNA from viral nucleic acid.
- **DNA virus** synthesize nucleic acid in host cell **nucleus** except pox which synthesis all their components in host cell cytoplasm.
- **RNA virus** synthesize nucleic acid in **cytoplasm** except orthomyxo, some paramyxo and retrovirus which synthesize partly in nucleus.
- **Viral protein** is synthesized only in cytoplasm.
- Herpes and adeno assembled in nucleus while picorna and pox are assembled in cytoplasm.
- **Envelop:** Lipoprotein envelop, proteins are synthesized in cytoplasm whereas lipid is derived from cell membrane.

ABNORMAL REPLICATIVE CYCLE

Von Magnus Phenomenon: High hemagglutinin but low infectivity due to defective assembly or incomplete virus e.g. *Influenza virus*.

Abortive Infection: Defect in the type of cell (non-permissive cell) not in the parental viruses, which lead to defective maturation or assembly.

Defective virus: Genetically defective virus which are incapable of producing infectious daughter virions without the helper activity of another virus, e.g. Rous sarcoma virus, Hepatitis D Virus, adeno-associated satellite virus (dependovirus), Measles virus from SSPE, etc.

VIRAL INTERACTION

- *Genetic Interaction* – occur in virus by:
  - *Mutation:* Occur during every viral infection. Most mutation are lethal.
  - *Recombination:* Occur when two different but related viruses (both active or both inactive or one active and one inactive) infect a cell simultaneously. It leads to cross reactivation/marker rescue; multiplicity reactivation and formation of pseudovirion.
- Non-Genetic Interaction
  - Phenotyping mixing: transcapsidation occurs
  - Genotyping mixing
  - *Complementation*
  - *Interference:* Infection of a cell by one virus inhibits simultaneous or subsequent infection by other virus. Most important mediator is Interferon, a soluble cellular product.
    - It is applied in controlling polio outbreaks by introducing live attenuated polio vaccine.
    - It can be produced by receptor destruction as in myxo and enterovirus or by autointerference.

INCLUSION BODIES

It is the most characteristic histological feature in virus infected cells. It is of following types:

a. Intracytoplasmic eosinophilic inclusions:

Negri bodies	–	Rabies
Guarnieri bodies	–	Variola (small pox), vaccinia
Bollinger bodies	–	Fowlpox
Henderson-Peterson bodies	–	Molluscum contagiosum

b. Intranuclear acidophilic inclusion bodies:

Cowdry type A	–	Herpes, Chicken pox, CMV, Yellow fever
Torres bodies	–	Yellow fever
Cowdry type B	–	Polio virus

c. Both Nuclear and cytoplasmic:

Warthin Finkeldey	–	Measles

d. Intranuclear basophilic inclusion bodies:

Cowdry type B	–	Adenovirus

RESPIRATORY VIRUSES

Viruses	Most frequent illness
Rhinoviruses	Common cold
Coronaviruses	Common cold
Respiratory syncytial virus	Pneumonia and bronchiolitis in young children
Parainfluenza viruses	Croup and lower respiratory tract disease in young children
Adenoviruses	Common cold and pharyngitis in children
Influenza A, B viruses	Influenza
Enteroviruses	Acute undifferentiated febrile illnesses
Herpes simplex viruses	Gingivostomatitis in children; pharyngotonsillitis in adults

VIRUS CAUSING LATENT INFECTION

• Measles	• Hepatitis B virus	• Hepatitis C virus	• Rabies virus
• Human T-lymphotropic virus	• Herpes virus	• Kuru	• Oncogenic virus
• Scrapie	• Human immunodeficiency virus		

REACTION TO PHYSICAL AND CHEMICAL AGENTS

- Stable at low temperature. So for long-term storage, they are kept by frozen at –70°C, by lyophilization or freeze drying but poliovirus do not stand freeze drying.
- All virus are disrupted under alkaline pH. Enterovirus are very resistant to acid pH while rhinovirus are very susceptible.
- Most active antiviral disinfectants are oxidising agents such as H_2O_2, $KMnO_4$ and hypochlorides.
- Chlorination kills most viruses except hepatitis virus and polio virus.

ONCOGENIC VIRUSES		
RNA VIRUSES	**Retroviruses**	
	• Avian leukosis viruses • Murine mammary tumour viruses • Human T-cell leukemia viruses	• Murine leukosis viruses • Leukosis-sarcoma viruses of various animals
DNA VIRUSES	**I. Papovavirus**	
	• Papillomaviruses of human beings, rabbits and other animals • BK and JV viruses	• Polyomavirus • Simian virus 40
	II. Poxvirus	
	• Molluscum contagiosum • Shope fibroma	• Yaba virus
	III. Adenovirus - *Not associated with human cancer*	
	IV. Herpes virus	
	• Marek's disease virus • Epstein-Barr virus • Herpes virus (pan, papio, ateles and saimiri)	• Lucke's frog tumour virus • Herpes simplex virus types 1 and 2 • Cytomegalovirus
	V. Hepatitis B and C viruses	

CHAPTER 3
Basics of Mycology

CLASSIFICATION OF FUNGI

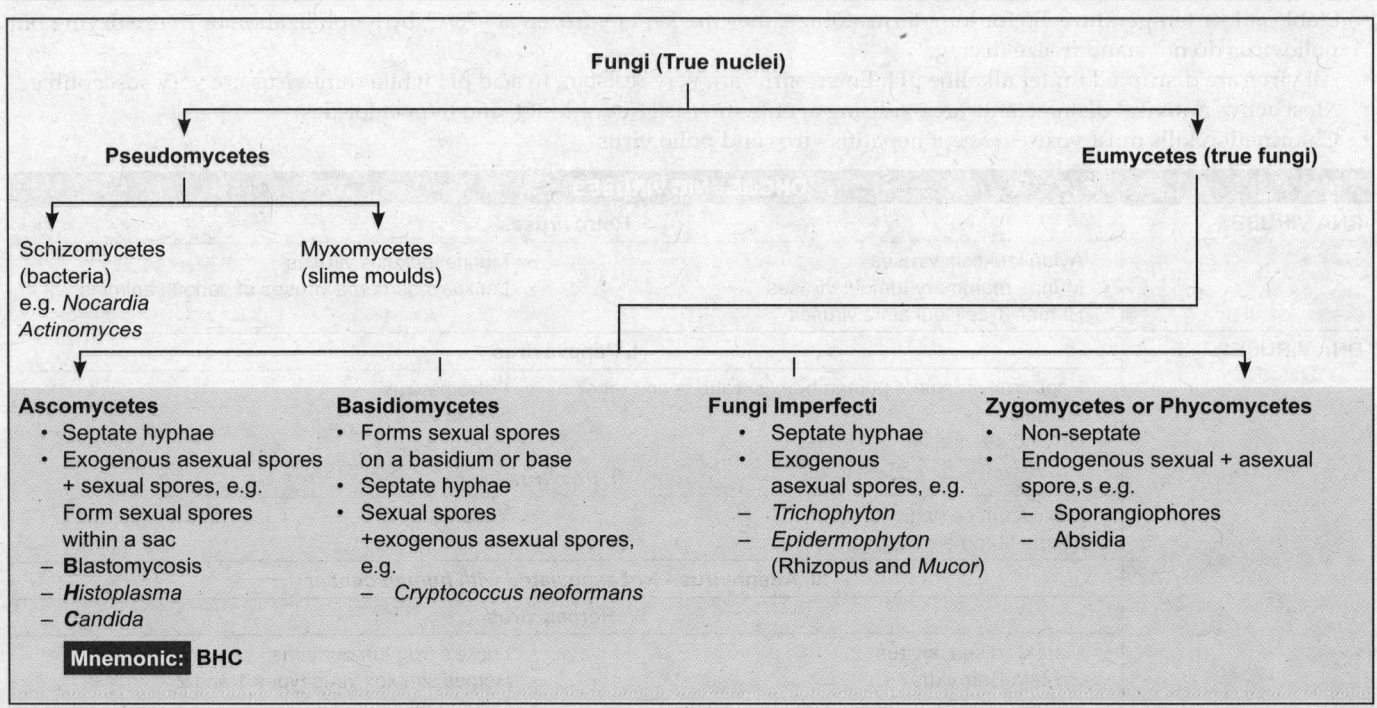

- Endogenous Asexual spores are called **'Sporangiospores'** while exogenous asexual spores are called **'Conidia'**.

Fungal stains	
• Gomori methenamine silver (Best)	• Giemsa
• Gridley fungus	• Alcian blue
• Periodic acid schiff	• Mayer's Mucicarmine

Fungal medias
• Sabouraud's glucose agar
• Corn meal agar
• Czapek-Dox medium

Morphological Classification			
Yeast	Yeast like fungi	Moulds/filamentous or Mycelial fungi	Dimorphic fungi
(No hyphae no mycelium) • Cryptococcus neoformans	Only hyphae in the form of pseudomycelium • Candida (forms blastopores) • Torulopsis (opportunistic)	Hyphae + mycelium forms • Dermatophytes (form arthrospores) • Aspergillus • Zygomycetes • Fusarium • Cephalosporium • Geotrichum • Scopulariopsis	• Candida albicans (not other candida) • Blastomyces dermatitidis • Paracoccidioides brasiliensis • Coccidioides immitis • Histoplasma capsulatum • Sporothrix schenckii • Penicillium marneffi

- Most fungi are soil saprophytes and human infection are mainly opportunistic.
- **Most** fungi causing *systemic infections* - Belong to Dimorphic fungi.
- **Most** fungi of medical importance belong to Fungi imperfecti group (Deuteromycetes or hyphomycetes).
- Aseptate fungi are called *Coenocytic fungi*.

Basics of Mycology

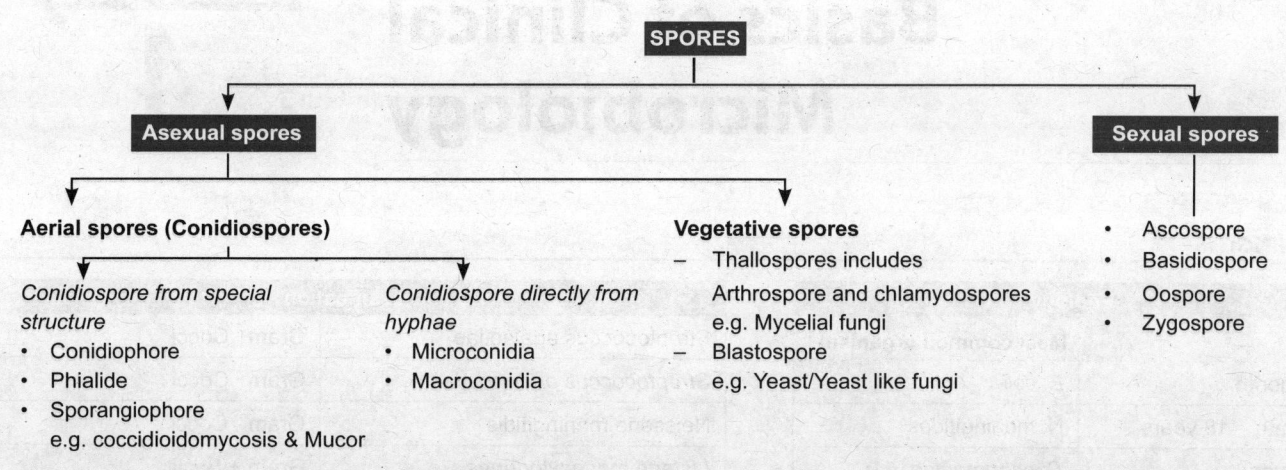

```
                            SPORES
                     ┌────────┴────────┐
               Asexual spores      Sexual spores
```

Asexual spores branches into:

Aerial spores (Conidiospores)

Conidiospore from special structure
- Conidiophore
- Phialide
- Sporangiophore
  e.g. coccidioidomycosis & Mucor

Conidiospore directly from hyphae
- Microconidia
- Macroconidia

Vegetative spores
- Thallospores includes
  Arthrospore and chlamydospores
  e.g. Mycelial fungi
- Blastospore
  e.g. Yeast/Yeast like fungi

Sexual spores
- Ascospore
- Basidiospore
- Oospore
- Zygospore

Fungal Disease in Man		
Superficial mycoses • Pityriasis versicolor • Tinea nigra • White piedra • Black piedra **Cutaneous mycoses** • Dermatophytes Microsporum, epidermophyton) • Candidiasis of skin, mucosa nails	**Subcutaneous mycoses** • Mycotic mycetoma • Sporotrichosis • Chromoblastomycosis • Rhinosporidiosis • Subcutaneous phycomycosis • Phaeohyphomycosis **Endemic (primary, systemic)** • Coccidioidomycosis • Histoplasmosis • Blastomycosis • Paracoccidiomycosis	**Opportunistic** • Systemic candidiasis • Cryptococcosis • Aspergillosis • Mucormycosis (Zygomycosis) • Penicilliosis

Basics of Clinical Microbiology

CHAPTER 4

MENINGITIS

Etiology	
Age	Most common organism
< 1 month	E. coli
1 month – 18 years	N. meningitides
> 20 years	S. pneumoniae

Classification	
Streptococcus agalactiae	Gram+ Cocci
Streptococcus pneumoniae	Gram+ Cocci
Neisseria meningitidis	Gram - Cocci
Listeria monocytogenes	Gram + Bacilli
Hemophilus influenzae	Gram - Cocco Bacilli

COMMON SYMPTOMS

Neisseria meningitidis	Symptoms	Hemophilus influenzae
• MC cause in 2-20 years age group. Transmission is via respiratory droplets. Pili allow the attachment to the nasopharyngeal mucosa from where it enters the blood stream causing meningococcemia. If it crosses the blood-brain barrier, it can infect the meninges, causing an acute inflammatory response that results in purulent meningitis. • Presence of petechiae or purpurial rash provides an important clue.	Headache Fever	• It is a normal resident of the human upper respiratory tract. Transmission is by respiratory droplets. • After attaching to the respiratory mucosa, the infection becomes systemic, with bacteria spreading via the blood to the central nervous system. It has been a leading cause of bacterial meningitis, especially in infants and very young children.
Streptococcus pneumoniae	Chills	**Streptococcus agalactiae**
• MC cause in > 20 years of age. It is carried in the nasopharynx of many healthy individuals. Infection can be either *endogenous* (in a carrier who develops impaired resistance to the organism) or *exogenous* (by droplets from the airway of a carrier). • S. pneumoniae infection can result in a bacteremia leading to infection of several sites in the human body, including the central nervous system. This meningitis has a high mortality rate.	Nausea and Vomiting	• It causes meningitis and septicemia in neonates. It is found normally in the vagino-cervical tract of female carriers, and the urethral mucous membranes of male carriers, as well as in the GI tract (especially the rectum). Transmission occurs during birth, and venereally among adults. • Infection of an infant occurs as it traverses the birth canal. Its infection is a leading cause of neonatal meningitis, and has a high mortality rate.
Listeria monocytogenes	Photo-phobia	
• It is common in neonates, pregnant women, elderly and in immunocompromised individuals for whom *Listeria* is one of the common causes of meningitis. *Listeria* infections are usually food borne, with the organism entering the body via the GI tract. • Newborns can become infected during birth, resulting in meningitis with a significant mortality rate, intrauterine infections can cause the fetus to spontaneously abort or be stillborn.		

URINARY TRACT INFECTION

Etiology

- **Non-catheter associated (community acquired):** E.coli, Proteus, Klebsiella.
- **Obstruction or calculi associated:** E.coli, Proteus, Klebsiella, Serratia and Pseudomonas.
- **Catheter associated (nosocomial):** E.coli, Proteus, Pseudomonas, Serratia, Staphylococcus saprophyticus.

COMMON SYMPTOMS

Escherichia coli

- *E.coli* is the most common cause of urinary tract infections (UTI), including cystitis and pyelonephritis. Women are particularly at risk for infection. Transmission is frequently from the patient's own flora.
- Uncomplicated cystitis (the most commonly encountered UTI) is caused by uropathogenic strains of *E. coli* characterized by *P. fimbriae* (an adherence factor). Complicated UTI (pyelonephritis) often occurs in settings of obstructed urinary flow, and may be caused by non-uropathogenic strains of *E.coli*.

Pseudomonas aeruginosa

- It is a major cause of hospital-acquired (nosocomial) infections such as UTI, particularly in patients who have been subjected to catheterization, instrumentation, surgery or renal transplantation, or to prior antibiotic therapy.
- Disease begins with attachment and colonization of host tissue. Pili on the bacteria mediate adherence, and glycocalyx capsule reduces the effectiveness of normal clearance mechanisms. Host tissue damage facilitates adherence and colonization.

Staphylococcus saprophyticus

- It is a frequent cause of cystitis in young sexually active women, probably due to its occurrence as part of normal vaginal flora. It is also an important agent of hospital-acquired infections associated with the use of catheters.
- It is a coagulase negative staphylococcal species. It is distinguished from other coagulase negative staphylococci by its *resistance to novobiocin*.

Common symptoms: Dysuria, Lumbar Pain, Fever, Chills, Hematuria

Proteus and Klebsiella

- *Proteus spp.* by virtue of urease production, and *Klebsiella spp.* through the production of extracellular slime and polysaccharides, predispose to stone formation and are isolated more frequently from patients with calculi.

Other enterobacteria

- Other genera of *Enterobacteriaceae,* such as Enterobacter and Serratia, which can be found as normal inhabitants of the large intestine, are primarily opportunistic and often nosocomial pathogens. They all frequently colonize hospitalized patients, especially in association with antibiotic treatment, indwelling catheters, or invasive procedures, causing extraintestinal infections such as those of the urinary tract.
- These organisms produce exotoxins. Wide spread antibiotic resistance among these organisms necessitates sensitivity testing to determine the appropriate antibiotic treatment.

Diagnosis

UTI is said when there is:	
	• Bacteriuria $\geq 10^5$/ml in *asymptomatic*
	• Bacteriuria of $> 10^4$/ml in *symptomatic*
	• Bacteriuria of $\geq 10^2$/ml in *catheterized* sample
	• Bacteriuria of *any degree* in *suprapubic* aspirate

Pyuria in the absence of bacteriuria (*sterile pyuria*) may indicate infection with *C. trachomatis, U. urealyticum,* and *Mycobacterium tuberculosis* or with fungi.

FOOD POISONING

Etiology

Onset : 1 – 6 hours	Onset : 8 – 16 hours	Onset : > 16 hours
• Bacillus cereus (vomiting) • Staphylococcus aureus	• Clostridium perfringens • Bacillus cereus (diarrhea)	• Vibrio cholerae • ETEC • EHEC • Campylobacter jejuni • Clostridium botulinum • Escherichia coli • Salmonella species • Shigella species • Vibrio parahemolyticus

COMMON SYMPTOMS

Staphylococcus aureus
MC cause of food poisoning in west.
• It is caused by ingestion of food containing the bacterial enterotoxin. Often contaminated by a food-handler, these foods tend to be protein-rich (e.g., egg, salad, cream, pastry).
• The toxin stimulates automatic nervous system by binding to neural receptors in the upper GI tract.
	Diarrhea
	
	Nausea and Vomiting
		Escherichia coli
		• It is part of the normal flora of the colon, but can be pathogenic both inside and outside of the GI tract. Transmission is by contaminated food (such as beef and unpasteurized milk) and water serving as the vehicles.
		• Several types of intestinal infections with *E.coli* have been identified.
		  – *Enteropathogenic E. coli*
		    - Diarrhea in infants and children
		  – *Enterotoxigenic E. coli*
		    - Traveller's diarrhea
		  – *Enteroinvasive E. coli*
		    - Diarrhea to dysentery similar to Shigellosis
		  – *Enterohemorrhagic E. coli*
		    - Hemorrhagic colitis
		  – *Entero aggregative E. coli*
		    - Persistent diarrhea

Campylobacter jejuni • Second MC cause of food poisoning in west. It also causes *traveller's diarrhea* and *pseudo-appendicitis*. • Transmitted to humans through exposure to contaminated meat (especially poultry). • It typically causes an acute enteritis after incubation period of 1-7 days. Symptoms may be both systemic (fever, headache, myalgia) and intestinal (abdominal cramping and diarrhea, which may or may not be bloody)	GI Disturbances	**Shigella species** • It causes shigellosis that occurs most commonly among young children. • It invades and destroys the mucosa of the large intestine resulting in bacillary dysentery which is characterized by diarrhea with blood, mucus, and painful abdominal cramping.
Clostridium species • *Cl. perfringens* food poisoning is caused by meat, chicken, fish. Typical episode involves cooking that fails to inactivate spores, followed by holding the food that allows bacterial germination and several cycles of growth. • It secretes a cytotoxin which acts on small intestine brush border altering its permeability. • Symptoms include diarrhea, abdominal cramp, nausea; fever is absent and vomiting is rare. • *Cl. botulinum* causes food poisoning without diarrhea. It produces a neurotoxin that results in flaccid paralysis. Contact with the organism itself is not required.	Fever Myalgia and Paralysis (in few cases)	**Salmonella species** • Non-typhoidal *Salmonella*, particularly *S. typhimurium* and *S. enteritidis*, cause a localized gastroenteritis where the symptoms result from the causative bacteria proliferating in the intestine of affected individuals. Transmission is usually via food, especially chickens, eggs, and egg products.

Culture and Sterilization

CHAPTER 5

Any chemical or method that aid growth of microbe in laboratory.
Louis Pasteur was the first person to use culture media, he used simple broth made up of urine or meat extract.
Robert Koch was the first to use solid media. He used potato piece to grow bacteria. After the suggestion of F. Elshemius wife of his assistant he used *agar to solidify culture media*, due to its high melting point.

The role of agar is to solidify the media.
It is used in 2% concentration

CULTURE MEDIAS

Type of medium	Name of medium	Laboratory use
Liquid media		
A. Basal (simple)	1. Peptone water	Routine culture, basal medium for sugar fermentation test
	2. Nutrient broth	Routine culture
B. Special (Complex) a. Enriched b. Enrichment	1. Glucose broth	Blood culture
	2. Robertson's cooked meat medium	Culture of anaerobic bacteria
	3. Tetrathionate broth	Enrichment culture for *Salmonellae*
	4. Selenite F broth	Enrichment culture for *Salmonella* & *Shigellae*
	5. Thioglycollate broth	Culture of anaerobic bacteria
	6. Alkaline peptone water	Enrichment culture for *Vibrio*
Solid media		
A. Simple	Nutrient agar (2-3% agar)	Routine culture
B. Special a. Enriched	1. Blood agar (also indicator media)	General culture, *Streptococcus*; **Most widely used medium**
	2. Chocolate agar	Culture of *H. influenzae, N. gonorrheae*
	3. Loeffler's serum	Culture of *C. diphtheriae*
	4. Dorsett's egg	Culture of *Mycobacteria*
b. Selective media (contains inhibitory substance)	1. MacConkey agar (also indicator and differential medium)	*Enterobacteria* (Lactose fermenters produce pink colonies)
	2. Deoxycholate citrate agar (DCA)	Selective medium for *Salmonella* and *Shigella*
	3. Lowenstein Jensen (LJ)	Culture of *Myco. tuberculosis*

Note: Agar is used in solid media due to its jellyfying property and it has no nutrient value.

Enriched Medium:
- Glucose broth (*Liquid*)
- Blood agar (*Solid*)
- Chocolate agar (*Solid*)
- Loeffler's serum (*Solid*)
- Dorsett's egg (*Solid*)

Selective Medium:
- MacConkey agar
- Deoxycholate citrate agar
- Lowenstein Jensen media

Indicator Media
- Wilson and Blair medium for *S. typhi*.
- Potassium tellurite in McLeod's medium for *diphtheria bacilli*.

Culture Medias of Important Bacteria	
Media	**Bacteria**
MacConkey Agar	Enterobacteria
Selenite F broth	Shigella and salmonella
Thioglycollate broth	Culture of anaerobic bacteria
BCYE Agar	Legionella
New York city Agar	Neisseria gonorrhoea
LJ Media	Mycobacterium
Charcoal yeast extract agar	Legionella

Enriched Media:
- Substances such as blood, serum or egg are added to basal medium

Enrichment Media:
- Liquid media containing substance that can promote the growth of desired bacteria or inhibit the growth of unwanted one.

Selective Media:
- Solid media containing inhibiting substances so as to depress the growth of unwanted bacterias.

Some Important Culture Medias
- ***Robertson's Cooked Meat Medium:***
  - Used for anaerobes
  - Consist of nutrient broth and pieces of fat free minced cooked meat of ox heart.
  - Unsaturated fatty acids present in meat utilize oxygen for auto-oxydation. Certain reducing substances such as glutathione and cysteine also utilize oxygen.
  - With growth of saccharolytic bacteria (*C. welchii*) color of meat turns red while proteolytic bacteria (*C. tetani*) turns it black.

- *MacConkey's Agar*
  - Selective and differential culture media for Gram-negative bacteria.
  - It contains bile salt, crystal violet dye, neutral red dye.
  - Crystal violet and bile salts inhibits the growth of Gram positive bacteria.
- *LJ Medium*
  - Specially used for Mycobacterium tuberculosis
  - Contains malachite green, glycerol, asparagine, potato starch.

STERILIZATION

Sterilization is the process by which article or medium is freed of all living microorganism either in the vegetative or spore state. Research of **Robert Koch** and his associates marks the beginning of science of disinfection and sterilization. Sterilizing agents are:
- Heat
- Radiation
- Filtration
- Sterilant gases, e.g. ethylene oxide
- Sterilant liquids.

DISINFECTION

Means destruction or removal of all pathogenic organism. Disinfecting agent (germicide) are:
- Substance interfere with membrane functions:
  - Surface active agents, e.g. quaternary ammonium compounds, tween - 80
  - Phenols, e.g. phenol, cresol
  - Organic solvents, e.g. chloroform, alcohols.
- Substance denaturing protein, e.g. organic acid, HCl, etc.
- Agents that destroy or modify functional group of proteins :
Heavy metals
  - Oxidizing agents, e.g. H_2O_2, chlorine, Iodine
  - Dyes, e.g. acriflovin, acridine
  - Alkylating agents, e.g. formaldehyde.

Heat
- Most reliable method of sterilization.
- It should be the method of choice unless contraindicated. It is of 2 types:

	Dry Heat	Moist Heat
Mechanism	Protein denaturation, oxidative damage and toxic effects of elevated levels of electrolytes	Denaturation and coagulation of proteins
Types	1. **Flaming** for sterilizing inoculating loop or wire tip of forceps and searing spatulas 2. **Burning or incineration** for contaminated cloth, animal carcasses and pathological materials, PVC and polythene (Polystyrene should autoclave) 3. **Hot air oven:** *Most widely used* method of sterilization by dry heat: • Holding period of 160°C for one hour is used to sterilize glassware, scalpels, forceps, scissors, all glass syringes, swabs, liquid paraffins, dusting powder, fats and grease. • For cutting instruments temperature of 150°C for 2 hours is required • **Drawback:** It has no penetrating power so not used for bulky articles such as mattresses	1. **Temperature below 100°C (for pasteurization of milk):** Holder method (63°C for 30 min) or **flash process** (72°C for 15 sec) destroy all nonsporing pathogens. Coxiella burnetii is relatively heat resistant and may survive holder method. Also used for vaccines of non-sporing bacteria, serum or body fluids containing coagulable proteins. **Inspissation:** Done between 75°C and 80°C. Purpose is to make the protein stiff without coagulation. Used for media containing serum or egg. 2. **Temperature at 100°C (Boiling):** Rolling boil (boiling for 5-10 minutes) will kill bacteria, but not spores or viruses 3. **Steam at atmospheric pressure 100°C:** Koch or Arnold steamer is usually used container and culture media are simultaneously sterilized. Single exposure of 20 min usually ensures sterilization; but for media containing sugars or gelatin an exposure of 100°C for 20 minutes on three successive days is used known as Tyndallization 4. **Steam under pressure = autoclave or steam sterilizer (>100°C)** - Most effective sterilizing agent for dressing, instruments, laboratory wares, media and pharmaceutical products; aqueous solutions. Sterilization control is by ***bacillus stearothermophilus***

Sterilization:
All organisms are removed.
Disinfection:
- Pathogenic organisms are removed

Moist heat sterilization:
- Pasteurization
- Boiling
- Tyndallization
- Autoclaving

- Sterilization control of dry heat is done by spore of non-toxigenic strain of Cl. tetani

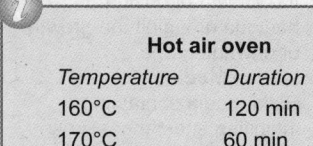

Hot air oven	
Temperature	Duration
160°C	120 min
170°C	60 min
180°C	30 min

- In autoclaving sterilization control is by bacillus stearothermophilus.
- Autoclaving is usually done at temperature of 121°C and chamber pressure of 15 psi for 15-20 minutes.

> **Note:** Autoclaving is usually done at temperature of 121°C keeping chamber pressure of 15lb per square inch for 15-20 min. It can also be done at 126°C (20 lbs psi) for 10 min on 133°C (30 lbs psi) for 3 min.

Filtration

Used to remove bacteria; virus isolation; testing water samples for Vibrio cholera or Typhoid bacilli; and obtaining bacterial toxins. Membrane filters is routinely used in water purification and analysis, sterilization and sterility testing and for preparations of solutions for parenteral use. Most widely used pore diameter is 0.22 µm.

Radiation

Bacterial vaccines are best sterilized by filtration.

Non-ionization	Ionizing radiation
1. Infrared radiation - Form of *hot air sterilization* used for rapid mass sterilization of prepacked items such as syringes and catheters	• X-rays, gamma rays (Commonly used) and cosmic rays referred to *as cold Sterilization* • Used for plastics, syringes, swabs, catheters, animal feeds, cardboard, oils grease, fabrics, metal foils, musculo-skeletal grafts catgut suture
2. Ultraviolet radiation - For entryways, operation theaters and laboratories	• Most effective but very costly

Cold Sterilization:
- Sterilization by ionizing radiation

Alcohols

- **Most commonly** used are ethanol and isopropyl alcohol *(better)*.
- Both used as skin disinfectant in 70% concentration.
- Non-sporicidal but active against non-sporing bacteria and viruses.
- Isopropyl alcohol is used for disinfection of clinical thermometers.
- Methyl alcohol, effective against fungal spores and is used for treating cabinets and incubators.
- Most effective skin antiseptic is alcoholic solution of chlorhexidine and iodine.

Aldehydes

- *Formaldehyde:* – Sporicidal (Slow activity), bactericidal, virucidal. Used for sterilizing instruments and heat sensitive catheters and for fumigating wards, sick rooms and laboratories.
- *Glutaraldehyde:* – Specially effective for *tubercle bacilli*, viruses and fungi.
  – 2% solution called *Cidex* used for cystoscope and bronchoscopes, face mask, plastic endotracheal tubes, corrugated anaesthetic tubes

- Cidex is used for sterilization of fiberoptic scopes (cystoscope, bronchoscope)
- Formaldehyde for fumigation
- Ethylene oxide for heart lung machine

Dyes

- Acridine and aniline dyes used as skin and wound antiseptic.
- More active against Gram positive organism.

Halogens

- Iodine in aqueous and alcoholic solution is used widely as skin disinfectant.
- Active against tubercle bacteria, viruses, spores (moderately).
- **Iodophores**^{Q} are compounds of iodine with non-ionic wetting or surface active agents. They are more active.
- Chlorine is used commonly as hypochlorites.

Ethylene Oxide

- Highly penetrating and highly active against all microorganism including viruses and spores^Q.
- Specially used for sterilizing **heart lung machine**^{Q} and commonly used for sterilizing disposable plastic syringes.

Formaldehyde Gas

- For fumigation of operation theaters and other rooms.
- Betapropiolactone is more efficient for fumigation than formaldehyde.

Sporicidal Agents:
- Ethylene oxide
- Formaldehyde
- Glutaraldehyde
- Halogens

Surface Active Agents

- Most important antibacterial agents are cationic surface active agents.
- Larks action on spores, tubercle bacilli and most viruses.
- Most active at alkalines pH.
- Soaps prepared from saturated fatty acids are more effective against G–ve bacilli while those prepared from unsaturated fatty acids are more active against G+ve and neisseria group.

Plasma sterilization

- Plasma consist of ions, electrons or neutral particles
- For sterilization, radiofrequency energy is applied to create an electromagnetic field. Hydrogen peroxide vapors are then introduced in the electromagnetic field. This results in generation of plasma containing free radicals of hydrogen and oxygen.
- Plasma sterilization is highly efficient and can be used for heat susceptible instruments too.
- Clinically it is used for sterilization of arthroscopes, uretheroscopes, etc.

> **Resistance of a living form to antiseptic:**
> Prions (Most resistant) > coccidia > Spores > Mycobacteria > cysts > Virus (non enveloped) > Gram negative bacteria > Fungi > Gram positive bacteria > Enveloped virus (Most sensitive)

Germicidal properties of chemical disinfectants and antiseptics

Agent	Bacteria	Mycobacteria	Bacterial spores	Fungi	Viruses
Disinfectants					
Alcohol	+	+	-	+	+/-
Formaldehyde	+	+	+	+	+
Phenolics	+	+	-	-	+
Chlorine	+	+	+/-	+/-	+
Iodine (iodophors)	+	+/-	-	-	+/-
Hydrogen peroxide	+	+	+	+	+
Glutaraldehyde	+	+	+	+	+
Quaternary ammonium compounds	+	-	-	-	+/-
Antiseptic agents					
Alcohol	+	+	-	+	+
Iodophors	+	+	-	+	+
Chlorhexidine	+	+	-	+/-	+
Parachlorometaxylenol	+/-	+/-	-	+	-
Triclosan	+	+/-	-	-	-

Biological controls of different sterilization methods

Methods of sterilization	Biological control
Steam	Bacillus stearothermophillus
Hot-air oven	Bacillus subtilis subsp. niger
Autoclave	Bacillus stearothermophilus
Ethylene oxide	Bacillus globigii (a red-pigmented variant of Bacillus subtilis)
Ionizing radiations	Bacillus pumilus
Filtration	Serratia marcescens, B. diminuta
Formaldehyde	B. stearothermophilus

- **Based on the efficacy disinfectant can be:**
- *High level disinfectant*: Chemical that kills all microbial pathogens except large number of spores, e.g., glutaraldehyde and hydrogen peroxide. They are used for *sub-critical* items like endoscopes and bronchoscopes.

- *Intermediate level disinfectant*: A chemical that kills all microbial pathogens including mycobacteria and non-enveloped viruses except spores, e.g., alcohol, phenolic compounds and iodophores. Used for some subcritical items like thermometer and BP cuffs for neonates.
- *Low level disinfectant*: A chemical that kills only vegetative bacteria, fungi and lipid enveloped viruses. Used for non critical items like bed rails, BP cuffs, bed side tables.

Note:

Critical Items:	Equipment/instruments that enters sterile tissue, e.g. surgical instruments, intravenous catheters. They should undergo sterilization.
Subcritical Items:	Equipment which came in contact with mucous membranes/non-intact skin
Non-critical Items:	These items came in contact with intact skin but not mucous membrane.

Remember: Some common terms:
- *Biocide:* A chemical or physical agent, usually broad spectrum, which inactivates microorganism
- *Bacteriostatic:* Property by which a biocide inhibits bacterial multiplication. Multiplication resumes, after removal of agent
- *Bactericidal:* Property by which a biocide kills bacteria (fungicidal, sporicidal, virucidal are analogous tems).

Multiple Choice Questions

Culture

1. Which of the following statement is true: [AI 07]
   a. Solid media are enrichment media
   b. Nutrient broth is basal media
   c. Agar adds nutrient to media
   d. Chocolate agar is selective media

Sterilization and Disinfection

2. Which of the following is most resistant to antiseptics?
   a. Spore   b. Prion   [AI 08]
   c. Cyst   d. Fungus

3. A chest physician performs bronchoscopy in the procedure room of the outpatient department. To make the instrument safe for use in the next patient waiting outside, the most appropriate method to disinfect the endoscope is by: [AI 03]
   a. 70% alcohol for 5 min
   b. 2% glutaraldehyde for 20 min
   c. 2% formaldehyde for 10 min
   d. 1% sodium hypochlorite for 15 min

4. Which of the following disinfectant is used to clean blood spill in OT: [AIIMS 2017]
   a. Chlorine based
   b. Phenol based
   c. Alcohol based
   d. Quaternary ammonium compound

5. All are true regarding disinfectants except:
   a. Glutaraldehyde is sporicidal [AIIMS 2011]
   b. Hypochlorites are virucidal
   c. Ethylene oxide is intermediate disinfectant
   d. Phenol usually requires organic matter to act

6. The operating temperature in an ethylene oxide sterilization during warm cycle is: [AIIMS 08]
   a. 20-35°C   b. 49-63°C
   c. 68-88°C   d. 92-110°C

7. The sterilization method for catgut suture: [PGI 2011]
   a. Steam   b. Radiation
   c. Boiling   d. Burning

8. Choose the correct ones for the decreasing order of resistance to sterilization: [PGI Dec. 07]
   a. Prions, bacterial spores, bacteria
   b. Bacterial spores, bacteria, Prions
   c. Bacteria, Prions, bacterial spores
   d. Prions, Bacteria, bacterial spores
   e. Bacterial spores, prions, bacteria

9. Decreasing order of resistance to sterilization: [PGI 07]
   a. Spores, prions, non-lipid of small virus
   b. Prions, spores, enveloped viruses
   c. Spores, mycobacteria, lipid or medium size virus

10. Sterilizing agents include: [PGI 02]
    a. Dry heat   b. Ethylene oxide
    c. Ether   d. Alcohol
    e. Chlorhexidine

11. Which of the following can be reliably used for hand washing: [PGI 00]
    a. Chlorhexidine   b. Isopropyl alcohol
    c. Lysol   d. Cresol
    e. Glutaraldehyde

12. Sporocidal agents are: [PGI June 09]
    a. Glutaraldehyde   b. Ethylene oxide
    c. Formaldehyde   d. Ether

13. Disinfection of sputum is done by: [PGI Dec 2008]
    a. Boiling   b. Autoclaving
    c. Sunlight   d. Burning
    e. Airing

14. Radiation can be used to sterilize all except:
    a. Bone graft   b. Suture   [AIIMS 2010]
    c. Bronchoscope   d. Artificial tissue graft

15. Which of the following is used as control during plasma gas sterilisation: [AIIMS 2010]
    a. B. subtilis
    b. B. stearothermophilus
    c. Cl. tetani
    d. Cl. perfringens

16. Sputum disinfection is done by all except:
    [AIIMS Nov. 2010, May 2012]
    a. Autoclaving   b. Cresol
    c. Boiling   d. Chlorhexidine

17. Which of the following is most resistant to the action of antiseptics and disinfectants: [AI 2012]
    a. Spores   b. Coccidia
    c. Prions   d. Mycobacteria

18. The indicator used in autoclave is: [AIIMS May. 2012]
    a. Clostridium tetani
    b. Bacillus stereothermophilus
    c. Bacillus pumilis
    d. Bacillus subtilis avarniger

19. Which is used in digestion and decontamination of sputum in smear preparation: [PGI May 2013]
    a. NaOH   b. KOH
    c. NaCl   d. KCl
    e. N-acetyl-L-cysteine

20. Plasma sterilization uses: [AIIMS May 2018]
    a. Ethylene oxide
    b. Hydrogen peroxide
    c. Formaldehyde
    d. Ozone

Explanations and References with Illustrative Answers

1. **Ans. (b) Nutrient broth is basal media** *Ref. Ananthanarayan 10/e, p 40, 9/e, p 40*

Media			
Simple media (basal media)	Complex media	Synthetic or defined media	Special media
• Nutrient broth • Nutrient agar	• Added ingredient	• Prepared from chemicals with defined composition e.g., simple peptone water medium	• *Enriched media* • Enrichment media • Selective media • Indicator media • Sugar media • Transport media

- **Enriched media:** Substance such as blood serum or egg are added to basal medium to promote growth, e.g. blood agar, chocolate agar, brain-heart infusion broth egg media.
- **Enrichment media:** In mixed culture usually the nonpathogenic or commensal bacteria tends to overgrow than pathogenic ones. In such circumstances, substances which has stimulating effect on pathogenic one or inhibitory effect on unwanted one are added to promote the growth of desired bacteria, if such substances are added to liquid medium. These media are called enrichment media, e.g. tetrathionate broth, selenite F broth, Alkaline peptone water.
- **Selective media:** As in enrichment media, if the inhibitory substance is added to solid medium, so as to supress the growth of unwanted one; the media is called *selective media* e.g., desoxycholate citrate medium.
- **Indicator media:** Changes colour on growth of bacteria e.g., Wilson Blair media; **McLeod** medium.
- **Differential media:** To differentiate different bacteria on the basis of characteristics, e.g. MacConkey's medium.
- **Sugar media:** – Here sugar means any fermentable substance.
  – Usual sugar media consist of 1% of the sugar in peptone water along with an appropriate indicator.
- **Transport media:** For delicate organism, e.g. Stuart media.

> **Remember Agar:** Contains long chain polysaccharide (mainly), organic salts and small quantities of protein like substances. It has no nutritive value. Its main role is to solidify the culture media. In solid media it is used in 2% concentration.

2. **Ans. (b) Prion** *See below*
   Resistance of organism to antiseptics in decreasing order is as follows:
   Prions > Coccidia > Spores > Mycobacteria > Cysts > Small non-enveloped virus > Trophozoites > Gram-negative bacteria (non-sporulating) > Fungi > Large non-enveloped virus > Gram-positive bacteria > Lipid enveloped/medium size virus (HIV, HBV)

3. **Ans. (b) 2% glutaraldehyde for 20 min** *Ref. Ananth. 10/e, p 33, 9/e, p 34; Chakorvarty 2/e, p 46*
   - 2% Glutaraldehyde also known as cidex (Aldehyde disinfectant), is specially effective against tubercle bacilli, fungi and viruses spores. It is most commonly used for cystoscope, endoscope, bronchoscopes, etc. which can't be disinfected by heat.
   - Also used to disinfect corrugated rubber anesthetic tubes and face masks, plastic endotracheal tubes, metal instruments and polythene tubing.

OTHER CHOICE		
• 70% alcohol is used as skin antiseptic • It acts by denaturing bacterial proteins • Methylated ethyl alcohol is MC alcohol preparation used for skin disinfection and hand washing	• 2-3 percent formaldehyde (20-30 ml of 40% formalin in one litre of water) is used for spraying rooms, walls, furniture and disinfecting blankets, beds, books • It is most effective at high temperature and relative humidity of 80-90%	• Sodium hypochlorite is recommended for sterilizing infant's feeding bottles • It acts in the same way as bleaching powder and is more strong.

Recommended Concentrations of Disinfectants Commonly used in the Hospitals

Disinfectant	Recommended concentration
Ethanol	70% (700 gm/litre)
Methylated spirit	70% (700 gm/litre)
Glutaraldehyde	2% activated (available commercially as cidex)
Bleaching powder (calcium hypochlorite)	14 g/litre of water
Sodium hypochlorite	1% solution, 0.1% solution
Hydrogen peroxide	3% solution
Lysol	2.5% solution
Savlon	2.0%, 5.0%
Dettol	4.0%
Betadine	2.0

4. Ans. (a) Chlorine based *Ref. CDC Recommendation Ministry of health website*

OSHA (Occupational safety and health standards) formulates a guideline in 1991 (amended in 1997) to eliminate or minimize occupational exposure to blood-borne pathogen.

As per the standard every blood stain has to be removed with hypochlorite solution or CPA registered tuberculocidal disinfectant.

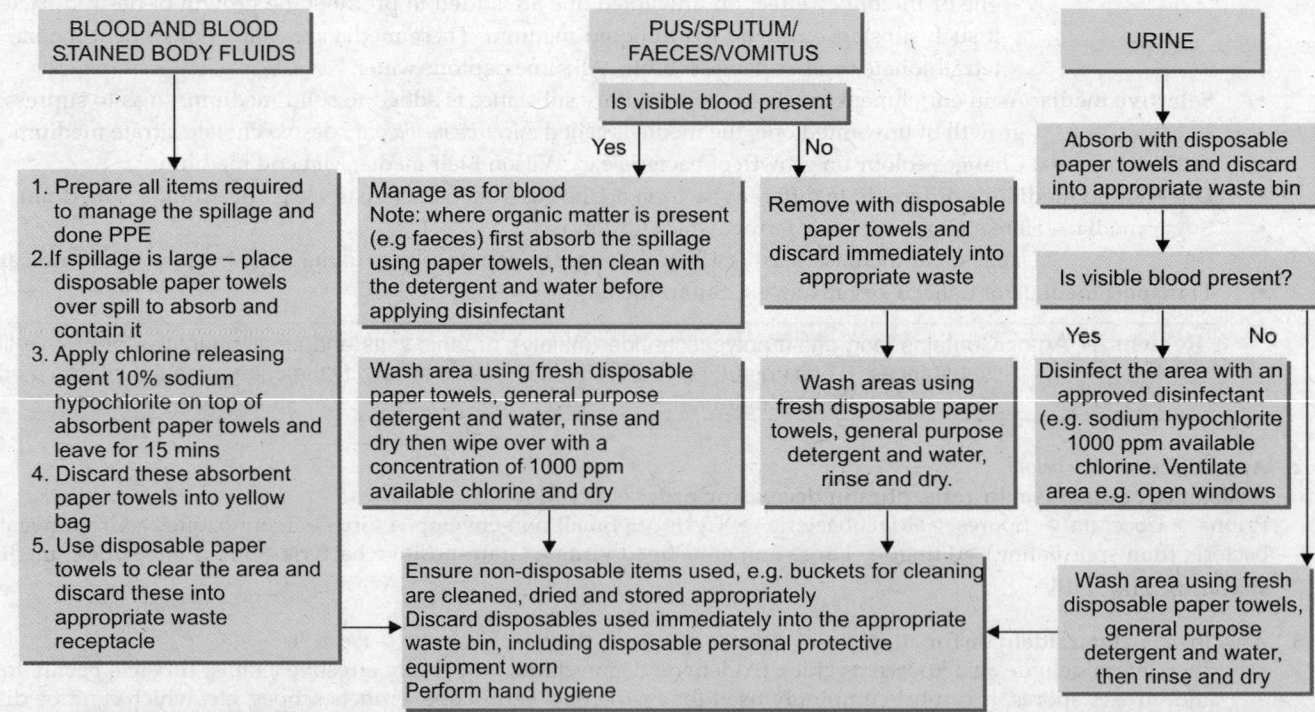

Clinical use	Commonly used disinfectant or method of sterilization
• Disinfect surgeon's hands prior to surgery	Chlorhexidine
• Disinfect surgical site prior to surgery	Iodophor
• Disinfect skin prior to venipuncture or immunization	70% ethanol
• Disinfect skin prior to blood culture or inserting vascular catheter	Tincture of iodine followed by 70% ethanol, or iodophor, or chlorhexidine
• Cleanse wounds	Thimerosal, chlorhexidine, hydrogen peroxide

Contd...

Contd...

Clinical use	Commonly used disinfectant or method of sterilization
• Cleanse burn wounds	Silver sulfadiazine
• Cleanup of blood spill from a patient with hepatitis B or C (disinfect area)	Hypochlorite (bleach, Clorox)
• Sterilize surgical instruments and heat-sensitive materials (e.g. endoscopes, respiratory therapy equipment)	Ethylene oxide or glutaraldehyde
• Sterilize non-heat-sensitive materials (e.g., surgical gowns, drapes)	Autoclave
• Sterilize intravenous solutions	Filtration
• Disinfect air in operating room (when not in use)	Ultraviolet light
• Disinfect floor of operating room	Benzalkonium chloride (Lysol)
• Disinfect stethoscope	70% ethanol
• Preservative in vaccines	Thimerosal

5. **Ans. (d) Phenol usually requires organic matter to act** *Ref. Ananthanarayan 10/e p34; 9/e p35*

   "Phenols are not readily inactivated by the presence of organic matter and are thus good general disinfectants".
   — *Ananthanarayan 10/e p 34*

   Phenols
   - Obtained by distillation of coal tar between temperature of 170 and 270°C.
   - Lethal effect is due to their capacity to cause cell membrane damage, precipitation of proteins and activation of membrane bound oxidases and dehydrogenases.
   - As they are not inactivated by organic matter, phenol can be used as general purpose disinfactant.
   - The related chlorphenols and chloroxyphenols are less irritant, active and more readily inactivated by organic matter.
   - Lysol and cresol are other phenolic disinfactants.

6. **Ans. (b) 49 - 63°C** *Ref. Park 22/e, p 121; Ananthanarayan 10/e p34*
   - Ethylene oxide is highly penetrating and highly explosive.
   - CO_2 or N_2 decrease its explosive tendency and water vapour increase its efficacy.
   - It acts as alkylating agent.
   - It is specially used for sterilizing heart-lung machines, sutures, dental equipment, books, fabrics, plastic equipment, cardiac catheters, clothing, glass, plastics, metal and paper surfaces.
   - *There are two types of cycles during ethylene oxide sterilization:*
     - Cold cycle operates at 37±5°C   Both cycles use Ethyle in oxide concentration of 700 mg/ltr. with
     - Warm cycle operates at 54±5°C   relative humidity 40-50%
   - It is unsuitable for fumigating room since it is explosive.

7. **Ans. (b) Radiation** *Ref. Ananthanrayan 10/e, p36, 9/e, p 33; Chakraborty 2/e, p 45-46*

Sterilization of Important Materials	
Materials	**Methods of sterilisation and disinfection**
1. Glasswares–syringes, Petri dishes, test tubes, flasks, surgical instrument; oily fluids and powders	Hot air oven
2. Serum, body fluids, bacterial vaccines	Waterbath, vaccine bath
3. Milk	Pasteurisation, 63°C × 30 min. or 72°C × 20 sec
4. Cystoscope and endoscope	Glutaraldehyde (Cidex-2%) or ethylene oxide
5. Most of the culture media	Autoclaving
6. Culture media containing egg, serum or sugar	Tyndallisation
7. Rubber, plastic and polythene tubes, disposable syringes	Glutaraldehyde, ethylene oxide gas
8. Dressings, aprons, gloves, catheters surgical instruments except sharp instruments.	Autoclaving
9. Sharp instruments	5% cresol
10. Suture materials except catgut	Autoclaving

Contd...

Contd...

Sterilization of Important Materials	
Materials	Methods of sterilisation and disinfection
11. Catgut	Ionising radiation
12. Rubber or plastic disposable goods, disposable syringes, bone and tissue graft, adhesive dressings	Ionising radiation
13. Faeces and urine, vomitus sputum	Bleaching powder, cresols, formalin, burning, autoclaving, boiling
14. Sterilisation of operation theatre	Formaldehyde gas
15. Wards and laboratory or operation theatre floor space	Formaldehyde gas and cresols (Lysol)
16. Skin	Tincture iodine, spirit (70% ethanol), Savlon (phenol derivative).

8. **Ans. (a) Prions, bacterial spores, bacteria**
   Already explained

9. **Ans. (b and c) Prions, spores, enveloped viruses and Spores, mycobacteria, lipid or medium size virus**
   Already explained

10. **Ans. (a and b) Dry heat and Ethylene oxide** *Ref. Chakraoborty 2/e, p 35, 41*
    Sterilization is the process by which an article, surface or medium is *freed of all living microorganism* either in vegetative or spore state.

Method of Sterilation		
Physical sterilants	**Gas Vapour sterilants**	**Chemical sterilants**
• Steam under pressure	• Ethylene oxide	• Glutaraldehyde
• Dry heat	• Formaldehyde vapour	• Peracetic acid
• Filtration	• Chlorine dioxide gas	
• UV radiation	• Hydrogen peroxide vapour	
• Ionizing radiation	• Plasma gas (highly ionized H_2O_2)	

Disinfection means "destruction or removal of *all pathogenic organism* which are capable of producing infection.

Disinfecting Agents	
• Heat (moist heat)	• Alcohols (ethyl and isopropyl alcohol)
• Dyes	• Halogens (Iodine, chlorine)
• Phenol derivatives (hexachlorophene, lysol, cresol)	• Biguanides (chlohexidine)
• Oxidising agents ($KMnO_4$, H_2O_2) peracetic acid.	• Quaternary ammonium compounds (cetrimide)
• Soaps	• Acids
• Aldehydes (formaldehyde, glutaraldehyde)	• Metallic salts
• U.V. radiation	

Remember: Ether is used as anaesthetic agent not as disinfectant or sterilizing agents.

11. **Ans. (a), (b) and (d) Chlorhexidine, Isopropyl alcohol and Cresol** *Ref. KDT 6/e, p 858-861; Chakarvarty 2/e, p 46*

Skin Disinfectants	
i. Chlorhexidine (Savlon)	vi. Cresol
ii. Alcohols (as spirit) - Isopropyl alcohol (preferred), ethyl alcohol	v. Chloroxylenol (Dettol)
iii. Iodine	vi. Hexachlorophene
	vii. Tincture iodine

12. **Ans. (a), (b) and (c) Glutarldehyde, Ethylene oxide, Formaldehyde** *Ref. Ananthanarayan 10/e, p 33*
    Sporicidal Agents:
    E – Ethylene oxide
    F – Formaldehyde

G – Glutaraldehyde
H – Halogens (moderate action on spores)
- Benzalkonium chloride is quaternary ammonium cationic, antiseptic which are not sporicidal. ...*KDT 6/e, p 860*
- Phenol and hexachlorophene are poor sporicidal

13. **Ans. (a, b and d) Boiling, Autoclaving, and Burning** *Ref. Park 22/e, p 122*

    Disinfection of sputum
    - Burning (best)
    - If amount is considerable as in TB, then disinfection is done by either boiling or autoclaving for 20 minutes at 20 lbs pressure or by 5% cresol.

14. **Ans. (c) Bronchoscope** *Ref. Ananthanarayan 7/e, p 35, 36; 9/e, p 34*
    - Rigid bronchoscopes are sterilized by autoclaving where as flexible bronchoscope and other flexible endoscopes are
    - sterilized by cidex (2% solution of glutarldehyde)
    - Bone graft and other salt tissue allograft (achilles tendon, fascialata) are sterilized by gamma irradiation.

Technique	Applications
Ionizing radiation	Rubber or plastic disposable items, bone grafts, tissue grafts, surgical catgut, culture media
Non-ionizing radiation	• Infrared radiation for rapid mass sterilization of syringes • Ultraviolate radiation for disinfection of OT, laboratories, entry ways.
Glutaraldehyde	Flexible endoscopes, face mask, anaesthesia breathing circuits, reusable plastic endotracheal tubes

Note:
- Red ruber (reusable) endotracheal tubes are sterilized by autoclaving
- Plastic endotracheal tubes (reusable) are sterilized by cidex (2% glutaratdehyde)
- PVC endotracheal tubes (disposable) are sterilized by ionizing radiation
- Spores and Gram positive bacteria are resistant to UV rays, that's why disinfection (not sterilization) is used in context to UV rays.

15. **Ans. (b) B. stearothermophilus** *Ref. Chakarvorty 2/e 41; Principles and practice of Disinfection and sterilization by A. P. Fraise, PA Lambert 4/e, p 423-428*

    Plasma Gas sterilization
    - This is a type of chemical sterilization using hydrogen peroxide
    - Hydrogen peroxide is vaporized which is then converted into plasma. For sterilizatiion only cold plasma is used.
    - When H_2O_2 vapours are energized into plasma, hydroxyl and hydroperoxyl free radicals are generated along with production or UV rays.
    - Microbicidal activity is via three mechanism:
      - Direct destruction by UV radiation
      - Free radical induced damage
      - Direct erosion of cells
    - The sterilization cycle of plasma is divided into five steps, viz:
      - Evacuation phase
      - Injection phase (until a 6 mg/L H_2O_2 level is obtained)
      - Diffusion phase
      - Plasma phase
      - Re-establishment of atmospheric pressure.
    - This plasma kills all spores, bacteria, fungi, virus. However prions are not killed at all.
    - Plasma sterilization is an alternative to ethylene oxide and is used for heat and water sensitive equipments.
    - *Sterrad sterilizers* is the only plasma gas sterilizer currently approved by FDA.

    Control: Bacillus stearothermophilus spores are used as biological indicator.

16. **Ans. (d) Chlorhexidine** *Ref. Park 22/e, p 120, 122*
    Already explained.

17. **Ans. (c) Prions** *Ref. Ananthanarayan 10/e p 560*

Already explained

18. **Ans. (b) Bacillus stereothermophilus** *Ref. Ananthanarayan 9/e p 32; 10/e p 30*
    Autoclave Quality Assurance
    Chemical and biological indicators are used to ensure than an autoclave reaches the desired temperature for the correct amount of time:
    (a) **Chemical Indicators:**
        - These indicators change colours when exposed to temperature equivalent to the autoclave desired temperature
        - Browne's tube, autoclave tapes are the chemical indicators commonly used.
        - Bowie dick tapes are used to test the vaccum obtained in the equipment.
    (b) **Biological Indicators:**
        - For determining the efficacy of autoclaving and other moist heat sterilization, spores of *Bacillus stearothermophilus* are used as test organism.
        - *B. Stearothermophilus* is a thermophilic organism with an optimum growth at 55 to 60°C. Spores of *B. stearothermophilus* require an exposure of 12 minutes at 121°C to be killed.
        - Paper strips impregnated with 10^6 spores are dried at room temperature and placed in paper envelope, along with the material to be sterilized.
        - After sterilization, the strips are inoculated at 55°C for five days, if growth is positive, than autoclave is faulty.

19. **Ans. (a, e) NaOH, N-acetyl-L-cysteine** *Ref. Ananthanarayan 9/e p 352, 10/e p 357*
    Decontamination of sputum
    - **Petroff's method**
        - Most commonly used method, here sputum is incubated with on equal volume of 4% NaOH solution at 37°C with frequent shakings till it become clear. It is then centrifuged and the sediment is neutralized with N/10 HCl
    - **N. acetylcysteine combined with 2% NaOH:**
        - This method is better than Petroff's. Here N acetylcysteine is used for liquification of sputum. NaOH kills the contaminating bacteria. The sample is then neutralized with buffer and concentrated by centrifugation.

20. **Ans. (b) Hydrogen peroxide** *Ref. Chakarvorty 2/e 41; Principles and practice of Disinfection and sterilization by A.P. Fraise, PA Lambert 4/e, p 423-428*
    Plasma Gas sterilization
    - This is a type of chemical sterilization using hydrogen peroxide
    - Hydrogen peroxide is vaporized which is then converted into plasma. For sterilization only cold plasma is used.
    - When H_2O_2 vapours are energized into plasma, hydroxyl and hydroperoxyl free radicals are generated along with production of UV rays.

    For details see answer no 15 of chapter 5.

Culture and Sterilization

NEET Pattern Questions

1. **Which is enrichment media:**
   a. Selenite F broth
   b. Chocolate media
   c. Meat extract media
   d. Egg media
   [Ref. Ananthanarayan, 10/e, p 40]

   Selenite F is an enrichment media for Sh. dysentery

2. **In nutrient agar concentration of agar is:**
   a. 1
   b. 2%
   c. 3%
   d. 4%
   [Ref. Ananthanarayan, 10/e, p 40]

   Nutrient agar is made by adding 2% agar to nutrient broth. Nutrient agar is the simplest and most common culture medium in routine

3. **Blood agar is an example of:**
   a. Enrichment media
   b. Indicator media
   c. Enriched media
   d. Selective media
   [Ref. Ananthanarayan, 10/e, p 40]

   Blood agar is a solid culture medium consisting of agar, peptones and blood

4. **Robert Koch assistant advised him to use agar instead of gelatine culture media for cultivation of bacteria as:**
   a. Agar has more nutrition
   b. Gelatin melts at 27°C
   c. Gelatin is not easily available
   d. Agar is cheaper
   [Ref. Ananthanarayan, 10/e, p 40]

   Gelatin liquids at 24°C whereas agar melts at 98°C

5. **Endoscope tube is sterilized by:**
   a. Glutaraldehyde
   b. Formalin
   c. Autoclaving
   d. Boiling
   [Ref. Ananthanarayan, 10/e, p 36]

6. **Brown's tube is used for:**
   a. Steam sterilization
   b. Radiation
   c. Chemical sterilization
   d. Filtration
   [Ref. Ananthanarayan, 10/e, p 30]

   Brown's tube: Chemical indicator of sterilization control. Green colour is produced after 60 minutes at 160°C or 115 minutes at 150°C

7. **Which of the following is a primary cell culture:**
   a. Chick fibroblast
   b. Hela
   c. HEP-2
   d. HL-8
   [Ref. Ananthanarayan, 10/e, p 442]

Cell Culture

Primary Cell culture
- Normal freshly taken cells e.g.
  - Monkey kidney
  - Human amnion
  - Chick embryo cell culture

Diploid Cell strains
- Cells that retain the original diploid chromosome number and karyotype
- Beside viral culture these cells lines are used for production of viral vaccine
  Example: Human fibroblast

Cutaneous Cell Lines
- Derived from cancer cells, they are capable of continuous serial cultivation indefinitely
  e.g. HeLa
  HEp-2
  KB Cell lines
  McCoy

8. **Prions are best killed by:**
   a. Autoclaving at 121°C
   b. 5% formaline
   c. Sodium hydroxide
   d. Sodium hypochloride
   [Ref. Harrison 20/e, p 3153]

   Autoclaving at 134°C for 5 hours or treatment with NaOH in 2N concentration is recommended for sterilization of prions

9. **Human fibroblast cell line is used for cultivation of:**
   a. Adenovirus
   b. Poliovirus
   c. HIV
   d. Measles
   [Ref. Ananthanarayan, 10/e, p 441]

   Diploid cell strain, Human fibroblast is used for cultivation of coxsackie, CMV, enterovirus, echovirus, HSV 1-2, Poliovirus, VZV.

1. **a.** Selenite F broth 2. **b.** 2% 3. **c.** Enriched media 4. **b.** Gelatin melts at 27°C
5. **a.** Glutaraldehyde 6. **a.** Steam sterilization 7. **a.** Chick fibroblast 8. **c.** Sodium hydroxide
9. **b.** Poliovirus

10. Chocolate agar is:
    a. Basal medium
    b. Enrichment medium
    c. Enriched medium
    d. Simple medium
    [Ref. Ananthanarayan, 10/e, p 40]

> Enriched media: Brain-heart infusion broth/agar, blood agar, chocolate agar, egg media.

11. Simple based media is:
    a. Simple nutrient agar
    b. Alkaline peptone water
    c. Glucose broth
    d. Blood agar
    [Ref. Ananthanarayan, 9/e, p 40]

> Nutrient agar made by adding 2% agar to nutrient broth is simplest and most common medium in routine microbiology

12. Triple iron sugar medium contains all, *except*:
    a. Lactose
    b. Sucrose
    c. Glucose
    d. Maltose

> Triple sugar iron agar (TSI) is a differential medium that contains lactose, sucrose and a small amount of glucose. It is used to differentiate enteric organism based on the ability to reduce sulfur and ferment carbohydrates.

13. Preferred urine specimen for anerobic culture should be:
    a. Mid stream urine sample
    b. First few drops at morning
    c. Sample by Foley's catheter
    d. Sample by suprapubic aspiration
    [Ref. Ananthanarayan, 10/e p 678]

14. Not an enrichment medium:
    a. Selenite F broth
    b. Tetrathionate broth
    c. Alkaline peptone water
    d. Loeffler's serum
    [Ref. Ananthanarayan, 10/e, p 40]

15. All selective media are correctly matched *except*:
    a. V cholerae-TCBS medium
    b. Pseudomonas-Cetrimide agar
    c. M tuberculosis-LJ medium
    d. Campylobacter-BCYE medium

> BCYE is the selective media for legionella.

16. Best specimen for anaerobic culture:
    a. Exudates from wound
    b. Pus aspirated in vial
    c. Swab from wound
    d. Mid-stream urine

> Best specimen for anaerobic culture is an aspirate obtained by needle & syringe, this is to prevent exposure of air.
> **Anaerobic specimen collection:**
> - Disinfect skin surface with 70% alcohol, allow to dry
> - Aspirate specimen directly into the syringe
> - If unable to aspirate, infect 0.9% saline and repeat aspiration
> - Remove air from syringe
> - Aseptically transfer material into an anaerobic transport vial for fluids

17. Aerobic blood culture should be incubated for how many days, before discarding:
    a. 2 days
    b. 3 days
    c. 10 days
    d. 14 days

> Incubation time
> 48 hours : Aerobic
> 72 hours : Anaerobic
> 7 days : Final report negative culture

18. Differential media is:
    a. Nutrient agar
    b. Chocolate agar
    c. MacConkey's agar
    d. Tetrathionate broth   [Ref. Ananthanarayan, 10/e, p 42]

19. New York agar is used for:
    a. Salmonella
    b. Clostridia
    c. Neisseria
    d. Bacillus Anthracis

> **New York city agar**, a peptone corn starch agar base buffered with phosphates supplemented with horse plasma, horse haemoglobin, dextrose and antibiotics. Peptone, haemoglobin provide nutrients for the growth of N. gonorrhoeae.

20. Laparoscope is sterilized by:
    a. 2% formaline
    b. 2% glutaraldehyde
    c. Autoclaving
    d. Boiling
    [Ref. Ananthanarayan, 10/e, p 36]

21. Gamma irradiation used for all of the following except:
    a. Syringes
    b. Catgut suture
    c. Grafts
    d. Endoscope
    [Ref. Ananthanarayan, 10/e, p 36]

22. Sterilization is defined as:
    a. Disinfection of skin
    b. Complete destruction of all microorganisms
    c. Destruction of pathogenic organisms
    d. Decrease bacterial count from objects
    [Ref. Ananthanarayan, 10/e, p 28]

23. Cold sterilization is:
    a. Sterilization by negative temperature
    b. Sterilization by ionizing radiation
    c. Sterilization by liquid CO_2
    d. Sterilization by non-ionizing radiation
    [Ref. Ananthanarayan, 10/e, p 32]

> Cold sterilization is a process in which sterilization is carried out at low temperature with the help of chemicals, radiation, membranous filters

24. Seitz filter is a:
    a. Candle filter
    b. Asbestos filter
    c. Membrane filter
    d. Sintered glass filters
    [Ref. Ananthanarayan, 10/e, p 32]

Ans.
10. b. Enrichment...   11. a. Simple nutrient...   12. d. Maltose   13. a. Mid stream...   14. d. Loeffler's serum
15. d. Campylobacter...   16. b. Pus aspirated...   17. b. 3 days   18. c. MacConkey's...   19. c. Neisseria
20. b. 2% glutaraldehyde   21. d. Endoscope   22. b. Complete...   23. b. Sterilization by...   24. b. Asbestos filter

Culture and Sterilization

Types of filters.
(a) *Candle filter*: Mainly used for purification of water for industrial and drinking purpose. E.g. Doulton and Chamberlon
(b) *Asbestos filter*: Disposable single use. The carcinogenic potential of asbestos has discouraged their use. E.g. Seitz and sterimat.
(c) *Sintered glass filter*: They are brittle and expensive
(d) *Membrane filter*: Made of cellulose esters. They are routinely used in water purification and analysis and have replaced other types of filters.

25. Best virucidal disinfectant is:
    a. Phenol
    b. Hypochlorite
    c. BPL
    d. Formaldehyde
    [Ref. Ananthanarayan, 10/e, p 436]

Virucidal Disinfectants
- The most active antiviral disinfectants are oxidising agents such as hydrogen peroxide, potassium permanganate and hypochlorite.
- Formaldehyde and beta propiolactone are actively virucidal but less effective than oxidising agents.
- Phenolic disinfectants are only weakly virucidal.

26. Lethal effect of dry heat is due to:
    a. Denaturation of proteins
    b. Oxidative damage
    c. Toxicity due to metabolites
    d. All of the above   [Ref. Ananthanarayan, 10/e, p 29]

27. Sterilization of culture media containing serum is by:
    a. Autoclaving
    b. Micropore filter
    c. Gamma radiation
    d. Centrifugation
    [Ref. Ananthanarayan, 10/e, p 36; 9/e p 37]

- Most of culture media are sterilized by Autoclaving at 121°C for 15 min at 15 lb pressure/inch^2.

28. Example of selective medium is:
    a. LJ medium
    b. Blood agar
    c. Selenite F broth
    d. Chocolate agar
    [Ref. Ananthanarayan, 10/e, p 42]

29. Principal of using Robertson cooked meat broth:
    a. Meat kills other bacteria
    b. Meat is utilized by anaerobes
    c. Content of meat extract utilize O_2
    d. All of the above   [Ref. Chakraborty 2/e, p56]

30. pH of Sabouraud's dextrose agar:
    a. 7.4
    b. 7.0
    c. 9.6
    d. 5.6
    [Ref. Ananthanarayan, 10/e, p 42]

Sabouraud Dextrose Agar
- Culture media for fungi
- Medium has low pH (about 5.0) which inhibits the growth of most bacteria
- Antibacterial agents can also be added to enhance antibacterial effect

31. Medium used for antibiotic sensitivity:
    a. CLED agar
    b. Hektoen agar
    c. Mueller-Hinton agar
    d. Salt milk agar
    [Ref. Ananthanarayan, 10/e, p 639]

Mueller-Hinton Agar is most frequently used culture media for antibiotic susceptibility testing.
Read antibiotic sensitivity testing in appendix.

32. Hot air oven is used to sterilize all *except*:
    a. Inoculating loop or wire
    b. Glassware
    c. Dusting powder
    d. Liquid paraffin
    [Ref. Ananthanarayan, 10/e, p 30]

33. Technique of sterilization was introduced by:
    a. Robert Koch
    b. Edward Jenner
    c. Louis Pasteur
    d. Lister

34. Inspissation is used for:
    a. Sputum
    b. Protein containing culture medium
    c. Serum containing culture medium
    d. Plasma sterilization
    [Ref. Ananthanarayan, 10/e, p 30]

35. High level disinfectant are used for:
    a. Stethoscopes
    b. Electronic thermometers
    c. Bronchoscopes
    d. Surgical instruments
    [Ref. Ananthanarayan, 10/e, p 37]

36. Hot air over holding time and temperature:
    a. 121°C for 15 minutes
    b. 160°C for 45 minutes
    c. 135°C for 5 minutes
    d. 190°C for 30 minutes
    [Ref. Ananthanarayan, 10/e, p 30]

Ans.
25. **b.** Hypochlorite
26. **d.** All of the above
27. **a.** Autoclaving
28. **a.** LJ medium
29. **c.** Content of meat extract utilize O_2
30. **d.** 5.6
31. **c.** Mueller-Hinton…
32. **a.** Inoculating loop…
33. **a.** Robert Koch
34. **b.** Protein containing…
35. **c.** Bronchoscopes
36. **d.** 190°C for 30 minutes

Bacterial Genetics

- Molecular genetics begins with central dogma in which DNA (deoxyribonucleic acid) carries genetic information which is transferred to RNA by *transcription* and then *translated* as a particular polypeptide.

$$DNA \rightarrow RNA \rightarrow Polypeptide$$

- This central dogma is seen in all eukaryotes and prokaryotes, however in some virus genetic material is stored in the form of RNA, as in HIV virus.

  Information in this case would be transferred as

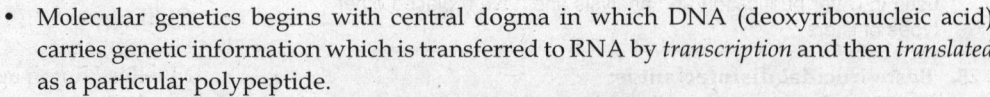

$$RNA \xrightarrow{\text{Reverse transcription}} ssDNA \rightarrow dsDNA \rightarrow \text{Integration with host chromosome}$$
$$\downarrow$$
$$\text{Viral polypeptide}$$

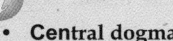

- **Central dogma:**→
- DNA → RNA → Polypeptide
- With few exceptions bacterial genes are haploid
- Most prokaryotes contain single circular DNA.

EXTRACHROMOSOMAL GENETIC ELEMENTS

- In addition to chromosomal DNA, most bacteria possess extrachromosomal genetic elements. These are not essential for life but provides additional properties such as drug resistance and toxigenicity
- Plasmids are circular DNA molecules present in the cytoplasm of bacteria capable of autonomous replication. They are seen in some eukaryotes also
- Plasmids encode properties such as drug resistance, toxin production
- Plasmids can be classified on the basis of:
  a. *Physical methods:* By restriction endonuclease enzyme (**enzyme that cut DNA molecule at or near to specific nucleotide sequence**). Similar plasmids produce similar restriction endonuclease finger prints
  b. *Genetic methods:* Genetic test can distinguish self transmissible plasmid from non-transmissible plasmids. Incompatibility typing is a specific genetic method in which plasmids are classified on the basis of compatibility. Closely related plasmids cannot co-exist in the same cell, hence are incompatible.

Properties encoded by plasmid:
- Resistance to antibiotics (R factor)
- Conjugation by coding for specialized fimbria (sex pilus)
- Bacitracin production, enterotoxin production
- Resistance to toxic metal ions
- Reduced sensitivity to mutagens
- Ability to degrade complex molecules.

TRANSMISSION OF GENETIC MATERIAL

Transformation

- Transfer of genetic material through the agency of **free DNA**[Q]
- Bacteria take DNA from outside, incorporate it with existing DNA through a process called recombination
- Seen in pneumococci[Q], *H. influenzae* and certain bacillus species.

Transduction

- Transfer of a portion of the DNA from one bacterium to another by a bacteriophage is known as transduction[Q]
- **MC** mode of gene transfer among prokaryotes
- Transduction happens through either the lytic cycle or lysogenic cycle:

- **Plasmids:**
  Extrachromosomal DNA molecules that are capable of autonomous replication. They are not essential for life, but provide some useful powers.
- **Episome:** Plasmid DNA integrated with chromosomal DNA

- *Lysogenic cycle*: The phage chromosome is integrated (*by covalent bonds*) to the bacterial chromosome where it can remain dormant for thousands of generation. This latent form of phage in which viral genes are present in the bacterium without causing disruption of bacterial cell is called as **Prophage**.
- *Lytic cycle*: In lytic or virulent cycle, large number of progeny phages are builtup inside the host bacterium which ruptures (lysis) to release them.

Note:	**Generalized transduction**: Transfer of any bacterial gene to another bacterium through bacteriophage **Specialized transduction**: Restricted set of bacterial genes is transferred to another bacterium. Transduction is not confined to chromosomal DNA episome and plasmid genes may also be transduced *Ananthanarayan 10/e p60*

Conjugation

- The process in which donor bacterium makes physical contact with female or recipient bacterium and transfers genetic element into it
- Male status or donor status is determined by the presence of a plasmid which codes for specialised fimbria.
- The plasmid responsible was termed as sex factor or F factor
- Other similar plasmids which can be transferred through conjugation are called transfer factor.

Factors Transferred by Plasmid

- F. factor: Factor containing information for synthesis of sex pilus (not for drug resistance)
- Col factor: Plasmid containing genes that synthesise colicins, an antibiotic like substance
- Resistance transfer factor: Transmit multiple drug resistance. This plasmid along with resistance determinant makes R. factor

```
                R. factor
                  |
        ----------+----------
        |                   |
Resistance transfer factor   Resistance determinant
```

- Can transmit resistance to as many as 8 drugs simultaneously. This mechanism of drug resistance is known as transferable, episomal or infectious drug resistance.

Genetic Mechanism of Drug Resistance

- Drug resistance may be acquired by mutation or by one of the method of genetic transfer
- Mutational resistance is mainly of two types:
  - *Step wise mutation*: As seen with penicillin where high level of resistance are achieved only by a series of small step mutation
  - *One step mutation*: As seen with streptomycin in which bacteria may become totally resistant to drug after one step mutation

GENETIC BASIS OF DRUG RESISTANCE

Mutation in gene = Chromosomal mutation

Gene transfer

Transformation
- Significance in nature is not known

Transduction
- Penicillin resistance in staphylococci
- Chromosomal DNA, plasmid and episomes all can be transduced
- Most widespread method of gene transfer

Conjugation
- **It is most important method of drug resistance.**
- Occurs by plasmid called R factor.
- It can promote chromosomal transfer from diverse bacteria including *Pseudomonas* species

---

Genetic Material is transmitted by:
Transformation: First example of genetic exchange to have been discovered. Involve transfer of information via **Free DNA**
Transduction: Transfer of DNA from one bacterium to other bacterium via demons, i.e. bacteriophage
Conjugation: Involve contact of two bacterium with one another.

> **Note:**
> - Transfer of drug resistance by conjugation of whole plasmid (RTF + r determinants = R factor) is known as transferable or episomal or infectious drug resistance.
> - Enterotoxin and hemolysin production in some enteropathogenic E. coli are also transmitted by RTF (resistance transfer factor).
> - Plasmid are genetic elements most frequently transferred by conjugation.

Few facts about HFr Strains

- In conjugation the male status or donor status is determined by presence of plasmid that codes for specialized fimbria. The prototype of this plasmid is called *F factor*
    - Cell containing F factor are called F$^+$ while lacking ones are called F$^-$
    - F factor is usually an episome which has got the ability to exist both in free state (as in F$^+$), as plasmid or integrated with host chromosome (HFR strains). It contains genetic information necessary for synthesis of sex pilus and for self transfer but is devoid of other markers such as drug desistance
    - Cells in which the F plasmid is inserted in to chromosome are called HFr strains as they can transfer the gene to recipient cell at a high frequency
    - In few HFr strains F plasmid can excise themself in to free state, but during excision they carry some of the neighboring gene. This F-plasmid which has picked up a small chromosome is called *F-prime (F')*
    - This F' when mates with F-transmit some additional gene in addition to F factor. This process resembles transduction and is called *sex duction.*

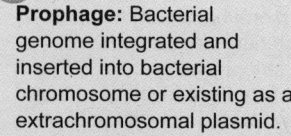

Prophage: Bacterial genome integrated and inserted into bacterial chromosome or existing as an extrachromosomal plasmid.

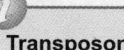

Transposons: Carry information from chromosome to plasmid and vice versa: (Analogous to "Naradhmuni')

Transposable Genetic Elements

- Certain structurally and genetically discrete segment of DNA, move between chromosomal and extrachromosomal DNA molecules within cells. These DNA of molecules are called *transposons (jumping genes)* and the process is called *transposition*.
- Unlike plasmids transposons are not self replicating and depend on chromosomal or plasmid DNA
- They can transfer DNA in molecules that have genetic homology and thus differ from recombination.

Biofilm Related Infections

Biofilm formation is a process whereby microorganisms irreversibly attach to and grow on a surface and produce extracellular polymers that facilitate attachment and matrix formation, resulting in an alteration in the phenotype of the organisms with respect to growth rate and gene transcription.

Biofilm Composition: Complex assembly of protein, polysaccharide, and DNA in a self-produced extracellular polymeric matrix of Glycocalyx.

Organism Involved: Broad types of organisms develop biofilms include a number of known pathogenic bacteria and fungi.

Indwelling medical device	Organisms
Central venous catheter	Coagulase-negative staphylococci, *Staphylococcus aureus*, *Enterococcus faecalis*, *Klebsiella pneumoniae*, *Pseudomonas aeruginosa*, *Candida albicans*
Prosthetic heart valve	Viridans *Streptococcus*, coagulase-negative staphylococci, enterococci, *Staphylococcus aureus*
Urinary catheter	*Staphylococcus epidermidis*, *Escherichia coli*, *Klebsiella pneumoniae*, *Enterococcus faecalis*, *Proteus mirabilis*

Contd...

Contd...

Indwelling medical device	Organisms
Artificial hip prosthesis	Coagulase-nagative staphylococci, β-hemolytic streptococci, enterococci, *Proteus mirabilis, Bacterioides species, Staphylococcus aureus,* viridans *Streptococcus, Escherichia coli, Pseudomonas aeruginosa*
Artificial voice prosthesis	*Candida albicans, Streptococcus mitis, Streptococcus salivarius, Rothia dentrocariosa, Candida tropicalis, Streptococcus sobrinus, Staphylococcus epidermidis, Stomatococcus mucilaginous*
Intrauterine device	*Staphylococcus epidermidis, Corynebacterium species, Staphylococcus aureus, Micrococcus species, Lactobacillus plantarum* group B streptococci, *Enterococcus species, Candida albicans*

Resistance Mechanisms of Biofilm

- *Capsules or Glycocalyx*: Glycocalyx is an integral part of the biofilms, this layer accumulates antibacterial molecule up to 25% of its weight. The adsorption sites of the matrix limit the transportation of biocides and served an adherent for exoenzymes
- *Enzyme-Mediated Resistance*: Enzymes present in biofilm detoxify the antimicrobial agents
- *Heterogeneity in Metabolism and Growth Rate*: Antibiotics are highly effective in killing rapidly dividing and metabolically active microbes, their effectivity is however reduced against dormant ones. The microbes present in centre of biofilm are metabolically more or less dormant.
- *Phenomenon of Persistence Shown by Cells*: Bacterial biofilm contains resistant persister cells that exhibit multidrug and bactericidal agent tolerance.
- *Genetic Adaptation*: The genetic adaptation imparted microbe a relatively protected and distinct phenotype.
- *Quorum Sensing (Cell to Cell Signaling)*: Quorum sensing (QS) is a process of the cell-to-cell interaction that regulates the behavior of bacteria. The bacteria by induction of a particular set of genes are capable of sensing and responding to increased cell population density. The role of signal molecule-mediated quorum sensing in biofilm formation has been demonstrated in many bacterial species.
- *Outer Membrane Structure*: Alteration/modification of cell envelope or adaptation is found to be responsible for bacterial cell resistance to antibiotics.
- *Efflux Pumps*: A set of efflux systems facilitates bacterial survival under extreme conditions, including antimicrobial agents. Efflux pumps exert both intrinsic and acquired resistance to different antibacterial agents that belong to same or different families

Treatment

The most effective strategy for treating these infections may be removal of the biofilm contaminated device wherever feasible.

Topical antibiotic route is preferred over parenteral route example antibiotic in aerosolized form for eradicating lung biofilms or endotracheal tube related infections.

Multiple Choice Questions

1. Virus mediated transfer of host DNA from one cell to another is known as: [AI 05]
   a. Transduction
   b. Transformation
   c. Transcription
   d. Integration

2. Biofilm cause antibiotic resistance by all of the following methods except: [AIIMS 2017]
   a. Mechanical barrier
   b. Adherence to a structure
   c. Decreased metabolism
   d. Increased antibiotic excretion

3. Lambda phage true is: [AIIMS May 11]
   a. Cause mad cow disease
   b. Lytic and lysogenic interconversion can't occur
   c. Lytic form incorporated within host DNA and multiply causing rupture of cell membrane
   d. Lysogenic form incorporates with host DNA and remains dormant

4. Intraspecies competition is the competition among:
   a. Species [AIIMS May 05]
   b. Individuals of a population
   c. Individuals of a community
   d. Populations and their regulatory factors

5. The following phenomenon is responsible for antibiotic resistance in bacteria due to slime production:
   a. Co-aggregation [AIIMS Nov 03]
   b. Biofilm formation
   c. Mutation evolving in altered target site for antibiotics
   d. Mutation evolving a target bypass mechanism

6. Shine-Dalgarno sequence in bacterial mRNA is near:
   a. AUG codon   b. UAA codon   [AI 03]
   c. UAG codon   d. UGA codon

7. Which of the following contains both DNA and RNA? [AIIMS May 14]
   a. Plasmids   b. Bacteria
   c. Prions   d. Viroids

8. True about bacteriophage is: [AIIMS May 11]
   a. Can transmit toxin to bacteria
   b. Bacteria which transmits DNA to another bacteria
   c. Causes transformation of bacteria
   d. Is a virus which invades bacteria

Explanations and References with Illustrative Answers

1. **Ans. (a) Transduction** *Ref. Ananthanarayan 10/e, p 59-61, 9/e, p 59-60*
   Transmission of genetic material = gene transfer = acquisition of characteristic occur by four process.
   a. *Transformation:* – Transfer of genetic information (about 10-50 genes) through the free DNA.
      – Seen mainly in pneumococci; bacillus species and *Haemophilus influenzae.*
      – Any characteristic may be transferred by transformation.
   b. *Transduction:* – Transfer of portion of DNA from one to other bacteria by agency of bacteriophage (*acts only as vehicle*).
      – It may be generalised (when it involves any segment of donor DNA) or restricted (when specific bacteriophage transduces only a particular genetic trait).
      – It is most widespread mechanism of gene transfer among prokaryotes.
      – Episomes and plasmids (e.g. plasmid determining Pn resistance in staphylococci) may also transduced.
      – It is used in *genetic engineering* in the treatment of some inborn errors of metabolism.
   c. *Conjugation* – *Bacterial equivalent of sexual mating*
      – Described by Lederberg and Tatum in strain of E. coli (K12), e.g. Transfer of episomes and plasmids of drug resistance.
   d. *Lysogenic conversion:* – Phage DNA becomes integrated with bacterial chromosome as the prophage which codes for new characteristic, e.g. toxin production in *C. diptheriae*.

2. **Ans. (b) Adherence to a structure** *Ref. Jawetz 27/e 58-59,165; Ananthanarayan 10/e 77; Open Microbiol J. 2017; 11: 53–62*
   Understanding the Mechanism of Bacterial Biofilms Resistance to Antimicrobial Agents
   Biofilms are well organized microcolonies of bacteria enclosed in self produced extracellular polymer matrices known as glycocalyx
   Reasons for the intrinsic antimicrobial resistance of biofilms:
   - Antimicrobial agents must diffuse through the biofilm matrix to contact and inactivate the organisms within the biofilm. EPSs retard diffusion either by chemically reacting with the antimicrobial molecules or by limiting their rate of transport.

- Biofilm-associated organisms have reduced growth rates, minimizing the rate that antimicrobial agents are taken into the cell and therefore affecting inactivation kinetics.
- The environment immediately surrounding the cells within a biofilm may provide conditions that further protect the organism. E.g. Decreased uptake of the antibiotic by the oxygen-deprived cells.
- Decreased bacterial metabolic activity and increased doubling times of the bacterial cells which enhances the number of more or less dormant cells that are responsible for some of the tolerance to antibiotics.
- Biofilm growth is associated with an increased level of mutations as well as with quorum-sensing-regulated mechanisms alteration in outer membrane proteins
- Conventional resistance mechanisms such as chromosomal beta-lactamase, upregulated efflux pumps (increased excretion) and mutations in antibiotic target molecules in bacteria also contribute to the survival of biofilms.

Treatment of Biofilm related infections
Removal of source wherever possible, flushing of catheter. Use of enzymes that can dissolve the biofilm matrix (e.g. DNase and alginate lyase) as well as quorum-sensing inhibitors that increase biofilm susceptibility to antibiotics are future promising strategy

3. **Ans. (d) Lysogenic form incorporates with host DNA and remains dormant** *Ref. Ananthanarayan 10/e, p 60; 9/e, p 60*
   Bacteriophage exhibits two different types of life cycle, i.e.
   - Lytic or virulent cycle
   - Temperate or lysogenic cycle

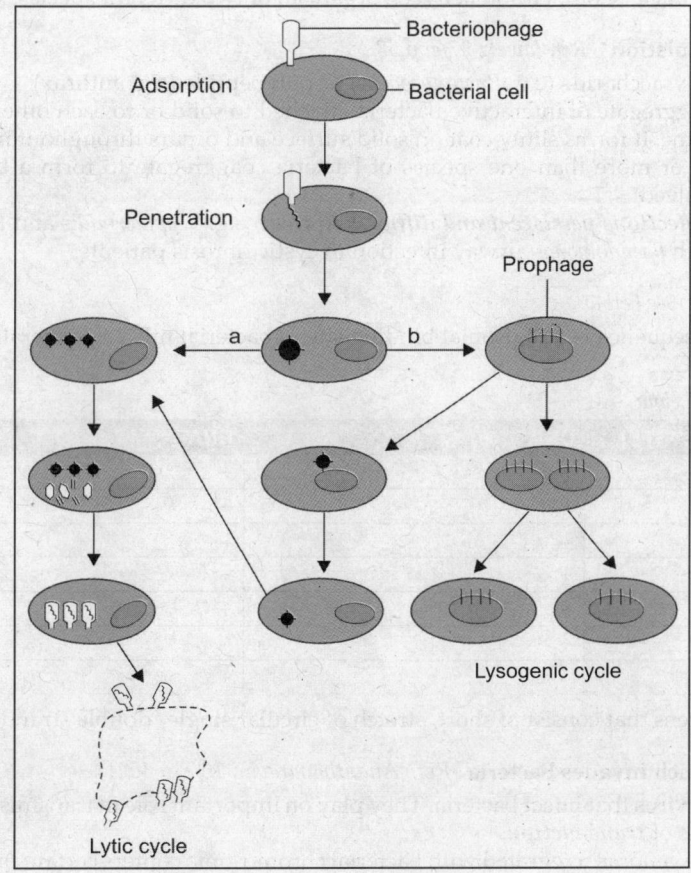

a. Lytic cycle **b.** Lysogenic cycle

a. **Lytic Cycle:** In this cycle bacteriophage enters bacteria, undergo intracellular multiplication, lyse the host bacterium which is followed by release of progeny. This cycle involves following steps:
   - Adsorption
   - Penetration
   - Synthesis of phage components
   - Assembly and maturation of phage particles

- Lyses of host bacteria
- Release of progeny

In this cycle phage genetic material never gets incorporated in host bacterial DNA.

> **Note:**
> - The interval between the entry of phage nucleic acid into the bacterial cell and appearance of the first infectious intracellular phage particle is known as eclipse phase.
> - The interval between the infection of bacterial cell and the first release of infectious phage particle is known as *latent period*.

b. **Lysogenic Cycle:** In this cycle following entry into the host cell. Phage nucleic acid integrates with bacterial chromosome. The integrated phase nucleic acid is known as **prophage** and this behaves like a segment of the host chromosome and replicates synchronously with it. Lysogeny does not upset the bacterial metabolism, in fact it imparts certain new properties.

During the multiplication of lysogenic bacteria sometimes prophage may get separated and starts lytic cycle *(Hence option b is wrong).*

> **Note:** Lambda phage infects *E. coli* and imparts it with property of fermenting glucose.

4. **Ans. (b) Individuals of a population.** *See below*
   - *Intraspecies competition:* Competition within a single population
   - *Interspecies competition:* Competition between organism of two different species

5. **Ans. (b) Biofilm formulation** *Ref. Jawetz 27/e, p 58*
   - Slime may be polysaccharide (e.g. *Pneumococcus*) or polypeptide (e.g. anthrax)
   - A **biofilm** is an aggregate of interactive bacteria attached to solid or to each other and encased in an exopolysaccharide matrix of slime. It forms slimy coat on solid surface and occurs throughout nature.
   - A single species or more than one species of bacteria coaggregate to form a biofilm. Fungi including yeasts are occasionally involved
   - *Biofilms make infections persistent and difficult to treat,* e.g. *S. epidermidis* and *S. aureus* infection of central venous catheters and with *Pseudomonas* airway infection in cystic fibrosis patients.

6. **Ans. (a) AUG codon** *See below*

   Shine-Dalgarno (SD) sequence is a ribosomal binding site in bacterial mRNA, generally located around 8 bases upstream of the start codon AUG.

7. **Ans. (b) Bacteria** *See below*

Microbe	DNA	RNA	Protein
Bacteria	+	+	+
Virus	+/−	+/−	+
Prion	−	−	+
Fungi	+	+	+
Parasites	+	+	+
Plasmids	+	−	−
Viroids	−	+	+

Viroids: Plant pathogens that consist of short, stretch of circular single/double stranded RNA.

8. **Ans. (d) Is a virus which invades bacteria** *Ref. Ananthanarayan 10/e, p 462*

   Bacteriophage are the virus that infect bacteria. They play on important role in transmission of genetic information between bacteria by the process of *transduction.*

   The presence of phage genome integrated with bacterial chromosome confers certain properties to the bacteria, this process is called *phage conversion.*

   > **Note:**
   > - Nucleic acid of phage is surrounded by a protein coat
   > - Some phage also contains lipid
   > - Most bacteriophage possess ds DNA as genetic material
   > - In diphtheria bacillus toxin production is determined by the presence of a bacteriophage prophage beta
   > - So option 'a' is also partially correct, as option 'd' is universal for bacteriophage it is taken as correct answer

Bacterial Genetics

NEET Pattern Questions

1. **Mechanism of direct transfer of free DNA:**
    a. Transformation
    b. Conjugation
    c. Transduction
    d. None   [Ref. Ananthanarayan, 10/e, p 59]

2. **Transfer of some chromosomal material from one bacteria to other can occur via:**
    a. F factor
    b. R factor
    c. Transfer factor
    d. All of the above   [Ref. Ananthanarayan, 10/e, p 59-61]

3. **R-factor in bacteria is transferred by:**
    a. Transduction
    b. Transformation
    c. Conjugation
    d. Vertical transmission [Ref. Ananthanarayan, 10/e, p 61]

> R factor: Whole plasmid with its two component resistance transfer factor (RTF) which is responsible for conjugational transfer and a resistance determinant (r) for each of several drugs
> R factor can transfer resistance to as many as 8 drugs simultaneously

4. **Multiple drug resistance is spread by:**
    a. Transformation
    b. Transduction
    c. Mutation
    d. Conjugation   [Ref. Ananthanarayan, 10/e, p 62]

> Multiple drug resistance is transferred by R plasmid through conjugation.

5. **Viral DNA is integrated into Bacterial DNA in:**
    a. Transduction
    b. Lysogenic conversion
    c. Transformation
    d. Conjugation   [Ref. Ananthanarayan 10/e, p 60]

6. **Prophage is defined as:**
    a. Insertion of viral nucleic acid into bacteria by bacteriophage
    b. First cycle of division of bacterial nucleic acid
    c. Last cycle of division of bacterial nucleic acid
    d. Integrated temperate bacteriophage genome into bacterial chromosome   [Ref. Jawety, 27/e, p109]

> **Prophage:** Bacteriophage integrated into a bacterial genome or episome
> **Provirus:** Viral DNA integrated into eukaryotic genome.

7. **Conjugation does not involve:**
    a. Bacteriophages   b. HFr
    c. Fr   d. Plasmids
    [Ref. Ananthanarayan 10/e p 61]

8. **Jumping gene is:**   [2016]
    a. Transposon   b. Episome
    c. Cosmid   d. Plasmid
    [Ref. Ananthanarayan 10/e p 63]

9. **Microbial killing below MIC is known as:**   [2016]
    a. Adverse effect   b. Post-antibiotic effect
    c. Both   d. None

> **Post-antibiotic effect**
> - Defined as the persistent suppression of bacterial growth after a brief exposure of bacteria to an antibiotic even in absence of host defense mechanism.
> - Mainly seen with antibiotics that inhibit protein and nucleic acid synthesis. Post-antibiotic effect is supposed to be due to alteration of DNA functions.

10. **Transfer of genetic material in transduction occurs through:**   [2016]
    a. Transposons   b. Plasmids
    c. Bacteriophage   d. Fungal elements
    [Ref. Ananthanarayan 10/e p 59]

> **Note:**
> | | | |
> |---|---|---|
> | Transformation | : | Free DNA |
> | Transduction | : | Bacteriophage |
> | Conjugation | : | Physical contact; mainly by plasmid |

1. a. Transformation   2. d. All of the above   3. c. Conjugation   4. d. Conjugation
5. b. Lysogenic conversion   6. a. Insertion of viral nucleic acid…
7. a. Bacteriophages   8. a. Transposon   9. b. Post-antibiotic..   10. c. Bacteriophage

SECTION B

UNIT I

Bacteriology

Gram-positive Cocci
- Staphylococci
- Streptococci

Gram-negative Cocci
- Neisseria

Gram-positive Bacilli
- Clostridium
- Corynebacterium
- Actinomycetes and Bacillus
- Listeria Monocytogenes
- Mycobacteria

Gram-negative Bacilli
- Enterobacteriaceae
- Vibrio
- Pseudomonas and Yersinia

Gram-negative Bacilli and Cocco-bacilli
- Hemophilus, Bordetella and Brucella
- Campylobacter and Helicobacter
- Legionella
- Rickettsiae and Chlamydiae

Others
- Spirochetes
- Mycoplasma

Staphylococci

CHAPTER 7

Catalase positive, nonmotile, aerobic and facultatively anaerobic organism, that do not form spores.

> **Gram-Positive Cocci:**
> - Staphylococci
> - Streptococci ⎤ anaerobic
> - Pneumococci ⎦ (–)ve

MORPHOLOGY

Staphylococci are spherical cells arranged in irregular clusters. Young cocci stain strongly Gram positive. On ageing, many cells become gram negative.

CULTURE

Staphylococci grow readily on most media. They grow most rapidly at 37°C but pigment production is maximum at room temperature (20–25°C). **S. aureus** forms gray to deep golden yellow colonies. **S. epidermidis** forms gray to white colonies. Under anaerobic condition there is no pigment production.

CLASSIFICATION

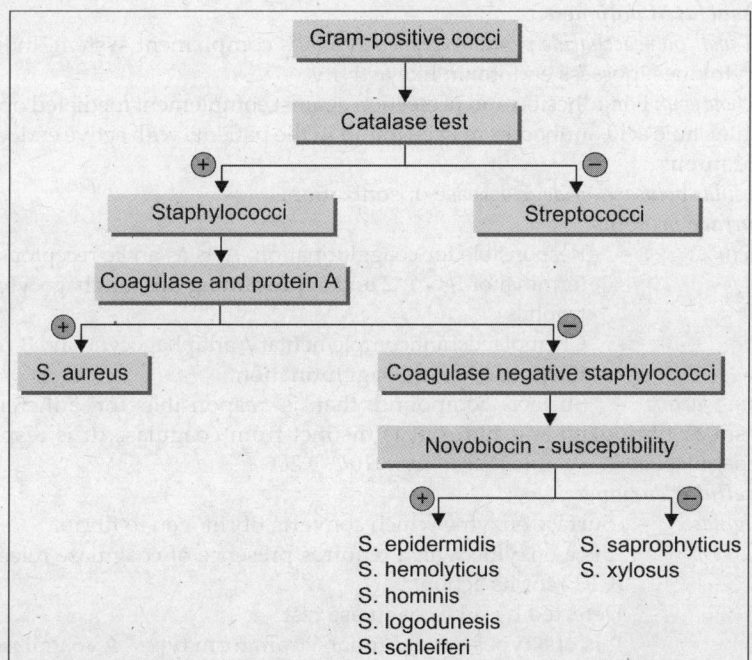

> **Site of colonization of S. aureus**
> - Anterior nares
> - Axillae
> - Perineum
> - Vagina

Classification of Staphylococci	
Coagulase +ve/Protein A +ve	**Coagulase –ve**
• More virulent	• Less virulent
• Form golden yellow colonies on solid media	• Form white colonies
• Usually pathogenic	• Usually less pathogenic
• Show hemolysis	• No hemolysis
• Ferments mannitol	• Do not ferment mannitol
• Produce nuclease	• Nuclease (-)ve

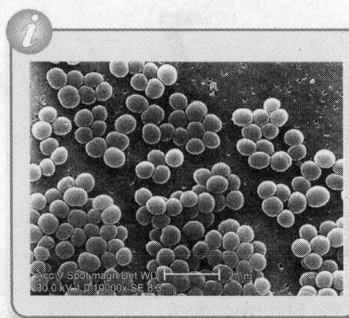

STAPHYLOCOCCUS AUREUS

- Part of normal human flora; 20-25% of healthy individuals may be persistently or transiently colorized. Anterior nares are the frequent site of human colonization.
- The colonization sites serve as a reservoir of strains for future infection and persons colonized with S. aureus are at higher risk for infection.
- *MC* route of infection—Skin.
- *MC* source of infection: Patients own colonizing strain. ... *Harrison 20/e, p1072*

Culture

- On nutrient agar, show characteristic *oil paint appearance*.
- Show β hemolysis which is marked on rabbit or sheep blood and weak on horse blood agar.
- Salt milk agar, salt broth and *Ludlam's medium* are selective medium ...*Ananthanarayan 10/e, p20*

Biochemical Reaction

- **Mannitol fermenter** anaerobically *(not by other species of Staphylococci)*
- **Phosphatase reaction**: – Gives prompt phosphatase reaction.
  – Useful screening procedure as *S.epidermidis is usually negative or only weakly positive.*

Virulence Factors

- Most constant association of *virulence* is production of enzyme *coagulase* and to a lesser extent with *mannitol fermentation*.
  a. **Cell associated polymers:**
    - *Cell wall polysaccharide peptidoglycan*: Activates complement system. Induce release of cytokines, possess endotoxin like activity.
    - *Teichoic acid:* For adhesion and protection against complement mediated opsonization. Antiteichoic acid antibodies may be found in the patients with active endocarditis due to S. aureus.
    - *Capsular polysaccharide*: Decrease opsonization.
  b. **Cell surface proteins:**
    - *Protein A:* – Responsible for coagglutination. Acts as an Fc receptor. Binds to Fc terminal of IgG 1, 2 and 4, preventing opsonophagocytosis by neutrophils.
      – Chemotactic, anticomplementary, antiphagocytic and B-cell mitogen.
      – Responsible for Coagglutination.
    - *Clumping factor:* – Surface compound that is responsible for adherence of the organism to fibrinogen and fibrin. It is distinct from coagulase. It is responsible for slide coagulase test. ...*Ananthanarayan, 10/e, p 206*
  c. *Extracellular enzymes*
    1. *Coagulase:* – Surface enzyme which converts fibrinogen to fibrin.
      – It is a enzyme which requires presence of coagulase releasing factor (CRF) for its action.
      – Detected by tube coagulase test.
      – It is of 8 types. Most human strain form type - A coagulase.

    > **Caution:** Initially clumping factor is supposed to be bound form of coagulase. Now it is clear that it is totally different. So, the concept of slide test for bound coagulase has diminished.

    2. *Nuclease:* A heat stable nuclease (DNAse) is **characteristic** of *S. aureus*
    3. *Protein receptors:* For mammalian proteins e.g. fibronectin, fibrinogen, IgG, C1q. Facilitates adhesion.
    4. *Lipases:* Helps in infecting skin and subcutaneous tissue
    5. Hyaluronidase ⎤
    6. Protease   ⎬ Helps in spread of infection
    7. Fibrinolysin (Staphylokinase) ⎦

Distinctive features of S. aureus:
– Coagulase
– Thermostable nuclease
– Clumping factor
– Shows β hemolysis

Source of infection
– Direct contact is the most important mode
– Airborne
– Through fomites

Toxin

A. Cytolytic Toxins:

- α Hemolysin:
  - Most important hemolysin
  - Protein inactive at 70°C, but reactivated paradoxically at 100°C.
  - Lyses rabbit erythrocyte but is less active against human erythrocytes.
  - Leukocidal, cytotoxic, dermonecrotic, neurotoxic and lethal.
- β Hemolysin — Shows 'hot cold phenomenon'. Sphingomyelinase, hemolytic for sheep cells.
- γ Hemolysin — Bicomponent protein.
- δ Hemolysin — Detergent like effect on cell membranes, plays role in S. aureus diarrheal disease ...*Jawetz,27/e, p 206*
- Leukocidin (Panton valentine Toxin): Bicomponent toxin associated with furunculosis. Important virulence factor in MRSA infection.

> **Note:** *Synergohymenotropic toxin:* Bicomponent toxin such as Leukocidin and γ Hemolysin.

> **Toxins:**
> **Staphylococcal enterotoxin:** Heat stable enterotoxin
> **TSST:** Superantigen
> **Leukocidin & γ Hemolysin:** Bicomponent toxin (synergohymenotropic toxin)

B. Enterotoxin: (A, B, C$_{1-3}$, D, E and H)

- Preformed, heat stable toxin, responsible for staphylococcal food poisoning which occur 2-6 hrs after consuming meat and fish, milk or milk products.
- *Source:* Usually food handler which is carrier.
- Mechanism: Toxin acts directly on autonomic nervous system (*Vagal stimulation*) and vomiting center.
- *Type A* toxin is responsible for *most* cases.

C. Toxic Shock Syndrome Toxin (TSST)

- Toxic shock syndrome is multisystem disease presenting with fever, hypotension, myalgia, vomiting, diarrhea, mucosal hyperemia, erythematous sunburn, rash, disorientation or altered consciousness seen mostly in menstruating women using highly absorbent vaginal tampons.
  - TSST-1 = Enterotoxin F = Pyrogenic Exotoxin; C is responsible for most cases.
  - TSST-1 binds to MHC class II molecules, yielding T-Cell stimulation.
  - Staph. Enterotoxin and TSST are *super antigen* leading to an excessive and non regulated immune response.

D. Exfoliative / Epidermatolytic Toxin / ET / Exfoliatin

- Cause staphylococcal scalded skin syndrome (SSS).
- Severe form is called Ritter's disease in **neonate** and *toxic epidermal necrolysis* in **elderly**.
- Milder form are pemphigus neonatorum and bullous impetigo.
- There are two type: **ETA** (chromosomal gene product, heat stable) and **ETB** (plasmid mediated, heat labile). Possess serine protease activity which triggers exfoliation.

Typing

- Staphylococci are typed on the basis of their susceptibility to bacteriophage.
- Phage typing is done by pattern method, Employing 1 over 28 phages. Most hospital epidemics are caused by group I.

> Toxic shock syndrome toxin. Mostly caused by TSST-1 = Pyrogenic exotoxin C.

Clinical manifestation

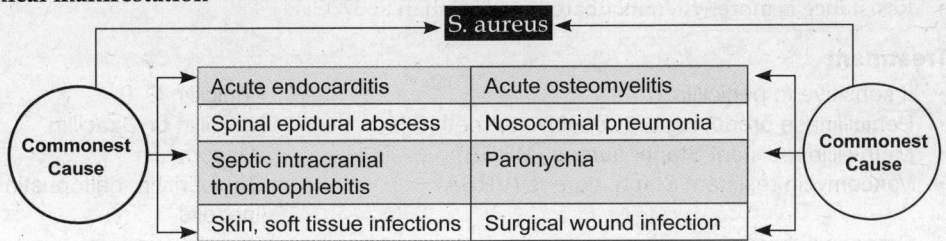

No antibiotic treatment is recommended in staphylococcal food poisoning.

- S.aureus is **MC** cause of acute endocarditis except early and late prosthetic valve endocarditis which are caused by Coagulase-ve staph. and Streptococci viridans respectively.
- Though rare, recently methicillin resistant S. aureus (MRSA) have been reported as primary cause of community acquired pneumonia. .... *Harrison 19/e, p 955*

Remember: Subacute endocarditis is typically caused by Strep. *viridans*.

Disease caused by Staph. aureus
Skin and Soft Tissue Infections
- Folliculitis   — Furuncle,   — Carbuncle   — Cellulitis
- Impetigo   — Mastitis   — Surgical wound infections   — Hidradenitis suppurativa

Musculoskeletal Infections
- Septic arthritis   — Osteomyelitis   — Pyomyositis   — Psoas abscess

Respiratory Tract Infections
- Ventilator-associated or nosocomial pneumonia   — Septic pulmonary emboli
- Postviral pneumonia   — Empyema

Bacteremia and Its Complications
- Sepsis, septic shock   — Metastatic foci of infection (kidney, joints, bone, lung)

Infective Endocarditis
Device-related Infections (e.g., intravascular catheters, prosthetic joints)
Toxin-mediated Illnesses
- Toxic shock syndrome   — Food poisoning
- Staphylococcal scalded-skin syndrome

Invasive Infections Associated with Community-acquired MRSA
- Necrotizing fasciitis   — Waterhouse-Friderichsen syndrome
- Necrotizing pneumonia

Lab Diagnosis

- Diagnosis is made by *culture*, specimen is plated on blood agar.
- Smears are examined from culture and coagulase test is done.
- Coagulase test is the standard criterion for S. aureus identification. It is done by two methods—tube and slide coagulase test. Slide coagulase test is simpler while tube coagulase test is more specific.
- *Serological Test*:   – Helpful in diagnosis of hidden deep infection.
    – Antistaphylolysin (antialphalysin) titre of more than two unit is important specially, when rising.
- Polymerase chain reaction (PCR) based assays have been applied for rapid diagnosis of S.aureus infection.   ... *Harrison 20/e, p 1074*

Methicillin Resistant Staph Aureus (MRSA)

- One of the emerging problem
- Both community acquired (CAMRSA) and can be hospital acquired (HAMRSA).
- Methicillin resistance is due to SCCmec gene–which synthesis PBP 2-α. SCCmec types 1–3 are associated with nosocomial infection where as types 4-6 have been associated with epidemic community acquired infection
- Gene for Pantone–Valentine leukocidin, arginine catabolic mobile element are specific virulence factors of MRSA   ... *Harrison 20/e, p 1073*
- Growth on cefoxitin disc diffusion agar and oxacillin screen agar is used to identify MRSA strains
- Resistance is more when incubated at 30°C than at 37°C

Treatment

• If sensitive to penicillin	→ Penicillin G
• Penicillinase producing but sensitive to methicillin	→ Naficillin or Oxacillin
• Methicillin resistant Staph. aureus (MRSA)	→ Vancomycin
• Vancomycin resistant Staph. aureus (VRSA)	→ Quinopristin, dalfopristin, linezolid
• Emperical therapy	→ Vancomycin

Special Cases

- TSS → Clindamycin (reduces toxin synthesis)
- Food poisoning → *No antibiotic* (as caused by preformed toxin)

COAGULASE (−) VE STAPHYLOCOCCI (CONS)

- **MC** pathogen complicating use of IV catheters, shunts and grafts, pacemaker wires, prosthetic valves, vascular grafts, CSF shunts, dialyser.

  Mnemonic—CoNS are **MC** source of infection on any exogenous implant (new substance).

Staph epidermidis / albus

- MC CoNS species associated with prosthetic device infection ... *Harrison 20/e, p 1077*
- Normally present on human skin. Not pathogenic ordinarily.
- Predilection for growth on implanted foreign bodies.
- Common source of stich abscess.
- *S. epidermidis* is adapted to colonize these devices by its capacity to elaborate the extracellular polysaccharide (glycocalyx or slime) that facilitates formation of protective biofilm on the device surface. This biofilm protects bacteria from antibiotics and host defence.
- The attachment is also facilitated by autolysis (AtlE), fibrinogen binding protein, and accumulation-associated protein (AAP).

> Coagulase (−) ve staphylococci
> – Staph. epidermidis (MC)
> – S. Saprophyticus (UTI)
> – S. lugdunensis (severe)

Staph. saprophyticus

- Non-pigmented, novobiocin resistant, and non hemolytic ....*Jawetz 27/e p 206*
- Present on normal human skin and periurethral area.
- Cause UTI in sexually active young women. This is due to its enhanced capacity to adhere to uroepithelial cells. A 160 KDA hemagglutinin/adhesin may contribute to this affinity ... *Harrison 20/e, p 1077*

S. lugdunensis and *S. schleiferi*

- Produces serious infections (native valve endocarditis and osteomyelitis) than do other CoNS.

Other CoNS are:

- *S. xylosus*, • *S. hominus*, • *S. haemolyticus* (shows β-hemolysis)

Micrococci

- Gram positive, catalase positive, oxidase positive aerobic bacteria that resemble staphylococci.
- Differentiated from staphylococci through Hugh and Leifson oxidation fermentation test.

Multiple Choice Questions

1. A diabetic patient developed cellulitis due to *S.aureus*, which was found to be methicillin resistant on the antibiotic sensitivity testing. All the following antibiotics will be appropriate *except*: [AI 06]
   a. Vancomycin
   b. Imipenem
   c. Teicloplanin
   d. Linezolid

2. Which of the following Staphylococcal infection is not toxin mediated? [AIIMS 2017]
   a. Toxic shock syndrome
   b. Scalded skin syndrome
   c. Food poisoning
   d. Septic shock

3. Which of the following statement is most correct regarding resistance to methicillin in MRSA:
   a. Resistance is produced as a result of alteration in penicillin binding protein [AI 2011]
   b. Resistance is produced by production of β lactamase
   c. Resistance is mediated by plasmids
   d. Expression of resistance is enhanced by incubating at 38°C during susceptibility testing

4. All of the following statements are true about Staphylococci *except*: [AIIMS 04]
   a. A majority of infection caused by coagulase (-) ve Staph. are due to *staph. epidermidis*
   b. b-Lactamase production is under plasmid control
   c. Expression of methicillin resistance in *Staphylococcus aureus* increases when it is incubated at 37°C on blood agar
   d. Methicillin resistance in *Staph. aureus* is independent of b-Lactamase production

5. Which one of the following Gram positive organism is most common cause of UTI among sexually active women? [AIIMS 04]
   a. *Staphylococcus epidermidis*
   b. *Staphylococcus aureus*
   c. *Staphylococcus saprophyticus*
   d. Enterococcus

6. The following is characteristic feature of *staphylococcus* food poisoning *except*: [AIIMS 04]
   a. Optimum temperature for toxin production is 37°C
   b. Intradietic toxin are responsible for intestinal symptoms
   c. Toxin can be destroyed by boiling for 30 minutes
   d. Incubation period is 1-6 hours

7. A patient in an ICCU is on CVP line. His blood culture shows growth of Gram-positive cocci which are catalase positive and coagulase negative. The most likely etiological agent is: [AIIMS 03]
   a. *Staph. aureus*
   b. *Staph. epidermidis*
   c. *Streptococcus pyogenes*
   d. *Enterococcus faecalis*

8. All of the following statements about staphylococcus aureus are true *except*: [AI 2010]
   a. Most common source of infection is cross infection from infected people
   b. About 30% of general population is healthy nasal carriers
   c. Epidermolysin and TSS toxin are superantigens
   d. Methicillin Resistance is chromosomally mediated

9. A cook prepares sandwiches for 10 people going for picnic. Eight out of them develop severe gastroenteritis within 4-6 hrs of consumption of the sandwiches. It is likely that on investigations the cook is found to be carrier of: [AIIMS 02]
   a. *Salmonella typhi*
   b. *Vibrio cholerae*
   c. *Entamoeba histolytica*
   d. *Staphylococcus aureus*

10. A 25-year-old IV drug abuser presents with fever for 3 weeks. ECHO shows tricuspid vegetation. The most likely organism associated with endocarditis in this case is: [AIIMS Nov 09, May 11]
    a. *Staph. aureus*
    b. *Candida albicans*
    c. *Pseudomonas*
    d. *Strep. viridans*

11. Synergohymenotropic toxin of staphylococci consist of: [PGI 2011]
    a. α toxin
    b. β toxin
    c. γ toxin
    d. δ toxin
    e. Panton valentine toxin

12. Staphylococcus in stool occurs in: [PGI 2012]
    a. Staphylococcal food poisoning
    b. Ischiorectal abscess
    c. Toxic shock syndrome
    d. May be a normal finding
    e. Pseudomembranous colitis

13. *Staphylococcus* can cause: [PGI 07]
    a. Ecthyma
    b. Erythrasma
    c. Furuncle
    d. Impetigo contagiosa
    e. Sycosis barbae

Explanations and References with Illustrative Answers

1. Ans. (b) Imipenem   *Ref. Harrison 20/e, p1079, 19/e, p962; Katzung 13/e, p781*

"Imipenem is not effective against Enterococcus faecium, MRSA, Clostridium difficile, Burkholderia cepacia as they produce metallobetalactamases." Though it is effective against methicillin sensitive staph. aureus.

Treatment of MRSA		
Drug of choice	**Alternative**	**Investigatory**
Vancomycin	TMP - SMX	Oritavancin
Daptomycin	Minocycline	Tigecycline
	Ciprofloxacine, Levofloxacin	Ceftobipirole
	Quinupristin/dalfopristin	
	Linezolid	
	Telavancin	
	Ceftaroline	

Antibiotic Resistance		
Agent	**Mechanism of resistance**	**Site**
Penicillins	β-lactamase	Plasmid
Methicilin	Altered binding protein	Chromosome
Cephalosporin		
Chloramphenicol	Acetyl transferase	Plasmid
Erythromycin	Methylation of ribosome	Plasmid
Streptomycin	Altered ribosomal protein	Chromosome
Vancomycin	Van A gene	Chromosome
Quinolones	Mutation in topoisomerase IV	

Note: Van A gene-Mechanism of vancomycin resistance involves Van A which produces replacement of the last D-alanine residue of peptidoglycan precursors with D-lactate or D-serine resulting respectively in high level and low level resistance.   ... *Harrison 20/e p 1078*

Remember:
- Ceftaroline: A novel cephalosporin with activity against MRSA
- Adjuvant drugs for MRSA include gentamycin, rifampicin, fusidic acid
- Teicloplanin is glycopeptide which is similar to vancomycin in both mechanism and spectrum of activity.
- **Drugs for VRSA (vancomycin resistant S. aureus):**
  – Daptomycin/dalfopristin   – Quinupristin   – Linezolid.   – TMP – SMX

Note: S. aureus is a member of ESKAPE; group of resistant bacterias which includes. Enterococcus faecium, S. aureus, Klebsiella sp, Acinetobacter baumannii, Pseudomonas aeruginosa, and enterobacter sp

2. Ans. (d) Septic shock   *Ref. Harrison 20/e p1074*

Toxin mediated illness of S. aureus	
Disease	**Toxin involved**
- Toxic shock syndrome	Toxic shock syndrome toxin
- Food poisoning	Enterotoxin
- Staphylococcal scalded skin syndrome	Exfoliative/epidermolytic toxin

Note: Septic shock is due to bacteremia.

3. Ans. (a) Resistance is produced as a result of alteration in penicillin binding protein

Ref. Katzung 13/e, p781; Harrison 20/e, p1078

"Production of novel penicillin binding protein (PBP 2a or 2') is responsible for methicillin resistance". Protein is synthesized by mec A gene which is part of a large mobile genetic element called *SCCmec*.

It is hypothesized that the genetic material was acquired via horizontal transfer from a related species, S. sciuri.

Drug resistance in staphylococcus

(A) Penicillin resistance:
1. Production of β lactamase:
   - Plasmid mediated inducible enzyme which is transmitted by transduction (more commonly) or conjugation. Now only <5% of strains of staph are sensitive to penicillin.
   - Hospital strains mostly form type A penicillinase.
   - Same plasmid carry genes for resistance to tetracycline, erythromycin, aminoglycoside too.
2. Altered penicillin binding protein:
   - Due to production of novel penicillin binding protein 'PBP2a', this protein is synthesized by mec A gene.
   - Chromosomally mediated, expressed more at 30°C than at 37°C.
   - Responsible for resistance against penicillinase resistant penicillin such as methicilin, cloxacillin. Strains are called **MRSA** (Methicillin resistant Staph. aureus).
   - MRSA escape methicillin by synthesizing an extra PBP called PBP-2A which carries out function of those PBP's that are inactivated by methicillin.
3. *Tolerance to penicillin:*
   - Bacteria only inhibited not killed.

(B) Vancomycin
1. *Intermediate susceptible strain:* Also known as **VISA** (*vancomycin-intermediate S. aureus*). For these VISA strain **MIC** (*minimal inhibitory concentration*) of vancomycin is 4-8 µg/mL. The mechanism of resistance is increased cell wall thickness and alteration in the cell wall.
2. *Resistant strain:* Also known as **VRSA** (*vancomycin resistant strain*): This is due to presence of van A gene

(C) Others
- Plasmid mediated resistance to teracycline, erythromycin, aminoglycosides

4. **Ans. (c) Expression of methicillin resistance in *Staphylococcus aureus* increases when it is incubated at 37°C on blood agar** *Ref. Ananthanarayan 10/e, p201, 9/e, p201; Jawetz, 27/e p 205*

"Methicillin resistance is expressed more when Staph. is incubated at 30°C than at 37°C."
Refer Ans. No. 3 for full explanation.

5. **Ans. (c) *Staphylococcus Saprophyticus*** *Ref. Harrison 20/e, p1077*

S. saprophyticus cause UTI in young women due to its enhanced capacity to adhere to uroepithelial cells. A 160 KDa hemagglutinin adhesins may contribute to this affinity.

> Note: S. Saprophyticus is novobiocin resistant.

6. **Ans. (c) Toxin can be destroyed by boiling for 30 minutes** *Ref. Harrison 20/e, p1076, 1074; Ananthanarayan 10/e, p204*

Staphylococcal food poisoning:
- Staphylococcal food poisoning is due to *heat stable preformed toxin* mostly after consuming milk products.
- Toxin is produced optimally at 35°C to 37°C and is resistant to the action of gut enzymes
- As disease is due to toxin, secondary spread is not there
- Main d/d is *B. cereus* food poisoning.
- IP- 1-6 hours.
- *Mechanism* - Acts by **stimulating vagus nerve and vomiting center of brain.** Also stimulates intestinal peristalsis
- *No antibiotics* are given for staphylococcal food poisoning.
- Treatment is conservative.

7. **Ans. (b) Staph. epidermidis** *Ref. Harrison 20/e, p1077*

Gram +ve, catalase +ve, coagulase -ve bacteria is **Coagulase-negative Staph.**

S. epidermidis is uniquely adapted to colonize prosthetic devices due to its capacity to elaborate the extracellular polysaccharide (*glycocalyx or slime*) that facilitates formation of protective biofilm on the device surface. This slime production also protect the bacteria against antibiotics.

Coagulase (–)ve *Staphylococcus*	
S. epidermidis	**S. saprophyticus**
• Novobiocin sensitive	• Novobiocin resistant
• Predilection for growth on implanted foreign bodies	• Not so
• *Most common* cause of *prosthetic valve endocarditis*	• Cause *UTI in sexually active young women*

> **Remember:** Both are present on normal skin and are not usually pathogenic.

8. **Ans. (a) Most common source of infection** ... *Ref. Jawetz 27/e p 171 ; Harrison 20/e, p 1072*
   Let consider each option
   Option 'a', 'b'
   Epidemiology of Staph aureus
   - Part of normal flora, nasal carriage occurs in 20-25% of humans. *Rate of colonization is higher among HIV patients, insulin dependent diabetes, patients undergoing hemodialysis, individuals with skin damage.* **Anterior nares** are the **most common** site of colonization; although skin, axilla, vagina, perinium may be colonized.
   - Most individual who develop S. aureus are infected with their own colonizing strain. Contact spread of infection is more common in hospitals, where transmission most frequently occurs through hands of hospital personnel. *Heavily colonized individual can transmit bacteria via aerosols of respiratory or nasal secretions.*

   Option 'c'
   - Toxic shock syndrome toxin (TSST-1), epidermatolytic toxin and other staphylococcal enterotoxin are superantigens.
   - These superantigens can bind MHC molecule outside the peptide binding cleft. Consequently super antigen can activate up to 10% of T-cell in nonspecific manner which in turn leads to release of large quantity of cytokines.

   Option 'd'
   - Resistance to methicillin (and nafcillin) is encoded and regulated by a sequence of genes located in a region of chromosome called ***staphylococcal cassette chromosome mec*** (*SCC mec*). This gene encodes for a low affinity penicilin binding protein.

9. **Ans. (d) Staphylococcus aureus** *Ref. Harrison 20/e, p262. 19/e p 266*
   Learn this table by heart, every year there is question on food poisoning.

Bacterial food poisoning		
Incubation Period, Organism	**Symptoms**	**Common food source**
1 to 6 H		
Staphylococcus aureus	Nausea, vomiting, diarrhea	Ham, poultry, potato or egg, salad, mayonniase, cream pastries
Bacillus cereus	Nausea, vomiting	Fried rice
8 to 16 H		
Clostridium perfringens	Abdominal cramps, diarrhea *(vomiting rare)*	Beef, poultry, legumes, gravies
B. cereus	Abdominal cramps, diarrhea vomiting	Meats, vegetables, dried beans, cereals
>16 H		
Vibrio cholerae	Watery diarrhea	Shellfish
Enterotoxigenic *Escherichia coli*	Watery diarrhea	Salads, cheese, meats
Enterohemorrhagic *E. coli*	Bloody diarrhea	Ground beef, raw vegetables
Salmonella spp.	Inflammatory diarrhea	Beef, poultry, eggs, dairy products
Campylobacter jejuni	Inflammatory diarrhea	Poultry, raw milk
Shigella spp.	Dysentery	Potato or egg salad, lettuce, raw vegetables
Vibrio parahaemolyticus	Dysentery	Mollusks, crustaceans

   - S. aureus is *MC* cause of food poisoning in west.

10. **Ans. (a) Staph. aureus** *Ref. Harrison 20/e p 922*

Endocarditis in IV drugs addicts	
Right sided (more common)	**Left sided**
Staph. aureus	Varied (Staph, aureus, enterobacter, polymicrobial)

11. **Ans. (c) and (e) γ toxin and Panton - Valentine toxin** *Ref. Ananthanarayan 10/e, p 204*
    Synergohymenotropic toxins are a family of bicomponent toxin that acts through the synergistic action of two non-associated secretory proteins. Staphylococcal leucocidin (Panton-Valentine toxin) and gamma hemolysin are the example of synergohymenotropic toxins. They enhance the virulence of MRSA.

12. **Ans. (a) and (d) Staphylococcal food poisoning and May be a normal finding** *Ref. Ananthanarayan 10/e, p206, 9/e, p204*
    - In case of staphylococcal food poisoning food remnant and faeces are inoculated on *selective medium* like **Ludlam's or salt milk agar** or **Roberson cooked meat medium** containing 10% NaCl.
    - Asymptomatic fecal carriage is seen in many nasal carriers.
    - TSS is due to systemic effect of absorbed toxin from site such as vagina, so there is no possibility of finding Staph. in case of TSS.

- Ischiorectal abscess is mostly due to *E. coli.*
- Normal intestinal flora usually do not contain *Staph. aureus.* So it is *not* a normal finding.
- Pseudomembranous colitis is caused by *Clostridium difficile.*

13. **Ans. (c) (d) and (e) Furuncle, Impetigo contagiosa and Sycobis barbae**   *Ref. Harrison 20/e, p 1074*
    Impetigo contagiosa is caused by S. aureus or Streptococcus or both. It is the most common type of impetigo.
    Skin and soft tissue infection of *S. aureus*
    - **Folliculitis:** Superficial infection of ostia of hair follicle.
    - **Furuncles (boils):** More extensive painful lesions that tends to occur in hairy moist region of body and extend from hair follicle to become a true abscess, e.g. buttock.
    - **Carbuncle:** Mostly located in lower neck and are even more severe and painful.
    - **Acute paronychia:** *MC* cause is *S.aureus.*
    - **Bullous impetigo:** Impetigo is *most frequently diagnosed bacterial infection. Almost always caused by S. aureus.*
    - **Ecthyma:** *It is deeper form of impetigo caused by Staph or Strep.*
    - **Cellulitis**
    - **Hidradenitis suppurativa:** Recurrent follicular infections in region such as axilla.
    - **Sycosis barbae** is *chronic folliculitis of beard hair follicle.*
    - **Botyromycosis** is a chronic granulomatous condition similar to mycetoma, usually involves the skin and characterized by granules in the pus, consisting of masses of bacteria generally *Staphylococcus aureus.*

    Remember:
    - *S. aureus* is most common cause of surgical wound infection and is second only to CoNS as a leading cause of primary bacteremia. ..... *Harrison 19/e, p 955*
    - Non-bullous impetigo, cellulitis and erysipelas is caused by Strep. pyogenes more commonly than *S.aureus.*
    - Ecthyma gangrenosum is caused by Ps. aeruginosa.
    - Erythema migrans is caused by Borrelia burgdorferi (Tick transmission).
    - Erythrasma is caused by corynebacterium minutissimum.
    - Impetigo contagiosa is usually caused by streptococci or mixed infections.
      – Most cases of impetigo are caused by *S. aureus.*

Staphylococci

NEET Pattern Questions

1. **Catalase positive, beta hemolytic staphylococcus:**
   a. S aureus
   b. S epidermidis
   c. S saprohyticus
   d. None
   [Ref. Harrison, 20/e, p1071]

   > On blood agar S aureus form golden β hemolytic colonies whereas CONS forms small white non-hemolytic colonies

2. **Catalase positive coagulase negative β-haemolytic bacteria:**
   a. Strep pyogenes
   b. Staph aureus
   c. Coagulase negative staph
   d. Enterococci [Ref. Ananthanarayan, 10/e, p208, 9/e, p206]

   > This denotes staph hemolyticus which is a coagulase negative staph.

3. **A cook is habitual of nose picking while cooking. His clients are at risk for food poisoning with:**
   a. Clostridia difficile
   b. Staph aureus
   c. Vibrio cholerae
   d. Bacillus cereus
   [Ref. Ananthanarayan, 10/e, p204]

4. **Staphylococcal scalded skin syndrome is caused by:**
   a. Hemolysin
   b. Coagulase
   c. Enterotoxin
   d. Epidermolytic toxin
   [Ref. Ananthanarayan, 10/e, p204]

5. **Blood culture is positive in which infection of staph. aureus?** [Ref. Ananthanarayan, 10/e, p205]
   a. TSS
   b. SSSS
   c. Infective endocarditis
   d. Impetigo

   > Blood culture is positive in endovascular infection of bacteremia septicemia, pyema and endocarditis.

6. **All cause Fournier gangrene except:**
   a. Staphylococcus
   b. Streptococcus
   c. Clostridium
   d. Bacteroides

   > Causative organisms of Fournier gangrene: S.aureus, S. pyogenes (B hemolytic streptococci), enterobacteriacae (E.coli Klebsiella, proters), enterococci, pseudomonas and anaerobes like bacteroides and peptostreptococcus

7. **Food poisoning case with diarrhea within 6 hours:**
   a. Staph aureus
   b. Cl. perfringens
   c. Cl. botulinum
   d. V. cholerae
   [Ref. Ananthanarayan, 10/e, p204]

8. **For phage typing, how many phages of Staphylococcus aureus are used?**
   [Ref. Textbook of Microbiology Chakarborty, 2/e, p242]
   a. 12
   b. 15
   c. 20
   d. 28

   > A set of over 28 bacteriophage are employed for typing of S. aureus. Most strain are lysed by more than one phage. In India most preventant phage type is 52/52A/80/81.
   > **Typing method of staphylococci**
   > - Genotypic: based on genetic composition of rRNA or pulse field gel electrophoresis
   > - Bacteriophage typing
   > - Molecular typing: Preferred method now.

9. **Protein A of staphylococcus binds to:**
   a. IgA
   b. IgG
   c. IgD
   d. IgE
   [Ref. Ananthanarayan, 10/e, p203]

   > Protein A binds to Fc terminal of all IgG subclass except IgG3 leaving Fab region free to combine with its antigen. This is the basic principle behind co-agglutination in which protein A bearing staphylococci coated with any IgG antiserum will be agglutinated if mixed with the corresponding antigen.

10. **Most common nosocomial infection is:**
    a. Staph aureus
    b. E. coli
    c. Legionella
    d. Strep pneumonia
    [Ref. Harrison, 20/e, p1072]

    > S. aureus is a leading cause of health care associated infections
    > - UTI is the commonest nosocomial infections
    > - CONS is the commonest cause of nosocomial bacteria

11. **Coagulase test differentiates:**
    a. Staphylococci from streptococci
    b. Streptococci from enterococci
    c. Staph aureus from Staph epidermidis
    d. Staph epidermidis from staph saprophyticus
    [Ref. Ananthanarayan, 10/e, p202]

12. **Staphylococcus aureus does not cause which of the following skin infection?**
    a. Ecthyma gangrenosum
    b. Bullous impetigo
    c. Botryomycosis
    d. Cellulitis
    [Ref. Harrison, 20/e, p1085, 1074]

    > **Note:** Though ecthyma gangrenosum is classically caused by pseudomonas and gram-negative rods. It can be due to methicillin resistant S. aureus.
    > **Botryomycosis** (Bacterial pseudomycosis): rare granulomatous bacterial infection that affects the skin and sometimes viscera. Staph aureus and Pseudomonas aeruginosa are the commonest associated bacteria.

Ans.
1. a. S aureus
2. c. Coagulase negative staph
3. b. Staph aureus
4. d. Epidermolytic toxin
5. c. Infective endocarditis
6. c. Clostridium
7. a. Staph aureus
8. d. 28
9. b. IgG
10. a. Staph aureus
11. c. Staph aureus from staph epidermidis
12. a. Ecthyma gangrenosum

13. **Best available option to prevent MRSA infection in a hospital:** [2015]
    a. Prophylactic antibiotics
    b. Fumigation of wards
    c. Proper hand washing
    d. Use of disinfectants [Ref. Harrison, 20/e, p1078]

14. **Most common site for staphylococcus carrier:** [2015]
    a. Skin   b. Nose
    c. Oropharynx   d. Perineum
    [Ref. Harrison, 20/e, p1072]

15. **Test to differentiate staphylococci from micrococci:**
    a. Catalase test   [2016]
    b. Coagulase test
    c. Novobiosin sensitivity
    d. Oxidation fermentation
    [Ref. Ananthanarayan, 10/e, p209]

16. **Most common cause of artificial heart valve infection in first 3 months:** [2016]
    a. Staphylococcus aureus
    b. Streptococcus mutans
    c. Staph epidermidis
    d. Pneumococcus   [Ref. Harrison, 20/e, p922]

> In initial 12 months MC cause is CoNS, after 12 months etiology is same as native valve endocarditis.

17. **Methicillin resistance in Staph. aureus is due to:**
    a. β-lactamase
    b. MECA gene
    c. AMPC gene
    d. Porin develop   [Ref. Jawetz 27/e 204]

> MeCA gene codes for altered penicillin binding protein which is not affected by methicillin, oxacillin and nafcillin.

18. **Pyomyositis is caused by:** [2016]
    a. Clostridium
    b. Staph. aureus
    c. Streptococcus
    d. E. coli
    [Ref. Harrison 19/e, 958, 18/e, p1068]

> Pyomyositis is usually caused by S. aureus while primary myositis is usually caused by Streptococcus pyogenes.

19. **Hot cold phenomenon is seen due to which toxin of staphylococci?** [2016]
    a. Alpha lysin
    b. Beta lysin
    c. Gamma lysin
    d. Theta lysin
    [Ref. Ananthanarayan 10/e, p203]

> **Hot cold phenomenon:** Hemolysis initiated at 37°C, but become evident only after chilling

20. **Most common mechanism of transfer resistance in Staphylococcus aureus is:** [2016]
    a. Conjugation
    b. Transduction
    c. Transformation
    d. Mutation   [Ref. Jawetz 25/e, p208]

Ans. 13. c. Proper hand washing   14. b. Nose   15. d. Oxidation fermentation   16. c. Staph epidermidis
17. b. MECA gene   18. b. Staph. aureus   19. b. Beta lysin   20. b. Transduction

CHAPTER 8

Streptococci

IMPORTANT STREPTOCOCCI AND THEIR CHARACTERISTICS

Species or common name	Lancefield group	Hemolysis	Laboratory test	Common diseases caused
S. pyogenes	A	beta	**Bacitracin sensitive;** PYR test positive; Ribose not fermented	Upper respiratory tract infections; pyoderma; rheumatic fever; glomerulonephritis
S. agalactiae	B	beta	**CAMP test,** hippurate hydrolysis	Neonatal meningitis, septicemia
S. equisimilis	C	beta	Ribose and trehalose fermentation	Pharyngitis, endocarditis
S. anginosus	A, C, F, G, untypable	beta (alpha, gamma)	Group A strains bacitracin resistant, PYR negative	Pyogenic infections
Enterococcus sp. (E. faecalis and E. faecium E. durans)	D	gamma (alpha, beta)	**Growth in 6.5% NaCl; PYR positive**	Urinary tract infections, endocarditis, suppurative infections
Nonenterococcal Group D species (S. bovis, S. equinus)	D	gamma	No growth in 6.5% NaCl	Endocarditis
Viridans streptococci	Not typed	alpha (gamma)	**Optochin resistant**	Endocarditis (Str. sanguis); dental caries (Str. mutans)

Hemolysis:
- α : S. viridans
- β : S. pyogenes
  S. agalactiae
  S. equisimilis
- γ : Enterococci

Mnemonic: Careless Lancefield And Manic Griffith
c-carbohydrate → Lancefield, Group A is classified by Griffith on the basis of M. Protein.

Note: **Hemolysis:**
Alpha: The agar under the colony is dark or greenish e.g. E. coli.
Beta: Complete hemolysis. Complete lysis of red cells in the media around and under the colonies.
Gamma: No hemolysis.

- Most streptococci that cause human infection are facultative anaerobe

... Harrison 20/e p1081

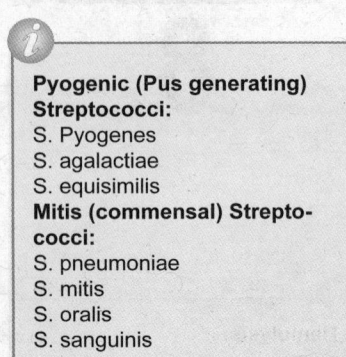

Pyogenic (Pus generating) Streptococci:
S. Pyogenes
S. agalactiae
S. equisimilis

Mitis (commensal) Streptococci:
S. pneumoniae
S. mitis
S. oralis
S. sanguinis

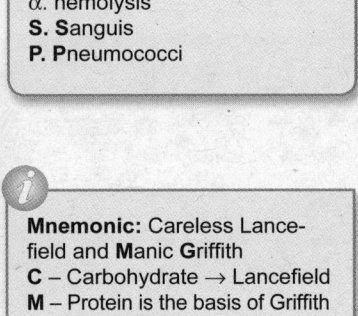

Mnemonic
α. hemolysis
S. Sanguis
P. Pneumococci

Mnemonic: Careless Lancefield and Manic Griffith
C – Carbohydrate → Lancefield
M – Protein is the basis of Griffith classification

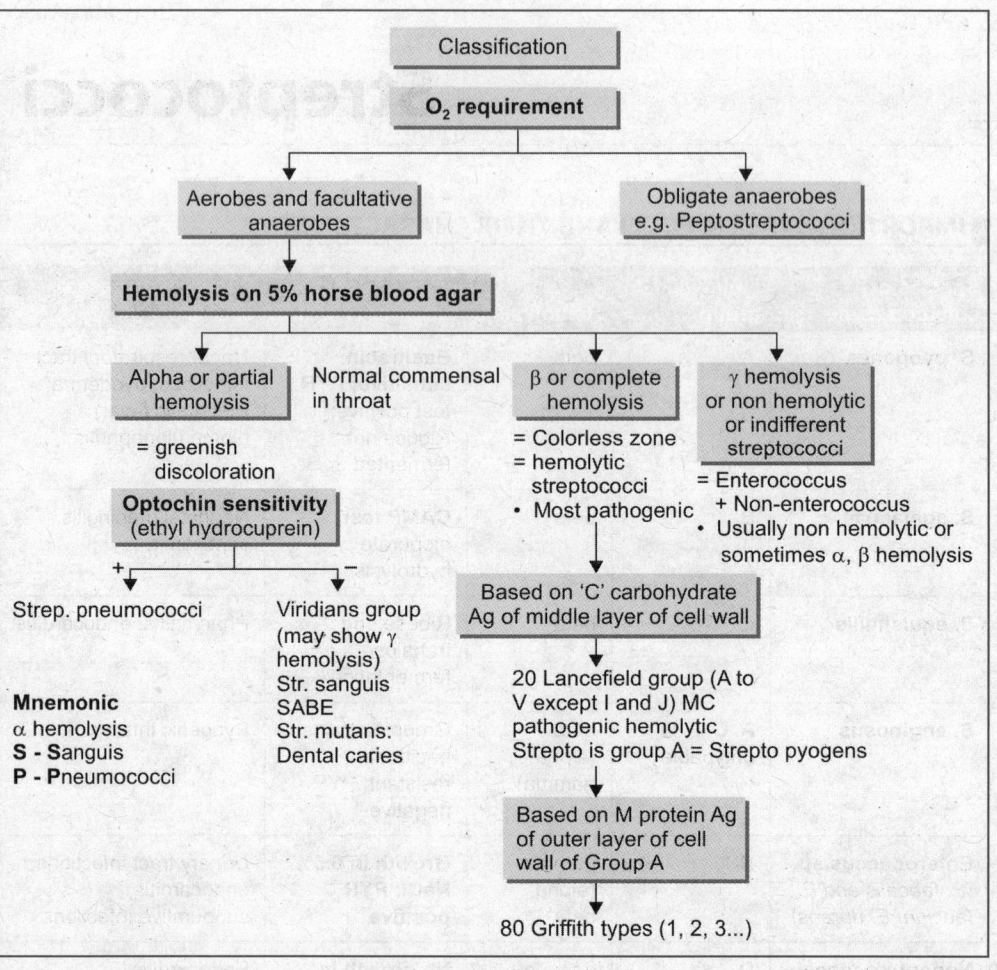

STREP. PYOGENES = LANCEFIELD GROUP A

- Can form *chain* as divide in one plane (*S. aureus* form grape-like cluster as it divide into three planes).
- *Longest chain* is produced by non pathogenic *Str. salivarius*.

Cultural Characteristic

- Growth occur only in media containing fermentable carbohydrate or enriched with blood or serum. Growth and hemolysis are promoted by 10% CO_2.

• Virulent strain	= Matt finely granular colonies
• Avirulent strain	= **Glossy** colonies
• Capsulated (virulent)	= **Mucoid** colonies

- Crystal violet agar is a selective medium.

Antigenic Structure

a. *Polysaccharide capsule:*
   - Group A streptococci (GAS) elaborates varying degree of polysaccharide capsule composed of hyaluronic acid. Capsular polysaccharide plays an important role in protecting GAS from ingestion and killing by phagocytosis. Capsular polysaccharide also plays a role in GAS colonization in the pharynx by binding to CD-44 (a hyaluronic acid binding protein) expressed on human pharyngeal epithelial cell.
   - However, hyaluronic acid capsule is a weak immunogen and antibodies to hyaluronate are not protective.

b. *Cell Wall:*
  - Inner layer made of peptidoglycan.
  - Middle layer made of carbohydrate (basis *of Lancefield classification*).
  - Outer layer made of protein and lipoteichoic acid e.g. M Protein, T, R.
    - **M protein is basis** of **Griffith typing**. *Act as virulence factor* by inhibiting phagocytosis. Antibody to M is protective.
    - T and R protein has no relation to virulence.
c. *Hair-like pilli (fimbria):* Important for attachment to epithelial cells.

Antigenic Similarity

Some antigens of streptococci are similar to normal human cells, because of which streptococcal infection is associated with autoimmune disease like rheumatic fever.

Capsular hyaluronic acid	→	Synovial fluid
Cell wall protein	→	Myocardium
Group A carbohydrates	→	Cardiac valves
Cytoplasmic membrane	→	Vascular intima
Peptidoglycan (mucoprotein)	→	Skin antigen

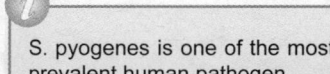

S. pyogenes is one of the most prevalent human pathogen

Toxins and Virulence Factors
a. **Hemolysin - Streptolysin:**

O [Oxygen labile]	S [Oxygen stable and serum soluble]
Activity only on pour plate	Hemolysis on surface
Antigenic specific	Non antigenic
Cardiotoxic	

  - ASO titre → Anti Streptolysin O titre used in retrospective diagnosis; > 200 units is significant; inhibited by cholesterol (but not by Normal sera).
b. **Pyrogenic Exotoxin = Erythrogenic = Dick = Scarlatinal Toxin:**
  - This is superantigen causing **TSS**.
  - *Dick test* used to identify children susceptible to scarlet fever by intradermal injection. *Schultz Charlton Reaction* is another historic test for diagnosis of scarlet fever.
  - **Three types** : Types A *(MC)* and Type C are coded by bacteriophage while type B is chromosomal.
c. **Streptokinase (Fibrinolysin):** Facilitates spread of infection.
d. **Spy Lep:** A serine protease that cleaves and inactivate IL-8, thereby inhibiting neutrophil recruitment to the site of infections.
e. **Deoxyribo nuclease (Streptodornase):** Responsible for thin serous character of strep exudates. Also called as DNAase.
  - Four subtypes. Type B is most antigenic. … AA 10/e, p214
f. **Nicotinamide Adenine Dinucleotidase** (*NAD-ase*).
g. **Hyaluronidase:** Favor spread of infection.
h. **Serum opacity factor:** Lipoproteinase.

Clinical Manifestations
1. *Respiratory:*
  - Sore throat *(pharyngitis)* is **MC** streptococcal infection.
  - Incubation period is 1–4 days.
  - Throat culture is the diagnostic gold standard.
2. *Scarlet fever:*
  - Streptococcal pharyngitis, accompanied by rash made up of minute papules giving a characteristic *"Sand paper"* feel to skin.
  - Associated with circumoral pallor, strawberry tongue.
  - Rash reflect hypersensitivity reaction to toxin.

Interaction with host fibronectin (a matrix protein on eukaryotic cells) is considered as the principal mechanism by which Str. pyogenes binds to epithelial cells of pharynx and skin.

3. **Skin and Soft tissue infection:**
   - *Impetigo*: Superficial infection of skin mainly by group A streptococci. Face and leg are MC site *(see image palette)*.
     – Bullous impetigo is caused by Staph. aureus.
   - *Cellulitis:* Diffuse spreading infection of skin and subcutaneous tissue especially of leg. Caused by *Str. pyogenes* (*MC*), *Staph, Cl. perfringens, E.coli.*
   - *Erysipelas*: Superficial form of cellulitis with bright red appearance of involved skin, seen classically on cheek. Skin assumes peau-d-orange texture due to involvement of superficial lymphatics.
   - *Necrotizing fascitis*: Caused by Group A streptococci called as *Hemolytic streptococcal gangrene.*
   - *In skin infection ASO titre is not high and so ASO estimation has not much clinical significance.*
4. **Genital infection:**
   - **Anaerobic streptococci** are most important cause of **puerperal sepsis.**
5. **Bacteremia, pneumonia, toxic shock syndrome.**
6. *Non suppurative complication:* Develop 1-3 weeks after acute infection.

> Catalase negative Gr(+) ve cocci from pus is likely to be streptococci.
> Bacitracin sensitivity test is the specific test for detection of Group A streptococci (i.e. Str. pyogenes)

Acute rheumatic fever	Acute glomerulonephritis
• Develop after throat infection by any serotype of S. pyogenes	• Develop after either sore throat or skin infection by serotype 49, 53-55, 59-64, 1 and 12
• Repeated attacks common	• No repeated attacks
• Penicillin prophylaxis indicated	• Not indicated
• Course is progressive or static	• Spontaneous resolution
• ASO titre always raised	• May or May not (after skin infection) raised
• Marked immune response with no change in complement level	• Moderate immune response with decrease in complement level

Lab Diagnosis

- In acute pharyngitis diagnosis is established by throat swab culture (diagnostics gold standard).
  - *Pike's medium* is used as *transport media.*
  - Sheep blood agar is recommended for isolation as it is inhibitory for *H. hemolyticus.*
- In Rheumatic fever and Glomerulonephritis retrospective diagnosis is needed.
  - *ASO titre* > 200 is indicative of prior streptococcal disease. After skin infection ASO titre is usually low. So useful only in retrospective diagnosis of rheumatic fever.
  - Organism are not detectable in acute rheumatic fever or acute glomerulonephritis. These lesions are believed to be due to hypersensitivity to some streptococcal component with antigenic cross reaction.
  - *In acute glomerulonephritis and pyoderma, Anti-DNAse and antihyaluronidase are used for retrospective diagnosis.*
- Streptozyme test: *Passive slide haemagglutination* test. Sensitive and specific test for all types of streptococcal infection.

> CAMP reaction is the specific test for detection of Group B streptococci.

Treatment of Group A Streptococci	
• *Pharyngitis, impetigo, erysipelas,* cellulitis	– **Penicillin (Pn)**
• *Necrotizing fascitis / myositis*	– **Surgical debridement + Pn + Clindamycin**
• *Pneumonia / Empyema*	– **Pn + empyema drainage**
• Streptococcal TSS	– **Penicillin + Clindamycin + iv Ig**

OTHER HEMOLYTIC STREPTOCOCCI (LANCEFIELD B HEMOLYTIC STREPTOCOCCI)

Group B (Strep. agalactiae)

- *S. agalactiae* is the *MC* cause of neonatal meningitis in west.

- It **does not** hydrolyse bile esculin agar, however, hydrolyse sodium hippurate and are bacitracin resistant.
- *Virulence factor* is **polysaccharide capsule.** *(Group A have hyaluronic acid capsule).*
- Identified by positive **CAMP** *(Christie, Atkins and Munch-Peterson)* **reaction (CAMP factor is a phospholipase).**
- 5–40% women are vaginal or rectal carries of Group B streptococci. ... *Harrison 20/e, p 1087*
- In infant it cause 2 types of infection:
  - *Early Onset:* More common, acquired from maternal vagina during birth.
  - Essentially all infants are bacteremic presenting with lethargy, respiratory distress and hypotension.
  - *Late Onset Infection:* Infection more often obtained from environment.
  - Meningitis is *the MC* manifestation and in most cases is associated with strain of *capsular type III.*
- In pregnant women it is the prominent cause of peripartum fever.
- *Treatment*
  Penicillin is *DOC* for all group B streptococcal infection.

> **Prevention of Neonatal GBS infection**
> - *Detection*: Screening for angenital colonization at 35–37 weeks of pregnancy by swab culture of lower vagina.
> - *Intrapartum chemoprophylaxis:* Indicated in patient who screen positive. Women whose culture status is unknown, who develop preterm labour.
> - Recommended regimen in 5 million units of Penicillin G followed by 2.5 million units every 4 hour until delivery cefazolin as an alternative in patients with Penicillin G.

GROUP C - STREP. EQUISIMILIS

- Predominant animal pathogen and is the source of streptokinase used for thrombolytic therapy.

GROUP D - STREPTOCOCCI (NON HEMOLYTIC)

Includes:

- Fecal streptococci/*Enterococcus.*
- Non enterococcal group D streptococci.
- Enterococci are now considered as separate genus on the basis of DNA homologous studies and 16S rRNA sequencing. ... *Harrison 20/e, p 1089*

> - Enterococci are identified by their ability to grow on bile containing medium.
> - E. faecalis and E. faecium are the important enterococci causing human disease.
> - Vancomycin resistance is seen in:
>   - 80% of E. faecium
>   - 7% of E. faecalis

Distinctive Features of *Enterococcus:*

- Grow in 40% bile and hydrolyse esculin ... *Jawetz 27/e, p 226*
- Grow in 6.5% NaCl at pH 9.6, 45°C and in 0.1% methylene blue milk
- Majority of clinically significant enterococci hydrolyze PVR. This is helpful in differentiating them from S. bovis.
- Heat resistant, surviving 60°C for 30 minutes
- Non-hemolytic to ovine or bovine RBC (commonly used in lab). However, some strains of E. faecalis can lyse human RBC ... *Harrison 20/e, p 1089*
- Majority of enterococcal species hydrolyze PYR, this feature distinguish them from organism of Str. bovis group.
- Present in intestine, genital tract and saliva
- Cause wound infection, UTI, nosocomial bacteremia in patient with IV catheters, endocarditis.
- Usually resistant to Penicillin, cephalosporin, etc
- In case of Vancomycin and β lactam resistance - Linezolid (against all enterococci) or quinupristin, dalfopristin (against E. faecium only) are given.

> Virulence factors of enterococci
> a. Enterococal secreted factors:
>   – Enterococcal hemolysin
>   – Enterococcal protease (GelE and SprE)
> b. Enterococcal surface components:
>   – Surface pili
>   – Surface protein
> c. E. faecalis stress protein

Distinctive features that distinguish Enterococci from Streptococci		
Characteristics	Enterococci	Streptococci
Shape	Oval cocci, sometimes at an angle to each other	Spherical
Length of chain	Short chains	Long chains
Growth on sheep blood agar	Generally non-haemolytic	Usually beta or alpha haemolytic
Growth on MacConkey medium	Tiny magenta pink colonies	Usually do not grow on MacConkey medium
Heat tolerance	Survive at 60°C for 30 minutes	Do not survive at this temperature

Non-enterococcal Group D Streptococci

- Grow in bile and hydrolyze esculin (bile-esculin positive)   ... *Jawetz 27/e, p 220*
- Unable to grow in 6.5% NaCl and PYR negative (*difference from enterococci*)
- Penicillin susceptible.
- Main species causing infection is *S.bovis*. *S.bovis* endocarditis is often associated with neoplasm of GIT, most commonly colon.

GROUP F - STREPTOCOCCI

- Called as minute streptococci.
- Includes *Streptococcus* MG.
- Isolated from cases of atypical pneumonia.

VIRIDANS STREPTOCOCCI

- Heterogenous group of organism that are the commonest agent causing bacterial endocarditis. These are part of normal flora of mouth.
- Species include:
  - *S. sanguis*: MC viridans streptococcus associated with endocarditis.
  - *S. mutans*: Important cause of dental caries.
  - *S. salivarus*.

PNEUMOCOCCUS

- Gram positive Lanceolate diplococci. *Possess polysaccharide capsule.*
- It is **MC** cause of *Lobar pneumonia, sinusitis, otitis media*.
- It is **MC** cause of *bacterial meningitis* in adults.

> Fermentation ability of pneumococci is tested in Hiss serum sugars

Characteristic	Pneumococci	Streptococci
Morphology	Capsulated	Mostly non capsulated
Quellung test	+ ve	– ve
Colonies	Draughtsman colonies	Dome-shaped colonies
Bile solubility	++	–
Inulin fermentation	++	–
Optochin sensitivity	++	–
Intraperitoneal Inoculation of mice	Fatal infection	Not pathogenic
Growth in liquid media	Uniform turbidity	Granular turbidity or powdery deposit

Morphology and Culture

- Capsule enclose a pair of flame shaped Lanceolate bacteria.
- Grow only in enriched media.
- Fastidios in nature. Grows best in 5% CO_2 ... *Harrison 20/e, p 1063*

- On blood agar they are α *hemolytic* and on prolong incubation colonies show *draughtsman or carrom* coin appearance. Under anaerobic conditions produce β hemolysis.
- Strains with **abundant capsular material (3, 7)** form large, mucoid colonies.
- Pneumococci readily undergo autolysis in culture due to presence of autolytic amidase which is activated by bile salts; hence *they are bile soluble*.
- *Bile solubility* is of *diagnostic importance*.
- *Inulin fermenter (useful test for differentiating from streptococci as they are unable to do so).*

Virulence Factors

- Capsular polysaccharide = specific soluble substance:
- *MC* antigen and virulent factor.
  - Protects against phagocytosis.
  - Type 3 pneumococci has abundant capsular material, *so more virulent.*
- *C substance ("cell wall" substance):*
  - Unique to pneumococci. It is a polysaccharide consisting of teichoic acid with a phosphoryl choline residue. These choline residue provide attachment to potential virulence factors such as pneumococcal surface protein A (PspA) and pneumococcal surface adhesin A (psaA).
- *Penumolysin:*
  - Membrane damaging toxin which has cytotoxic and complement activating properties.
- *Autolysin.*
- *IgA_1 Protease:*
  - Pneumococci produce an extracellular protease, that specifically cleaves human IgA_1. IgA1 protease enable pneumococci to establish infection in upper respiratory tract, where IgA predominates.
- *Pili, Biofilm, LytA.*

Quellung Reaction

On mixing pneumococci with specific or polyvalent antipolysaccharide serum the capsule becomes apparently swollen, sharply delineated and refractile. This reaction is used for *rapid identification.*

Risk factor for pneumococcal infection	
• **Respiratory infection Inflammation**	• **Defective complement function**
– Influenza, other viral respiratory infection	• **Defective clearance of pneumococcal bacteremia**
– Allergies	– Congenital asplenia, hyposplenia
– Cigarette smoking	– Splenectomy
– Chronic obstructive pulmonary disease	– Sickle cell disease
• **Anatomical disruption of meninges (dural tear)**	• **Other conditions**
• **HIV infection**	– Alcoholism
• **Defective antibody formation**	– Malnutrition
– Selective IgG subclass deficiency	– Glucocorticoid treatment
– Multiple myeloma	– Cirrhosis of the liver
– Chronic lymphocytic leukemia	– Renal insufficiency
– Lymphoma	– Diabetes mellitus
	– Anemia
	– Coronary artery disease

> **Quellung reaction:** Rapid identification of pneumococci

Manifestations

- *Most common* pneumococcal infection are **otitis media** and **sinusitis.**
- *Meningitis* is ***most serious*** pneumococcal infection. Pneumococci is the most common cause of meningitis in alcoholics.

- Pneumonia: Mostly due to types 1 to 8 strains.
  - *Type 3 strain is **most virulent**.*
  - *MC complication of pneumococcal pneumonia—**Empyema***
- *S. pneumoniae* are *MC* cause of sepsis in splenectomized patient.
- *Austrian syndrome:* Concurrence of pneumococcal pneumonia, endocarditis and meningitis.

Diagnosis

- Gram's staining and culture of sputum or CSF.
- *Gold standard* for diagnosis of pneumococcal pneumonia is pathologic examination of lung tissue.
- **Biomarkers** – CRP: testing by passive agglutination
  - Raised procalcitonin level is another biomarker which gets elevated in invasive pneumococcal disease.

Most common pneumococcal infection:
- Otiis media\
- Sinusitis

Most serious pneumococcal infection: Meningitis

Most virulent pneumococcal strain type 3 strain

Treatment

- *Otitis media/Sinusitis/Pneumonia*—**Amoxicillin**.
- *Meningitis*—**Ceftriaxone + vancomycin**.
- *Endocarditis*—**Ceftriaxone or cefotaxime + vancomycin**.
- Penicillin resistance is due to alteration in penicillin binding protein (not due to production of β lactamase).

Pneumococcal Vaccine

Two types are available:
a. Polyvalent polysaccharide vaccine:
   - Contains capsular antigen of *23 most prevalent serotypes.*
   - *Protection rate—80 - 90%*

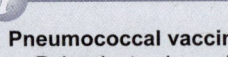

Pneumococcal vaccine:
- Polyvalent polysaccharide vaccine
- Polysaccharide protein conjugate vaccine

PNEUMOCOCCAL VACCINE	
Indication	**Contraindication**
In patient with absent or dysfunctional spleen	< 2 yr child
Sickle cell disease	Lymphoreticular malignancies and immunosuppressive therapy
Coeliac disease	CSF leak
Chronic renal, lung, heart and liver disease	Alcoholic cirrhosis
Diabetes mellitus	Multiple myeloma
Immunodeficiencies including HIV	Chronic glucocorticoid therapy
Routinely as ≥ 65 years of age	'Hodgkin's' disease
	Organ transplant recipient

b. Polysaccharide protein conjugate vaccine:
   - As infants and young children responds poorly to polysaccharide vaccine, protein conjugate vaccines were developed.
   - Till 2010, three PCV products containing 7, 10 and 13 serotypes were commercially available.
   - PCV are recommended by WHO for inclusion in routine childhood immunization schedule worldwide.

> **Splenectomy**
> - Splenectomy increase the risk of following infections: streptococcus pneumococcal, Hemophilus influenzae and some Gram negative enteric organisms.
> - Splenectomized patient should be vaccinated against Pneumococi Haemophilus influenzae, Meningococci
> - In splenectomized individual any unexplained fever is medical emergency.

Multiple Choice Questions

General

1. Which is false regarding gram-positive cocci? [AI 08]
   a. *Staph. saprophyticus* causes UTI in females
   b. Micrococci are oxidase positive
   c. Most enterococci are sensitive to penicillin
   d. Pneumococci are capsulated

2. A patient of RHD developed infective endocarditis after dental extraction. Most likely organism causing this is: [AIIMS 01, 13]
   a. *Streptococcus viridans*
   b. *Streptococcus pneumoneae*
   c. *Streptococcus pyogenes*
   d. *S. aureus*

3. In a case of neonatal meningitis, the etiologic bacteria was found to have properties of b-hemolysis, bacitracin resistance, CAMP positive. Which of the following is most likely causative agent? [AI 2010]
   a. S. pyogenes
   b. S. agalactiae
   c. S. pneumoniae
   d. E. faecalis

4. Eight months after prosthetic valve replacement, most common organism causing infective endocarditis is: [AIIMS Nov 10]
   a. Staph. epidermidis
   b. Strep. viridans
   c. Staph. aureus
   d. HACEK

Streptococcus Pyogenes

5. Which component of *St. pyogenes* has cross reactivity with synovium of human? [AI 08]
   a. Capsular hyaluronic acid
   b. Cell proteins
   c. Group A carbohydrate antigens
   d. Peptidoglycan

6. A boy with skin ulcer on leg, culture revealed beta hemolysis. School physician said that similar hemolysis was seen in organism from sorethroat, what is the similarity between both? [AIIMS Nov 10]
   a. A protein is same for both
   b. C carbohydrate antigen is different
   c. C carbohydrate antigen is the same
   d. Strain causing both are same

7. A person from village is complaining of development of pustules. Extract from pus has shown gram positive cocci, showing hemolysis, catalase –ve, identified as a group of streptococci. Following test is used:
   a. Bacitracin sensitivity [AI 07; AIIMS Nov 06]
   b. Novobiocin sensitivity
   c. Optochin sensitivity
   d. Hemolysis

8. All are true about *Streptococcus* except: [AI 01]
   a. M-protein is responsible for production of mucoid colonies
   b. M- protein is responsible for virulence
   c. Mucoid colonies are virulent
   d. No resistance to penicillin has been reported

9. Toxin involved in the streptococcal toxic shock syndrome is: [AI 01]
   a. Pyrogenic toxin
   b. Streptokinase
   c. Hemolysin
   d. Neurotoxin

10. True statement about antistreptolysin 'O' titre is: [AIIMS, 011, AI 97]
    a. In normal people the titre is < 200
    b. In acute glomerulonephritis the titre is low
    c. ASO titre >200 indicate rheumatic fever
    d. Streptozyme test is an active hemagglutination test

11. Lance field grouping of streptococci is done by using:
    a. M protein [AIIMS 07]
    b. Group C peptidoglycan cell wall
    c. Group C carbohydrate antigen
    d. M antigen

12. An outbreak of Streptococcal pharyngitis has occurred in a remote village. In order to carry out the epidemiological investigations it is necessary to perform the culture of the throat swab of the patient suffering from the disease. The transport media of choice would be:
    a. Salt manitol media [AIIMS 02]
    b. Pike's media
    c. Stuart media
    d. Carry Blair media

13. The commonest organism causing cellulitis is:
    a. *Streptococcus pyogenes* [AI 09]
    b. *Streptococcus faecalis*
    c. *Streptococcus viridans*
    d. Microaerophilic streptococci

14. Streptococcus all are true *except*: [AIIMS 10, 11]
    a. Streptodornase cleaves DNA
    b. Streptolysin O is active in reduced state
    c. Streptokinase is produced from serotype A, C, K
    d. Pyrogenic toxin A is plasmid mediated

15. Antigenically similar to Streptolysin O:
    a. Clostridial perfringenes toxin [PGI 2010, 2009]
    b. Tetanolysin
    c. Botulinum toxin
    d. Erythrotoxin

16. A 5-year-old child presents with pustular lesions on the lower legs. The culture from the lesion showed hemolytic colonies on blood agar which were Gram-positive cocci. Provisional diagnosis of Group A streptococcal pyoderma can be done by: [AI 2012]
    a. Catalase positivity
    b. Optochin sensitivity
    c. Bile solubility
    d. Bacitracin sensitivity

17. Group A streptococci is best diagnosed by:
    a. Optochin sensitivity   [AIIMS Nov 2011]
    b. Bacitracin sensitivity
    c. Catalase negative
    d. Bite solubility

Enterococci

18. Which of the following is not true regarding enterococcus ? [AI 08]
    a. Common species are *E. faecalis* and *E. faecium*
    b. It is a cause for peritonitis
    c. It is universally susceptible to penicillins
    d. Can cause intra-abdominal abscess

19. A beta hemolytic bacteria is resistant to vancomycin, shows growth in 6.5% NaCl, is non bile sensitive. It is likely to be: [AI 09]
    a. *Strep. agalactiae*
    b. *Strep. pneumonia*
    c. *Enterococcus*
    d. *Strep. bovis*

20. A patient admitted to an ICU is on central venous line for the last one week. He is on ceftazidime and amikacin. After 7 days of antibiotics he develops a spike of fever and his blood culture is positive for gram positive cocci in chains which are catalase - negative. Following this vancomycin was started but the culture remained positive for same organism even after 2 weeks of therapy. The most likely organism causing infection is:
    a. *Staphylococci aureus*   [AI 07; AIIMS 06]
    b. *Viridans streptococci*
    c. *Enterococcus faecalis*
    d. Coagulase negative *Staphylococcus*

21. Which of the following organism, when isolated in the blood, requires the synergistic activity of penicillin + amino glycoside for appropriate therapy: [AIIMS 04]
    a. *Enterococcus faecalis*
    b. *Staph. aureus*
    c. *Streptococcus pneumoniae*
    d. *Bacterioides fragilis*

Pneumococci

22. An infant had high grade fever and respiratory distress at the time of presentation to the emergency room. The sample collected for blood culture was subsequently positive showing growth of α-hemolytic colonies. On Gram staining these were Gram-positive cocci. In the screening test for identification, the suspected pathogen is likely to be susceptible to the following agent:
    a. Bacitracin   [AI 07, AIIMS May 2012]
    b. Novobiocin
    c. Optochin
    d. Cloxacillin

23. The sputum specimen of a 70-year-old male was cultured on a 5% blood agar. The culture showed the presence of α-hemolytic colonies next day. The further processing of this organism is most likely to yield: [AIIMS 05]
    a. Gram-positive cocci in short chains, catalase negative and bile resistant
    b. Gram-positive cocci in pairs, catalase negative and bile soluble
    c. Gram-positive cocci in clusters, catalase positive and coagulase positive
    d. Gram-negative coccobacilli, catalase positive and oxidase positive

24. A 65-year-old man presents with complaints of chest pain, fever, cough with sputum. Sputum examination reveals pus cells with Gram positive cocci. Blood agar showed positive results. How will you differentiate this from other Gram positive cocci? [AIIMS Nov 2009]
    a. Bacitracin sensitivity   b. Optochin sensitivity
    c. Bile solubility   d. Positive coagulase

25. An eight year old child with history of pain and discharge from right ear presents with fever, neck rigidity and a positive Kerning's sign. Discharge was stained with Gram stain which revealed gram positive cocci. Which of the following is the most likely organism? [AI 2011]
    a. H. influenzae
    b. Staphylococcus
    c. Pneumococcus
    d. Pseudomonas

26. All are true about streptococcus pneumoniae *except*:
    a. Capsule aids in infection   [AI 2011]
    b. Commonest infection is otitis media
    c. Respiratory tract of carriers is most important source of infection
    d. Meningitis caused by S. pneumoniae is milder than others

27. A person presents with pneumonia. His sputum was sen for culture. The bacterium obtained was gram positive cocci in chains and alpha haemolytic colonies on sheep agar. Which of the following will help in confirming the diagnosis: [AIIMS 2012]
    a. Novobiocin   b. Optochin
    c. Bacitracin   d. Oxacillin

28. A 6-year-old unimmunized child present with fever, neck stiffness, vomiting. Lumbar puncture was performed and the Gram staining shows the following picture:

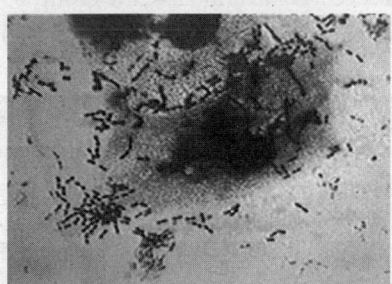

   Identify the causative agent: (2019)
   a. Streptococcus pneumoniae
   b. Klebsiella
   c. Neisseria meningitidis
   d. Haemophilus influenzae
   [Ref. Harrison, 20/e, p 1068, 1001]

29. True about group B streptococcus infection in pregnancy:
   a. Not harmful to mother (2019)
   b. Intrapartum antimicrobial prophylaxis is given to positive cases
   c. Screening is performed in 2nd trimester
   d. Cause cardiac and limb defects in fetus
   [Ref. Harrison, 20/e, p 1088]

30. Bacitracin sensitive streptococci: [AIIMS 2018]
   a. Steptococcus agalactiae
   b. Streptococcus pyogenes
   c. Enterococcus
   d. Streptococcus viridans

Explanations and References with Illustrative Answers

1. **Ans. (c) Most enterococci are sensitive to penicillin**   Ref. Harrison 20/e, p 1092; Ananthanarayan 10/e, p 219, 223
   - Unlike streptococci, enterococci are not reliably killed by penicillin or ampicillin alone at concentration achieved clinically in the blood or tissues.
   - Antimicrobial susceptibility testing should be performed routinely on enterococcal isolates.

   Enterococci resistance to penicillin is via two mechanism:

Penicillin Resistance	
Penicilase production	**Altered penicillin binding protein**
• Seen in *E. faecalis*	• Common in *E. faecum*
• Vancomycin, ampicillin/sulbactam, amoxicillin/clavulanate, imipenem may be used in combination with gentamycin	• Vancomycin plus gentamycin is used

   Other options
   Option 'a'
   - *Staph. saprophyticus* specially causes UTI in sexually active young women.

   Option 'b'
   - Micrococci are catalase and oxidase positive Gr +ve cocci. They are strict aerobes and are non-pathogenic.
   - Micrococci are differentiated from Staphylococci by Hugh and Deifson oxidation fermentation test in which micrococci shows oxidative pattern while staphylococci show fermentative pattern.

Anaerobic Cocci		
Features	**Gram +ve**	**Gram –ve**
Organism	• **Peptostreptococci** • **Peptococcus**	***Veillonellae***
Inhabitation	• Intestine, vagina and mouth	Mouth, intestine and genital tract
Diseases	• **Puerperal sepsis** • Visceral abscess • UTI, wound infection • Gangrenous apendicitis	No disease is identified till now.
Treatment	• Sensitive to penicillin, chloramphenicol and metronidazole	

2. **Ans. (a) *Streptococcus viridans*** *Ref. Harrison 20/e, p 922, 923, Ananthanarayan 10/e, p271*
   This is case of **subacute bacterial endocarditis (SABE)** as patient has rheumatic heart disease (so damaged heart valves).

   Subacute endocarditis is typically caused by Viridans streptococci, enterococci, CoNS and HACEK group.

   Among viridans S. sanguinis (a normal commensal of oral cavity) produce endocarditis in at risk individual (like damaged heart valves) after dental procedures.

Endocarditis					
	Native valve		**Prosthetic valve**		**Injection drug users**
	Community associated	Nosocomial	Early (<12 Month)	Late (>12 month)	
Most common organism	Staph. aureus	Staph. aureus	Coagulase (–)ve staph	Viridans Streptococci	*Staph. aureus* (usually right sided)

   Remember
   - Staph. aureus is now the leading cause of native valve endocarditis
   - MC cause of SABE — S. viridans
   - MC cause of acute bacterial endocarditis — S. aureus
   - MC cause of prosthetic valve endocarditis — S. epidermidis
   - MC cause of endocarditis in iv drug users — S. aureus

3. **Ans. (b) S. agalactiae** *Ref. Ananthanarayan 10/e, p 218, 9/e, p 216*
   - *S. agalactiae* is the **MC** cause of neonatal meningitis in west.
   - It does not hydrolyse bile esculin agar, however hydrolyse sodium hippurate and are bacitracin resistant.
   - Identified by **CAMP** (*Christie, Atkins and Munch - Peterson*) **reaction.**
   - In infant it cause 2 type of infection:
     a. **Early Onset:** – More common, acquired from maternal vagina during birth.
        – Essentially all infants are bacteremic presenting with lethargy, respiratory distress and hypotension.
     b. **Late Onset Infection:** – Infection more often obtained from environment.
        – Meningitis is the **MC** manifestation and most cases are associated with strain *capsular type III.*
   - Other Group B infections in neonates include arthritis, osteomyelitis, conjunctivitis, peritonitis, omphalitis, and endocarditis.
   - Adult infection include puerperal sepsis and pneumonia.
   - **Treatment:** Penicillin is **DOC** for all group B streptococcal infection.

4. **Ans. (a) Staph. epidermidis** *Ref. Harrison 20/e p 1077*
   - Coagulase negative staphylococci is the most common cause of endocarditis in posthetic value recepients with in one year of surgery. *For full explanation refer previous answers.*

5. **Ans. (a) Capsular hyaluronic acid** *Ref. Ananthanarayan 10/e, p 213; Harsh Mohan 5/e, p 330*

Cross reactivity of Streptococcal antigen	
Bacterial antigen	**Cross reacting human component**
Capsular hyaluronic acid	Human synovial fluid
Group A carbohydrate antigen	Cardiac valves
Cytoplasmic membrane antigen	Vascular intima
Cell wall protein	Myocardium
Peptidoglycan	Skin antigen
Membrane antigens	Sarcolemma of smooth and cardiac muscle, dermal fibroblasts and neurons of caudate nucleus

6. **Ans. (c) C-carbohydrate antigen is the same** *Ref. Jawetz 27/e, p 215, Ananthanarayan 10/e, p 210*

   β hemolytic streptococci causing both skin infection and sore throat can be none other than Group A streptococci.
   - The basis by which Lancefield classified streptococci in to groups A-H and K-V is c carbohydrate. So, different Group A streptococci have same c carbohydrate. In group A, c carbohydrate is rhannose – N-acetyl glycosamine.

- Based on the M protein Griffith divided Group A carbohydrate in to 80 subtypes. Sore throat strains and skin strains of streptococci differ in their M-protein. Skin infection is usually caused by M-types 49,57, 59-61.

7. **Ans. (a) Bacitracin sensitivity** *Ref. Ananthanarayan 9/e, p 210; 10/e, p 218*

   "Sensitivity to bacitracin is employed as a convenient method for differentiating Str. pyogenes from other hemolytic streptococci."

   Hydrolysis of PYR and failure to ferment ribose also differentiate S. pyogenes from other.

   Pustule – A vesicle filled with leukocyte. MC cause is virus. MC bacterial cause is *Strep. pyogenes*.

   > **Remember:**
   > - Str. pyogenes is the etiologic agent in most of the streptococcal skin infection.
   > - Vancomycin is the drug of choice.
   > - Optochin sensitivity and bile solubility is used to differentiate pneumococci from *Strep. viridans* group.

8. **Ans. (a) M-protein is responsible for production of mucoid colonies** *Ref. Ananthanarayan 10/e, p 212, 218*

   "Mucoid colonies are due to production of capsule of hyaluronic acid not due to M-protein." .... Harrison 20/e, p 1081

   Growth characteristic of Strep. pyogenes:
   - On blood agar *virulent stains* forms **matt or mucoid colonies** while *avirulent* form **glossy colonies**.
   - M, T, R are proteins found on outer part of cell wall and forms the basis of **Griffith classification**.
     – **M protein** - Acts as virulence factor and antibody against it are protective.
     – **T and R protein** - No relation to virulence
   - Streptococci (except enterococci) are usually susceptible to penicillin. Now enterococci is taken as separate genus. So option "d" is correct.

9. **Ans. (a) Pyrogenic toxin** *Ref. Jawetz 25/e, p 198, 27/e 218*

   "Streptococcal TSS is caused by pyrogenic exotoxin."

   Pyrogenic exotoxin = Erythrogenic toxin = Dick = Scarlatinal toxin
   - Produced by group A streptococci (type 1, 2, 3, 12 and 28)
   - Associated with streptococcal toxic shock syndrome and scarlet fever.
   - There are 3 type of pyrogenic exotoxin: A, B, and C
   - A (*MC* cause of streptococcal TSS) and C are coded by bacteriophage gene, while B is chromosomal
   - Acts as superantigen
   - Associated with streptococcal toxic shock syndrome and scarlet fever
   - *DOC* for streptococcal TSS is — **Clindamycin** ..... Harrison 20/e, p 1087

10. **Ans. (b) In acute glomerulonephritis the titre is low** *Ref. Ananthanarayan 10/e, p 216*

    Retrospective diagnosis of streptococcal infection
    - *ASO (Anti Streptolysin 'O') titre:*
      – Estimation of antibody against streptolysin is a standard serological test for retrospective diagnosis of streptococcal infection.
      – ASO titre > 200 are indicative of prior streptococcal infection.
      – Raised after throat infection only
      – *Acute rheumatic fever:* – High level of ASO titre are usually found
        – Titres > 300 or 350 are taken as significant.
      – *Acute glomerulonephritis:* – ASO titres are often low.
    - *Streptozyme test*
      – Passive slide hemagglutination test
      – Becomes positive after nearly all types of streptococcal infection whether of throat or skin.
    - *Anti DNA ase B and Antihyaluronidase*
      – Useful for retrospective diagnosis of streptococcal pyoderma or for acute glomerulonephritis for which ASO titre is of much less value.

70 Self-Assessment and Review of Microbiology and Immunology

11. **Ans. (c) Group C carbohydrate antigen** *Ref. Ananthanarayan 10/e, p 211*

    Lancefield classification: Classification of β-hemolytic streptococci into Group A to V (except I, J) on the *basis* of **group specific C carbohydrate**.

    Griffith classification: Serological typing of group A streptococcus pyogenes on the *basis* of **M proteins into types 1, 2, 3, etc.**

    Group C Carbohydrate
    - Present in middle layer of cell wall.
    - This antigen is an integral part of cell wall.
    - Serological grouping of streptococci depend on C carbohydrate for which it has to be extracted from cell wall.
    - *Method for extraction are:*
      - Lancefield's acid extraction method (organism are grown in Todd Hewitt broth)
      - Fuller's method
      - Maxted's method
      - Rantz and Randall's method (Autoclaving).

Streptococcal Group C Carbohydrate	
Group A	Rhamnose N-acetyl glucosamine
Group B	Rhamnose glusamine Polysaccharide
Group C	Rhamnose N-acetylgalactosamine
Group D	Glycerol teichoic acid

12. **Ans. (b) Pike's media** *Ref. Ananthanarayan 10/e, p 216*

    "Pike's media is transport media for Streptococci."
    Throat culture is the gold standard for diagnosis of streptococcal pharyngitis

    Diagnosis of Streptococcal Pharyngitis
    - **Specimen:**
      - Throat specimen collected by vigorous rubbing of a sterile swab over both tonsillar pillars
    - **Culture**
      - Throat culture is diagnostic gold standard for pharyngitis.
      - Swab are either plated immediately or sent to laboratory in Pike's medium (used as transport media).
      - Specimen is plated on blood agar and incubated at 37°C anaerobically or under 5-10% CO2.
      - Sheep blood agar is recommended for primary isolation because it is inhibitory for Haemophilus.
    - Latex agglutination or enzyme immunoassay of swab specimen is a useful adjunct to throat culture. These rapid diagnostic tests are highly specific but less sensitive. So, a positive result is an indication for treatment, but negative result should be confirmed by throat culture.

    > **Remember:**
    > - Stuart's medium is transport media for Gonococci.
    > - Cary - Blair medium is transport media for V. cholera.
    > - Crystal violet added to blood agar is a selective media for *S. pyogenes*.

13. **Ans. (a) *Streptococcus pyogenes*** *Ref. Harrison 19/e, p 967; 20/e, p 1085*

    Cellulitis:
    - Diffuse spreading infection of skin (dermis and subcutaneous tissue) especially of lower leg.
    - Caused by *Strep pyogenes* **(MC)**, Staph, *Cl perfringens*, *E.coli*.
    - Major portal of entry for lower leg cellulitis is toe web *tinea pedis* with fissuring of skin.
    - Skin become peud orange in appearance; recurrent attack may sometimes affect lymphatic vessels producing permanent swelling called as *solid edema*.
    - Streptococcus cellulitis tends to develop at sites where lymphatic drainage is disrupted.

14. **Ans. (d) Pyrogenic toxin A is plasmid mediated** *Ref. Ananthanarayan 10/e, p 213*

    Let us cnsider each option

Option 'a'

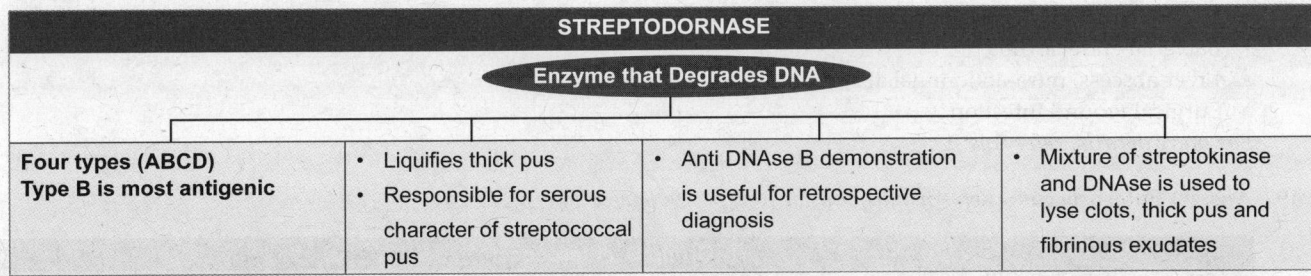

Option 'b'

STREPTOCOCCI HEMOLYSIN	
Streptolysin O	**Streptolysin S (Serum soluble)**
• Oxygen labile	• Oxygen stable
• Activitiy only on pour plate not on surface	• Responsible for hemolysis seen around streptococcal colonies on surface
• Antigenic protein	• Non Antigenic protein elaborated in presence of serum
• Active only is reduced state	

Note: Lysins similar to streptolysin O are also produced by S. pneumonia (Pneumolysin), Clostridium tetani (tetanolysin), C. perfringens (Q toxin), Bacillus cereus (cereolysin) and Listeria monocytogens (listeriolysin).

Option 'c' *Ref. Textbook of Mirobiology by D.R Arora, 3/e p 228*

Streptokinase (Fibrinolysin)

- Streptococci of group 'A', C and G produce a substance called streptokinase which is actively fibrinolytic for human fibrin. Streptokinase is produced maximally in the early stage of growth.
- Streptokinase converts plasminogen to plasmin, which in turn lyse fibrin.
- Streptokinase facilitates the spread of infection by breaking down fibrin barrier arund the lesion.
- Therapuitically it is used for the treatment of early myocardial infarction and other thromboembolic phenomenon.

Option 'd'

There are three types of pyrogenic exotoxin. Exotoxin A & C are encoded by bacteriophage while type B is coded by chromosome.

15. **Ans. (a), (b) Clostridium perfringenes toxin ; Tetasolysin** *Ref. Textbook of Microbiology by DR Arora, 1/e p 228*

    Already explained

16. **Ans. (a) Catalase positivity** *Ref. Harrison 20/e, p 1084*

    Pyoderma (Impetigo) (see image palette)
    - Superficial infection of the skin, caused primarily by Group A Streptococci and Staphylococci
    - Usual site of infection are face (particularly around nose and mouth) and the legs
    - Diagnosis is based on the culture and staining of indeginous lesion.
    - Gram positive cocci if catalase positive, than it is most likely to be Staphylococci and if catalase negative than it is Streptococci.

17. **Ans. (b) Bacitracin sensitivity** *Ref. Greenwood 18/e, p 195*

    "Species identification of Pyogenic streptococci is based largely on serological detection of group antigen by immune precipitation or co-agglutination techniques".
    An additional test that is useful in the presumptive identification of Str. pyogenes **(Group A Streptococci) is bactracin sensitivity test.** In contrast to most of other streptococci, Str. pyogenes is uniformly sensitive and large inhibition zones are formed around bacitracin discs on blood agar.
    - Str. agulactiae, the other pyogenic streptococci is identified presumptively by the CAMP reaction.

18. **Ans. (c) It is universally susceptible to penicillins** *Ref. Harrison 20/e, p 1091*

    Enterococci are resistant to penicillin

Disease caused by Enterococci
- UTI (particularly who are on antibiotic treatment)
- Bacterial endocarditis
- Liver abscess, intra-abdominal abscess
- Surgical wound infection.

For more details, refer Ans. 1

19. **Ans. (c) Enterococcus** *Ref. Ananthanarayan 10/e, p 219; Jawetz 24/e, p 243-244*

Group D enterococci	
Enterococci (E. faecalis, E. faecium)	**Non enterococci (Strep. bovis)**
• Able to grow in 6.5% NaCl	• Can't grow
• PYR positive	• PYR negative
• May shows α hemolysis	• Non hemolytic
• Penicillin resistant	• Penicillin susceptible
• Causes UTI and other nosocomial infection	• Causes UTI, endocarditis in patients with GI neoplasm

- Both enterococci and non enterococci group D stereptococci can grow in presence of bile and hydrolyze esculin (bile esculin positive). ... *Jawetz 25/e, p 202, 207, 27/e 226*

20. **Ans. (c) *Enterococcus faecalis*** *Ref. Harrison 20/e, p 1091*
    - Enterococci are catalase negative and grow in chains and above all resistant to cephalosporins.
    - Enterococci is a frequent cause of nosocomial bacteremias and many of these enterococci are resistant to vancomycin.
    - Enterococcal bacteremias is characteristically seen in ICU in patient taking cephalosporin as antibiotic.
    - Enterococci are resistant to all cephalosporins, aminoglycosides and resistant to vancomycin is also becoming common.

Treatment of antibiotic resistant enterococcal infection	
Resistance pattern	**Recommended therapy**
β-lactamase production	Gentamicin plus ampicillin/sulbactam, amoxicillin/clavulanate, imipenem, or vancomycin
β-lactam resistance, but no β-lactamase production	Gentamicin plus vancomycin
High-level gentamicin resistance	***Streptomycin-sensitive isolate:*** Streptomycin plus ampicillin, or vancomycin
	Streptomycin-resistant isolate: Continuous-infusion ampicillin
Vancomycin resistance	Ampicillin plus gentamicin
Vancomycin and β-lactam resistance	No uniformly bactericidal drugs; linezolid (all enterococci) or quinupristin/dalfopristin (*E. faecium* only)

Note: Linezolid is the antibiotic approved by USFDA for treatment of vancomycin resistant enterococci.

- Three phenotypes of vancomycin resistant enterococci have been identified viz. Van A; Van B; Van C. Van A is associated with high grade resistance to vancomycin and teicoplanin. Van B and Van C are susceptible to teicoplanin.

Other options:
- *Staph. aureus* and coagulase negative staph. are catalase positive.
- *Streptococci viridans* are sensitive to vancomycin.

Remember: Whole streptococci group forms chains while staphylococci group forms bunch similar to grapes.

21. **Ans. (a) *Enterococcus faecalis*** *Ref. Harrison 19/e, p 1093*
    See the following line.
    "Unlike streptococci, enterococci are not reliably killed by penicillin or ampicillin alone. Because in vitro testing has shown evidence of synergistic killing by combination of penicillin or ampicillin with an aminoglycoside, combined therapy is recommended for enterococcal endocarditis and meningitis."
    - Enterococci are resistant to all cephalosporins

22. **Ans. (c) Optochin** *Ref. Ananthanarayan 10/e, p223*
    Infant is suffering from pneumococcal pneumonia (*Gram-positive α-hemolytic cocci*).

Pneumococci is differentiated from other α hemolytic Gram-positive cocci by its susceptibility to optochin and bile solubiliy.

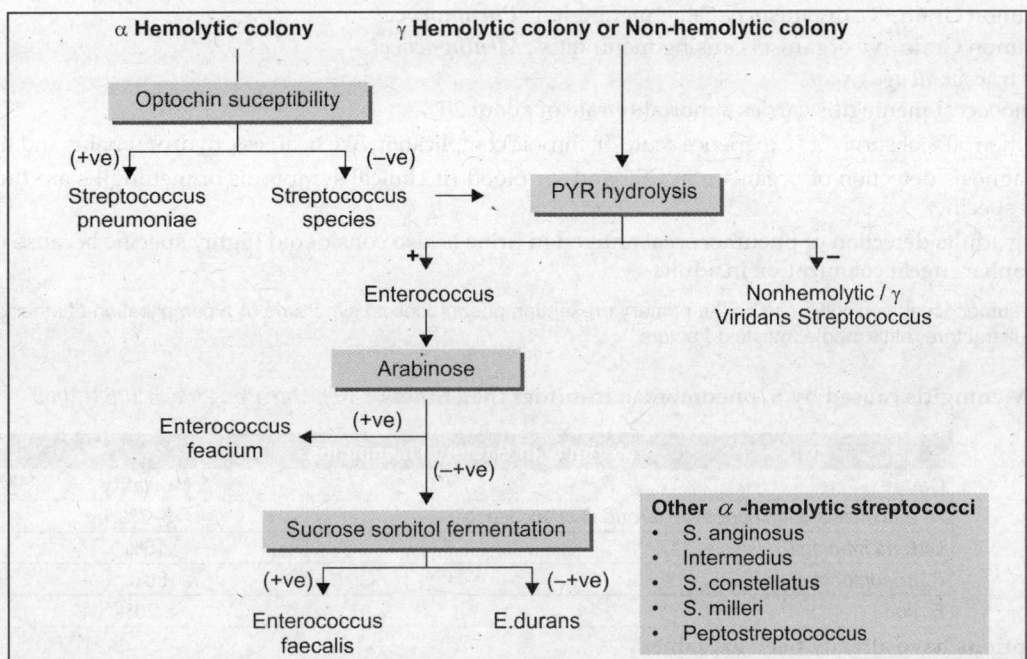

23. **Ans. (b) Gram-positive cocci in pairs, catalase negative and bile soluble** *Ref. Ananthanarayan 10/e, p 223*

    Bacteria which shows α or partial hemolysis includes:

Species	Common disease caused
a. *Strep. viridans*	
S. sanguis,	SABE
S. mutans	Dental caries
b. Pneumococci	Lobar pneumonia, otitis media
c. *S. anginosus*	Pyogenic infections
d. Enterococcus including *S.faecalis*	UTI, endocarditis
e. Peptostreptococus	Abscesses

    - As in question, sputum specimen is taken which is required in the diagnosis of respiratory tract infection (e.g. pneumonia).
    - *So, it is clear that most probable* answer is Pneumococci which is: diplococci; bile soluble; catalase negative.
    - *Choice 'a'* points towards *S. viridans* but it rarely cause pneumonia.
    - *Choice 'c'* points towards *S. aureus* which shows β hemolysis not α hemolysis.
    - *Choice 'd'* points towards *Legionella*. Though it cause pneumonia but it does not shows hemolysis.

    Note: All streptococci is catalase negative while staphylococci is catalase positive:

24. **Ans. (c) Bile solubility** *Ref. Harrison 20/e, p 1063*

    This is a classic presentation of pneumococcal pneumonia *(The most common community acquired pneumonia)*
    - *There is confusion between optochin sensitivity and bile solubility as both are unique features of pneumococci.*
      - Bile solubility has got more diagnostic importance as suggested by following lines of *Harrison:*
      - "More than 98% of pneumococcal isolates are susceptible to ethyl hydrocupreine (optochin) and virtualy all pneumococcal colonies are dissolved by bile salts". *...Harrison 17/e 865*
      - Bile solubility of pneumococci is due to the presence of autolytic amidase which are activated by surface active agents (bile salts).
      - *Inulin fermentation is the other test used to differentiate pneumococci and streptococci.*
      - Pneumococci can ferment inulin, while streptococci don't. This is tested in Hiss's serum water or serum agar slopes

    Note: Pneumococci are catalase and oxidase negative gram-positive cocci showing α hemolysis

25. **Ans. (c) Pneumococcus** *Ref. Harrison 20/e, p 1066; Nelson 18/e, p 2632-2633*

Most common Gram +ve organism causing meningitis : ***Pneumococci***
Most common Gram –ve organism causing meningitis : ***Meningococci***
This holds true for all age group
- Pneumococcal meningitis carries a mortality rate of about 20%.
- In addition 50% of survivors experience acute or chronic complication like deafness, hydrocephalus and mental retardation.
- For diagnosis detection of organism in CSF and/or blood (if clinical symptoms of meningitis are there) is considered highly specific.
- Among adults detection of pneumococcal antigen in urine is also considered highly specific because of low prevalence of nasopharyngeal colonization in adults.

> **Note:** Pneumococcal meningitis can be the primary presenting pneumococcal syndrome or a complication of other conditions such as skull fracture, otitis media, mastoid fracture.

26. **Ans. (d) Meningitis caused by S. pneumoniae is milder than others** *Ref. Harrison 20/e, p 1068, 1069*

Mortality in Bacterial Meningitis	
Cause	Mortality
H. Influenzae, Meningococci, Group B streptococci	3–7%
Listeria meningitis	15%
S. pneumococci	20%
E. coli	> 20%

Others options have already been explained.

> **Note:**
> - Pneumococci is the most common cause of pneumonia, meningitis, otitis media.
> - Otitis media is the most common infection of Pneumococci.

27. **Ans. (b) Optochin** *Ref. Greenwood 18/e, p 195*

Pneumococci are distinguished from other a hemolytic stroptococci by their characteristic senstivity to optochin.

28. **Ans. (a) *Streptococcus pneumoniae*** *Ref. Harrison 20/e, p 1068, 1001*
- Meningitis with Gram (+)ve cocci can be none other than Pneumococci.
- Pneumococci and Meningococci are most common cause of bacterial meningitis, pneumococci being Gram (+)ve (violet) where as meningococci being Gram (–)ve (pink).
- Definitive diagnosis of meningitis relies on CSF examination. Gram staining PCR or antigen testing aids in identification of organism.
- A positive blood culture for S. pneumonia in conjunction with clinical manifestation of meningitis is also confirmatory.

29. **Ans. (b) Intrapartum antimicrobial prophylaxis is given to positive cases** *Ref. Harrison 20/e, p 1088*
- Chemoprophylaxis (5 million units of penicillin followed by 2.5 million units every 4 hours) is indicated antenatally in patients-
    - Who screen positive (screening is done at 35–37 weeks)
    - Who preterm labour (< 37 weeks)
    - Prolong rupture of membrane
    - Intrapartum fever.
- Chemoprophylaxis should be given 24 hours prior to delivery and atleast 4 hours prior to delivery.

30. **Ans. (b) *Streptococcus pyogenes*** *Ref. Ananthanarayan 8/e, p 207, 9/e, p 210*

"Sensitivity to bacitracin is employed as a convenient method for differentiating Str. pyogenes from other hemolytic streptococci."

For details see answer no 20 of chapter 8.

NEET Pattern Questions

1. **Necrotizing fasciitis is caused by, all except:**
   a. Staphylococcus aureus
   b. Beta haemolytic streptococci
   c. Clostridium perfringens
   d. Pneumococcus [Ref. Harrison, 20/e, p 1086]

   > Necrotizing fascitis may be caused by Group A streptococcus or mixed aerobic anaerobic bacteria or may occur as part of gas gangrene caused by Cl. perferingens. Strains of MRSA that produce panton valentine leukociclin (PVL) toxin have also been reported to cause necrotizing fascitis.

2. **Virulence factor of group. A beta haemolytic streptococci:** [Ref. Ananthanarayan, 10/e, p 213]
   a. Protein M
   b. Protein T
   c. Protein R
   d. Lipotechoic acid

3. **Which group of streptococcus grow at > 60°C:**
   a. A
   b. B
   c. C
   d. D [Ref. Ananthanarayan, 10/e, p 219]

   > Enterococcus species are relatively heat resistant can tolerate 60°C for 30 minutes.

4. **False regaruing streptococcurs pyogenes:**
   a. Causes necrotizing fascitis
   b. Beta hemolytic [Ref. Ananthanarayan, 10/e, p 211]
   c. M. protein is virulence factor
   d. Resistant to bacitracin

5. **Post-splenectomy patient is in need of — vaccination:**
   a. Pneumococcal
   b. Rota virus
   c. BCG
   d. MMR [Ref. Harrison, 20/e, p 1070]

   > Pneumoccocal vaccine should be administered to all patients two weeks before electrive splenectomy. Repeat vaccination should be performed five years post splenectomy.

6. **Most common post splenectomy infection is:**
   a. Pneumococcus
   b. Meningococcus
   c. Staphy lococcus
   d. Corynebacterium [Ref. Harrison, 20/e, p 416]

Splenectomy increase risk of following infections	
Bacterial	• Pneumococcal • H. influenzae • Some Gram –ve enteric organism
Parasitic	• Babesia
Viral	• Risk of viral infection is not increased

   > **Remember:** MC cause of septicemia in asplenic patient - Pneumococci.

7. **Streptococcal cell wall polysacharide cross reacts:**
   a. Myocardial muscle
   b. Cardiac valve
   c. Ednocardium
   d. Synovial fluid [Ref. Ananthanarayan, 10/e, p 213]

   > Cell wall protein mimics myocardium where as C-carbohydrate (present in middle layer of cell wall) mimics cardiac valves.

8. **Not true regarding the mimcry of Str. pyogenes:**
   a. Peptidoglycan and skin antigen
   b. Cell wall protein and myocardium
   c. Hyaluronic acid and synovial fluid
   d. Group A carbohydrate and vascular intima [Ref. Ananthanarayan, 10/e, p 213]

9. **Most common infection caused by streptococcus pneumonia:**
   a. Otitis media
   b. Sore throat
   c. Meningitis
   d. Pneumonia [Ref. Harrison, 20/e, p 1069]

   > **Remember:**
   > • MC - infection of pneumococci: Otitis media
   > • Pneumococci is MC cause of lobar pneumonia, acute sinusitis, adult meningitis
   > • MC cause of bronchopneumonia: Staphylococci
   > • MC cause of atypical pneumonia: Mycoplasma pneumoniae.

10. **Streptococcus pyogenes shows pathogenicity by all except:**
    a. M protein
    b. Pyrotoxin
    c. Pili
    d. Streptolysin O [Ref. Ananthanarayan, 10/e, p 212]

11. **Bile esculin agar is used for:**
    a. Group A streptococcus
    b. Group B streptococcus
    c. Group C streptococcus
    d. Enterococcus [Ref. Jawety, 27/e, p 226]

    > Enterococcus grows well in presence of bile and hydrolyze esculin (bile esculin positive).

12. **Dental carries is caused by:**
    a. Streptococcus salivarius
    b. Streptococcus mutans
    c. Streptococcus pyogenes
    d. Streptococcus equisimulus [Ref. AA, 10/e, p 271]

    > **S. mutans:**
    > • It is member of viridans streptococci (α-hemolytic) which is part of the normal flora of the oral cavity.
    > • It assumes bacillary form in acid environment.
    > • Can synthesize acid and large polysaccharide (adhesive dextran or levan) from sucrose.

Ans.
1. d. Pneumococcus 2. a. Protein M 3. d. D 4. d. Resistant to bacitracin
5. a. Pneumococcal 6. a. Pneumococcus 7. b. Cardiac valve 8. d. Group A carbohydrate and vascular intima
9. b. Sore throat 10. b. Pyrotoxin 11. d. Enterococcus 12. b. Streptococcus mutans

13. Infective endocarditis after tooth extraction is probably due to:
    a. Streptococcus viridans
    b. Streptococcus pneumoniae
    c. Streptococcus pyogenes
    d. Streptococcus aureus
    [Ref. Ananthanarayan, 20/e, p 220]

> Following tooth extraction or other dental procedures, S.sangius produce transient bacteremia and get implanted on damaged or prosthehtic value or in a congenitally diseased heart and grow to form vegitation. Thus, under such conditions prophylactic antibiotic cover is advisable before tooth extraction.

14. Bullous impetigo is caused by:
    a. Streptococcus   b. Staphylococcus
    c. Pseudomonas   d. Clostridium
    [Ref. Harrison, 20/e, p 1085]

> For impetigo also, S.aureus is a prominant cause.

15. Most common cause of cellulitis:
    a. Streptococcus
    b. Staphylococcus
    c. Pseudomonas
    d. E. coli
    [Ref. Harrison, 20/e, p 1085]

> Staphylococcal cellulitis usually occur around wound or ulcer.

16. Most common organism implicated in causation of necrotizing fascitis: (2016)
    a. Staphylococcus aureus
    b. Streptococcus pyogenes
    c. Clostridium perfringens
    d. Pneumococcus
    [Ref. Harrison, 20/e, p 1086]

> Necrotizing fascitis caused by S. pyogenes has increased in frequency and severity since 1985.

17. Crystal violet blood agar is used for which bacteria?
    a. Corynebacterium diphtheriae   (2016)
    b. Staph aureus
    c. β-hemolytic streptococcus
    d. Meningococcus   [Ref. Ananthanarayan, 10/e, p 214]

> S. pyogenes is resistant to crystal violet than any other bacteria. Thus addition of crystal violet to blood agar makes a good selective medium.

18. Which streptodornase is most antigenic in human beings: (2016)
    a. A   b. B
    c. C   d. D
    [Ref. Ananthanarayan, 10/e, p 214]

> Type B streptodornase is most antigenic and demonstration of anti DNA as B antibody is useful in retrospective diagnosis

19. Antibiotic used to for sensitivity in identification of streptococcus pyogenes: (2016)
    a. Bacitracin
    b. Novobiocin
    c. Penicillin
    d. Optochin   [Ref.Ananthanarayan, 9/e, p 211]

> Streptococcus pyogenes is bacitracin sensitive.

20. Streptococcal toxic shock syndrome is due to liberation of:
    a. TSST-1
    b. Enterotoxin   (2016)
    c. Pyrogenic exotoxin
    d. Endotoxin
    [Ref. Ananthanarayan 10/e, p 214]

21. True statements about pneumococcus are all except: (2016)
    a. Pneumolysin a thiolactivated toxin, exerts a variety of effects on ciliary and PMN's action
    b. Autolysin may contribute to the pathogenesis of pneumococcal disease by lysing bacteria
    c. Anticapsular 'antibodies are serotype specific
    d. The virulence of pneumococci is dependent only on the production of the capsular polysaccharide
    [Ref. Ananthanarayan, 10/e, p 224]

> Virulence of pneumococci depends on its capsule, toxin called pneumolysin and autolysin.

Virulence factors of Pneumococci	
Capsule:	• Polysaccharide in nature • Protects against phagocytosis • Type 3 pneumococci has abundant capsular material and is more virulent • Antibody against capsule are type specific and protective.
Pneumolysin:	• Cytotoxin, exerts variety of effects on ciliary cells and PMN. .... *Harrison 18/e, p 1151* • Complement activating and cytotoxic properties • Immunogenic
Autolysin:	• By lysing the bacteria and releasing bacterial components contributes to virulence
IgA1 protease	• Cleaves IgA1 and hence decreases the function of this immunoglobulin.
C-substance and peptidoglycans.	

Ans.
13. a. Streptococcus ...   14. b. Staphylococcus   15. a. Streptococcus   16. b. Streptococcus pyogenes
17. c. β-hemolytic ...   18. b. B   19. a. Bacitracin   20. c. Pyrogenic ...   21. d. The virulence...

Streptococci

22. True about Streptococcus pyogenes are all except:
   a. Causes only localized infection (2016)
   b. Rheumatic fever is non-supporative complications
   c. Erythrogenic toxin causes scarlet fever
   d. Glomerulonephritis is due to antigenic cross-reactivity

   [Ref. Jawetz, 27/e, p 217]

> Nonsuppurative complications of streptococci:
> - Acute rheumatic fever.
> - Acute glomerulonephritis.

23. Causative agent of acute rheumatic fever: (2016)
   a. Group 'A' β-hemolytic streptococcus
   b. Group -B β-hemolytic streptococcus
   c. Group -C β-hemolytic streptococcus
   d. Group -D β-hemolytic streptococcus

   [Ref. Ananthanarayan, 10/e, p 211]

24. Lancefield classification of beta hemolytic streptococci is based on: (2016)
   a. Protein percent
   b. Cell wall carbohydrate antigen
   c. Cell membrane M protein
   d. Hemolytic properties

   [Ref. Ananthanarayan, 10/e, p 211]

25. Griffith classification is based on: (2016)
   a. Cell wall carbohydrate
   b. M protein
   c. Hemolytic R properties
   d. None of the above

   [Ref. Ananthanarayan, 10/e, p 211]

26. Capsule of pneumococcus is: (2018)
   a. Polypeptide
   b. Polysaccharide
   c. Lipopolysaccharide
   d. Not a Virulence factor

   [Ref. Ananthanarayan, 9/e, p 220]

27. Culture medium used for Streptococcus pneumoniae:
   a. Human blood agar (2016)
   b. Sheep blood agar
   c. MacConkey's agar
   d. Deoxycholate agar

   [Ref. AA, 10/e, p 224]

28. A chronic alcoholic is presenting with clinical features of meningitis. Most likely organism which will grow on CSF culture: (2016)
   a. Streptococcus pneumoniae
   b. N. meningitidis
   c. Listeria monocytogenes
   d. E. coli

   [Ref. Harrison, 20/e, p 1068]

> **Risk factors for pneumococcal meningitis:** sinusitis, otitis media, alcoholism, diabetes, splenectomy, hypogamma globulinemia, CSF rhinorrhea, complement deficiency and head trauma.

29. Heating at 60°C for 30 minute would isolate: (2018)
   a. Staphylococci
   b. Enterococci
   c. Micrococci
   d. Streptococci

   [Ref. Ananthanarayan, 10/e, p 220]

Ans.
- 22. **a.** Causes only localized infection
- 23. **a.** Group 'A' β-hemolytic streptococcus
- 24. **b.** Cell wall carbohydrate antigen
- 25. **b.** M protein
- 26. **b.** Polysaccharide
- 27. **b.** Sheep blood agar
- 28. **a.** Streptococcus pneumoniae
- 29. **b.** Enterococci

Neisseria

CHAPTER 9

- Genus consist of *Gram-negative, aerobic, nonmotile, oxidase +ve diplococci* [i.e. grow in pairs].
- Oxidase test is the key test for identifying *Neisseria*.
- Can grow both intracellularly and extracellularly.
- It includes:
  a. *N. meningitidis*: Causative agent of:
     1. Meningococcal meningitis
     2. Purpura fulminans (Fulminant meningococcemia)
  b. *N. gonorrhoeae*: Causative agent of gonorrhoea
- Nonpathogenic neisseriae grow on ordinary nutrient media, but pathogenic ones require the addition of heated blood (or ascitic fluid) and incubation at 35-37°C in moist atmosphere containing 5-10% CO_2

> **Meningococci:**
> - Lives commensally in the nasopharynx and is transmitted via close kissing contact.

N. meningitidis [meningococci]	N. gonorrhoeae [gonococci]
Lens shaped	Kidney shaped
Capsulated	Noncapsulated
Ferment both glucose and maltose	Ferment glucose only
Rarely have plasmid	Plasmid usually present
Possess polysaccharide capsule	Do not possess

N. MENINGITIDIS [MENINGOCOCCI] (See color plate, pg xxii for related image)

- Categorize as β proteobacterium on basis of genome sequencing.
- Natural habitat is human nasopharynx.
- Colonizes human only.
- Catalase and oxidase positive organism that utilizes glucose and maltose to produce acid.

> In India Group A is the most common strain.

Classification

- On *basis* of *capsular polysaccharide* classified into 13 serogroups.
- 5 serogroups A, B, C, W, Y are responsible for most meningococcal disease.

Group A	Epidemic (MC strain in India)
Group B	Both epidemic and outbreak, most prevalent in developed world
Group C	Localized outbreaks
Group Y	Sporadic
Group W	Sporadic, Epidemic in subsaharan Africa

Beneath the capsule meningococci are surrounded by an outer phospholipid membrane containing Lipopolysaccharide (LPS, endotoxin) and multiple outer membrane protein.

... Harrison 20/e, p 1114

> **Meningococci:**
> - Nonpathogenic neisseria can grow on ordinary media, whereas pathogenic one require addition of heated blood and incubation at 35-37°C.

Virulence Factors

Important virulence factors are:
- *Capsular polysaccharide*: Major virulence factor that imparts antiphagocytic and antibacteriocidal properties. Acapsular strains very rarely cause invasive disease.
- *Outer membrane proteins*: Pilli are complex OMP based organelles that facilitates adhesion.
- *Lipoligosaccharide LOS (endotoxin)*: Morbidity and mortality of meningococcal bacteremia and meningitis is directly proportional to amount of circulating meningococcal endotoxin.

Pathogenesis

- Meningococci causes invasive disease in susceptible individuals only. Principal determinant of disease susceptibility is age (peak incidence is in first year).
- Deficiency of terminal or alternate complement pathway C_5-C_9 increase risk of meningococcal infection.
- Other factors increasing the risk are cigarette smoking, recent viral respiratory tract infection, overcrowding, infection with mycoplasma species.
- Infants are particularly susceptible to serogroup B. ... *Harrison 20/e, p 1116*
- Humans are the only natural hosts for whom meningococci are pathogenic.

- Lipid A moiety of lipo-oligosaccharide is the main factor responsible for septic shock syndrome.
- A Gr(–)ve diplococci with positive urease test suggest diagnosis of meningococci.

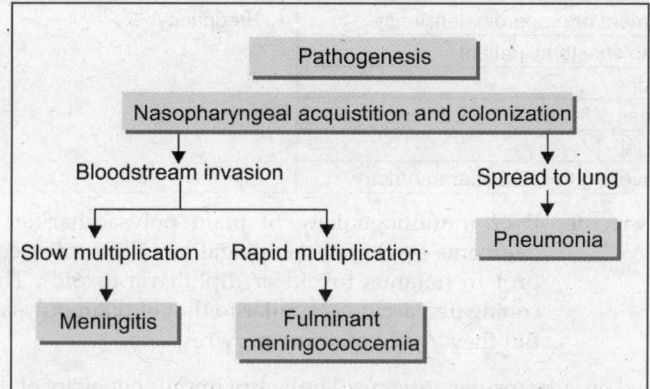

Thus, *meningitis* is result of blood borne dissemination and not direct invasion.
... *Harrison 20/e, p 1116*

- Meningitis and for bacteremia are the most common presentation.
- Meningococcal meningitis usually left permanent sequelae like intellectual impairment, cranial nerve deficit.

Clinical Features

a. *Fulminant meningococcemia [Purpura fulminans]*
   - Most rapid lethal form of septic shock.
   - Differs from other septic shock by *prominence of hemorrhagic skin lesions* (petechiae, purpura) and development of DIC. *Rash* is most distinctive feature.
   - Lab findings include hypoglycemia, acidosis, hypomagnesemia, hypophosphatemia, anemia and coagulopathy.
   - LOS (endotoxin) is responsible for most cases.
   - CSF may be normal and CSF culture may be –ve which is poor prognostic sign.
   - Due to its rapidity acute phase reactant, may remain normal.
   - May progress to **Waterhouse-Friderichsen syndrome**–DIC induced microthrombi, *hemorrhage, tissue injury and circulatory collapse.*
   - Endotoxin of meningococci are capable of producing both generalized and localized Schwartzman reactions. These reactions are involved in the pathogenesis of petechial hemorrhage and Waterhouse-Friderichsen syndrome
b. *Meningitis* - Common in age between 3 months and 5 years.
c. *Other manifestation* - Arthritis, conjuctivitis, urethritis, rarely endocarditis.

Lab Diagnosis

- Diagnosis is established by recovering meningococci from sterile body fluids (such as blood, CSF, etc.) or from Petechial aspirate.
- PCR amplification of DNA in buffy coat or CSF samples is the most sensitive method.
- They grow best on *Muller-Hinton* or chocolate agar at 35^0 C in 5 to 10% CO_2.
- **Thayer Martin media** is selective media used for culturing throat or nasopharyngeal specimen, as it suppress the competing oral flora.
- Culture media containing sodium polyethanol sulfonate, which may inhibit meningococcal growth, should be avoided.
... *Harrison 20/e, p 1118*

> - Gonococci is the MC cause of PID globally.

Treatment
- 3rd generation cephalosporin such as cefotaxime or ceftriaxone is *DOC* for initial therapy.
- Prophylaxis—Rifampin is *DOC* for meningococcal prophylaxis.

Prevention
- *Vaccine* - Quadrivalent meningococcal polysaccharide vaccine [serogroup *A, C, W, Y*].
- *There is no vaccine against serogroup B* as its capsule is nonimmunogenic.
- Vaccine is ineffective in age < 2 years so, given after 2 years.

Indication	Contraindication
Late complement or properdin deficiency	Pregnancy
Asplenia or splenectomy patient	
Military persons	
Epidemic areas	
Pilgrims on Haj	
Individual travelling to sub-Saharan Africa	

- **Conjugate vaccine:** Poor immunogenicity of plain polysaccharide vaccine has been overcome by chemical conjugation of the polysaccharide to a carrier protein (tetanus toxoid or diphtheria toxoid). The rectogenicity of conjugate vaccine is similar to that of plain polysaccharides vaccine. But they yeild better memory response.
- Vaccine based on subcapsular antigens: The lack of immunogenicity of the group B capsule has led to the development of vaccines based on subcapsular antigen. Outer membrane vesicles have been used for this purpose.

N. GONORRHOEAE [GONOCOCCI] (See color plate, pg xxii for related image)

- *MC* cause of PID worldwide [*MC* cause of PID in India is TB].
- *MC* cause of septic arthritis in adult [*MC* joint knee].
- Cause *most severe* type of ophthalmia neonatorum.
- Strains are characterized by auxotyping which recognizes requirement of nutrients
- Exclusively a human pathogen.

> - Both gonococci and meningococci produce IgA$_1$ protease that inactivates IgA

Culture

– More difficult to grow than meningococci	– Essential to provide 5-10% CO_2
– Four types of colonies recognised - T_1 to T_4	– Type 1 and 2 = P$^+$ and P^{++} respectively.
– Type 3 and 4 = P$^-$ and are avirulent	– They are piliated and virulent.

Biochemical Reactions
- Gonococci ferment only glucose (not maltose)
- Rapid carbohydrate utilisation test (RCUT): This is a rapid, sensitive and specific test for detection of gonococci.

Pathogenic Factors

> - Gonococcal infection is usually limited to superficial mucosal surfaces lined with columnar epithelium.

- **Outer-membrane protein:**
  - Pilli – Piliated strains adhere better to cells and are more virulent.
- Opacity associated protein (Protein II) – Important for adhesion.
- Porin (Protein I, III) – *Most abundant* gonococcal surface protein ... *Harrison 20/e, p 1123*
- H.8 Lipoprotein – Excellent target for antibody based diagnostic testing.
- Transferrin and lactoferrin binding protein.
- IgA1 protease (also produced by meningococci).

> **Remember:** IgA-1 protease is also produced by S. pneumoniae, H. influenza; some streptococci.
> ...*Jawetz 27/e, p 283*

- **Lipooligosaccharide = Endotoxin**
  - Resemble human glycosphingolipid, contributes to the local cytotoxic effects.
- **Host factors**
  - Deficiency of terminal complement components.

Clinical Features

- Mode of infection is almost exclusively veneral except ophthalmia neonatorum.
- *Incubation period:* 2-8 days
- Terminal complement component [C_5-C_9] deficiency predispose to gonococcal infection.
- Higher incidence of gonorrhea occur in blood group B.
- Gonococcal infection in *males*: **Acute urethritis** is *MC* clinical manifestation of gonorrhea *in males.*
- Gonococcal infection in *females*: Cervicitis is *MC* manifestation. Adult vagina is resistant to gonococcal infection.
- Gonorrhea in *pregnant woman*: Salpingitis and PID can occur during 1st trim and can cause abortion. In 2nd and 3rd trim, relative impermeability of cervical mucous prevent ascending infection.
- Gonococcal infection in *neonates*: MC is ophthalmia-neonatorum while *septic arthritis* is MC manifestation of systemic infection.
- In *children vulvovaginitis* is *MC* gonococcal infection.

- MC gonococcal manifestation:
  Males: Acute urethritis
  Females: Cervicitis

Diagnosis

- Rapid diagnosis by gram's staining of urethral exudates, organism appear as diplpcocci predominantly with in the polymorphs
- Part of sample should be inoculated on ***Thayer Martin*** Media. Detection of gram-negative diplococci or monococci is usually specific.
- It is important to process all samples immediately because gonococci do not tolerate drying.
- If processing is to occur within 6h, transport of specimens may be facilitated by the use of non-nutritive swab transport systems such as *Stuart* or *Amies medium.*
- For longer holding periods culture media with self-contained CO_2 generating systems (such as the JEM BEC or Gono-Pak system may be used).

Treatment

- 3rd generation cephalosporins cefixime and ceftriaxone are *DOC*.
- Penicillin is *DOC when sensitive (But most isolates are resistant to penicillin)*

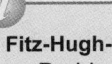

Fitz-Hugh-Curtis Syndrome:
- Peri-hepatic inflammation secondary to transperitoneal spread of gonococci

Prevention and Control

- Gonorrhea is transmitted from males to females more frequently than in opposite direction.
- Condoms provide effective protection against transmission.

Multiple Choice Questions

Meningococci

1. The following bacteria are most often associated with acute neonatal meningitis *except*: [AI 05]
   a. Escherichia coli
   b. Streptococcus agalactiae
   c. Neisseria meningitidis
   d. Listeria monocytogenes

2. The following statements about meningococcal meningitis are true *except*: [AI 03]
   a. The source of infection is mainly clinical cases
   b. The disease is more common in dry and cold months of the year
   c. Chemoprophylaxis of close contacts of cases is recommended
   d. The vaccines is not affective in children below 2 years of age

3. Xavier and Yogender stay in the same hostel of same university, Xavier develops infection due to group B meningococcus. After few days Yogender develops infection due to Group - C meningococcus. All the following are true statement *except*: [AI 02]
   a. Educate students about meningococcal transmission and take preventive measures
   b. Chemoprophylaxis to all against both group B and group C
   c. Vaccine prophylaxis of contacts of Xavier
   d. Vaccine prophylaxis of contacts of Yogender

4. Conjugate vaccine are available for the prevention of invasive disease caused by all of the following bacteria *except*: [AIIMS 04]
   a. H. influenzae
   b. Strep pneumoniae
   c. Neisseria meningitidis (Group-C)
   d. Neisseria meningitidis (Group-B)

5. Young female with 3 day fever presents with headache, BP 90/60 mmHg, Heart rate of 114/min, and pin point spots developed distal to BP cuff. Most likely organism is:
   a. Brucella abortus
   b. Brucella suis
   c. N. meningitidis
   d. Staphylococcus aureus

6. A man presented with a 3 day H/o lacrimation redness and discharge from left eye. Later on he developed perforation. Discharge from his eye demonstrated gram negative cocci which were oxidase positive. Which of the following can be the probable organism?
   a. Pseudomonas
   b. Acinetobacter
   c. Neisseria gonorrhoea
   d. Moraxella catarrhalis

7. The best site to obtain a swab in asymptomatic gonorrhea is: [AI 95, 02]
   a. Endocervix
   b. Urethra
   c. Lateral vaginal wall
   d. Posterior fornix

8. The virulence factor of Neisseria gonorrhoeae includes all of the following *except*: [AIIMS 03]
   a. Outer membrane proteins
   b. IgA protease
   c. M protein
   d. Pilli

9. All are true about Neisseria gonorrhoea *except*: [AIIMS 01]
   a. Gram-positive cocci
   b. Causes stricture urethra
   c. Involves seminal vesicles and spreads to epididymis
   d. Drug of choice is ceftriaxone

10. Which of the following is not true about Neisseria gonorrhoeae? [AIIMS Nov 09]
    a. It is an exclusive human pathogen
    b. Some strains may cause disseminated disease
    c. Acute urethritis is most common manifestation in males
    d. All strains are highly sensitive to penicillin

11. Which is the true statement regarding gonococcal urethritis? [PGI 06, 200]
    a. Symptoms are more severe in females than in males
    b. Rectum and prostate are resistant to gonococci
    c. Most patients present with symptoms of dysuria
    d. Single dose of ciprofloxacin is effective in treatment
    e. Commonly leads to arthritis

12. Which deficiency would cause neisseria infection? [PGI 09]
    a. C9
    b. C8
    c. C7
    d. C6
    e. C5

Explanations and References with Illustrative Answers

1. **Ans. (c) N. meningitidis** *Ref. Forfar and Arneils - Textbook of Paedia, p 319, 1338*
   Causes of Meningitis
   - Neonatal (< 1 month)
     1. **Bacterial causes:**

Organism	E. coli >	Gp B streptococci >	Other gram-negative bacilli >	L. monocytogenes
Frequency	34%	30%	8%	6%

   - *Other bacterias are:* Staph, other Streptococci, Pneumococcus, Pseudomonas, Haemophilus, Meningococcus.
     2. **Viral and protozoal infections:** TORCH, Varicella zoster and HIV.
     3. **Spirochetal and fungal infections**
   - **1-11 months:** *N. meningitidis > Strep pneumoniae > H. influenza*
   - **1-20 years:** *N. meningitidis > Strep pneumoniae > H. influenza*
   - **More than 20 years :** Strep pneumoniae (MC) ..... *Harrison 20/e, p 1001*

2. **Ans. (a) The source of infection is mainly clinical cases** *Ref. Harrison 20/e, p 1117*

   Source of infection are carriers not cases.
   Meningococcal meningitis or cerebrospinal fever.
   - It is caused by *N. meningitides*, a *gram-negative diplococci*.
   - Fatality of typical untreated cases is about 80%.
   - *Agent:* Group A and C and to lesser extent Group B cause major epidemics.
   - *Source:* Carriers are the most important source of infection. Clinical cases present only a negligible source of infection.
   - **Environmental Factors:** Seasonal variation is well established. Outbreaks occur more frequently in the dry and cold months.
   - *Mode of Transmission:* Mainly by droplet infection.
   - *Incubation Period:* Usually 3-4 days
   - *Diagnosis:* Recovering gram-negative diplococci (within pus cells) from sterile body fluids such as CSF, blood
   - *Treatment:*   – Antibiotics save the lives of 95% of patients provided that it is started during the first 2 days of illness.
     – *Cases:* [3rd generation cephalosporins are DOC].
     – *Carriers:* Rifampicin
   - *Chemoprophylaxis:*   – Rifampicin (the **DOC** unless the organism is known to be sensitive to sulfadiazine).
     – It is suggested for close contacts. Mass chemoprophylaxis is restricted to closed and medically supervised communities.
   - *Vaccinization:* Immunity last for 3 years

3. **Ans. (c) Vaccine prophylaxis of contacts of Xavier** *Ref. Park 22/e, p 157, Jawetz 27/e 288*

   For group B meningococcal infection no vaccine is available, as polysaccharide of Group B meningococci is *sialic acid homopolymer* that is poorly immunogenic in humans.

Meningococcal Vaccine	
Tetravalent polysaccharide vaccine	**Tetravalent conjugated vaccine**
• Contains purified polysaccharide capsule of A, C, W, Y	• Contains capsular polysaccharide of A, C, W, Y conjugated to diphtheria toxoid.
• Poorly immunogenic in children under 18 months	• Induce T-cell dependent response resulting in enhanced primary response among infants too.
• Doesn't confer long lasting immunity (< 3 years)	• Immunity is relatively long lasting
• Nasopharyngeal carriage is not affected	• Reduce carriage

   Contd...

Contd...

Tetravalent polysaccharide vaccine	Tetravalent conjugated vaccine
• Use is limited to control of epidemics and in individuals who are at high risk (asplenia, complement deficiencies, laboratory workers, travellers to highly endemic areas, military persons)	• Licensed for routine use in persons 11-55 years of age and for high risk individuals.

Note: Now subcapsular antigens of serotype B are being used as vaccine. Two such vaccine have been licensed in USA.

4. **Ans. (d)** *Neisseria meningitidis* (Group B) *Ref. Ghai 6/e, p 197 - 198; Harrison 19/e, p 1001*
   Already explained

   Note: Conjugate vaccines are available for:
   a. Hemophilus influenza B.
   b. meningococcal serotypes A, C, Y and W-135.
   c. Streptococcal pneumoniae (pneumococcus).

5. **Ans. (c).** *N. meningitidis* *Ref. Harrison 20/e, p 1118*
   - The patient here is under state of shock (hypotension, tachycardia) in conjunction with meningitis (headache fever) and rash.
   - Meningococcal meningitis is the most common meningitis complicated by shock.

Clinical Manifestation of Meningococcal Disease	
Rash	A nonblanching rash (petechial or purpuric) develops in >80% of cases of meningococcal disease. Rashes are initially blanching in nature but within hours become non-blanching. In severe cases large purpuric lesions (purpura fulminans) develops.
Meningitis	Commonly present as fever, vomiting, headache, irritability, petechial or purpuric rash occurs in 2/3 of cases. Headache is seen in adults usually. In upto 40% of cases there are some features of septicemia too.
Septicemia	Can be isolated or as a accomplication of meningitis. The condition may cause death within hours. Purpura fulminans is a specific feature.
Chronic meningococcemia	Present as repeated episodes of petechial rash associated with fever joint pain, arthritis and splenomegaly. The main differential diagnosis is acute rheumatic fever. This condition has been associated with complement deficiently and with inadequate sulfonamide therapy. If left untreated chances of progression to meningococcal septicemia are high.
Post-meningococcal reactive disease	In small proportion of patients, an immune complex disease develops 4-10 days after the onset of meningococcal disease with manifestations that include a maculopapular or vasculitic rash, arthritis, pericarditis and/or polyserositis associated with fever.

6. **Ans. (c)** *Neisseria gonorrhoea* *Ref. Harrison 19/e 1006; 20/e, p 1126,*
   Gram negative oxidase positive bacteria can be none other than neisseria, and here in this case it is N. gonococci.
   Occular gonorrhea in adults
   - Results from autoinoculation from an infected genital site
   - Manifestations range from mild to very severe
   - Severe signs include markedly swollen eyelid, chemosis, profuse purulent discharge. Occasionally there may be corneal ulceration and rarely perforation.
   - Diagnosis is confirmed by culture of purulent discharge.

7. **Ans. (a) Endocervix** *Ref. Harrison 20/e, p 1126; Ananthanarayan 8/e, p 229, 9/e, p 232*
   Diagnosis Of Gonococcal Infection

Specimen	
In acute gonorrhea	In chronic gonorrhea
Endocervical culture—80-90% sensitivity	• Morning drop secretion
Urethral discharge—50% sensitivity	• Exudate after prostatic massage
High vaginal swab are not satisfactory	• Centrifuged deposits of urine when no urethral discharge
Rectal wall swab—if there is history of rectal sex	

Contd...

Contd...

In acute gonorrhea	In chronic gonorrhea
Microscopy	Presence of gram-negative diplococci inside polymorphs is suggestive. Fluorescent antibody technique, increase the sensitivity of microscopy
Transport media	Stuart's or Amies media. For longer holding period culture media with self CO_2 generating system (such as JEMBEC or Gono-pak systems) may be used.
Culture media	Acute → Chocolate agar or Muller-Hinton agar.
	Chronic → Selective media like Thayer-Martin medium.
Serology	CFT: Done in chronic case or with metastatic lesion.
Chemiluminescent DNA Probe	In high-risk patient undergoing screening for STD's.
Blood Culture (e.g. of synovial fluid)	In suspected cases of disseminated infection.

- Preferred method for diagnosis of gonococcal infection in children is a standardized culture, from urethera and cervix. However, cervical specimen are not recommended in prepubertal girls unless necessary.
- Rapid diagnosis of gonococcal infection in men may be obtained by Gram staining of urethral exudates.

8. **Ans. (c) M protein** *Ref. Harrison 20/e, p 1123; Ananthanarayan 10/e, p 234*

   M protein is the virulence factor of *Strept. pyogenes* not of gonococci.

Virulence Factors of Neisseria Gonorrhea	
1. Capsular polysaccharide	
2. Outer Membrane Proteins	
• Pili • Porin (Protein I and III) • IgA1 protease	• Opacity associated protein (Protein II) • Lipoprotein H. 8 • Transferrin and lactoferrin binding protein
3. Lipooligosaccharide (endotoxin)	

9. **Ans. (a) Gram-positive cocci** *Ref. Harrison 20/e, p 1125*

Gonococcal Infection in Males	
MC Clinical manifestation	• Acute urethritis.
Major symptoms	• Urethral discharge and dysuria usually without urinary frequency or urgency.
Other features	• Epididymitis (uncommon)
	• Prostatitis (rare).
	• Edema of penis and balanitis.
	• Urethral stricture and Periurethral abscess or fistulae (= Watering-can perineum)
	• Inflammation or abscess of Cowper's gland.
	• Seminal vesiculitis
DOC	• 3rd generation cephalosporin—cefixime and ceftriaxone

Remember:	• All cocci are gram-positive except GMC, i.e N. gonorrhoeae, N. meningococci, N. catarrhalis. • All important bacilli are gram-negative except **ABC, CML**, i.e **A**ctinomycetes, **B**acillus, **C**lostridia, **C**orynebacteria, **M**ycobacteria, **L**isteria. • Testicular involvement is very rare.

10. **Ans. (d) All strains are highly sensitive to penicillin** *Ref. Harrison 20/e, p 1128*

    Let us consider each option

    Option 'a'
    - *N. gonorrhoeae* is an exclusive human pathogen. The bacteria contains three genome copies per coccal unit; this polyploidy permits a high level of antigenic variation and the survival of organism

    Option 'b' ...*Ananthanarayan 10/e p 235*
    - Few strains of *N. gonorrhoea* disseminate through blood stream causing arthritis, skin lesions, endocarditis, meningitis (rare)

    Option 'c'
    - **Commonest presentation of gonococcal infection**
        - **Males:** Acute urethritis
        - **Female:** Mucopurulent urinitis

    Option 'd'
    - **Gonococcal resistance to antimicrobial agents**
        - Gonococci has acquired resistance to sulfonamides, penicillin, fluoroquinolones
        - They acquire resistance either by chromosomal mutation or by acquisition of R factors (plasmid):
            (a) Chromosomal mutation: *Two types of chromosomal mutation have been described:*
                1. Single step drug specific mutation, leading to high level resistance
                2. Mutation involving several chromosomal loci that determine the level as well as pattern of resistance.
            (b) Plasmid borne resistance: Gonococci contains several plasmid. 95% gonococci have a small, cryptic plasmid of unknown function. Two other plasmids contain gene that codes for β lactamase, hence resistance to penicillin. *Tetracycline resistance is also acquired by plasmid.*
        - Alteration in DNA gyrase and topoisomerase IV have been implicated as mechanism of fluoroquinolone resistance.

11. **Ans. (c) and (d) Most patients present with symptoms of dysuria and Single dose of ciprofloxacin is effective in treatment**
    Ref. Harrison 20/e, p 1128; Ananthanarayan 10/e, p 235

    Gonococcal infection in Females:
    - Initial infection involves urethra and cervix uteri.
    - Cervicitis is *MC* manifestation.
    - Vaginal mucosa is resistant due to stratified squamous epithelium but can involve in an estrogenic women (prepubertal, postmenopausal).
    - Infection spreads to endometrium, fallopian tube, bartholin gland, peritoneum with perihepatic inflammation (Fitz-Hugh-Curtis syndrome).
    - Clinical disease (as a rule, is less severe in women).
    - Proctitis occur in both sexes.
    - **Disseminated gonococcal infection (DGI) or Arthritis,** occurs in very few patient.
    - DGI can cause skin lesion, meningitis, endocarditis, etc.

    Treatment: (For both males & females)
    - 3rd generation cephalosporin cefixime and ceftriaxone.
    - Single dose ciprofloxacin, ofloxacin, levofloxacin, etc. also affective.

    > **Remember:** Incubation period of gonococcal infection is 2-8 days.

12. **Ans. (a, b, c, d, e) All options are correct** *Ref. Harrison 20/e, p 1124*
    - Complement is required for bactericidal activity and for efficient opsonophagocytosis. Individuals deficient in any of the late complement components (C5-C9) can not assemble the membrane attack complex (MAC) which is required to kill Neisseria. Thus the incidence of meningococcal disease is higher among these patients.
    - Surprisingly these patients typically develop less severe disease than complement sufficient individuals; and tends to have disease due to uncommon sero-groups.

    > **Remember:** Properdin deficiency is another risk factor for Neisseria infection.

NEET Pattern Questions

1. **Virulence of gonococci is due to all *except*:**
   a. Pili
   b. Endotoxin
   c. Exotoxin
   d. Opacity associated protein
   [Ref. Harrison 20/e, p 1123]

2. **Where does gonococci initially infect:**
   a. Vagina
   b. Cervix
   c. Uterus
   d. Fallopian tubes
   [Ref. Ananthanarayan, 10/e, p 235]

   - In men gonococci initially infects urethra
   - In females urethra and cervix are first to get involved.

3. **Meningococci differ from gonococci in that they:**
   a. Are intra-cellular
   b. Possess a capsule
   c. Cause fermentation of glucose
   d. Are oxidase positive *[Ref. Ananthanarayan, 10/e, p 231]*

   Important difference between meningococci and gonococci is the presence of polysaccharide capsule in meningococci and of plasmids (see color plate pg xxii for related image).

4. **Waterhouse-Friderichsen syndrome is seen in:**
   a. Pneumococci
   b. N. meningitidis
   c. Pseudomonas
   d. Yersinia
   [Ref. Ananthanarayan, 10/e, p 232]

   Fulminant meningococcimea is called as Waterhouse-Friderichsen syndrome, which is characterized by shock, DIC and multisystem failure.

5. **Genus Neisseria is:**
   a. Gram positive diplococci
   b. Gram negative diplococci
   c. Gram negative coccobacilli
   d. Gram positive bacilli *[Ref. Ananthanarayan, 10/e, p 230]*

6. **Which of the following can be used for obtaining specimen for isolation of microorganism in laboratory diagnosis?**
   a. Meningococcal rash
   b. Blood in staphylococcal food poisoning
   c. Throat swab in Rheumatic fever
   d. Blood in post-streptococcal GN
   [Ref. Ananthanarayan, 10/e, p 232]

   Meningococci can be sometimes demonstrated in petechial lesions by microscopy and culture
   - Rheumatic fever and glomerulonephritis requires retrospective diagnosis.

7. **Differentiation of *Neisseria gonorrhoeae* and *Neisseria meningitidis* is by:** (2018)
   a. Glucose fermentation
   b. Maltose fermentation
   c. V. P. reaction
   d. Indol test
   [Ref. Ananthanarayan 10/e, p 231]

8. **The diagnosis of gonorrhea is established by:**
   a. Complement fixation tests (2016)
   b. Pili agglutination tests
   c. Hem agglutination tests
   d. All of the above tests
   [Ref. Ananthanarayan 10/e, p 236]

   CFT is useful in diagnosing chronic cases of gonorrhea and gonococcal arthritis. Many other serological tests have been attempted, but no test have been found useful for routine diagnosis.

9. **CSF in meningococcal meningitis shows:** (2018)
   a. Gram-positive Diplococci, in pus cells
   b. Gram-negative Diplococci in pus cells
   c. Gram-negative bacilli
   d. Gram-positive bacilli
   [Ref. Ananthanarayan 10/e, p 232]

   Gram-negative diplococci – *Neisseria*
   Gram-positive diplococci – *Pneumococcus*

Ans
1. c. Exotoxin
2. b. Cervix
3. b. Possess a capsule
4. b. N. meningitidis
5. b. Gram negative diplococci
6. a. Meningococcal rash
7. b. Maltose fermentation
8. a. Complement fixation tests
9. b. Gram-negative Diplococci in pus cells

Clostridium

CHAPTER 10

- *Anaerobic* obligatory *Gram positive spore* bearing bacilli.
- *Motile* except *Cl perfringens* and *Cl tetani type VI*. Motility is slow and described as stately.
- *Cl. perfringens* and *Cl. tetani* are found normally in intestine.
- Spores may be:
  - Spherical and terminal (=*Drumstick*) in *Cl. tetani, Cl. tetanomorphum, Cl. sphenoides.*
  - Oval and terminal (= *Tennis racket*) *Cl. difficile, Cl. tertium, Cl. cochleurum.*
  - Others have either central (*spindle shape*) or sub-terminal (club-shaped) spores.
- Useful *medium* for *Clostridia* – Robertson's cooked meat broth.
- Important members – *Cl. difficile, Cl. perfringens, Cl. tetani, Cl. botulinum.*
- Non-capsulated except *C. perfringens* and *C. butyricum* which are capsulated.

> Anaerobic Gram(+)ve bacilli motile (except perfringenes)
> Non-capsulated (except perfringenes and butyricum)

Spores

The shape & position of spores varies in different spp. & thus useful in their identification.
spores may be:

- **Central or equatorial** in *C. bifermentans* (Spindle shaped)
- **Sub-terminal** in *C. perfringens* (club shaped)
- **Oval and terminal** in *C. tertium* (resembling tennis racket)
- **Spherical and terminal** in *C. tetani* (drum sticks)

> Spores of C. tetani resist:
> - Dry heat at 160°C for 1 hour
> - 5% phenol for 2 weeks
> - Iodine for few hours

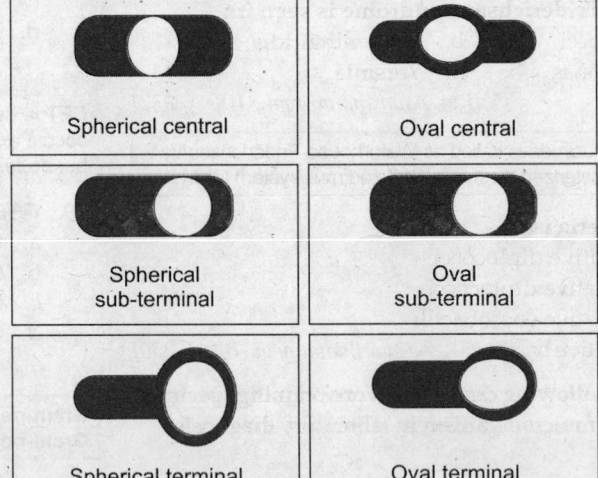

Spherical central | Oval central
Spherical sub-terminal | Oval sub-terminal
Spherical terminal | Oval terminal

I. CLOSTRIDIUM TETANI (See color plate, pg xxiii for related image)

- Causative Agent of Tetanus
- Motile, straight, slender, Gram positive drum stick shaped rod

Culture

- Marked tendency to *swarm*. Extremely fine translucent film of growth enables its separation from mixed cultures.
- Show α hemolysis which later develops into β hemolysis.
- It is strict anaerobe and forms surface growth only when O_2 tension is less than 2 mm Hg.
- Spores are resistant to various disinfectants and to boiling for 20 min. Vegetative cells, however, are easily inactivated. Glutaraldehyde is the only sure sporicidal.

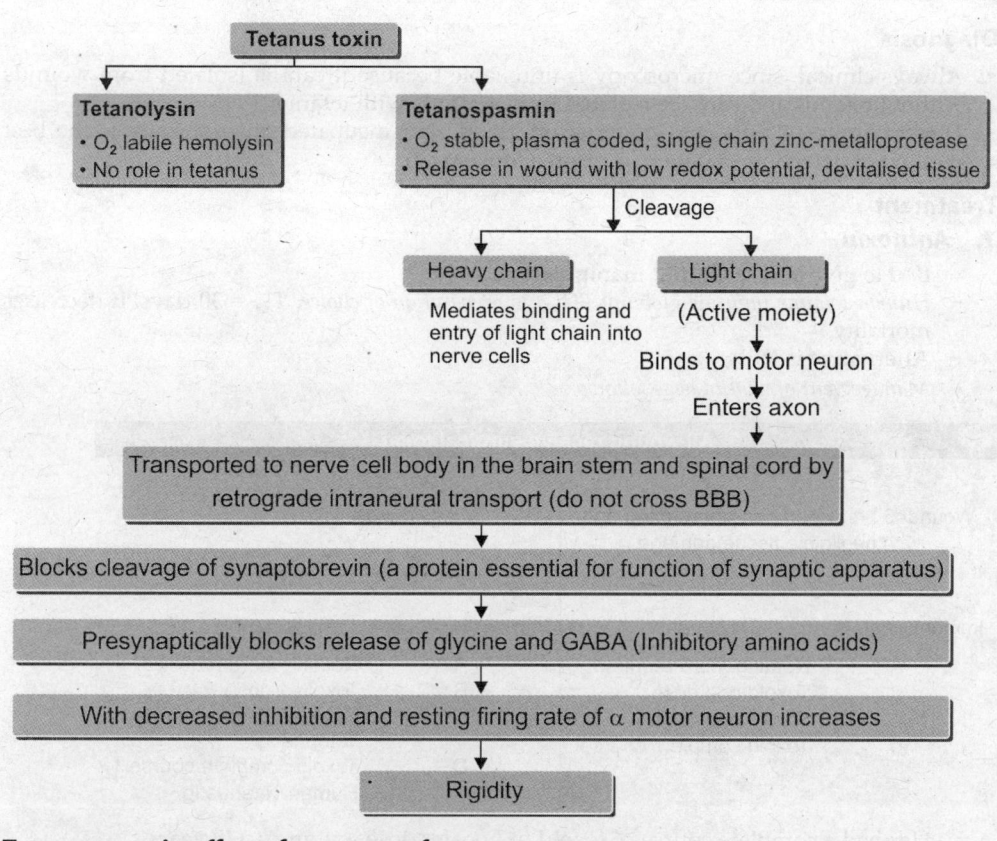

- Gene encoding tetanospasmin is located on plasmid
- In tetanus nerves of head and neck are affected initially as they are short.
- Tetanospasmin exerts its effect on the spinal cord, brainstem, peripheral nerves, at neuromuscular function and directly on muscles

Commonest initial symptoms are trismus, muscle pain and stiffness.

Pain and tingling at the site of inoculation is the earliest symptom of tetanus.

Tetanospasmin affects four areas of nervous system:
- Spinal cord (Mainly)
- Motor end plate in skeletal muscle
- Sympathetic system (resulting sympathetic overactivity)
- Brain

Note: Strychinine acts post-synaptically

Clinical Manifestations

- *Cl. tetani* has little invasive property. Symptoms are due to the effect of toxin.
- *MC* form of tetanus is *Generalized tetanus in which toxins enter the lymphatics and blood stream.*
- Median time of onset after injury is 7 days.
- *First symptom*   – *Pain and tingling at the site of inoculation*   ....CMDT 2014, p 1382
- *Early signs*   – Increased tone in masseter muscles called as *trismus or lock jaw*, followed by sequential involvement of nerves of head, trunk and extremities (*Descending tetanus*) since *short nerves are affected earlier. Hands and feet are relatively spared. Sustained contraction of facial muscles results in sinus sardonius.*
- Mentation remains unimpaired.
- *Deep tendon reflex increase.*
- Autonomic dysfunction (sympathetic increase), sudden cardiac death may occur.
- *Short Incubation period = Grave prognosis.*
- Neonatal tetanus usually occurs as generalized form.
- In local tetanus, only the nerves supplying the affected muscles are involved.
- Cephalic tetanus is a rare form with high mortality, it may occur after head injury or ear infection.

Invasiveness
Cl. tetani: Rarely invasive
Cl. botulinum: Non invasive
Cl. perfringens: Invasive
Cl. novii: Invasive
Cl. histolyticum: Invasive

Remember: Tetanus patients are not infectious and there is no person to person transmission. Tetanospasmin like botulinum toxin block neurotransmitter release and may produce paralysis, however, this effect is seen in cephalic tetanus only.

Diagnosis

- Always clinical, since microscopy is unreliable because it can be isolated from wounds without tetanus and can't be isolated from wounds with tetanus.
- Direct culture of unheated material on blood agar incubated anaerobically is the best method of detecting Cl. tetani. in source (dust, iron).

Serum antitoxin level ≥ 0.1 IU/mL are considered protective.

Treatment

1. Antitoxin
- *Best to give before wound manipulation.*
- *Human tetanus immune globulin (TIG) is preparation of choice.* $T\frac{1}{2}$ = 30 days. It decreases mortality.
- Alternative is IV Ig
- *Management of wound is as follows:*

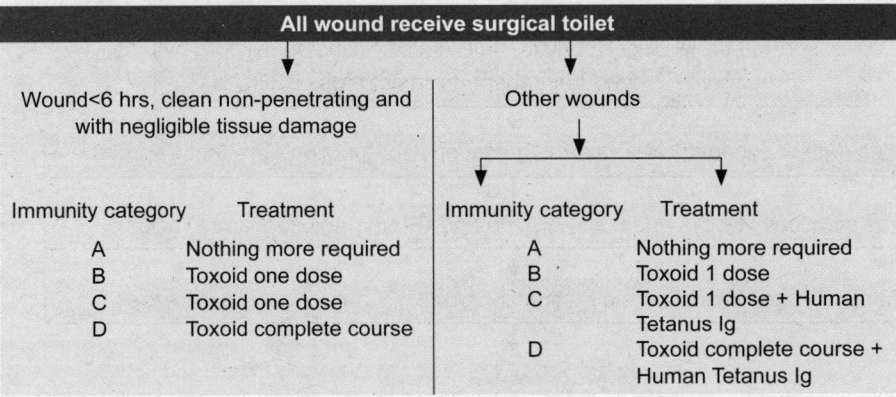

A = Has had a complete course of toxoid or booster dose within past 5 years.
B = Has had a complete course of toxoid or booster dose within past > 5 years and <10 years.
C = Has had a complete course of toxoid or booster dose within past >10 years.
D = Has not had complete course of toxoid or immunity status is unknown.

2. Antibiotic
- Penicillin or metronidazole eradicate source of toxin, i.e. vegetative cells.
- Alternative clindamycin or erythromycin.
- It is of no role if given > 6 hours.

Prevention
- Best prevented by *active immunization*. Protective level of antitoxin > 0.01 IU/ml serum
- WHO guidelines for tetanus vaccination consist of primary course of three doses in infancy, boosters at 4–7 and 12–15 years of age and one booster at adulthood.
- Passive immunization – Human tetanus hyperimmunoglobulin (TIG) is *best* prophylactic to use. Toxin already bound to neural tissue is not affected.
- Combined active and passive immunization – Patient is given TIG in one arm and TT in other arm followed by another dose of TT 6 weeks later and third dose 1 year later.
- As per expanded immunization programme of India tetanus vaccine is routinely offered to infants in combination with Diphtheria vaccine and killed β pertussis organisms as DPT vaccine. According to schedule, the primary course of immunization consists of 3 doses of DPT, at interval of 4-8 weeks starting at 6 weeks of age followed by a booster at 18 months of age and a second booster (only DT) at 5-6 years of age and a third booster (only TT) after 10 years of age.

Botulinum toxin is characterized as biothreat level A biological warfare agent
All type can cause human disease but type A, D (both associated with soil) and type E (marine origin) are the most common one.

Type E strain: Marine source
Type A & B strain: Soil

II. CLOSTRIDIUM BOTULINUM

- Strict anaerobic Gram positive bacillus that causes botulism
- Motile, possess oval and subterminal spores
- It is agent of bioterrorism
- Classified into type A to G based on immunological difference in the toxins.
- Optimal growth temperature is about 35°C but some strains can grow at temperature as low as 5°C

Botulinum toxin differs from other exotoxin in that it is not released during the life of organism.

Toxin

- Botulinum toxin is *most potent bacterial toxin known.*
- Produces 8 distinct toxin (A, B, C1, C2, D, E, F, G).
  - All toxins except C2 are neurotoxin. C2 is cytotoxin of unknown clinical significance.
- Acts on *peripheral cholinergic nerve endings* including Neuromuscular junctions, post-ganglionic parasympathetic nerve endings and peripheral ganglion, *CNS is not involved.* Where it blocks release of Acetylcholine.
- A, B, E and rarely F cause human disease. Type G (from *C. argentinense*) has been associated with sudden death. ..... Harrison 19/e, p 987, 18/e, p 1200
- Type A toxin used for treatment of strabismus, blepharospasm, cervical dystonia.

Clinical Features

- Cause noninvasive botulism of three types:
  1. *Food borne botulism:* –Due to *preformed toxin* of canned food. With incubation period of 18-36 hrs. Nausea vomiting, abdominal pain and *characteristic symmetric cranial nerve palsies followed by descending flaccid paralysis occurs.*
     - The source of botulism is usually preserved food, meat and meat products, canned vegetables.
     - Symptoms begin with Cranial Nerve involvement producing diplopia, dysphagia, ptosis, diminished pupillary reflex.
     - Deep tendon reflexes usually decreases but may remain normal, *severe constipation* no fever, no sensory finding, mentally intact.
     - Death is due to respiratory failure.
  2. *Wound botulism:* Toxin is produced in wound. It resembles food borne illness except IP is longer (~ 10 days) and gastrointestinal symptoms are lacking.
  3. *Infant or intestinal botulism:* –Due to ingestion of subterminal spores
     - Toxin is produced inside.
     - Source of infection is usually honey
     - Occur in infant < 6 months.
     - Results in floppy child syndrome.

> *Remember:*
> - Botulism is a food poisoning that do not cause diarrhea.
> - Infant botulism is most common form of botulism.

Diagnosis

- Demonstration of organism in serum by bioassay in mice is definitive.
- Diagnosis must be considered in patient with symmetric descending paralysis who are mentally intact.

Treatment

- Food borne botulism: – No role of antibiotics
  – Guanidine hydrochloride and bivalent antitoxin given
- Wound botulism: – Antitoxin
- Infant botulism: – Supportive care and human botulism immunoglobulin

III. CLOSTRIDIUM DIFFICILE

- Motile, possess oval and subterminal spores
- Cause CDAD (clostridium difficile associated disease)
- *MC* diagnosed diarrheal illness *acquired* in the hospital, which results from ingestion of spores.
- This infection is acquired almost **exclusively** in association with **Antimicrobial use** (*MC clindamycin*).
- **Risk factors** for CDAD: Old age, severe illness, use of electronic rectal thermometer, enteral tube feeding, antacid treatment and gastrointestinal surgery.
- Acquired exogenously and carried in stool of symptomatic and asymptomatic patients.

> C. difficile is found normally in the faeces of neonates and babies until the age of weaning, but it is not generally found in adults.
> C. difficile is the most common cause of hospital acquired diarrhea.

> Worldwide epidemic of fluoroquinolone resistant ribotype 027 Cl. difficile is due to excessive use of fluoroquinolones

> Treatment of choice for CDAD: Metronidazole.

Cl. Welchi: Stormy fermentation.

- Asymptomatic faecal carriage is very common in healthy neonates.
- It releases toxin A (enterotoxin) and toxin B (cytotoxin), both **glucosylate the GTP binding proteins** and disrupt cell cytoskeleton, so fluid is leaked leading to whitish yellow plaque formation over, colon, known as *Pseudomembranous colitis*. Data shows that toxin B is the essential virulence factor.
- *MC* symptom caused by *Cl. difficile* - **Diarrhea**
- *Complication* - Toxic megacolon and sepsis.
- Infants don't develop symptomatic CDAD as they lack receptors for mucosal toxin, which develop later in the life.
  .... *Harrison 18/e, p 1092*

Diagnosis

- Diagnosis of CDI is based on a combination of clinical criteria:
  - 1 (Diarrhea with no other recognized cause
  - 2 Toxin A or B detected is stool
- Demonstrating toxin in faces by its characteristic effect on Hep-2 and human diploid cell culture (Tissue culture) is *gold standard*. .... *Harrison 19/e, p 859*
- ELISA – Rapid and easy but has less sensitivity.
- Stool culture for clostridium difficile is most sensitive.
- Endoscopy is a rapid diagnostic tool in seriously ill; which demonstrates pseudomembrane.

Treatment

- *Doc* – Metronidazole
- *Doc even* for relapse is Metronidazole
- If not respond for >48 hours, give vancomycin
- Rifampin, Bacitracin, *Saccharomyces boulardii* or *lactobacillus* GG, colonization with nontoxigenic strain of *Cl. difficile*, anion exchange binding resin, cholestyramine, IV lg can also given.

IV. CLOSTRIDIUM PERFRINGENS = CL. WELCHII

- Relatively large with fluent ends.
- Capsulated, non-motile, shows **Stormy fermentation**
- Causative agent of gas gangrene, enteritis necroticans (*caused by Cl. perfringens type C*)
- Toxigenic as well as invasive.
- Absence of its central or subterminal spore in artificial media or pathological tissue is the characteristic feature.
- Classified on the basis of toxin, they produced.
- It is the *MC* clostridial species isolated from tissue infection and bacteremia.
- *Clostridia* are present in the normal colonic flora, *Clostridia ramosum* is the most abundant and is followed by *C.perfringens*.
- Spores are usually destroyed within five minutes by boiling but those of food poisoning strains of Type A and certain Type C strains resist boiling for 1–3 hours.

Toxins

- Produce twelve distinct toxin. Four major enterotoxins are: α, β, ε and ι.
- **α Toxin** = Phospholipase C = lecithinase: Associated with gas gangrene.
  - Hemolytic, Hot-cold variety toxin produced by all *Cl. perfringens* but most abundantly by Type A.
  - Shows Nagler reaction in which zone of opacity is formed where there is no antitoxin.
  - Lecithinase also produced by *Cl. novyi, Cl. bifermentans*, some vibrios.
  - It initiates muscle infection that may progress to gas gangrene.
- **β and iota (ι) toxin** also have lethal and necrotizing properties. Increase capillary permeability.
- **θ (theta) toxin** - Hemolysin, antigenically related to streptolysin O. Also known as *Perfringolysin O.*
- Also produce neuraminidase, histamine - bursting factor, etc.
- **Nagler Reaction**: When C. perfringens is grown on a medium containing 6% agar, 5% fildes peptic digest of sheep blood, colonies with antitoxin exhibit no opacity. In colonies without antitoxin there would be opacity. *This is due to lecithinase effect of α–toxin.*

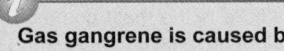

Gas gangrene is caused by:
- C. perfringens
- C. Septicum
- C. novyi type A
- C. histolyticum
- C. sordellii

Clinical Features

It causes following diseases:

1. **Skin and soft tissue infection:**
   a. *Gas gangrene = Clostridial myonecrosis:*
      - Most commonly caused by *Cl. perfringens* Type A. Also caused by *Cl. septicum, Cl. novyi, Cl. histolyticum, Cl. sordellii* etc.
      - Characteristic pathology – *Near absence of PMNs despite extensive tissue destruction.*
      - Essential factor - Trauma particularly deep muscle laceration.
      - Incubation period usually short: *10-48 hours* with *Cl. perfringens*, *2-3 days* with *Cl. septicum*, *5-6 days* with *Cl. novyi*.
      - Pain and *crepitus* present and death is due to circulatory failure.

      ### Diagnosis
      - Frozen section biopsy of muscle.
      - Gram's staining: - Showing gram-positive bacilli *without spores*: *Cl. perfringens*
      - Showing *citron* bodies and *boat or leaf shaped* pleomorphic bacilli - *Cl. septicum*
      - Showing large bacilli with oval or subterminal spores - *Cl. novyi*.

      ### Treatment
      - Surgery - mainstay of therapy
      - **Doc** Clindamycin + penicillin   .... *Harrison 20/e, p 1113*
      - Hyperbaric O_2 may also used.

   b. *Non-traumatic gas gangrene:*
      - Spontaneous gas gangrene generally occurs via hematogenous seeding of normal muscle with histotoxic Clostridia principally C. perfringens, C. septicum and C. novyi.
      - Bacteria reaches blood via GIT (as in colonic malignancy, inflammatory bowel disease, diverticulitis, necrotizing enterocolitis).
      - The first symptom of spontaneous gas gangrene is confusion, which is followed y sudden onset of severe pain in absence of trauma. Mortality rate is very high (67-100%)

      ...... *Harrison 20/e, p 1113*

2. **Intestinal disorders:**
   a. *Food poisoning:*
      - *Cl. perfringens* (type A) is 2nd or 3rd **MC** cause of food poisoning. It is mediated by Cytotoxin which act on small bowel brush border and induces Ca^{2+} dependent alteration in permeability.
      - Usually caused by cold or warmed up meat dish after 8-24 hours. It is self-limited.
      - C. perfringens strains associated with food poisoning possess the gene (CPe) which codes for enterotoxin.   ..... *Harrison 20/e, p 1110*
   b. *Enteritis necroticans (Pigbel)*
      - Caused by β toxin of type C strain.
      - Following ingestion of high protein meal with trypsin inhibitors (sweat potato) by host who have limited proteolytic activity in small intestine. Patient present with acute abdominal pain, bloody diarrhea, vomiting, signs of peritonitis.
   c. *Necrotizing enterocolitis:*
      - Disease resemble *enteritis necroticans* but associated with C. perfringens type A. Affect previously healthy individual.
   d. *Neutropenic enterocolitis*

> Cl. perfringens food poisoning is mediated by cytotoxin which induces Ca^{2+} dependent alteration in permeability.

CLOSTRIDIUM SORDELLI

- Rare cause of endometritis and toxic shock syndrome following child birth.

  .....*CMDT 2014, p 1381*

- Fatal cases of uterine infection following medically induced abortion with mifepristone have been reported.
- Illness occur within 4-5 days of ingestion of mifepristone.
- Emergent surgical depridement along with C. sordellii susceptible antibiotics is the treatment of choice.

Multiple Choice Questions

1. The following statements are true regarding *Clostridium perfringens* except: [AI 05]
   a. It is the commonest cause of gas gangrene
   b. It is normally present in human feces
   c. The principal toxin of *C. perfringens* is the alpha toxin
   d. Gas gangrene producing strains of *C. perfringens* produces heat resistant spores

2. Gas gangrene is/are caused by: [PGI 2011]
   a. Cl. novyi
   b. Cl. septicum
   c. Cl. histolyticum
   d. Cl. perfringens
   e. Cl. tetani

3. Gastrointestinal enteritis necroticans caused by: [PGI 07]
   a. Cl. difficile
   b. Cl. perfringens
   c. Botulinum
   d. C. jejuni
   e. Pseudomonas

4. Which species of clostridium does not cause gangrene? [AIIMS, 09]
   a. Cl. perfringens
   b. Cl. histolyticum
   c. C. novyii
   d. C. sporogenes

5. Regarding *Clostridium perfringens* gas gangrene, all are true, except: [AIIMS, 10]
   a. Commonest cause of gas gangrene
   b. Naegler reaction positive
   c. Most common toxin is hyaluronidase
   d. Food poisoning strain of *Clostridium perfringens* produced heat resistant spores.

6. Which of the following regarding *Clostridium tetani* is false? [AIIMS, 10]
   a. Soil and intestine of human and animals are the reservoirs
   b. Predominantly seen in dry and winter season
   c. Transmission through contaminated wounds
   d. No herd immunity or seen

7. True about gas gangrene: [PGI 2013]
   a. Underlying skin and muscle are normal
   b. Caused by tetanospasmin toxin
   c. Muscle rigidity and spasm are characteristic
   d. Most common organism implicated is Cl. Perfringens
   e. Passive immunization does not help

8. A person has received complete immunization against tetanus 10 years ago. Now he presents with a clean wound without any lacerations from an injury sustained 2.5 hours ago. He should now be given: [AIIMS 16]
   a. Full course of tetanus toxoid
   b. Single dose of tetanus toxoid
   c. Human tet. globulin
   d. Human tet. globulin and single dose of toxoid

9. The most effective way of preventing tetanus is: [AIIMS 07]
   a. Surgical debridement and toilet
   b. Hyperbaric oxygen
   c. Antibiotics
   d. Tetanus toxoid

10. True about clostridium tetani: [PGI 17]
    a. It is Gram +ve bacilli
    b. Drum stick appearance
    c. Grows in aerobic environment
    d. It is Gram –ve cocci
    e. Produces endotoxin

11. All are true regarding *Clostridium tetani* except: [AI 2011, AIIMS, 2011]
    a. Produces heat resistant spores
    b. Incubation period 6-11 days
    c. 3 primary doses of vaccine needed for full protection
    d. Man-to-man transmission is seen

12. True regarding pseudomembranous colitis are all *except*: [AIIMS 07]
    a. It is caused by *Clostridium difficile*
    b. The organism is a normal commensal of gut
    c. It is due to production of phospholipase A
    d. It is treated by vancomycin

13. An 18-year old male presented with acute onset descending paralysis of 3 days duration. There is also a history of blurring of vision for the same dura-tion. On examination, the patient has quadriparesis with areflexia. Both the pupils are non-reactive. The most probable diagnosis is: [AIIMS 06]
    a. Poliomyelitis
    b. Botulism
    c. Diphtheria
    d. Porphyria

14. A patient of acute lymphocytic leukemia with fever and neutropenia develops diarrhea after administration of amoxicillin therapy, which of the following organism is most likely to be the causative agent? [AIIMS 05]
    a. Salmonella typhi
    b. Clostridium difficile
    c. Clostridium perfringens
    d. Shigella flexneri

15. The following statements are true regarding botulism *except*: [AIIMS 03]
    a. Infant botulism is caused by ingestion of performed toxin
    b. *Cl. botulinum* A, B, E and F cause human disease
    c. The gene for botulinum toxin is coded by bacteriophage
    d. *Cl. baratii* may cause botulism

16. Not true about Botulinum toxin: [PGI 07]
    a. Short life span
    b. Increased acetyl-choline release
    c. Used for treatment in Blepharospasm, static and dynamic wrinkles
    d. Effective for 3-4 months
    e. Irreversibly decreases Ach in NM junction

17. Subterminal spores are found in: [PGI Dec 2008]
    a. Clostridium sordellii   b. Clostridium sporogenes
    c. Clostridium difficile   d. Clostridium tertium
    e. Clostridium botulinum

18. Most important and potential agent that can be used for bioterrorism. [AI 2011]
    a. Plague   b. Small pox
    c. TB   d. Clostridium botulinum

19. A 47-year-old hospitalized man who received multiple antibiotic in last 10 days develop diarrhea. A faecal sample is sent to the laboratory which of the following test is used to establish clostridium difficile as a causative agent:
    a. Immunofluorescence [AIIMS 2017]
    b. PCR for toxin genes
    c. ELISA for toxin
    d. Culture

Explanations and References with Illustrative Answers

1. **Ans. (d) Gas gangrene producing strains of *C. perfringens* produces heat resistant spores** *Ref. Ananthanarayan 10/e, p 257*

   "Spores of C. perfringens are heat sensitive":
   - Gas gangrene is caused by *Cl. perfringens* (**MC** by type A), *Cl. novyi*, *Cl. septicum*, *Cl. histolyticum* and *C. sordellii*
   - Most important toxin for gas gangrene is Alpha toxin = lecithinase which is responsible **Nagler's Reaction.**
   - *Cl. perfringens* is found in feces and contaminates the skin of perineum, buttocks, thigh.
   - Its spores are used as remote indicator of fecal contamination of water.
   - Spores are usually destroyed within 5 minutes by boiling but those of food poisoning strains of Type A and certain type C strain resist boiling for several hours.
   - Spores are destroyed by autoclaving at 121°C for 20 minutes.
   - Spores are resistant to antiseptics and disinfectants in common use.

   Resistance of Clostridia spores
   - Spores of C. botulinum survive boiling for 3-4 hours and even at 105°C they are not killed completely in less than 100 minutes
   - Spores of C. perfringens: Destroyed by boiling in less than 5 minutes except food poisoning type A strains which can survive after boiling.
   - Clostridia titani spores resist boiling for 15-90 minutes
   - However all species spores are killed by autoclaving at 121°C
   - Among disinfectants clostridia spores are sensitive to halogens and glutaraldehyde.

2. **Ans. (a, b and d) Cl. novyi, Cl. septicum, Cl. perfringens**
   Ref. Harrison 19/e, p 992; 20/e, p 1111; Ananthanarayan 10/e, p 259

Clostridium Causing Gas Gangrene		
Common	**Less pathogenic**	**Doubtful**
• Cl. perfringens	• Cl. histolyticum	• Cl. bifermentans
• Cl. septicum	• Cl. fallax	• Cl. sporogenes
• Cl. novyi	• Cl. tertium	• Cl. tetani
		• Cl. sordellii

3. **Ans. (b) Cl. perfringens** *Ref. Harrison 20/e, p 95; Ananthanarayan 10/e, p 260*

   "Necrotizing enteritis (enteritis necroticians, or pig bel) is caused by β toxin (located on plasmid) produced by type C strains of C.perfringens following ingestion of a high protein meal in conjunction with trypsin inhibitors by a susceptible host who has limited intestinal proteolytic activity". Source of organism is patient own intestinal flora.

   Clinical Features
   - Acute abdominal pain, diarrhea, vomiting, shock and peritonitis, 40% of patient die.
   - Pathological studies show an acute ulcerative process of the bowel restricted to small intestine.

4. **Ans. (d) C. sporogenes** *Ref. Harrison 20/e, p 1111; Ananthanarayan 10/e, p 261*
   Already explained

5. **Ans. (c) Most common toxin is hyaluronidase** *Ref. Ananthanarayan 10/e, p 261-262*
   Already explained

6. **Ans. (b) Predominantly seen in dry and winter season** *Ref. Ananthanarayan 10/e, p 266; Park 22/e, p 261*
   "Tetanus is more common in developing countries where the climate is warm and in rural area where soil is fertile".
   Epidemiology of Tetanus
   - Natural habitat of Clostridium tetani is soil and dust. Bacilli can be found in intestine of herbivorous animals, e.g. cattle, horses. The spores can survive for years.
   - Infection is acquired by contamination of wound with spores.
   - *Sequence of events are:* introduction of spores; germination, *elaboration of exotoxin* and binding to the receptor.
   - It is not transmitted from person to person.

7. **Ans. (d) Most common organism implicated is Cl. Perfringens** *Ref. Harrison 20/e, p 1111*
   Gas gangrene
   - Rapidly spreading, edematous myonecrosis occurring characteristically in association with wound contamination.
   - Clostridium perfringens is the most common organism associated, C. septicum and C. tertium are aerotolerant cause of gas gangrene
   - The major C. perfringenes toxin implicated in gas gangrene are α toxin and θ toxin
   - In case of C. septicum four toxins have been implicated:
     – *α toxin* (lethal, hemolytic, necrotizing activity), *β toxin* (DNase) *γ toxin* (hyaluronidase) and *Δ toxin* (septicolysin)
   - Radical surgical debridement along with antibiotic therapy is treatment of choice
   - Penicillin plus clindamycin is the preferred antibiotic. If C. tertium is suspected, vancomycin should be used
   - Hyperbaric oxygen may be considered after surgery
   - Passive immunization with anti gas gangrene serum has not yield any beneficial result and is now not recommended

8. **Ans. (b) Single dose of tetanus toxoid** *Ref. Park 22/e, p 287*
   Management of wound depends on nature of wound and immune status of person.
   - All wounds should receive surgical toilet.

Category	Immunization status	Clean wound of < 6 hrs and with negligible tissue damage	Other wounds, e.g. (contaminated wound)
A	Complete immunization within past 5 yrs	Nothing	Nothing
B	Complete immunization within 5-10 years	1 dose of toxoid	Toxoid 1 dose
C	Complete immunization more than 10 years	Toxoid 1 dose	Toxoid 1 dose + Human Tet. Ig
D	Has not had complete immunization or immunity status is unknown	Toxoid complete course	Toxoid complete course + Human Tet Ig

   Patient in question falls in category B.

9. **Ans. (d) Tetanus toxoid** *Ref. Park 21/e, p 287; 22/e, p 287*

Remember:	**Best** way of prevention	=	Active immunization	=	TT
	Best passive immunization	=	Antitoxin	=	Human tetanus immunoglobulin.

10. **Ans. (a) and (b) It is gram +ve and Drum stick appearance** *Ref. Ananthanarayan 10/e, p 257*
    - Clostridium is obligatory anaerobic gram-positive spore bearing bacilli.

Spores of Clostridia		
Spherical and terminal spore (= Drum stick appearance)	**Oval and terminal (= Tennis racket)**	**Central or subterminal**
• Cl. tetani • Cl. tetanomorphum • C. sphenoides	• Cl. difficile • Cl tertium • Cl. cochleurum	• Cl. botulinum • Cl. perfringenes • Cl. septicum • Cl. novyl • Cl. histolyticum • Cl. sporgenes • Cl. sordellii • Cl. chauvoei

Clostridium

11. **Ans. (d) Man-to-man transmission is seen** *Ref. Park 21/e, p 285; 22/e p 285*

   There is no man to man transmission or a tetanus patient is not infectious.

   Other Options
   Option 'a'
   - Cl. Tetani produce terminal spores which are highly resistant to boiling, cresol, autoclaving for 15 min at 120°C.
   - Spores are best destroyed by steam under pressure at 120°C for 20 minutes or by gamma irradiation.

   Option 'b'
   - I.P. of tetanus is usually 6-10 days however it may be as short as one day or as long as several months.

   Option 'c'
   - Tetanus is best prevented by active immunization with tetanus toxoid.
   - The aim is to ensure a life long antitoxin level ≥ 0.01 IU/ml. This can be accomplished either by combined vaccine (DPT) at interval of 48 weeks starting at 6 weeks of age followed by booster at 18 months of age, and a second booster (only DT) at 5-6 years of age
   - For monovalent vaccine a primary course of immunization consists of two doses of TT given at interval of 1-2 months. This is followed by a booster dose 1 year after the initial dose. Second booster dose is advised after 5 year. Thus, total 4 doses of monovalent vaccine ensure life long protection in an adult.

12. **Ans. (c) It is due to production of phospholipase A** *Ref. Harrison 20/e, p 965; Ananthanarayan 10/e, p 270*

   "Cl. difficile cause pseudomembranous colitis (PMC) due to the production of toxin A (enterotoxin) and toxin B (cytotoxin) not phospholipase A."
   - Toxin A is potent neutrophil chemoattractant and both toxin A and B glucosylate the GTP binding protein of Rho subfamily resulting in disruption of cytoskeleton causing loss of cell shape adherence with consequent fluid leakage.
   - Asymptomatic fecal carriage of Cl. difficile in healthy neonates is very common. It also colonizes the colon of 3% of healthy adults.
   ..... CMDT
   - For Cl. diffcle associated diarrhea (CDAD) three events are essential:

   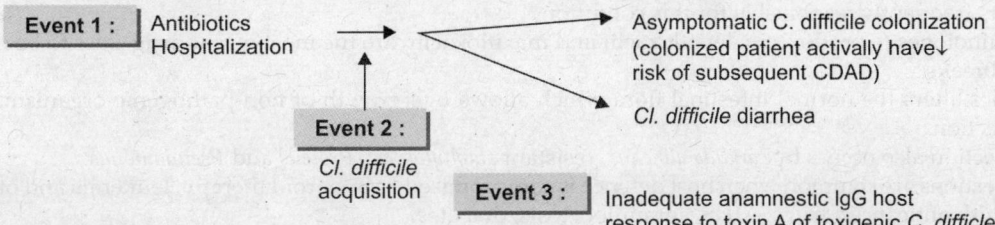

   Diagnosis
   - Diagnosis of CAD is based on combination of clinical criteria:
     - Diarrhea (≥ 3 unformed stools per 24 hours for > 2 days)
     - Toxin A or B detected by stool culture or pseudomembrane seen in colon.
   - Endoscopy is a rapid diagnostic tool in seriously ill patient with suspected PMC but a negative result does not rule out CDAD.

   Treatment
   - Discontinue offending antibiotic
   - *Drug of Choice*: Metronidazole
   - *Drug of Choice* for relapse: Metronidazole
     If not respond > 48 hrs, give Vancomycin.

   > **Note:** Patients colonized with C. difficile were initially thought to be at high risk for CDI. However four prospective studies have shown that colonized individual actually have a decreased risk of subsequent CDI.

13. **Ans. (b) Botulism** *Ref. Harrison 20/e, p 1107; Madell's infectious disease 6/e, p 2824*
   Diagnosis of botulism should be considered in patient with symmetric descending paralysis with bilateral cranial neuropathies in addition of following features:
   - Absent fever
   - Patient remain responsive

- Heart rate normal or slow
- Sensory deficits don't occur except for blurred vision.

Neurologic signs and symptoms of botulism:			
• Dysphagia	• Diplopia	• Dysarthria	• Dry mouth
• Upper limb weakness	• Lower limb weakness	• Burred vision	• Dyspnea

Important Points:
- *Cl. botulinum* produce exotoxin which differs from other exotoxin in that it is produced intracellularly and appears in the medium only on death/autolysis of cell.
- Toxin production is determined by bacteriophage at least in types C and D toxin.
- All toxins are neurotoxin except C_2 which is cytotoxin.
- Toxin acts by blocking production or release of Ach. at synapse and Neuromuscular junction (= parasympatholytic = effect of atropine) so cause constipation, paralysis, etc.
- Human disease is caused by type A, B, E and rarely F.
- *MC* Type of botulism is 'Infant botulism' which is produced by eating of honey containing spores of Cl. botulism which grows and produce toxins.
- *Food borne botulism and wound botulism are produced by preformed toxin.*
- Diagnosis may be confirmed by demonstration of bacillus or toxin in food or feces.
- A retrospective diagnosis may be made by detection of antitoxin in the patient serum but it may not be seen in all cases.

Remember: Polio present with asymmetric descending paralysis.

14. Ans. (b) Clostridium difficile *Ref. Greenwood 18/e,p 255; KDT 6/e, p 672 - 73*
- It is a typical presentation of CDAD (*Cl. difficile* associated diarrhea).
- *Historically, MC* antibiotics causing CDAD - clindamycin, ampicillin and cephalosporins.   ...*Harrison 10/e, p 964*
- Now second and third generation cephalosporins particularly cefotaxime, ceftriaxone cefuroxime and ceftazidine are the agents frequently responsible for this condition.   ... *Harrison 20/e, p 964*
- Fluoroquinolones (ciprofloxacin, levofloxacin and maxifloxacin) are the most recent drug class to be implicated in hospital outbreaks.
- Antibiotics alters the normal intestinal flora which allows overgrowth of non-pathogenic organism. This is called as superinfection.
- Superinfection also occurs by *candida albicans*, resistant *staphylococci*, *Proteus* and *Pseudomonas*.
- Superinfections are common when host defence is compromised as in steroid therapy, leukemia and other malignancies treated with anticancer drugs, AIDS, agranulocytosis, diabetes.

15. Ans. (a) Infant botulism is caused by ingestion of preformed toxin   *Harrison 20/e, p 1105*
- Infant botulism is caused by toxin produced in situ by toxigenic clostridia colonizing the intestine of infant
  - Most of these infants recover with supportive therapy alone.
  - Spores of botulinum are highly resistant to heat, and can withstand 100°C for several hours.

16. Ans. (a) and (b) Short life span; Increased acetyl-choline release *Ref. Harrison's 20/e p 1106*
Botulinum toxin (a zinc metalloprotease) decreases the release of acetylcholine by proteolysis of SNARE proteins. The SNARE proteins are synaptobrevin SNAP-25 and syntaxin. The toxin of C.botulinum types A and E cleaves SNAP-25 while type B toxin cleaves synaptobrevin.
- Though botulinum toxin is the most lethal toxin known (lethal dose 1-2 μg) it is used therapeutically for many conditions.

Therapeutic uses of Botulinum toxin	
Muscular disorders	**Ophthalmic disorders**
Myoclonus	Strabismus
Palatal myoclonus	Lower lid entropion
Focal dystonias	Acquired nystagmus
Tics, tremor	Thyroid ophthalmopathy
Hemi-facial spasm	Dwayne's syndrome
Tourette's syndrome	Oscillopsia

Contd...

Contd...

Therapeutic uses of Botulinum toxin	
Muscular disorders	**Ophthalmic disorders**
Synkinesis	Apaxia of eyelid opening
Tardive disorders	Hyper-lacrimation
Rigid akinetic syndromes	
Parkinson's progressive supranuclear palsy	
Hallervorden-Spatz	
Stiff person syndrome	
Plastic surgery	**Otolaryngology**
Wrinkles	Vocal cord polyps
Masseter hypertrophy	Stuttering
Facial asymmetry (post Bells)	Hypersalivation
Muscle flap paralysis during healing	
Genitourinary	**Gastroenterology**
Detrusor - sphincter dyssynergia	Achalasia
Vaginismus	Cricopharyngeal spasms
	Rectal fissures
Rehabilitation Medicine	
Disorders of Painful Muscular Spasm Spasticity: Focal myofascial pain TMJ associated muscle spasm.	

Note: Botulinum toxin once bound leads to permanent dysfunction of that neuron. Recovery (or duration of action) takes 10-20 weeks (usually 3 months) when dysfunctioned nerve terminals are replaced as a result of sprouting.

17. **Ans. (a) (b) and (e) Clostridium sordelli, Clostridium sporogenes and Clostridium botulinum**

    Ref. Ananthanarayan 10/e 257

    Already explained

18. **Ans. (d) Clostridium botulinum** *Ref. Harrison 18/e, p 1769, 20/e chapter S2*

    Cl. botulinum belong to category A of potential bioterrorism agents
    Category A bioterrorism agents:
    - Anthrax *(Bacillus anthracis)*
    - Botulism *(Clostridium botulinum toxin)*
    - Plague *(Yersinia pestis)*
    - Smallpox *(Variola major)*
    - Tularemia *(Francisella tularensis)*
    - Viral hemorrhagic fevers

    Category A agents are the highest priority pathogens because they:
    a. Can be easily disseminated or transmitted from person to person
    b. Possess high mortality rates
    c. Require special action for public health preparedness.

19. **Ans. (c) ELISA for toxin** *Ref. Harrison 20/e, p 966*

    Diagnosis of Clostridia difficle infection
    - Based on combination of clinical criteria:
      a. Diarrhea ≥ 3 unformed stools per 24 h for ≥ 2 days plus
      b. Detection of toxin A on B in the stool or detection of toxin producing C. difficile in the stool by nucleic acid amplification testing (PCR) or by culture or by visualization of pseudomembrane in the colon. (by endoscopy)
    - **Tests for detection of toxin**
      - Demonstration of toxin in feces by its effect on Hep-2 cells and human diploid cell culture is gold standard but time consuming and available only in reference laboratories
      - Enzyme immunoassay: Specific but sensitivity is low

NEET Pattern Questions

1. **Tetanospasmin encoding genes are located on:**
   a. Chromosome
   b. Plasmid
   c. Both
   d. Transposon [Ref. Ananthanarayan, 10/e, p 265]

2. **Main site of action of tetanus toxin:**
   a. Presynaptic terminal of spinal cord
   b. Postsynaptic terminal of spinal cord
   c. Neuromuscular junction
   d. Muscle fibers [Ref. Ananthanarayan, 10/e, p 265]

3. **Nagler reaction is shown by:**
   a. Cl. difficle
   b. Cl. perfringens
   c. Cl. tetani
   d. Cl. butyricum [Ref. Ananthanarayan, 10/e, p 259]

4. **Botulism is most commonly due to:**
   a. Egg
   b. Milk
   c. Meat
   d. Pulses [Ref. Ananthanarayan, 10/e, p 269]

   > The source of botulism is usually preserved food meat and meat products

5. **Mechanism of action of tetanospasmin:**
   a. Inhibition of GABA release
   b. Inhibition cAMP
   c. Inactivation of Ach receptors
   d. Inhibition of cGMP
   [Ref. Ananthanarayan, 10/e, p 265; Greenwood 18/e p250]

   > Tetanus toxin prevents the release of neurotransmitter γ-aminobutyric acid in presynaptic cells.

6. **Botulism causes:**
   a. Descending flaccid paralysis
   b. Descending spastic paralysis
   c. Ascending paralysis
   d. Ascending spastic paralysis
   [Ref. Harrison 20/e, p 1107]

   > Distinctive feature of botulism is symmetrical cranial nerve palsies followed by symmetric descending flaccid paralysis that may progress to respiratory arrest.

7. **Most common cause of gas gangrene:**
   a. Cl welchii
   b. Cl septicum
   c. Cl novyi
   d. Cl histolyticum [Ref. Ananthanarayan, 10/e, p 259]

   > *Etiologic agents of gas gangrene:*
   > C. perfringenes (= C.welchii) (60% of cases)
   > C. novyi and C. septum (20–40% of cases)
   > C. histolyticum

8. **Which of the following is false about Botulism:**
   a. It is a type food poisoning
   b. Botulinum toxin is a potent neurotoxin
   c. It is an infection and not intoxication
   d. The causative organism is clostridium botulinum
   [Ref. Harrison, 20/e, p 1105]

9. **Virulence factor for clostridium tetani:**
   a. Endotoxin
   b. Tetanolysin
   c. Tetanospasmin
   d. Bacteremia [Ref. Ananthanarayan, 10/e, p 265]

   > Tetanospasmin is the main toxin responsible for tetanus.

10. **Spores of clostridium perfringens are located:**
    a. In the middle of cells
    b. At the poles of cells
    c. Between middle and pole of cells
    d. None of the above [Ref. Ananthanarayan, 10/e, p 257]

    > Spores of Cl. perfringens are subterminal

11. **Not true about gas gangrene:**
    a. Most common cause is Cl perfringens
    b. Extensive necrosis of muscles
    c. Cl perfringens produce heat-labile spores
    d. Metronidazole is the drug of choice
    [Ref. Harrison 20/e, p 1112]

    > C. perfringens spores can be heat labile or heat resistant
    > Except for infection caused by C. tertium, antibiotic treatment of traumatic or spontaneous gas gangrene is combination of penicillin and clindamycin
    > For C. tertium combination of vancomycin and metronidazole is used

Ans.
1. b. Plasmid
2. a. Presynaptic...
3. b. Cl. perfringens
4. c. Meat
5. a. Inhibition of...
6. a. Descending ...
7. a. Cl welchii
8. c. It is an infection ...
9. c. Tetanospasmin
10. c. Between middle...
11. d. Metronidazole...

12. Tetanus is caused by:
    a. Gram positive bacilli
    b. Gram negative bacilli
    c. Gram positive cocci
    d. Gram negative cocci
    [Ref. Ananthanarayan, 10/e, p 256]

Treatment of Gas gangrene
- Emergent Surgical exploration and thorough debridement is most important
- Penicillin G 4 million units IV plus Clindamycin, 600-900 mg IV. If patient is allergic to penicillin then Cefoxitin is used along with Clindamycin.
- Hyperbaric oxygen therapy may be considered after surgery and antibiotics have been initiated.

Note: Closure of traumatic wounds or compound fracture should be delayed for 5-6 days until it is certain that these sites are free of infection.

13. Which of following clostridia is non-invasive:
    a. Clostridium novyi
    b. Clostridium botulinum
    c. Clostridium perfringens
    d. Clostridium tetani   [Ref. Ananthanarayan, 10/e, p 256]

C. botulinum are virtually non-invasive and non-infectious
C. tetani has little invasive property.
C. perfringens is both invasive and toxigenic

14. Most common symptom of tetanus is:
    a. Tonic-clonic seizures
    b. Hemiplegia
    c. Lock-jaw
    d. Opisthotonos   [Ref. Harrison, 20/e, p 1103]

15. True about Cl perfringens are all except: [2016]
    a. Invasive as well as toxigenic
    b. Alpha toxin is detected by Naegler's reaction
    c. Beta toxin is important in gas gangrene
    d. Theta toxin is perfringolysin
    [Ref. Ananthanarayan, 10/e, p 259]

16. All clostridia cause myonecrosis except: [2016]
    a. C septicum   b. C difficile
    c. C novyi   d. C welchii
    [Ref. Harrison, 20/e, p 1111]

17. Naegler's reaction is due to: [2016]
    a. Coagulase   b. Hyaluronidase
    c. Lecithinase   d. None of the above
    [Ref. Ananthanarayan, 10/e, p 259]

Naegler's reactions is due to a toxin which is phospholipase C

18. Spore rorming anaerobic gram positive bacilli: [2016]
    a. Bacillus Anthracis
    b. Clostridia
    c. Corynebacterium
    d. Peptostreptococcus
    [Ref. Ananthanarayan 10/e, p 257]

Note: Spore forming aerobic Gram positive bacilli: Bacillus anthracis

19. Among the toxin produced by botulinum, the non-neurotoxic one is: [2016]
    a. A   b. D
    c. Cl.   d. C2
    [Ref. Ananthanarayan 10/e, p 269]

Ans.
12. a. Gram positive ...   13. b. Clostridium ...   14. c. Lock-jaw   15. c. Beta toxin...
16. b. C difficile   17. c. Lecithinase   18. b. Clostridia 19. d. C2

Corynebacterium

CHAPTER 11

Gram-positive nonmotile rods with *high G+C (guanine + cytosine)* content.
It includes: *C. diphtheriae, C. ulcerans* and other coryneform bacteria like *Arcanobacterium, Rhodococcus*.

> **Corynebacterium**
> - Club shaped bacteria contains Babes Ernst or volutin granules
> - Cesteine-Tellarite blood agar is a selective medium.

CORYNEBACTERIUM DIPHTHERIAE (KLEBS-LOEFFLER BACILLUS)

Morphology

- Characteristically *club shaped* pleomorphic, noncapsulated, nonsporing nonmotile bacilli.
- Arranged in pairs, palisades, clusters (*Chinese letter or cuneiform arrangement*).
- Contain Granules known as *Babes Ernst or volutin granules* which are composed of **polymetaphosphate** and are **more strongly gram-positive.**
- On staining with *Loefler's methylene blue,* granules show *metachromatism.*
- *Special stain to see granules clearly* – Albert's, Neisser's and Ponder's. Granules are also called as *polar bodies* since they are arranged on poles.

Culture

- Enrichment is necessary. Grows best on a blood or serum containing medium at 35-37°C with or without CO_2 enrichment. Optimum pH is 7.2.
- *Selective medium*: **Cysteine-Tellurite blood agar (grow in 2 days) or Tinsdale** medium.
- For rapid growth (6-8 hours) - **Loeffler's serum slope** used (also used for Mycobacteria TB).
- Mcleod classified *Corynebacterium* into 3 types:

> - Toxigenicity is under the control of phage gene, invasiveness is under the control of bacterial genes.

Feature	C. gravis	C. intermidius	C. mitis
Colony on tellurite	Daisy head	Frog's egg colony	Poached egg colony
Hemolysis	Variable	Non-hemolytic	Usually hemolytic
Glycogen and starch fermentation	Positive	Negative	Negative
Most common complication	Paralytic and hemorrhagic	Hemorrhagic	Obstructive lesion in air passage
On broth medium	Form pellicle and a granular deposit	No pellicle only granular deposits	Diffuse turbidity

Diphtheria Toxin

- *Heat Labile single chain three domain Polypeptide exotoxin,* production depends on iron concentration.
- Composed of 2 fragments: Fragment B for binding and fragment A (enzymatic activity) for inactivating elongation factor (EF-2) on nucleus in presence of NAD. Hence, *inhibits protein synthesis.*
- Toxin has special affinity for myocardium, adrenals and nerve endings.
- *Fragment B binds to host cell membrane proteins CD-9 and heparin binding epidermal growth factor and triggers the entry of toxin into all through receptor mediated endocytosm.*
- Toxin is synthesized in precurser form (inactive) in the pseudomembranous lesion.
- Toxin acts both locally and systemically (mainly) while bacilli remain localized. Hence, Diphtheria is *toxemia not bacteremia.*
- Genes coding diptheria toxin are present on corynebacteriophage beta, and a family of closely related corynebacteriophages are responsible for toxigenic conversion of tox- phenotype to tox + phenotype. This is called as *lysogenic conversion.*

> - Diphtheria toxin is an exotoxin made-up of two fragments which inhibits protein synthesis.
> - The standard strain used for toxin production is the Park Williams 8' Strain

- The strain almost universally used for toxin production is the *'Park William 8' Strain*.
- Exotoxin is also produced by *C. ulcerans, C. pseudotuberculosis*.
- Both tox + and tox– strains are infectious.
- Growth under iron limiting condition leads to optimal expression of diptheria toxin.
- Toxin has a special affinity for myocardium, adrenals nerve endings.

Clinical Features

- Cause diphtheria which is localized infection of mucous membrane or skin. It primarily involves respiratory tract.
- The incubation period is 3-4 days, but it can be as short as one day.
- Diphtherias are of following types:
    1. **Respiratory Diphtheria**
        - *MC* type Tonsillopharyngeal (Faucial)
        - *MC* symptoms: Fever, sore throat and weakness.
        - Also cause malignant or hypertoxic or bull neck appearance
        - Laryngeal involvement leads to obstruction of lower larynx and lower airways.
        - **Complications of Respiratory Diphtheria**
            - Mechanical complication (Asphyxia) due to membrane.
            - Systemic effects due to toxin, e.g. myocarditis, peripheral polyneuropathy of descending type.
            - *Myocarditis and neuropathy are the most common and most serious systemic complications.*
              ...Ref CMDT 2014, p 1386
            - Risk is greater when involves larynx or tracheobronchial tree and in children (because of small airway size).
            - Neurologic complication appear during first or second week of illness and begins with dysphagia.
            - Cardiac damage is permanent while recovery of nerve damage is the rule.
            - 1st muscle involve in paralysis - palatopharynges.
            - Ciliary paralysis occur but not pupillary paralysis, i.e. blurred vision with preserved light reflex.
            - System manifestation of diphtheria toxin include weakness and cardiac arrhythmia
              ...Ref Harrison 20/e, p 1098
            - Cause of death is circulatory failure.
    2. **Cutaneous Diphtheria**
        - Punched out ulcers commonly caused by non-toxigenic strains (tox-).
    3. **Invasive Infection**
        - (Rare) Risk factors are pre-existing cardiac abnormality, IV drug abusers, alcoholic cirrhosis.

Diagnosis

- Diagnosis of respiratory diphtheria is usually clinical while cutaneous diphtheria requires lab confirmation.
- Lab diagnosis can be either by demonstration of organism or demonstration of toxigenicity by *in vivo* or *in vitro* test.
    a. **Demonstration of organism:** – By Gram-staining of throat swab.
        - Smear examination in special stain (Neisser's or Albert's stain)
        - Culture in specified media (Loeffler slant, tellurite plate).
    b. **Test for toxigenicity**

In vivo	In vitro
• Done on guinea pigs (can be intra-cutaneous or subcutaneous)	• Elek's gel *ppt.* test
	• PCR for detection of toxigene
	• ELISA
	• Immunochromatographic strip assay (fastest, with in hours)

... *Jawetz 27/e, p 194*

- Matrix-assisted laser desorption/ionisation time of flight (MALDI-TOF) is also a reliable tool for rapid diagnosis of potentially toxigenic corynebacterium species.

- MC type of diphtheria is tonsillopharyngeal
- For treatment initiation, diagnosis is purely clinical
- Elek's precipitation test is a test for toxigenicity

- The pseudomembrane is caused by diphtheria toxin mediated necrosis of respiratory epithelial layer, producing fibrinous coagulative exudate

Treatment

- Most important element in treatment of respiratory diphtheria is antitoxin however, it does not prevent colonization nor eradicates carrier state.
- The recommended dose is 20,000–100,000 units for serious cases; half of the dose to be given intravenously.
- Antitoxin treatment is not indicated in cutaneous diphtheria
- Antibiotics **DOC** Erythromycin or procaine penicillin G. Alternative is Rifampicin or clindamycin.
- Sedatives or hypnotics are contraindicated.
- Glucocorticoids do not reduce the risk of myocarditis or polyneuropathy.

Prevention

- Active immunization by Toxoid is best method to prevent diphtheria. Though active immunization can prevent manifestation of Diphtheria, it cannot prevent carrier stage.
- Active immunization - Combined DPT is used most commonly.
- Pertussis component in DPT increase potency of diphtheria toxoid.
- Toxoid of diphtheria shows Danysz phenomenon and Ehrlich phenomenon.

- Schick test is an intradermal test which provide information regarding immune status of patient
- Pertusis component in DPT increase the potency of diphtheria toxoid.

Schick Test

Intradermal test which provide information regarding:
a. Immune status
b. Hypersensitivity to diphtheria toxin.

In one arm toxin is injected, in other arm heat inactivated toxin is injected and following reaction may be seen.

a. *–ve reaction*	–	No reaction in both arm. Suggest patient is immune to diphtheria.
b. *+ve reaction*	–	Red flush of 10-50 mm within 24-36 hours, reaching its maximum by 4th to 7th day. Control arm shows no change. Patient is susceptible to diphtheria.
c. *Pseudopositive reaction*	–	Red flush equally on both arm, reaction fades very quickly. This is an allergic type of reaction interpreted as Schick's negative.
d. *Combined reaction*	–	Test arm shows +ve, and control arm shows pseudo (+) ve. Dose of vaccine should be reduced.

C. ULCERANS

Transmitted by cow's milk, usually present as pharyngitis and can mimic respiratory diphtheria. Produce a toxin 95% identical to the diphtheria toxin. Transmitted by dog or cat.

C. PSEUDOTUBERCULOSIS (PREISZ NOCARD BACILLUS)

Typically present as suppurative granulamatous lymphadenitis.
Primarily an animal pathogen.

C. MINUTISSIMUM

Cause *Erythrasma* and exhibits coral-red fluorescence under wood's light.

C. PARVUM

Used as immunomodulator.

C. UREALYTICUM

- Frequent skin colonizer mainly in hospital patients.
- Associated with UTI

DIPHTHEROIDS

- Corynebacterium resembling C. diphtheriae occur as natural commensal in throat, skin, conjunctiva
- Stain more uniformly than diphtheria bacilli, possess few or no metachromatic granules
- Common diphtheroids are C. pseudodephtheriticum (C. hofmanni) and C. xerosis.
a. C. hofmanni
   - Urease positive diphtheroid found in throat
   - Occasionally associated with respiratory tract infection, pneumonia and long abscess
   - It has been reported to cause endocarditis
b. C. xerosis
   - Found in conjunctival sac

> - C. minutissimum cause erythrasma

Multiple Choice Questions

1. The following statements are true about DPT vaccine *except*: [AI 04]
   a. Aluminium salt has an adjuvant effect
   b. Whole killed bacteria of *Bordetella pertussis* has an adjuvant effect
   c. Presence of acellular pertussis component increases its immunogenicity
   d. Presence of *H. influenza* type B component increases its immunogenicity

2. Positive Schick's test indicates that the person is:
   a. Immune to diphtheria [AIIMS 07]
   b. Hypersensitive to diphtheria
   c. Susceptible to diphtheria
   d. Susceptible and hypersensitive to diphtheria

3. A child presents with a white patch over the tonsils; diagnosis is made by culture in: [AI 01]
   a. Loeffler medium   b. LJ medium
   c. Blood agar   d. Tellurite medium

4. True about *Corynebacterium diphtheriae* are all *except*:
   a. Iron is required for toxin production [AI 98]
   b. Toxin production is responsible for local reaction
   c. Nonsporing, noncapsular and nonmotile
   d. Toxin production is by lysogenic conversion

5. Ehrlich phenomenon is seen in: [PGI 2011]
   a. Mycobacterium TB   b. Proteus
   c. Staphylococcus   d. Corynebacterium
   e. Mycoplasma

6. True about corynebacterium diphtheria includes all of the following *except*: [AIIMS 07]
   a. Deep invasion is not seen
   b. Elek's test is done for toxigenicity
   c. Metachromatic granules are seen
   d. Toxigenicity is mediated by chromosomal change

7. False about C. diphtheriae [AI 2011]
   a. Toxin production is chromosome mediated
   b. Toxic production is phage mediated
   c. Toxic to heart and neuron
   d. Toxin inhibits protein synthesis

8. In a completely and adequately immunized child against diphtheria, the throat swab was collected. It showed the presence of C. diphtheriae organisms on Albert staining. These organisms can have one of the following properties on further processing: [AIIMS 04]
   a. It can grow on potassium tellurite media
   b. It would show a +ve Elek's gel precipitation test
   c. It can be pathogenic to experimental guinea pig
   d. It can produce cytotoxicity in tissue culture

9. A 12 years old child presents with fever and cervical lymphadenopathy. Oral examination shows a grey membrane on the right tonsil extending to the anterior pillar. Which of the following medium will be ideal for the culture of the throat swab for a rapid identification of the pathogen? [AIIMS 02, 09]
   a. Nutrient agar   b. Blood agar
   c. Loeffler's serum slope
   d. LJ medium

10. Clinical diphtheria is caused by: [PGI June 09]
    a. Corn. diphtheria   b. C. pyogenes
    c. C. ulcerans   d. Streptococcus pyogens
    e. Pseudodiphtheriticum

11. A child with fever and pharyngitis which of the following investigation should not to be done: [AIIMS 00]
    a. Widal test
    b. ASO
    c. Throat swab and culture
    d. Chest X-ray

12. Which of the following is true about diphtheria *except*:
    a. Faucial diphtheria is more dangerous than laryngeal diphtheria [PGI 05]
    b. Laryngeal diphtheria mandates tracheostomy
    c. Child is infectious with faucial diphtheria
    d. Myocarditis may be a complication
    e. Palatal paralysis is irreversible

13. Metachromatic granules are found in: [PGI 00]
    a. Diphtheria   b. Mycoplasma
    c. Gardenerella vaginalis
    d. Chlamydia
    e. Staphylococcus

14. Unimmunized female present with low grade fever and sore throat. Oral examination shows of lesion as shown: [NEET Pattern 2019]

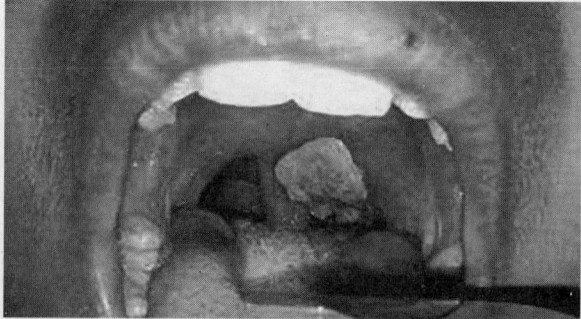

    What is the diagnosis:
    a. Candidiasis   b. Diphtheria
    c. Aphthous ulcer   d. Membranous tonsillitis

15. Dose of diphtheria antitoxin [NEET Pattern 2019]
    a. 2000–5000   b. 5000–1000
    c. 10,000–15,000   d. 20,000–1 Lakh

Explanations and References with Illustrative Answers

1. **Ans. (d) Presence of *H. influenza* type B component increases its immunogenicity**
   Lets consider each choice one by one.

Option 'a':	Two types of diphtheria toxoid are in use now. *Ref. Ananthanarayan 10/e, p 245*
	1. Fluid toxoid (Also known as Formol toxin): Prepared by incubating the toxin with formalin
	2. Adsorbed toxoid : Adsorbed toxoid is purified toxoid adsorbed into insoluble aluminium compounds usually aluminium phosphate or less often hydroxide.
	: Adsorbed toxoid is much more immunogenic than fluid toxoid.
Option 'b':	Pertussis component in DPT (whole killed bacteria of bordetella pertussis) vaccine enhances the potency of the diphtheria toxoid. Most serous complication of DPT is neurological which is primarily due to pertussis component. Duration of immunity after whole cell pertussis vaccination is short lived, with little protection remaining after 10-12 years.
Option 'c':	To reduce complications of whole killed bacteria of pertussis in DPT, acellular vaccine developed. • Protection against pertussis by vaccines correlated best with the production of antibody to pertactin, fimbriae and pertussis toxin. • All acellular pertussis vaccines currently available contain pertussis toxoid. • Acellular vaccine is more immunogenic has less adverse effects. It is given as DTaP. • DTaP has replaced DTP in 1997. DTaP is a tetanus toxoid, reduced diptheria toxoid and acellular pertusis vaccine formulated for adolescent and adults. *.... Harrison 20/e, p 1058*
Option 'd':	Quadriple vaccine of DPT with H. influenza B is available in India but conjugate vaccine (e.g. Hib vaccine) do not interfere with immunogenicity of simultaneously given other vaccines. *.... Ghai 6/e, p 197*

2. **Ans. (d) Susceptible and hypersensitive to diphtheria** *Ref. Ananthanarayan 10/e, p 86, 245*

   ### Schick Test
   - Intradermal test which provide information regarding:
     a. Immune status,
     b. Hypersensitivity and susceptibility to diphtheria toxin before giving active immunization.
   - In one arm toxin is injected (test arm) and in other arm heat inactivated toxin is injected (control arm).

	Type of reaction	Observation	Inference
i.	Negative reaction	No reaction in both arm (toxin is neutralized by circulating antitoxin)	No susceptibility. No hypersensitivity Patient is immune to diphtheria
ii.	Positive reaction	No change in control arm. Red flush in test arm that persist	No hypersensitivity Susceptibility present
iii.	Pseudopositive reaction (Schick's negative)	Red flush equally on both arm that fades very quickly	Hypersensitivity present No susceptibility
iv.	Combined reaction	Test arm shows positive and control arm shows pseudo- positive reaction	Hypersensitivity present Susceptibility present Dose of vaccine should be reduced

   Remember:
   - Antitoxin level of 0.1 IU unit or more per ml of blood is considered as index of immunity. *.... AA 10/e, p 245*
   - Schick test is no longer in use. The level of antitoxin, is assesed by passive hemagglutination or by neutralization in cell culture.

3. **Ans. (a) Loeffler medium** *Ref. Ananthanarayan 10/e, p 242*
   In a child with white patch over tonsils, probable diagnosis is diphtheria.
   Culture media for corynebacterium are:
   i. *Loeffler serum slope:* Growth is very rapid and colonies *seen in 6-8 hr*, before other bacteria grows. It is also used for *M. tuberculosis*. Diphtheria is emergency condition, so Loeffler's slope is preferred media in this child.
   ii. *Tellurite blood agar media:* Selective media but growth is delayed and may take about 2 days to appear.

> **Remember:**
> - LJ media, is for Mycobacteria TB.
> - McLeods and Hoyle's are modified Tellurite media.

Diagnosis of Diphtheria

i. *Microscopy:* Stained smear examination. Smears are stained with Neisser's or Albert's stain (bacilli with metachromatic granules) Loeffler Methylene blue, Gram- or Leishman stained smear (to rule out spirochetes)
ii. *Isolation by culture:*
   - Swabs are inoculated on:
   - Loeffler's serum slope (growth is rapid): For rapid diagnosis.
   - Tellurite blood agar (growth is delayed but it is particularly important in isolation of bacilli from convalescent, contacts, carriers): Selective media.
   - Blood agar (for differentiating staphylococcal and streptococcal pharyngitis).
iii. *Demonstration of toxicity of isolated strain:*
   In vivo test – done by infected broth emulsion of culture subacutaneously (animal will die) and intracutaneously into (animal will not die) guinea pigs.
   In vitro test – Elek's gel precipitation test, tissue culture test on agar overlay of cell culture monolayer.
   – ELISA
   – PCR for detection of toxigene

Control of Diphtheria

i. *Cases*
   - Antitoxin + penicillin or erythromycin   ... *Park 22/e, p 152*
ii. *Carriers*
   - Erythromycin
iii. *Contacts*
   a. When primary immunization or booster dose was received within the previous 2 years.
      - No further treatment.
   b. When primary immunization or booster dose was received more than 2 years ago.
      - Only a booster dose of diphtheria toxoid.
   c. Nonimmunized close contacts:
      - Prophylactic penicillin or erythromycin
      - 1000-2000 units of diphtheria antitoxin
      - Active immunization against diphtheria.
iv. *Community*
   - Only effective control is by active immunization with diphtheria toxoid of all infants with subsequent booster doses every 10 years thereafter.

> **Remember:** Vaccine 'being a toxoid' is not directed against organism and hence immunization does not prevent carrier state which is due to organism not due to toxin

4. Ans. (b) Toxin production is responsible for local reaction   *Ref. Ananthanarayan 10/e, p 241; Jawetz 27/e, p 194*
"*Mechanical complications of diphtheria are due to the membrane while the systemic effects are due to the toxin.*"
- Toxin acts *mainly systemically though there are partial local effects.*
- It has affinity for myocardium, adrenals and nerve endings.
- Toxin acts by inactivating EF-2 *thus inhibiting protein synthesis*.
- Toxin production is influenced by *iron* concentration in the medium. Toxin production is optimal at 0.14 µg/ml and is suppressed at 0.5 µg/ml.
- Toxigenicity of diphtheria bacillus depends on symbiotic bacteriophages, so it shows *lysogenic or phage conversion* i.e. nontoxigenic strain → toxigenic strain by infecting with beta phage.

> **Remember:**
> - Corynebacteria are gram-positive, non-acid fast, non-sporing, non-capsulated, non-motile bacteria.
> - It contains polar bodies or volutin or Babes-Ernst or metachromatic granules of poly-metaphosphate which are more gram-positive.
> - Granules are also stained by Loeffler's methylene blue, Albert's, Neisser's and Ponder's stain.

5. **Ans. (d) Corynebacterium** *Ref. Internet sources*
   - Diphtheria toxin undergoes spontaneous denaturation into toxoid. This toxoid also combines equally with antitoxin. So, in any sample, it would be difficult to estimate the level of toxin as sample will contain a variable amount of toxoid which will vitiate standardisation of antitoxin.
   - Due to the above mentioned issue, two other units for measurement of toxin have been introduced, the Lo and L+ doses.
     - Lo (Limes nul) dose of diphtheria toxin is the largest amount of toxin that when mixed with one unit of antitoxin and injected subcutaneously into a 250 g guinea pig, will on an average cause no observable reaction.
     - L+ (Limes tod) dose of diptheria toxin is the smallest amount of toxin that when mixed with one unit of antitoxin and injected subcutaneously into a 250g guinea pig will on an average kill the animal with in 96 hours.
   - It would be expected that the difference between the L+ dose and Lo dose would be equal to 1 MLD. But when the estimations are actually made, it is found to vary from 10 to 100 MLD or more. This discrepancy is due to the presence of varying amount of toxoid in toxin preparation. This is called as *Ehrlich phenomenon*.

6. **Ans. (d) Toxigenicity is mediated by chromosomal change** *Ref. Ananthanarayan 10/e, p 240*
   "*Corynebacteriophage beta carries the structural gene (tox+) encoding diphtheria toxin and a family of closely related corynebacteriophage are responsible for toxigenic conversion of tox– C.diphtheria to tox+ phenotype.*"
   - Elek's gel precipitation test is in *vitro* test for toxin detection.

7. **Ans. (a) Toxin production chromosome mediated** *Ref. Ananthanarayan 8/e, p 233, 9/e, p 238; Jawetz 27/e, p 193*
   Already explained

   Note: Toxicity of corynebacterium is under control of phage gene, but the invasiveness is under control of bacterial gene.

8. **Ans. (a) It can grow on potassium tellurite media** *Ref. Ananthanarayan 10/e, p 242*
   This child is carrier of diphtheria.
   - Postassium tellurite is selective media for isolation of diphtheria bacillus from convulescent contact, carriers.
   - Other three tests are done for testing virulence only when isolated strain is *C. diphtheriae*.

9. **Ans. (c) Loeffler's serum slope** *Ref. Ananthanarayan 10/e, p 242*
   Already explained

10. **Ans. (a) Corn. diphtheria** *Ref. Harrison 17/e 890; 893; 19/e 980*
    Clinical diphtheria is caused only by *C. diphtheria*.
    C. ulcerans can cause diphtheria like lesions (but not diphtheria)

11. **Ans. (a) Widal test** *Ref. Ananthanarayan 10/e, p 242*
    Widal is test for diagnosing typhoid which is not a cause of pharyngitis, so there is no need to perform widal in this child.

12. **Ans. (a) and (e) Faucial diphtheria is more dangerous than laryngeal diphtheria; and Palatal paralysis is irreversible**
    Ref. Harrison 20/e, p 1096

Diphtheria

- *Causative agent* – Corynebacterium diphtheriae (Gram positive bacillus)
- *Incubation period* – 2-6 days
- *Depending on site diptheria is classified as:*
  - Nasal diphtheria: Mildest, Toxemia is minimal.
  - Faucial diphtheria (most common) = Nasopharyngeal diphtheria: More severe than nasal diphtheria.
  - Laryngotracheal diphtheria: Most severe, maximum obstructive symptom, tracheostomy may be essential.
- *Complications:*
  - Myocarditis—Occurs towards the end of 1st or begining of 2nd week.
  - Peripheral neuropathy of descending type.
  - Renal failure.

> **Remember:**
> - Cardiac damage is permanent while recovery of nerve damage is rule.
> - Myocarditis and neuropathy are the most common complication.
> - Most common site of pseudomembrane is tonsillopharyngeal region

13. Ans. (a) Diphtheria *Ref. Ananthanrayan 8/e, p 232, 9/e, p 236*
Metachromatic Granules

- It is type of *intracytoplasmic* inclusions characteristically seen in diphtheria bacilli.
- Also known as *volutin* or *metachromatic* or *Babes-Ernst granules*.
- Strongly *basophilic* bodies consist of polymetaphosphate.
- These granules are composed of polymetaphosphate. They are reservoir of energy and phosphate.
- They are more frequent in cells growing under nutritional deficient condition.

> **Remember:**
> - Dorset egg media is for *M. tuberculosis*.
> - McConkey is for differentiating between lactose and non-lactose fermenters of Enterobacteriacea.
> - Metachromatic granules also seen in *B. pertussis*.

14. Ans. (b) Diphtheria *Ref. Harrison 20/e, p 1096, Dhingra ENT 6/e p 260*

This is the characteristic pseudomembrane on fauces and soft palate. "
The presence of pharyngeal pseudomembrane or an extensive exudate should prompt consideration of diphtheria"
Ref. Harrison 20/e, p 1096

Diphtheria should be considered in patients with severe pharagngitis particularly when there is difficulty in swallowing respiratory compromise or sign of systemic disease

- Treatment: Prompt administration of diphtheria antitoxin
    - Antitoxin dose depends on the site involved and is in the range of 20,000–100,000.
    - Dose is 20,000–40,000 for diphtheria in less than 48h or when membrane is confined to tonstil only.
    - 80,000–100,000, if disease is more than 48h old or membrane is extensive
    - Penicillin and erythromycin are the antibiotics of choice

15. Ans. (d) 20,000–1 lakh *Ref. Ananthanrayan 10/e, p 245; Dhingra ENT 6/e.p 260*
Already explained

NEET Pattern Questions

1. True about corynebacterium diphtheriae:
   a. All types produce toxin
   b. Toxin production is dependent upon critical concentration of iron
   c. Heat stable toxin
   d. Inhibit cAMP
   [Ref. Ananthanarayan, 10/e, p 240]

> Toxigenicity of diphtheria depends on the intracellular presence of corynephages (tox+)
> Optium Ionc. of iron for toxin production is 0.1 mg/l while a concentration of 0.5 mg/l inhibits toxin formation

2. Lysogenic conversion is seen:
   a. Diphtheria
   b. Salmonella
   c. Staphylococcus
   d. E coli   [Ref. Ananthanarayan, 10/e, p 240]

3. A child come with fever, cold, cough, membrane over tonsils; nasal swab is taken, culture should be done on which medium for earliest diagnosis:
   a. Loffelers serum slop
   b. L.J. media
   c. MC Conkey's Agar
   d. Citrate media   [Ref. Ananthanarayan, 10/e, p 242]

4. Commonest complication of diphtheria:
   a. Myocarditis   b. Neuropathy
   c. Endocarditis   d. Pericarditis
   [Ref. CMDT 2014, p 1386]

5. C. diphtheriae is also called as:
   a. Koch's bacillus
   b. Roux bacillus
   c. Klebs-Loeffler bacillus
   d. Yersin bacillus   [Ref. Ananthanarayan, 10/e, p 238]

> Diphtheria bacillus was first observed by Klebs and was first cultivated by Loeffler, so the name Klebs Loeffler bacillus.
> Roux and Yersin discovered the diphtheria exotoxin

6. Receptor for diphtheria toxin lies at:
   a. Cell membrane
   b. Mucous membrane
   c. Nucleus
   d. None   [Ref. Jawetz, 27/e, p 193]

> B subunit of diphtheria toxin binds to host cell membrane protein CD-9 and HB-EGF which triggers the entry of A subunit into the cell through endocytosis.

7. Schick test is for:
   a. Susceptibility to diphteria
   b. Susceptibility to tetanus
   c. Susceptibility to scarler fever
   d. Susceptibility to RF   [Ref. Ananthanarayan 10/e, p 245]

> The test is no longer used due to availability of effective and safer toxoid preparation.

8. Confirmatory tests for C. diphtheriae:
   a. Serological tests
   b. Isolation in selective media
   c. Tests for toxin   [Ref. Ananthanarayan, 10/e, p 242]

9. True about diphtheria toxin:
   a. Heat stable
   b. Acts through cGMP
   c. Consists of three polypeptides
   d. Special affinity for brain   [Ref. Javetz, 27/e, p 193]

10. True about Corynebacterium diphtheriae:
    a. Schick test is done for resistance
    b. Gram positive organism
    c. Schick test is an intramuscular test
    d. Most important treatment is antibiotic
    [Ref. Ananthanarayan, 10/e, p 239]

11. Earliest growth of diphtheria is detect on which media:
    a. Potassium tellurite media with iron
    b. McConkey's agar
    c. Dorset egg medium
    d. Loeffler's serum slope   [Ref. Ananthanarayan, 10/e, p 242]

12. Chinese letter configuration is seen in: (2016)
    a. Cl tetani
    b. Cl perfringens
    c. Strept salivarius
    d. C. diphtheriae   [Ref. Ananthanarayan, 10/e, p 238]

> Bacilli are arranged in characteristic pairs, palisades. They often appears at various angles to each other resembling the letters 'V' or 'Y'. This has been called as Chinese letter on cuneiform arrangement.

 Ans.
1. b. Toxin...   2. a. Diphtheria   3. a. Loffeler's   4. a. Myocarditis   5. c. Klebs-Loeffler bacillus
6. a. Cell membrane   7. a. Susceptibility... 8. b. Isolation in... 9. c. Consists of... 10. b. Gram positive...
11. d. Loeffler's ... 12. d. C. diphtheriae

13. **Most dangerous type of diptheria:** (2016)
    a. Facial
    b. Laryngeal
    c. Nasal
    d. Cutaneous
    [Ref. Dhingra ENT 6/e, p 260]

14. **Erythrasma is caused by:** (2018)
    a. S. pyogenes
    b. Corynebacterium miniutissimum
    c. S. aureus
    d. Ricketessiae
    [Ref. Ananthanarayan 7/e, p 240, 9/e, p 242]

> **Erythrasma is a localized infection of the stratum corneum usually affecting the axilla and grain.**
> - It is caused by a lipophilic Corynebacterium, C. miniutissimum.
> - Bacteria can be grown readily in media containing 20% fetal calf serum.

15. **Corynebacterum other than diphtheriae carrying toxin:**
    a. Corynebacterium ulcerans (2016)
    b. Corynebacterium xerosis
    c. Corynebacterium striatum
    d. Corynebacterium urealyticum
    [Ref. Greenwood 18/e, p 203; AA 10/e, p 246]

> C. ulcerans produce two types of toxin one identical to diphtheria toxin whereas the other one resemble C. pseudotuberculosis.

16. **Beta phage is seen in:** (2016)
    a. Bacillus anthracis
    b. Corynebacterium diphtheriae
    c. Clostridium botulinum
    d. Peptostreptococci
    [Ref. Jawetz, 27/e, p 193]

Ans.
13. b. Laryngeal
14. b. Corynebac...
15. a. Corynebacterium...
16. b. Corynebacterium diphtheriae

Actinomycetes and Bacillus

CHAPTER 12

ACTINOMYCETES

- Transitional forms between bacteria and fungi.
- Gram-positive, nonmotile, nonsporing, noncapsulated filaments.
- It includes:
  a. Actinomyces
  b. Nocardia

ACTINOMYCES

- Anaerobic Gram-positive bacillus cause: Lumpy jaw (in cattle) and actinomycosis in human.

> - Branching Gram positive bacilli.
> - Grows best under anaerobic or micro-aerophilic conditions with the addition of 5–10% CO_2
> - Actinomyces israelii is the most common cause of human actinomycosis.

Actinomycosis

- **It is endogenous** infection since Actinomyces normally present in mouth, intestine, vagina.
- MC causative agent A. israelii.
- A. israelii is differentiated from other atinomyces species by gel diffusion and immunofluorescence.
- Usually a cooperative disease, i.e. Actinomycosis is usually accompanied by other associate bacteria which may enhance the pathogenic effect.
- Characterized by indurated swelling (mainly in connective tissue), suppuration, multiple sinuses towards skin with discharge of sulphur (black) granules.

Types of Actinomycosis

- **MC type cervicofacial**
  - MC site of cervicofacial is lower jaw (lumpy jaw) often adjacent to carious tooth.
- **Abdominal** – Usually around caecum.
- Thoracic
- **Pelvic** – In association with **IUCDs**.
- Mycetoma

> Most common type of actinomycosis: Cervicofacial.
> MC site of cervicofacial actinomycosis: Lower jaw

Mycetoma

- Painless localized woody induration without systemic symptoms. Granulomatous involvement of subcutaneous and deeper tissue induced by traumatic inoculation of saprophytic fungi or bacteria.
- **MC site foot,** present as tumor with multiple discharging sinus called as **Madura foot.**
- **MC cause** is fungi called as eumycotic mycetoma/Maduramycosis/Madura foot. Black granules, stout filament seen on microscopy.
- Fungal agents of mycetoma:
  - *Pseudallescheria boydii*
  - *Madurella mycetomatis*
  - *Madurella grisea*
  - *Exophiala jeanselmei*
  - *Acremonium falciforme*
- Bacterial mycetoma are usually caused by *Actinomyces, Nocardia, Streptomyces, Nocardiopsis*.
- Even *S. aureus* and other pyogenic bacteria may cause mycetoma like lesion called **botryomycosis.**
- In actinomycotic mycetoma - Granules are white to yellow and thin filaments seen on microscopy.

  Treatment
  - *Actinomycetoma:* Streptomycin + Dapsone or cotrimoxazole
  - *Eumycetoma of Madurella mycetoma:* Keto/Itra-conazole
  - *Other Eumycetoma:* rarely responds to chemotherapy.

> **Actinomycetoma**
> **Mycetoma** caused by filamentous branching bacteria. The most common causes of actinomycetoma are actinomodura madurae, streptomyces somaliensis, Actinomodura pelletieri, Nocardia asteroides and Nocardia brasiliensis.

- Most common site of actinomycetoma is foot   ...*Harrison, 20/e, p1222*

Diagnosis of Actinomycosis

- Specimen
  - Sputum, aspirations, biopsies
  - Shake it in test tube with saline - Sulphur granules can be seen by naked eyes in some case and by microscope in remaining (see color plate pg xxiv for related image).
- Microscopy
  - Granules are in fact, bacterial colonies
  - Gram-positive filaments in the form of radiating *club shaped = sun ray appearance* seen.
  - Club is formed due to antigen-antibody reaction
  - Culture on solid media-shows spidery colonies which later develop into "molar tooth" colonies.

> **Note:** Though sulfur granules are characteristic of actinomycosis, also they can be seen in mycetoma and botyromycosis.

Treatment
- **Penicillin** is *drug of choice*

NOCARDIA

> **Nocardia**
> - Gram positive, branched, strictly aerobic bacteria, that resemble rapidly growing mycobacteria.
> - **MC cause of pulmonary nocardiosis:** N.asteroides.
> - MC cause of cutaneous nocardiosis is N. brasiliensis.

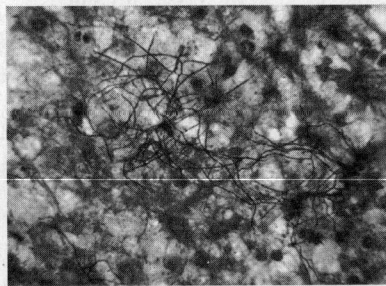

- Filamentous, nonsporing, acid fast, rod shaped bacteria.
- **Aerobic, partially urease positive, catalase positive, partially acid fast**, causing exogenous infection, Nocardiosis (which refers to invasive disease).
- *MC* species associated with invasive disease **N. asterodes.**
- *MC* **risk factor** - Contact with soil or vegetable matter.
- Cell mediated immunity is important as neutrophil limit its growth but not kill them efficiently.
- Nocardiosis is usually initiated by inhalation and there is no person to person transmission.
    ... *Jawetz 27/e, p 299*

Clinical Manifestation

- *MC* manifestation is **pneumonia** and disseminated disease which follows inhalation of bacteria.
- *So, manifestation can be divided into:*
  a. *Respiratory tract disease* – *MC* **is pneumonia.** Prominent cough, small amount of thick purulent sputum that is odourless.
  b. *Extrapulmonary dissemination* – *MC* site **brain.** Typical manifestation is subacute abscess usually **supratentorial.**
    ... *Harrison 20/e, p 1217*

c. *Disease following transcutaneous inoculation* – Cellulitis, lymphocutaneous syndrome (most cases associated with *N. brasiliensis*), actinomycetoma (old fistula disappear with appearance of new fistula) (see color plate pg xxiv for related image).

Diagnosis

- **First step:** Examine sputum or pus for crooked, branching (See color plate, pg xxv for related image), beaded, Gram-positive, acid fast (with weak acid) filaments, It also takes silver stains.
- In nocardial pneumonia sputum smears are often negative and diagnosis may require sampling through bronchoscopy or lung aspiration.
- Transtracheal aspiration should be avoided as it frequently leads to cellulitis in tissue around puncture wound.
- *Culture:*
  - It use paraffin as carbon source *so paraffin baiting is used for isolation.*
  - Relatively slow to grow colony may take up to 2 weeks to appear.
  - *Selective media* (Colistin-nalidixic acid agar, modified Thayer-Martin Agar or buffered charcoal yeast agar) improves recovery from mixed flora ... Harrison 20/e, p 1218
  - Nocardia grow relatively slowly; colonies may take up to 2 weeks to appear
  - Selective growth is favored by inoculation at 45°C
  - Species is identified by analysis of 16S r RNA gene sequences.

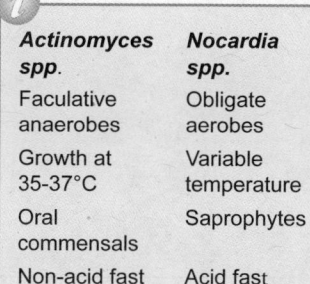

Actinomyces spp.	*Nocardia spp.*
Facultative anaerobes	Obligate aerobes
Growth at 35-37°C	Variable temperature
Oral commensals	Saprophytes
Non-acid fast	Acid fast

Treatment

- **DOC** Trimethoprim - Sulfamethoxazole
- **Best** alternative oral drug minocycline
- **Best** parenteral drug amikacin.

Bacillus

- Genus consist of **sporogenous aerobic** Gram-positive bacilli.
- They are generally *motile* with peritrichous flagella *except* anthrax bacilli.
- Spores are heat resistant and constitute the most common contaminants of bacteriological culture media.
- Its important species are:
  1. Bacillus anthracis
  2. B. cereus.

B. anthrax:
- Large nonmotile, sporing bacillus that grows on all media forming colonies with ground glass surface appearance.
- Capsule and toxin are encoded by plasmid PXO_2 and PXO_1 respectively.

BACILLUS ANTHRACIS

- *First* pathogenic bacteria to be observed under microscope.
- *First* bacterium used for preparation of attenuated vaccine.
- *First* communicable disease shown to be transmitted by inoculation of infected blood.
- *First* bacillus to be isolated in pure culture and shown to possess spores.

Morphology

- Nonmotile, capsulated sporing Gram-positive bacilli.
- Aerobic and facultative anaerobic
- Capsule is *polypeptide* in nature (*exception since usually capsule is of lipopolysaccharide in nature*).
- Bacilli arranged in Bamboo stick/box car like appearance.
- Colonies of *B. anthracis* are round and have a *"cut glass"* appearance in transmitted light.
- On staining with polychrome methylene blue, it shows M'Fadyeans reaction; which represents capsular material.
- *Spores* – Used in biological warfare or **bioterrorism.** Formed in culture or soil but never in animal body. Not stained by ordinary methods. Not cause bulging of vegetative cells (in comparison of clostridia spores).

Mc-Fadyean's Reaction, Strings of pearls reaction: Differentiate between B. cereus and B. anthracis

Culture

- **Selective** medium: **PLET** medium.
- On *Agar plates* – frosted glass appearance seen.
- On microscopy it has Medusa head appearance.
- On *Gelatin stab* – characteristic Inverted Fir tree appearance.
- *Solid Media* with penicillin – String of pearl reaction.
- **Cut glass appearance** – In transmitted light.

Resistance

- Bacilli remain viable in bone marrow for a week and in skin for 2 weeks.
- Spores are destructed by oxidizing agents H_2O_2, 4% $KMnO_4$, formaldehyde (called as *Duckering*)

Virulence Factor

i. *Capsular poly - D-glutamic acid:*
   - Plasmid mediated, inhibit phagocytosis. Loss of plasmid cause loss of virulence (basis of live attenuated anthrax spore vaccine).
ii. **Toxin:** Plasmid coded, complex of **three fractions:**
   - *Factor I or edema factor (EF)* – Activated only intracellularly increases cAMP.
   - *Factor II or protective antigen factor (PA)* – It is the fraction that binds to receptors on target cell surface and provides attachment sites for EF and LF. *Antibody* to PA is protective because it blocks first step in toxin activity i.e. binding to target cells.
   - Lethal factor (LF) or factor III - cause cell death. The lethal toxin stimulates macrophages to produce IL-1β and INF α.
   - EF + PA = Edema toxin
   - LF + PA = Lethal toxin

- Cutaneous anthrax is the commonest type of anthrax.
- It is characterized by malignant pustule.

Disease

- Cause anthrax which occurs primarily in herbivores (*zoonosis*).
- *Humans* are *more resistant* to anthrax than herbivores.
- Transmitted by spores, by contact with infected animals or contaminated animal products, insects bites, ingestion or inhalation.
- *Human anthrax is of 3 types:*
  a. *Cutaneous anthrax* (Hide Porter's disease): *MC* (95%);
     - Characterized by *malignant pustule,* i.e. central eschar surrounded by nonpitting edema.
     - Toxemia always present.
     - Smear of vesicle fluid is used to confirm diagnosis by culture and animal inoculation.
  b. *Pulmonary/inhalational anthrax/Wool Sorter's disease:*
     - Typically cause hemorrhagic mediastinitis. Characteristic X-ray finding is *symmetric mediastinal widening.*
  c. *Gastrointestinal anthrax:*
     - Rare form

B. anthracis:	B. cereus
Nonmotile	Motile
Capsulated:	Non-capsulated
Susceptible to γ phage	Non-susceptible

Laboratory Diagnosis

- *Microscopy:*
  - Gram-positive bacilli with M'Fadyean's reaction - presumptive diagnosis made.
  - Immunofluorescent microscopy can confirm identification.
- If sample is putrid, *Ascoli's thermoprecipitin (ring precipitin)* test is done which demonstrate anthrax antigen in tissue extract.
- Test for *antibody by immunoassays* are useful in *confirming* diagnosis.

Treatment

- **DOC** Penicillin
- **In Penicillin allergy** – Ciprofloxacin, erythromycin, tetracycline or chloramphenicol.

BACILLUS CEREUS

- Resembles *B. anthrax except* that it is *motile (Swarming), non-capsulated, not susceptible to gamma bacteriophage, not show 'string of pearls' reaction.*
- Isolated from feces and other sources on **MYPA** (mannitol, egg yolk, phenol red polymyxin agar).
- It causes two type of food poisoning manifest as nausea, vomiting and abdominal cramps (seen in both emetic and diarrheal types).

Features	Diarrheal type	Emetic type
Incubation period	8-16 hr	1-5 hr
Food	Cooked meat and vegetables	Exclusively by rice
Enterotoxin	Resemble heat labile toxin of **E. coli** Either preformed or produced in intestine	Resemble heat stable toxin of **S. aureus** Already preformed in rice
Clinical features	Fever, vomiting rare	Diarrhea is not common
Serotype	2, 6, 8, 9, 10, 12	1, 3, 5

Remember:

- Presence of B. cereus in patient stool is not sufficient for diagnosis since it may be present in normal stool specimen; concentration of 10^5 or more bacteria per gram of stool is considered diagnostic.
  ... *Jawetz 27/e, p 182*
- It also causes eye infections; localized and systemic infections (occur in patient with medical device or IV drug users).

Note: In 2001 there were may cases of anthrax in USA. At that time, B. anthrax was used as bioterrorism agent. Spores of bacillus in powdered form were packed in envelop and posted. After this experience CDC (Center for Disease Control) have prepared guidelines for identification of anthrax. Any large non-motile Gram (+)ve bacteria which is non-hemolytic and catalase positive is presumed to be anthrax bacilli for treatment purpose.

Multiple Choice Questions

Baccilus

1. An abattoir worker developed pustule which later progress to necrotic ulcer. Which of the following stain is useful demonstration of organism from smear made from pustule? [AI 07; AIIMS May 2012, 06]
   a. Polychromic methylene blue
   b. Chalkofluor white
   c. Geimsa
   d. Modified kinyon stain

2. A man, after skinning a dead animal, developed a pustule on his hand. A smear prepared from the lesion showed the presence of gram-positive bacilli in long chains which were positive for McFadyean's reaction. The most likely aetiological agent is: [AI 04]
   a. Clostridium tetani   b. Listeria monocytogenes
   c. Bacillus anthracis   d. Actinomyces sp

3. An abattoir worker presented with a malignant pustule on his hand that progressed to form an ulcer. Smear was taken from the ulcer and sent to laboratory for investigation. The diagnosis is: [AIIMS Nov 2012]
   a. Cutaneous anthrax
   b. Carbuncle
   c. Ulcerating melanoma
   d. Infected rodent ulcer

4. Characteristic of Bacillus cereus food poisoning is:
   a. Presence of fever   [AIIMS Nov 10]
   b. Presence of abdominal pain
   c. Absence of vomiting
   d. Absence of diarrhoea

5. Which of the following is true regarding anthrax:
   a. M'Fadyean reaction shows capsule   [PGI 01]
   b. Humans are usually resistant to infection
   c. Less than 100 spores can cause pulmonary infection
   d. Gram stain shows organism with bulging spores
   e. Sputum microscopy helps in diagnosis

6. Noninvasive diarrhea can be caused by the following?
   a. Shigella   b. B. cereus   [AI 09]
   c. Salmonella   d. Y. enterocolitica

7. A patient present with vomiting he had eaten rice 6 hour before. The most probable cause is: [PGI 07]
   a. Bacillus cereus   b. Staph. aureus
   c. Cl. difficle   d. All

8. Malignant pustule is caused by: [AIIMS Nov. 10]
   a. B. anthracis   b. Leishmaniasia
   c. Basal cell carcinoma   d. Pyoderma

9. Malignant pustule is/are seen in infection with:
   a. Treponema pallidum   [PGI 11]
   b. Compylobacter granulomatosis
   c. Bacillus anthracis
   d. H. ducreyi
   e. Pseudomonas aeruginosa

Actinomycosis

10. Which of the following is the most predominant constituent of sulfur granules of Actinomycosis:
    a. Organisms   [AIIMS 04, 02]
    b. Neutrophils and monocytes
    c. Monocytes and lymphocytes
    d. Eosinophils

11. A farmer present with multiple discharging sinuses in the leg not responding to antibiotics. Most likely diagnosis is: [AIIMS 02]
    a. Madurella   b. Actinomycetoma
    c. Nocardia   d. Sporothrix

12. Actinomycotic mycetoma is caused by: [PGI 05]
    a. Actinomyces   b. Nocardiasis
    c. Streptomyces   d. Madura mycosis
    e. Staphylococcus

13. Which of the following is/are true about actinomyces:
    a. Causes Actinomycetoma   [PGI 17]
    b. Most commonly causes cervico-facial actinomycosis
    c. Can be detected directly from sample by FISH
    d. Drug of choice is penicillin
    e. It is aerobic and acid fast

Nocardia

14. Characteristic infection of Nocardia asteroides is:
    a. Diarrhea   [AI 2012]
    b. Secondary dissemination to liver
    c. Brain abscess
    d. Colonic diverticula

15. The causative organism of Mycetoma is: [PGI 02]
    a. Nocardia   b. Dimorphic fungus
    c. Aspergillus   d. Dermatophytes

16. Nocardia is stained by: [AIIMS 08]
    a. Acid fast stain   b. Kiram's stain
    c. Alcian blue   d. Mucin stain

17. A clinical specimen was obtained from the wound of a patient diagnosed as nocardiosis. For the selective isolation of Nocardia sp. which one of the following would be the best method: [AIIMS 04]
    a. Paraffin bait technique
    b. Castaneda's culture method
    c. Craige's culture method
    d. Hair bait technique

18. Nocardia is differentiated from Actinomyces by:
    a. Gram stain   [PGI 02]
    b. ZN stain
    c. Nocardia causes mycetoma, Actinomyces do not
    d. Nocardia is faculative anaerobe

19. True about Madura foot?   [PGI Dec 2008]
    a. Can erode bones
    b. Spread to lymph nodes
    c. Most commonly occur in hand
    d. Slow growing
    e. Antibiotic has no role

20. A patient comes with history of unresponsive fever and cough. X-ray revealed pneumonia. Sputum examination showed gram positive, partially acid fast bacteria with branching filaments that grows on sheep blood agar. The most likely etiologic agents is: [AI 2011]
    a. Actinomycetes   b. Nocardia
    c. Aspergillosis   d. Pneumococci

21. Identify the organism in the Slide?   [AIIMS 2017]
    a. Nocardia species
    b. Mycobacterium tuberculosis
    c. Mycobacterium leprae
    d. Actinomyces species

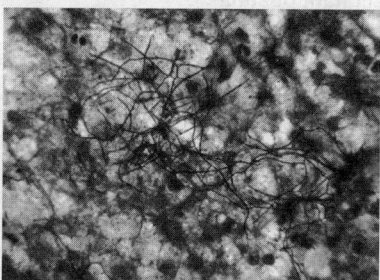

Explanations and References with Illustrative Answers

1. **Ans. (a) Polychromic methylene blue** *Ref. Ananthanarayan 10/e, p 249*

   It is case of cutaneous anthrax in abattoir worker (slaughter house worker).
   - Cutaneous anthrax is also common in dock workers (who carry loads of hides and skin on their bare backs), butchers, farmers, veterinarians, workers involved in meat packing.
   - Pulmonary anthrax is common in workers of wool factories.
   - Intestinal anthrax occur in communities who eat carcasses of animals dying of anthrax.
   - Stains used in case of anthrax:
     – Gram's stain
     – Sudan black B
     – Polychrome methylene blue (stains capsule = M'Fadyean reaction).

2. **Ans. (c) Bacillus anthracis** *Ref. Ananthanarayan 10/e, p 249; Harrison 20/e, p 1769; 20/e 936*

   This is typical presentation of cutaneous anthrax.

   ### Bacillus Anthracis
   - Gram-positive, aerobic, catalase positive, non-motile, capsulated **(polypeptide in nature),** spore forming bacilli.
   - Spore are formed in culture or in the soil but never in the animal body during life and do not cause bulging of vegetative cell (In comparison of Clostridium spores).
   - Spores are highly stable and can remain viable for decades. This remarkable stability makes them an ideal bio-weapon.
   - Chain of bacilli have bamboo stick or box car like appearance.
   - When blood film containing anthrax bacilli is stained with polychrome methylene blue and then examined under microscope, amorphous purplish material representing capsular material is noticed around bacilli. This is called **M'Fadyean's reaction (characteristic of anthrax bacilli)** and is used for presumptive diagnosis of anthrax in animals.

   ### Cultural Characteristic
   - Agar   : **Frosted glass** appearances
   - Microscopy   : **Medusa head** appearance
   - Gelatin stab   : **Inverted fir tree** appearance
   - **String of perals reaction** : **For differentiating B. anthrax from B. cereus and other aerobic spore bearers.**

Clinical Features

- Anthrax is zoonotic disease primarily of herbivores. Humans are more resistant than animals.
- Human become infected when spores are introduced into body by contact with infected animal or contaminated animal products, insect bites, ingestion, inhalation.

TYPES OF HUMAN ANTHRAX		
Cutaneous anthrax (Hide Porter's disease) (= Malignant pustule)	**Pulmonary anthrax (Wool Sorter's disease) (= Inhalation anthrax)**	**Gastrointestinal anthrax**
• *MC* type of anthrax	• *Earliest symptom* are typically viral like prodrome with fever, malaise, abdominal or chest symptoms	• Rare form
• Usual sites arms, hand, face, neck	• 100% fatal though with prompt treatment, survival is possible	• High mortality rate
• Characterized by presence of malignant pustule – Central necrotic painless lesion covered by black eschar surrounded by satellite lesions	• Characteristic X-ray mediastinal widening, hemorrhagic pleural effusion	• Primary lesion is most often located on tonsil
• Generally resolved spontaneously but 10-20% patients develop fatal septicemia		

Remember:
- 10,000 spores are required to produce lethal disease in 50% of animals (LD_{50}). Though sometime few as minimum as one to three spore may be adequate to produce disease.
- Incubation period of cutaneous anthrax is 1 to 7 days while that of pulmonary anthrax may be as long as 6 weeks...... *Jawetz 25/e, p 166*

3. **Ans. (a) Cutaneous anthrax** *Ref. Ananthanarayan 8/e, 242, 9/e, p 247*

   Cutaneous anthrax is also known as Hide Porter's disease or malignant pustule

   Remember: Carbuncle is infection of 2-3 hair follicles

4. **Ans. (b) Presence of abdominal pain** *Ref. Ananthanarayan 10/e, p 253*

   Abdominal pain is seen in both emetic and diarrheal type of B. cereus food poisoning.

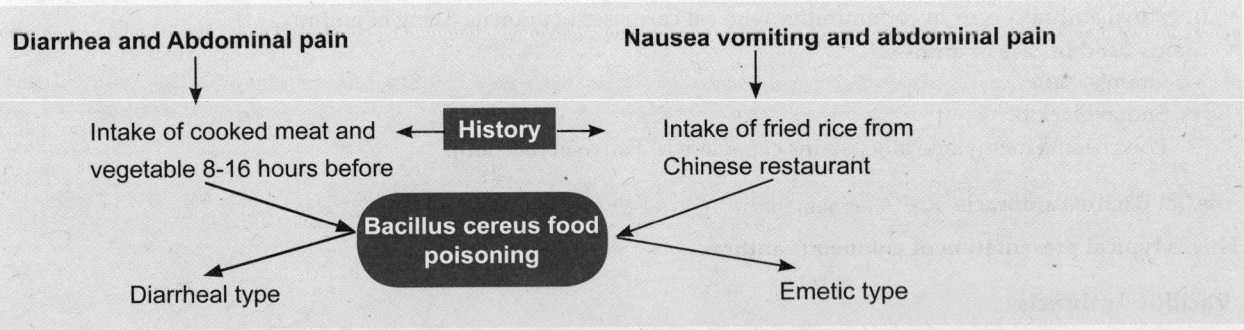

   Remember: A special media mannitol - egg yolk - phenol red-polymyxin agar (MYPA) medium is useful for isolating B. cereus from feces. Fever is common in invasive diarrhea and is rare in toxin mediated diarrhea.

5. **Ans. (a, b and e) M'Fadyean reaction shows capsule, Humans are usually resistant to infection and Sputum microscopy helps in diagnosis** *Ref. Harrison 15/e, p 914; Ananthanarayan 10/e, p 250*

   Diagnosis of Anthrax
   1. **Microscopy:**
      – Examination of cut piece of ear or swab soaked in blood of animals, it reveals gram-positive bacilli and positive M'Fadyean reaction; presumptive diagnosis is made.
      – Immunofluorescent microscopy confirms the diagnosis.
   2. Any large gram-positive bacillus with morphology and cultural features of anthrax, i.e. non-motile, non-hemolytic on blood agar, catalase positive - presumptive report of anthrax can be given.

Diagnosis of Anthrax		
Initial confirmation	**Further confirmation**	**For epidemiological studies and strain characterization**
Lysis by gamma phage and direct fluorescent antibody test (DFA) for capsule specific staining and for polysaccharide cell wall antigen	By PCR for bacillus specific chromosomal markers	MLVA (multiple locus variable number tandem repeat analysis) and **AFLP** (amplified fragment length polymorphism) can be done

Remember: For Animal suspected to have died due to anthrax, autopsy is not permitted as the split blood can contaminate soil.

6. **Ans. (b) Bacillus cereus**   *Ref. Ananthanarayan 10/e, 254*

   Diarrhea of *B. cereus* is mediated by enterotoxin which resemble *E. coli* LT. *The incubation period is 8-16 hours.*

   Bacteria causing invasive diarrhea
   - Shigella
   - Salmonella
   - Enteroinvasive E. coli
   - Campylobacter jejuni

7. **Ans. (a) Bacillus cereus**   *Ref. Ananthanarayan 10/e, p 254*

   This is a characteristic presentation of B. cereus food poisoning (emetic type).
   Bacillus cereus food poisoning
   - *Produces two type of food poisoning:*
       a. *Emetic type*   : It is associated with contaminated frid rice; the organism is common in uncooked rice, and its heat-resistant spores survive boiling. It is mediated by staphylococcal type of enterotoxin.
       b. *Diarrheal type* : Mediated by enterotoxin resembling E. coli. IP of diarrheal type is more in comparison to emetic type
   - *Diagnosis:* The presence of B cereus in patient's stool is not sufficient to make a diagnosis of B cereus disease, since the bacteria may be seen in normal stool specimens; a concentration of 10^5 bacteria or more per gram of food is considered diagnostic.

8. **Ans. (a) B. anthracis**   *Ref. Ananthanarayan 10/e, p 250*

   Already explained

9. **Ans. (c) Bacillus Anthracis**   *Ref. Ananthanarayan 10/e, p 250*

   Already explained

10. **Ans. (a) Organisms**   *Ref. Ananthanarayan 10/e, p 399*

    Actinomycetes are true bacteria (possess cell wall, prokaryotic nuclei, etc.) bearing superficial resemblance to fungi (form mycelium or branching filaments).
    - Actinomyces cause actinomycosis in human.
    - **MC** cause is **A. israelii**
    - **MC** type of actinomycosis — Cervicofacial (lower jaw).

    Diagnosis of actinomycosis is made by:
    1. *Demonstrating organism in the lesion by microscopy:*
        - Specimen: Pus/sputum containing sulphur granules.
        - Granules are crushed, gram-positive filaments seen as 'sun-ray appearance'.
        - These granules are infact bacterial colonies.
    2. *Isolation in culture:*
        - In thioglycollate liquid media   : A. israelli as **fluffy ball** at bottom of tube.
        - Solid media   : **Spidery colonies** of A. israelii

11. **Ans. (a) Madurella**   *Ref. Harrison 17/e, p 1266, 18/e, p 1325*

    Actinomycetoma, usually responds to antibiotics.

Mycetoma
- Localized chronic granulomatous involvement of the subcutaneous and deeper tissue.
- Two types:

Eumycotic mycetoma = Fungal (More common)	Actinomycotic mycetoma = Bacterial
• Madurella mycetomatis	• Actinomyces
• Pseudollescheria boydii	• Nocardia
• Madurella grisea	• Streptomyces
• Acremonium falciforme	• Nocardiasis
• Exophiala jeanselmei	

Treatment of Mycetoma	
Actinomycetoma	**Eumycetoma**
Prolonged combination chemotherapy, e.g. with streptomycin and either dapsone or cotrimoxazole, cotrimoxazole + amikacin	Rarely responds to chemotherapy, some cases caused by Madurella mycetomatic respond to ketoconazole itraconazole, posaconazole

12. **Ans. (a, b and c) Actinomyces, Nocardiasis and Streptomyces** *Ref. Jawetz 27/e, p 673*

    Remember:
    - Most common site of mycetoma - foot - (Called as Madura foot)
    - Staphylococcus is causative agent of botryomycosis.

13. **Ans. (a, b and c) Causes Actinomycetoma, Most commonly causes cervico-facial actinomycosis and Can be detected directly from sample by FISH** *Ref. Harrison 19/e, p 1088, Jawetz 27/e, p 200*
    Already explained see previous answer.

    Note: Antinomycetoma is caused by Actinomodura, Streptomyces and nocardia.

14. **Ans. (c) Brain abscess** *Ref. Harrison 20/e, p 1217*
    - Subacute abscess is the typical extrapulmonary manifestation of nocardia, the most common site of dissemination is brain.
    - Nocardial brain abscess are usually supratentorial, multiloculated, may be single or multiple. Brain abscess tend to burrow into ventricles and may extend out into subarachnoid space. Otherwise Meningitis is uncommon and is usually due to spread from nearby abscess.

    Remember: Other common site of dissemination skin, kidney, bone, muscle.

15. **Ans. (a) Nocardia** *Ref. Ananthanarayan 10/e, p 401; Jawetz 27/e, p 673*

    Mycetoma
    - Chronic granulomatous disease.
    - Involve subcutaneous and deeper tissues destructing the contagious bone and fascia.
    - **Site: Foot (MC), hand, gluteal region and thigh often called as *Madura foot*.**
    - It was first described from Madurai (South India).
    - Presents as abscess, tumors with multiple sinuses discharging pus with sulphur granules.
    - Granules are tightly clumped colonies of causative agent.

    Diagnosed by:
    A.

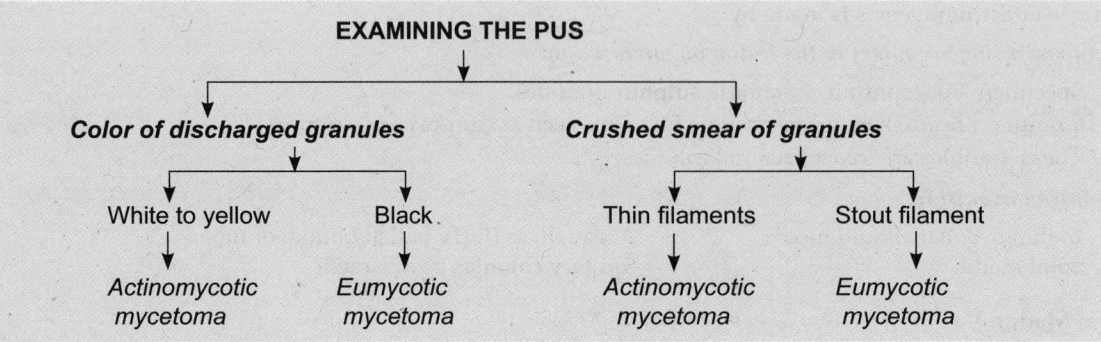

    B. Isolation of agent by culture.

16. **Ans. (a) Acid fast stain** *Ref. Jawetz 27/e, p 199*

    Nocardia is urease positive, catalase positive partially acid fast organism.

    Stains for Nocardia

    - **Acid fast staining** – Nocardia cell wall contains mycolic acid that are shorter chain than mycobacteria. If they are stained with routine acid fast reagant (carbol-fuchsin) and decolorized with 1-4% sulfuric acid instead of the stronger acid decolorant, most isolate will stain acid fast.
    - **Silver stains.**

17. **Ans. (a) Paraffin bait technique** *Ref. Harrison 18/e, p 1324; Harrison 19/e 1086; Jawetz 27/e p 199*

    ### Diagnosis of Nocardiosis

    - **Specimen** – Sputum or pus or spinal fluid or urine or biopsy material. In case of pneumonia, sampling done by bronchoscopy or lung aspiration. Transtracheal aspiration should, however, be avoided as it frequently leads to nocardial cellulitis around the puncture wound.
        i. Microscopy – Crooked, branching, beaded, gram-positive filament seen.
        ii. Stain – They are **Acid fast** and also take silver stains.
        iii. Isolation – Paraffin baiting mixed culture's done as it use paraffin as carbon source
           – Selective media are Thayer Martin agar, Colistin-nalidixic acid buffered charcoal yeast extract agar.
    - If brain involved – CT or MRI
    - In actinomycetoma – granules are examined.

    > **Remember:**
    > - Castaneda culture is method of blood culture (e.g. S. typhi, Brucella).
    > - Craigie's tube is used for the separation of motile from non-motile bacteria and also used to obtain phase variants in Salmonella species.
    > - Recently Molecular methods such as—t RNA sequencing and RFLP analysis are approved for identification.

18. **Ans. (b) ZN stain** *Ref. Ananthanarayan 10/e, p 401; Harrison 17/e, p 994; Harrison 19/e 1084; Greenwood 18/e 235*

    Both are gram-positive filaments causing mycetoma.

Features	Actinomyces	Nocardia
Morphology	Nonacid fast	Acid fast (Ziehl and Neelsen stain); Fite Faraco Method
Growth in media	Anaerobes	Aerobic
Mode of infection	Endogenous	Exogenous
Diseases	**MC** is cervicofacial actinomycosis (Lumpy Jaw)	**MC** is pneumonia and disseminated disease
Treatment	Penicillin G	Sulfonamides
Paraffin	Can't use	Can use

19. **Ans. (a) and (d) Can erode bones and Slow growing** *Ref. Ananthanarayan 8/e 393, 9/e, p 394; Harrison 17/e p 1265, 1266*
    Already explained

20. **Ans. (b) Nocardia** *Ref. Harrison 20/e, p 1217, 1218; Jawetz 27/e, p 199*
    Already Explained

21. **Ans. (a) Nocardia species** *Ref. Harrison 19/e, p 1086*
    Filamentous rod shaped acid fast bacilli seen in this slide can be none other than nocardia species.

NEET Pattern Questions

1. **Bacillus anthracis toxin rediates its action through all except:**
   a. cAMP
   b. Stimulating macrophages
   c. TNFα
   d. cGMP
   [Ref. Greenwood, 18/e, p 238]

Anthrax toxin (three components) (plasmid coded).	
Protective antigen	Binds to host cell
Edema toxin	↑cAMP
Lethal factor (metalloprotienases)	Inactivate mitogen-activated protein kinase in macrophages. Raise IL-1β and TNFα

2. **A person developed severe vomiting after eating food from chinese restaurant, 3 hours before. Most likely causative agent is:**
   a. Staph. aureus
   b. B. cereus
   c. C. difficle
   d. Pseudomonas
   [Ref. Ananthanarayan, 10/e, p 253]

3. **Color of granule of actinomycetes:**
   a. Black
   b. Yellow
   c. Red
   d. Brown *[Ref. Ananthanarayan, 10/e, p 398]*

   Granules are bacterial colonies consist of a dense network of thin Gram positive filaments. Surrounded by a peripheral zone of swollen, club shaped structures presenting a sun ray appearance. The clubs are antigen antibody complex.

4. **Actinomycosis most common site:**
   a. Cervicofacial   b. Thorax
   c. Abdomen   d. Brain
   [Ref. Harrison 20/e, p1220]

5. **A patient is suffering from pneumonia. Laboratory study shows acid-fast filamentous bacterium. The causative organism is:**
   a. M. tuberculosis
   b. Actinomyces
   c. Nocardia
   d. Mycobacterium Avium intracellulare
   [Ref. Harrison 20/e, p1218]

6. **Mc fadyean reaction seen with which organism:**
   a. Clostridium perfringens
   b. Clostridium botulinum
   c. Bacillus cereus
   d. Bacillus anthracis
   [Ref. Ananthanarayan, 10/e, p 251]

   Demonstration of capsular material through staining with polychrome methylene blue is called Mc Fadyean's reaction

7. **Medusa head colonies on nutrient agar is seen in:**
   a. Pneumococcus   b. Legionella
   c. Brucella
   d. Anthrax   *[Ref. Ananthanarayan, 10/e, p 251]*

   On agar plates: The edge of colony is composed by long, interlacing chains of bacilli resembling matted hair called as Medusa head colonies.

8. **True about anthrax toxin are all except:**
   a. Has three fractions
   b. Increase cAMP
   c. Coded by plasmid
   d. Inhibits protein synthesis
   [Ref. Ananthanarayan, 10/e, p 249]

   Anthrax toxin acts by increasing cAMP

9. **Capsule of Bacillus anthracis is formed of:**
   a. Polysaccharide
   b. Lipopolysaccharide
   c. Polypeptide
   d. Long chain fatty acids
   [Ref. Ananthanarayan, 10/e, p 249]

10. **Actinomyces differs from bacteria in that:** (2016)
    a. Gram positive
    b. Filamentous organism
    c. Non-motile
    d. Non-acid fast
    [Ref. Ananthanarayan, 10/e, p 398]

    This is emetic type of food poisoning of B. cereus

11. **A patient with sulphur granules discharging from sinus, suggestive of infection with:** (2016)
    a. Staphylococcus
    b. H. ducryei
    c. Mycetoma
    d. Sporotrichosis
    [Ref. Ananthanarayan, 10/e, p 401]

Ans.
1. d. cGMP   2. b. B. cereus   3. a. Black   4. a. Cervicofacial
5. c. Nocardia   6. d. Bacillus anthracis   7. d. Anthrax   8. d. Inhibits protein synthesis
9. c. Polypeptide   10. b. Filamantous...   11. c. Mycetoma

Actinomycetes and Bacillus 125

12. Most common cause of actinomycetoma in India: (2016)
    a. Nocardia braziliensis
    b. Actinomadura madure
    c. Piedra
    d. Tinea crurin

    [Ref. Jawetz 24/e, p 220; AA, 10/e, p 401]

- MC cause of mycetoma is fungi.
- MC cause of Actinomycetoma are:
  - Nocardia brasiliensis
  - Streptomyces somaelinsis and
  - Actinomadura madurae

13. Anthrax bacilli differs from anthracoid bacilli by being: (2018)
    a. Non-capsulated
    b. Strict aerobe
    c. Non-motile
    d. Hemolytic colonies on blood

    [Ref. Ananthanarayan 10/e, p 253]

Differentiating features between anthrax and anthracoid bacilli

Anthrax Bacilli	Anthracoid Bacilli
– Nonmotile	– Generally motile
– Capsulated	– Noncapsulated
– Grow in long chains	– Grow in short chains
– Medusa head colony	– Not present
– No growth in penicillin agar (10 units/ml)	– Grow usually
– Hemolysis absent or weak	– Usually well marked
– Inverted fir tree growth and slow gelatin liquefaction	– Rapid liquefaction
– No turbidity in broth	– Turbidity usual
– Salicin fermentation negative	– Usually positive
– No growth at 45 °C	– Grows usually
– Growth inhibited by chloral hydrate	– Not inhibited
– Susceptible to gamma phage	– Not susceptible
– Pathogenic to laboratory animals	– Not pathogenic

Ans. 12. a. Nocardia...   13. c. Non-motile

Listeria Monocytogenes

CHAPTER 13

- Catalase positive, Gram positive non-spore forming coccoid rod (coccobacilli) with tendency to occur in chains.
- Shows slow tumbling motility at *20°-25°C* and is non-motile at 37°C.
- Humans are accidental host.
- Monocytogenes is of interest not only to clinicians but also to scientist as a model intracellular pathogen that can be used to study basic mechanism of microbial pathogenesis and host immunity.

Culture

- Grows on ordinary media. (*Mueller-hinton agar*).
- Growth is better in blood agar or if material is stored in tryptose phosphate or thioglycollate broth at 4°C called *cold enrichment*.
- Growth is improved when cultures are incubated at reduced oxygen tension and with 5-10% CO_2
- *Listeria monocytogenes can be differentiated from other Listeria by:*
  - β hemolysis on sheep blood agar.
  - Production of acid from glucose and mannose but not from D. xylose.
- *Listeria monocytogenes* is divided into serotypes on the basis of somatic [O] or flagellar [H] antigen.
- Most human infections are caused by 1/2a, 1/2b, 4b.
- Human disease due to L.monocytogenes generally occurs in pregnancy or immuno-suppression.

- Catalase (+)ve
- Gram (+)ve
- Shows tumbling motility at 20-25°C and is nonmotile at 37°C
- Growth is better on cold enrichment

Mode of Transmission

Food borne [Ready to eat food are most likely].
Human to human transmission is not seen (except vertical transmission from mother to fetus.)

Pathogenesis

- Intracellular pathogen [so, no role of humoral immunity] hence immunity is primarily cell - mediated.
- Lack of gastric acidity increase risk.
- Most important determinant of pathogenesis is its β hemolysin listerolysin O.
  - ... *Harrison 20/e, p 1100*
- **Life-cycle of *Listeria monocytogenes* in host macrophages includes following step.**

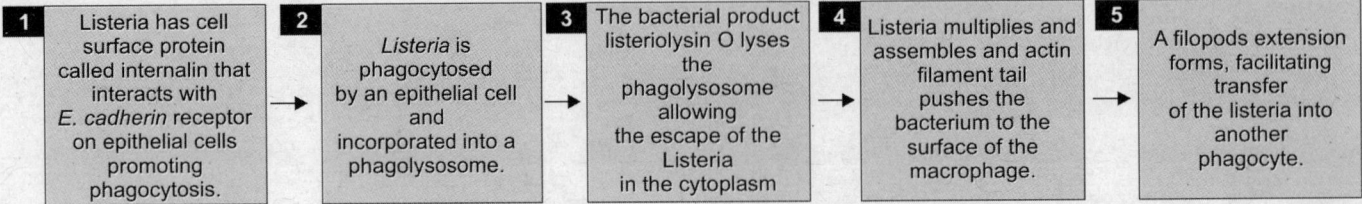

- Though the name *L. monocytogenes* is suggestive of monocytosis, monocytosis is not a hallmark of human infection, it is seen only in rabbits.

Clinical Presentation

1. ***Pregnancy Associated Listeriosis***
   - Most infections detected in 3rd trimester.
   - Woman experiences mild illness characterized by fever, myalgia, backache.
   - Transplacental spread results in chorioamnionitis, premature labor, intrauterine fetal death, stillbirth, early onset disease of newborn, recurrent spontaneous abortion.

2. ***Neonatal Listeriosis***

   A. *Early onset disease:*
   - Occur within 7 days of birth. Most infants are symptomatic by 2nd day.
   - Transmitted by aspiration of infected amniotic fluid.
   - Present as:
     a. Intrauterine sepsis
     b. Respiratory distress
     c. Skin lesions
     d. ***Granulomatosis infantisepticum:*** –Characterized by abscesses involving liver, spleen, adrenal gland and other sites.
   - Mostly follow complicated labor.

   B. *Late onset disease:*
   - Occur between 7-21 days.
   - Mostly present as meningitis
   - Born at term by uncomplicated labor
   - Transmitted during passage through birth canal.

3. ***Listeriosis not associated with pregnancy***
   - **MC** underlying conditions are *chronic glucocorticoid therapy*, diabetes, solid and hematologic *malignancy (particularly fludarabine treated), liver disease, AIDS*
   - Bacteremic infection without evident focus is **MC** clinical manifestation while infection in CNS ranks **2nd** in which meningitis is **MC**. It can directly invade brain parenchyma producing *cerebritis or focal abscess.*
   - *L. monocytogenes* is **MC** cause of *meningitis* in kidney *transplant* patient after **1 month.**
   - *Listeria* meningitis must be considered in chronically ill patient with aseptic meningitis particularly when presentation is subacute. It is also related to 5-10% of community acquired meningitis.
   - **Gastroenteritis**
     - Can be seen in immunocompetent individual within 48h of ingestion of contaminated food such as milk meat and salad.
     - Manifestation includes fever, diarrhea, headache.
   - It is also associated with basilar meningitis of cattles and sheep.
   - Meningoencephalitis: Listeria can directly invade the brain parenchyma.

> **Listeria:**
> - Human listeriosis is almost always caused by L. monocytogenes.
> - Non motile at temp ≥ 37°C and exhibit characteristic tumbling motility at 25°C
> - Listeria is an intracellular bacteria
> - Most infection are food borne.
> - Fetal infection is acquired from mother

Diagnosis

- Invasive listeriosis is diagnosed when organism is cultured from blood, CSF or amniotic fluid.
- *Listeria* may be confused with diptheroids or pneumococci in Gram stained CSF or may be Gram variable and confused with *Hemophilus* sp.
- Antibody to listeriolysin O:
  - For epidemiological purpose.
  - For diagnosis of culture negative CNS infection.
- **Antons test** – Instillation into rabbit eye cause conjunctivitis.

Treatment

- IV administration of ***Ampicillin (DOC)*** or penicillin often in combination with aminoglycoside.
- ***Cotrimoxazole*** in case of pencillin allergy.
- Cephalosporins are not effective.

Multiple Choice Questions

1. A 30-year-old woman with a bad obstetric history presents with fever. The blood culture from the patient grows Gram-positive small to medium coccobacilli that are pleomorphic, occurring in short chains. Direct wet mount from the culture shows tumbling motility. The most likely organism is:
   a. Listeria monocytogenes [AI 08]
   b. Corynebacterium sp.
   c. Enterococcus sp
   d. Erysipelothrix rhusiopathiae

2. A 3-week-old child presented to the pediatrician with meningitis. A presumptive diagnosis of late onset of perinatal infection was made. The CSF culture was positive for gram-positive bacilli which of the following characteristics of this bacteria would be helpful in differentiating it from other bacterial agents?
   a. Ability to grow on blood agar [AIIMS 05]
   b. Ability to produce catalase
   c. Fermentative attack on sugars
   d. Motility at 25°C

3. Gram (+)ve bacilli causing meningitis:
   a. Pneumococci [AIIMS Nov 2014]
   b. Listeria
   c. E. coli
   d. Meningococci

4. A major step in the pathogenesis of listeriosis is:
   a. The formation of antigen-antibody complex with resultant complement activation and tissue damage
   b. The release of hyaluronidase by L. monocytogenes, which contributes to its dissemination from local sites [AIIMS 05]
   c. The antiphagocytic activity of the L. monocytogenes capsule
   d. The survival and multiplication of L. monocytogenes within mononuclear phagocytes and host epithelial cells

5. In patient with Listeria meningitidis who is allergic penicillin the treatment of choice is: [AIIMS 12]
   a. Vancomycin
   b. Gentamicin
   c. Trimethoprim - sulfamethoxazole
   d. Ceftriaxone

6. Which of the following is not true regarding transmission? [AI 09]
   a. Legionella – Through water aerosols
   b. Listeria – Refrigerated food
   c. Leptospirosis – Rat urine
   d. Tetanus – Droplets/Dust

7. Listeria culture media: [AIIMS May 09]
   a. Baker
   b. Korthoff
   c. Tinsdale
   d. Blood agar

8. A 28-year-old lady presented with, headache, kernigs sign positive, culture showed gram positive bacilli, most probable organism is: [AI 2011]
   a. Listeria monocytogenes
   b. H. influenza
   c. Meningococci
   d. Streptococcus pneumoniae

Explanations and References with Illustrative Answers

1. **Ans. (a) Listeria monocytogenes** *Ref. Ananthanarayan 10/e, p 403*

   Tumbling motility is characteristic of Listeria monocytogenes - (other three are non-motile).

   ### Listeria monocytogenes
   - Catalase positive, non-sporing-gram positive, Cocco bacilli.
   - Tendency to occur in chains.
   - Characteristicly **show tumbling motility at 25°C and at 37°C** is non-motile because Peritrichous flagella are produced optimally at 20 to 30°C but only scantily or not at all at 37°C.
   - Grows best between 30°C and 37°C (temperature range is 1 to 45°C).
   - Aerobic or microaerophilic.
   - Intracellular as well as able for direct cell to cell spread so not eliminate by antibodies and cause infection in deficient cell mediated immunity.

   ### Lab diagnosis of Listeria Monocytogenes
   - **Specimen:** Blood, pus, CSF, swab from cervical and vaginal secretion, cord blood.
   - **Microscopy:** Usually negative. In rare case extra and intracellular coccobacilli may be seen.
   - **Culture:** – Listeria can grow on ordinary media, but growth is better on blood agar or tryptose phosphate agar. On blood agar, Listeria form small colonies surrounded by a narrow zone of β hemolysis. The bacilli are actively motile (tumbling motility) when grown at 25°C. Biochemical tests are required to differentiate L. monocytogenes from other Listeria species.
     – Growth is improved when cultures are incubated at reduced oxygen tension.
   - **Biochemical test:** L. monocytogenes is always D. xylose negative and d-methyl-D-mannoside positive.
   - **Rapid detection:** Selective enrichment broths based on immunoassays are commercially available for rapid detection of Listeria from food species.
   - **Serology:** Serological test and PCR assays are not useful in diagnosing clinical infection at present.

   > **Remember:**
   > - E. rhusiopalthae is α-hemolytic non-motile Gram-positive bacillus with tendency to form long filaments.
   > - Its **MC** infection in humans is called erysipeloid = Seal finger = whole finger.

2. **Ans. (d) Motility at 25° C** *Ref. Ananthanarayan 10/e, p 403*
   - This is a case of **'Late onset neonatal meningitis'** of Listeria monocytogenes as culture reveals Gram-positive bacillus.
   - Bacterial cause of neonatal meningitis are:
     – E. coli > Group b streptococci (Strep. agalactiae) > other gram-negative bacilli > L. monocytogenes.

     ..... *Forfar and Anelus textbook of pedia 319, 1338*
   - E. coli is Gram-negative bacilli while group b streptococci is gram-positive cocci.

Important bacterias causing meningitis					
Features	Listeria	E. coli	Streptococci	Staphylococci	H. influenzae
Ability to grow on blood agar	+	+	+	+	+
Production of catalase	+	+	–	+	+
Fermentation of sugars	+	Both acid and gas are produced	+	+	+
Motility at 25°C	+	–	–	+	–
Gram staining	+	–	+	+	–

   > **Remember:**
   > - Catalase production and β hemolysis is used to differentiate Listeria monocytogenes from other Listeria not from other bacterias.
   > - Only Listeria and E.coli are motile in above mentioned bacterias.

3. **Ans. (b) Listeria** *Ref. Harrison 20/e, p 1101*

   Already explained

4. **Ans. (d) The survival and multiplication of *L. monocytogenes* within mononuclear phagocytes and host epithelial cells**
   Ref. Jawetz 27/e, p 196 – 198

   Pathogenesis of Listeria Monocytogenes

   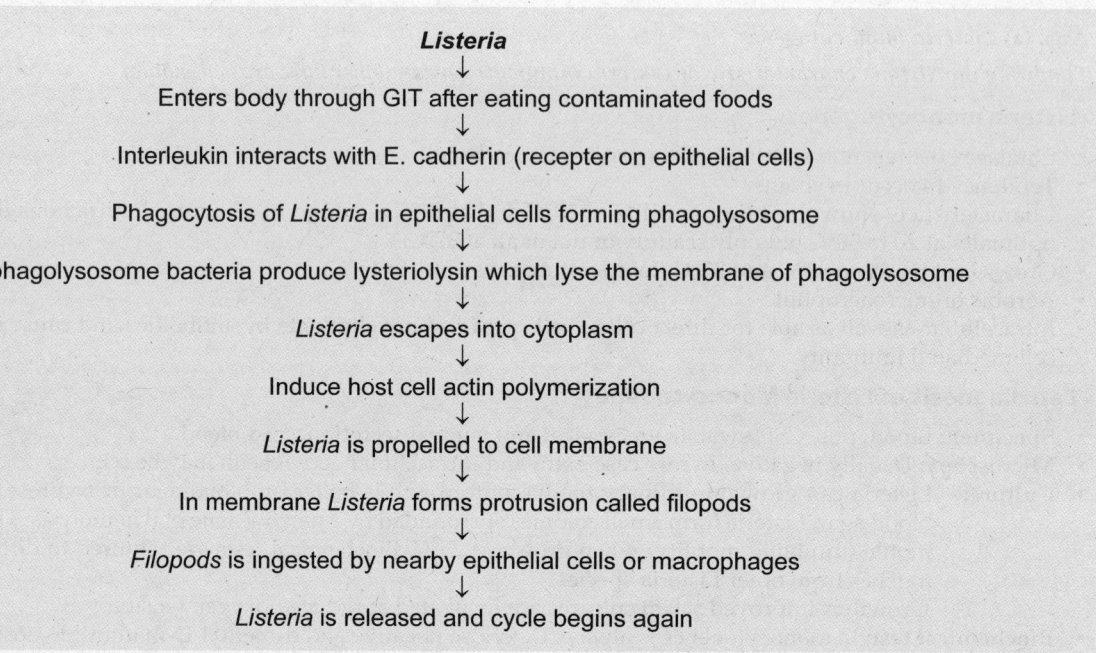

   So, in this way Listeria can move from cell to cell without being exposed to antibodies, complement or polymorphs.

   Remember:
   - Iron is important virulence factor of Listeria
   - Shigella flexneri and rickettsia also use the host cell actin and contractile system to spread infection.

5. **Ans. (c) Trimethoprim - sulfamethoxazole** *Ref. Harrison 20/e, p 1102*
   - **DOC** for listeriosis (non-pregnant, neonate, pregnant) is ampicillin or penicillin often in combination with aminoglycosides.
   - During last month of pregnancy (in case of penicillin allergy), may be treated with erythromycin.
   - Otherwise in all cases of penicillin allergy **DOC** is trimethoprim-sulfamethoxazole.

6. **Ans. (b) Listeria: Refrigerated food** *Ref. Harrison 20/e, p 1110; Chakoraborty 2/e, p 453*
   Mode of transmission of listeriosis
   - Food borne by ready to eat food, milk, deli meat, salad.
   - Through birth canal at the time of delivery
   - Nosocomial through contaminated resuscitation equipments of newborn.

7. **Ans. (d) Blood agar** *Ref. Ananthanarayan 8/e, p 395, 9/e, p 395*
   Already explained, in Ans. 1

8. **Ans. (a) Listeria monocytogenes** *Ref. Harrison 20/e, p 1101*
   Among options provided listeria is the only Gr positive bacilli. Listeria accounts for 10% of cases of community acquired bacterial meningitis.
   Diagnosis should be considered in all older or chronically ill patients with "aseptic meningitis". The presentation is usually subacute and nuchal rigidity and meningeal signs are less common.

Listeria Monocytogenes

NEET Pattern Questions

1. **True statement about Listeria:**
   a. Gram negative bacillus
   b. Motile by peritrichous flagella
   c. Commonest cause of community acquired meningitis
   d. Only one serovar is known
   [Ref. Ananthanarayan, 10/e, p 402]

2. **Anton test is used for:**
   a. Listeria monocytogenes
   b. Ligaonella
   c. Brucella
   d. Bordetella
   [Ref. Ananthanarayan, 10/e, p 402]

   > **Anton's test:** Instillation of culture containing listeria into the eye of rabbit or guinea pig produces severe kerato conjunctivitis

3. **Most common serotype of listeria causing infections:**
   a. 1/2a   b. 1/3a
   c. 1/3b   d. 1/2c
   [Ref. Ananthanarayan, 10/e, p 402]

4. **Tumbling motility is shows by:**
   a. Listeria monocytogenes
   b. Proteus vulgaris
   c. Borrelia
   d. Clostridla
   [Ref. Ananthanarayan, 10/e, p 402]

5. **Mode of transmission of listeria:**
   a. Ingestion   b. Inhalation
   c. Skin inoculation   d. None
   [Ref. Harrison, 20/e, p 1100]

6. **All are true about listeria except:** (2016)
   a. Gram positive
   b. PALCAM agar is used for isolation
   c. Characteristic tumbling motility at 37°C
   d. Umbrella shaped growth
   [Ref. Ananthanarayan, 10/e, p 402]

   > Listeria is nonmotile at 37°C

7. **Listeria resists phagocytosis in phagosomes (phagolysosomes) due to:** (2016)
   a. β-hemolysin
   b. Caspases
   c. Cell membrane adhesion molecules
   d. Opacity associated protein (OAP)
   [Ref. Harrison, 20/e, p 1100]

   > Listeriolysin O, a β-hemolysin is largely responsible for mediating the rupture of phagosomal membrane that forms after phagocytosis of L. monocytogenes.

8. **Granulomatous infantisepticum is caused by:** (2016)
   a. HSV-1
   b. HSV-2
   c. Listeria
   d. Group B streptococcus
   [Ref. Harrison, 20/e, p 1101]

   > Granulomatous infantisepticum is an overwhelming fetal infection with miliary microabscess and granuloma in skin, liver and spleen.

UNIT-I: Bacteriology

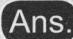
1. b. Motile by peritrichous flagella
2. a. Listeria monocytogenes
3. a. 1/2a
4. a. Listeria monocytogenes
5. a. Ingestion
6. c. Characteristic…
7. a. β-hemolysin
8. c. Listeria

Mycobacteria

CHAPTER 14

> Gram positive acid fast
> Nonmotile
> Noncapsulated

Gram-positive, **Aerobic**, acid fast, nonmotile, noncapsulated and non sporing fungus like bacteria.

Classification of mycobacteria is as follows:
1. **Tubercle bacilli** - *M. tuberculosis, M. bovis, M. africanum*
2. **Lepra bacilli** - *M. leprae*
3. **Mycobacteria causing skin ulcers** - *M. ulcerans, M. haemophilum, M. marinum* or balnei
4. **Atypical mycobacteria** = Nontuberculous = Paratubercle = MOTT (Mycobacteria other than Tuberculosis)

Classification of Atypical Mycobacteria	
Group I	Photochromogenes e.g. M. kansasii, M. marinum, M. simiae, M. asiaticum
Group II	Scotochromogens e.g. M. scrofulaceum, M. gordonae, M. szulgai, M. flavescens.
Group III	Nonphotochromogens e.g. M. avium, M. intracellulare, M. xenopi, M. ulcerans, M. malmoense, M. celatum, M. hemophilum, M. gastri, M. genavense, M. shimoidei, M. trivale, M. terrae, M. nonchromogenicum.
Group IV	Rapid growers – M. fortuitum, M. chelonae Chromogenic rapid growers are saprophytes e.g. M. smegmatic, M. phlei.

5. **Johne's bacillus** - *M. paratuberculosis*

MYCOBACTERIA LEPRAE (HANSEN BACILLUS) (See color plate, pg xxvi for related image)

Morphology

> **M. leprae:**
> - Gram positive, acid fast, obligate intracellular parasite.
> - Phenolic glycolipid acts as a virulence factor.
> - O-diphenol oxidase is an enzyme characteristic of leprosy bacilli.
> - **Generation time** - 12-13 days

- Obligate intracellular bacilli with polar bodies and intracellular elements, resist decolorization with 5% H_2SO_4 (acid fast).
- Live bacilli in tissue appear solid and uniformly stained.
- *Morphological index (MI)* is a measure of number of viable *M. leprae*.
- Dead bacilli – fragmented and granular appearance.
- *Bacteriological index (BI)* – number of *bacilli* in tissue, include both live and dead.
- Increasing BI and MI suggests relapse/drug resistance.
- Bacilli can be seen as single or multiple intracellular or lying free outside the cell.
- They frequently appear as agglomerates, the bacilli being bound together by lipid like substance, the glia. These masses are known as globi.
- The parallel row of bacilli in the globi imparts a cigar bundle appearance
- The globi appear in Virchow's lepra cells or foamy cells which are large undifferentiated histiocytes
  ...*Ananthanarayan 10/e, p 371*
- Strain variability is demonstrated recently.
- (PGL-I) phenolic glycolipid act as virulence factor.

Culture

> - Principal target is Schwann cells.
> - First sign of leprosy is a non-specific indeterminate skin lesion which often heal spontaneously.

- Unique in exhibiting dopa oxidase activity and acid fastness that is pyridine extractable.
- *Not grow in artificial media* but multiply in foot pad of mice at low temperature of 20°C.
- Nine banded **armadillo** (*Dasypus novemcinctus*) is highly *susceptible* to it.
- Grows **best in** cooler tissues (skin, peripheral nerves, anterior chamber of eye, upper respiratory tract, testis) **sparing** warmer areas (axilla, groin, scalp, midline of back, ovary).

Mycobacteria

Transmission
- Nasal droplet, contact with infected soil and amoeba insect vectors. Skin to skin contact is not an important route. Physicians and nurses caring for leprosy patient are not at risk.
- Leprosy is associated with poverty and rural residence. It appears not to be associated with AIDS, parhaps because of Leprosy's long incubation period. ...Harrison 19/e, p 1260
- Aerosolized M. leprae can cause infection in immunocompromise mice.

> M. leprae cannot be cultivated in vitro due to loss or disruption of many genes in artificial media

Clinical Features
- It causes Leprosy (Hansen's disease) having spectrum of manifestations.
- Incubation period generally varies from 5-7 years.
- Two extremes or polar form of disease are the lepromatous or tuberculoid types.

> **Note:** Sneeze from an untreated lepromatous leprosy contains >10^{10} AFB T- helper lymphocyte response to M. leprae determine whether an individual has tuberculoid or lepromatous leprosy

Tuberculoid Leprosy (See color plate, pg xxvi for related image)
- Symptoms confined to skin and peripheral nerves.
- **MC nerve involved-** Ulnar, posterior auricular, peroneal and posterior tibial nerve.
- Invasion and destruction of nerves in dermis by T1 cells (by bacilli in LL) are **pathognomic for** leprosy.
- Medial popliteal **nerve** never involved.

Lepromatous Leprosy (See color plate, pg xxvi for related image)
- Bacilli are present in blood and in all organ system **except lungs and CNS**. Even than patient are afebrile and not susceptible to opportunistic infection.
- Leprosy bacilli are numerous in the skin where they are often found in large clumps (*globi*) and in peripheral nerves where they initially invades Schwann cells.

Other important clinical features are as follows:

Clinical & Histologic features	Tuberculoid (TT) Borderline	Borderline Tuberculoid (BT) Leprosy	Mild-Borderline (BB) Leprosy	Borderline Lepromatous (BL)	Lepromatous Leprosy (LL)
	MC type in India		Most unstable leprosy		
Skin lesions	Up to 3 in number; sharpy defined, hypopigmented asymmetric macules or plaques with tendency toward central clearing, elevated borders	Smaller or larger than in TT; potentially more numerous than in TT; usually annular lesions with sharp margination on exterior & interior borders; borders not as elevated as in TT	Dimorphic lesions intermediate between BT & BL	LL-type lesions; ill-defined plaques with an occasional sharp margin; few or many in number, shiny appearance	Symmetric, poorly marginated, multiple infiltrated nodules & plaques or diffuse infiltration; xanthoma-like or dermatofibroma papules; leonin facies and eyebrow alopecia, Granzee zone seen
Nerve lesions	Skin lesions anesthetic early; nerve near lesions sometimes enlarged	Skin lesion anesthetic early; nerve trunk palsies asymmetric; nerve abscesses most common in BT	Anesthetic skin lesions; nerve trunk palsies	Skin lesions usually hypoaesthetic, may be anesthetic; nerve trunk palsies common and frequently symmetric	Hypesthesia a late sign; nerve palsies variable; acral, distal, symmetric anesthesia common
Acid fast bacilli (BI)	3	0-1+	3-4+	4-5+	4-6+
Lymphocytes	3+	2+	1+	1+	0-1+
Macrophage differentiation	Epithelioid	Epithelioid	Epithelioid	Usually undifferentiated; epithelioid foci sometimes present; may show foamy change	Foamy change is the rule; may be undifferentiated in early lesions

Contd...

Contd...

Clinical & Histologic features	Tuberculoid (TT) Borderline	Borderline Tuberculoid (BT) Leprosy	Mild-Borderline (BB) Leprosy	Borderline Lepromatous (BL)	Lepromatous Leprosy (LL)
Langhan's giant cells	1-3+	2+	-	-	-
Lepromin test	+++	+++	-	-	-
Lymphocyte transformation test	95%	40%	10%	1-2%	1-2%
CD4+/CD8+-T cell ratio in lesions	1.35	1.11	NT	0.48	0.50
M. leprae PGI-1 antibodies	1 + (60%)	2+	2+	3+	3+ (95%)

> - Type I lepra-reaction: Type IV hypersensitivity seen in borderline leprosy
> - Type II lepra reaction: Type III hypersensitivity seen in multibacillary (BL and LL) leprosy.

Reactional States

I. **Type I Lepra reaction/Jopling Type I:**
   - *Type IV hypersensitivity* seen in *Borderline* leprosy not in polar form.
   - If *precede* therapy then termed *down grading* reaction i.e. towards LL.
   - If *after* therapy then termed *Reversal reaction* i.e. towards more tuberculoid.
   - Manifestations include classic signs of inflammation within previously involved macules, papules and plaques. Ulnar nerve trunk is the most commonly involved.
   - Most characteristic microscopic feature of type I reaction is *Edema*.
   - It is associated with increased T cells bearing γ/δ receptors, a unique feature of leprosy.
   - MC nerve trunk involved - *Ulnar at elbow*
   - **Treatment:**
     - **DOC** glucocorticoids
     - Clofazimine also given
     - Thalidomide - ineffective.
   - If patients are not treated promptly with steroids, irreversible nerve damage may result in as little as 24 h. The most dramatic manifestation is foot drop d/t involvement of common peroneal nerve.

II. **Type II lepra reaction – Erythema Nodosum Leproticum/Jopling Type II:**
   - *Type III hypersensitivity* occurs exclusively in BL, LL
   - Usually follows therapy (sulfone syndrome) but may precede therapy.
     MC feature - crops of painful erythematous papules that resolve spontaneously in a few days to weeks but may recur.
   - Central role in pathobiology: TNF
   - **Treatment:**
     - Mild - antipyretics alone
     - Moderate to severe - Ist drug to be used glucocorticoids
       DOC thalidomide
       Clofazimine - More active than in Type I.

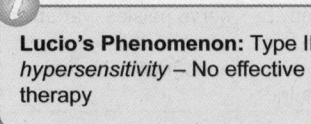

Lucio's Phenomenon: Type III *hypersensitivity* – No effective therapy

III. **Lucio's Phenomenon:**
   - **Type III Hypersensitivity** exclusively in diffuse lepromatosis form of LL, usually in untreated patient.
   - **Treatment:**
     - Neither glucocorticoid nor thalidomide is effective.
     - Wound care and therapy for bacteremia.

Complications

- MC complication of leprous neuropathy is *plantar ulceration* particularly at metatarsal heads.
- *Nerve abscess:*
  - **MC** site is ulnar nerve.
  - Treatment is rapid surgical decompression.

Mycobacteria

Diagnosis
Usually clinical in patient of low socioeconomic status with characteristic lesion
...Harrison 20/e, p1263

- Biopsy of advancing edge of lesion in TT but in LL, biopsy of normal skin is also taken.
- In lepromatous leprosy, nodules plaques and indurated areas are optimal biopsy site.
- In tuberculoid leprosy, lesional areas preferably the advancing edge must be biopsied.
- If M antibodies to PGL-1 are found in 95% of patients with untreated lepromatous leprosy and <65% of tuberculoid leprosy patients. Titre decreases with treatment.
- Hyperglobulinemia in LL.
- *Lepromin test* – Type IV delayed hypersensitivity which is biphasic.
- *Early reaction of Fernandez* – read in **24 - 48 hours (analogous to tuberculin reaction).**
- *Late reaction of Mitsuda* – peak in **4 weeks.** More meaningful.
- It is of little diagnostic value but has more prognostic importance.

Lepromin test: Type IV hypersenstivity

Treatment

Form of leprosy	More intensive regimen	WHO recommended regime
i. Tuberculoid (paucibacillary)	Dapsone 100 mg/d × 5 years	Dapsone 100 mg/d + Rifampin 600 mg/month for 6 months
ii. Lepromatous (Multibacillary) or > 6 skin lesions	Rifampin 600 mg/d for 3 years + dapsone 100 mg/d indefinitely	Dapsone 100 mg/d + Clofazimine 50 mg/d and Rifampin 600 mg + clofazimine 300 mg monthly for 1year

- Single lesion paucibacillary leprosy - Single dose of ROM - rifampin, ofloxacin, minocycline.

Remember: Mycobacterium lepraemurium is a causative agent of rat leprosy.

MYCOBACTERIA TUBERCULOSIS

Morphology
- Belong to family mycobacteriaceae and the order Actinomycetales.
- M. tuberculosis comprises 8 subgroups commonest being M. tubeculosis.
- Other subgroups are M. bovis, M. caprae, M. africanum, M. microti, M. pinnipedi, M. mungi, M. orgis. ..... *Harrison 20/e, p1236*
- Mammalian tubercle, isolated by Koch is stained by Ziehl - Neelsen method or by **fluorescent dyes (auramine O, rhodamine).** They cannot be classified as Gram positive or negative.
- When strained with carbol fuschin they resist decolorization by 20% H_2SO_4 and absolute alcohol for 10 minutes. Hence acid and alcohol fast.
- Acid fastness is due to unsaponifiable wax (mycolic acid) or to a semipermeable membrane.
- It has thick cell wall; shows spheroplast and L forms.

Mycobacterium tuberculosis complex:
Group of closely related mycobacteria that can cause tuberculosis, includes:
- M. tuberculosis
- M. bovis
- M. africanium
- M. caprae
- M. pinnipedi
- M. microti
- M. carnetti

Constituents of Tubercle Bacilli
a. **Lipids:** Mycobacteria are rich in lipids, which include mycolic acid, waxes and phosphatides. Muramyl dipeptide complexed with mycolic acid is involved in granuloma formation, while phospholipids induce caseous necrosis.
b. **Proteins:** Mycobacterium contains several proteins that elicit the tuberculin reaction.
c. **Polysaccharides:** Mycobacterium contains variety of polysaccharides. These polysaccharides can induce immediate hypersensitivity.

Culture
- Generation time 14-15 hours.
- Colonies appear in about **2 weeks (may take up to 8 weeks).**
- Grows **luxuriantly in culture (Eugonic)** and addition of 0.5% glycerol and CO_2 improves its growth but has no effect on **M. bovis** (causative agent of bovine tuberculosis) **which is dysgonic (grows sparsely).**
- Solid medium most widely employed for routine culture is Lowenstein - Jensen (LJ) medium without starch.

Stains for Mycobacterium tuberculosis:
- Ziehl-Neelsen stain
- Auramine O rhodamine

M. bovis stains more uniformly

- Liquid media are not generally used routinely, but used for sensitivity testing, chemical analyses and preparation of antigens and vaccines. e.g. Middle brook, MGIT system.
- In liquid culture grow as twisted rope like colonies *(mimicing serpentine cords)*.
- *M. tuberculosis* is an obligate aerobe, while *M. bovis* is microaerophillic in primary isolation.
- When incorporated in soft agar media M. tuberculosis grows on the surface whereas M. bovis grows as a band a few mm below the surface.
- *Virulent strains forms long serpentine cords in liquid media while avirulent strain grow in dispersed manner. Cord formation is correlated with virulence.* ... Jawetz 27/e, p 312
- A cord factor (trehalose 6.6' dimycolate) has been extracted from virulent bacilli. It inhibits migration of leukocytes causes chronic granuloma and can serve as a immunologic adjuvant.

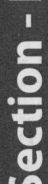

- Tubercle bacilli are non-motile, non-sporing, non-capsulate, straight or slightly curved
- L J medium: Egg glycerol based medium to which malachite green dye is added, so as to inhibit the growth of other contaminating bacteria and to provide contrasting colour.

Biochemical reaction	Positive in	Negative in
Niacin test : N	Human tubercle	Bovine tubercle
Aryl sulphatase : A	Only with atypical mycobacteria	
Neutral red test : N	Virulent strain of tubercle	Avirulent strain
Peroxidase test : P	Tubercle bacilli	Atypical mycobacteria
Catalase test : C	Most atypical mycobacteria	Weakly positive in tubercle
Nitrate reduction test : N	M. tuberculosis	M. bovis

- *Catalase and peroxidase activities are lost when tubercle bacilli become INH resistant.*
- Urea test is positive in *M. tuberculosis, M. bovis* and most of the atypical mycobacteria except MAIC complex.
- Mycobacteria are susceptible to alcohol, formaldehyde, glutaraldehyde and, to a lesser extent hypochlorites and phenolic disinfectants.

Virulence Factors
- **Kat-G gene:** encodes for oxidase, catalase enzyme.
- **rpoV:** main sigma factor initiating transcription of several genes.
- **Erp gene:** encodes for protein required for multiplication.
- **Strains of Beijing/w genotype family.**
- **Cord protein:** Control rRNA transcription required for replication and persistance in host cell.

Antigenic Property
- Group specificity is due to polysaccharide while type specificity is due to protein antigen.
- Antibodies are not useful for diagnosis and immunity.

Pathogenicity

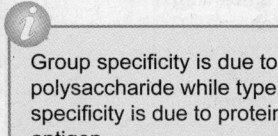

Group specificity is due to polysaccharide while type specificity is due to protein antigen.

- Majority of inhaled bacilli are trapped in upper airways, 10% reach the alveoli. There antigens of mycobacteria processed through APC activates T-cell. Activated T-cells secrete IFN γ which together with calcitriol, activate macrophages. Macrophage engulf bacteria but does not kill them. ...Greenwood 18/e, p214
- It is due to escape killing by macrophages and induction of type IV hypersensitivity.
- *Following factors contribute in pathogenesis:*
  - Cord factor
  - Lipoarabinomannan
  - Complement system
  - *M. TB* heat shock protein.
- Risk of ***acquiring*** infection is determined mainly by *exogenous* factors while risk of developing *disease* depends largely on *endogenous* factors.
- Most potent risk factors - HIV coinfection.

Clinical Features
- Divided into two categories: Pulmonary and extrapulmonary TB.
  1. **Pulmonary TB:** Divided into two:
     a. **Primary Disease:** Usually localized in middle and lower zones.
        Primary focus is usually peripheral in subpleural region and is accompanied by draining lymphatics, inflamed regional lymph nodes which are collectively called *Primary complex/Ghon's facus*.

> **Note:** When the bacilli enters through mouth as in case of M. bovis primary complex involve the tonsil and cervical nodes or the intestine often the ileocaecal region and the mesenteric nodes. In occupational exposure (pathologist) primary focus may be in skin called as prosector's wart.

Depending on the host immune response development of complex can follow healing by fibrosis/calcification; cavitation or progressive primary TB in form of consolidation; obstructive emphysema or atelactasis; TB bronchitis; miliary TB; occult hematogenous dissemination to apex of lung (**Simons Focus**).

b. *Post primary disease* (adult type or reactivation or secondary tuberculosis or chronic pulmonary TB).
   – Usually localized to apical and posterior segments of upper lobe due to high O_2 concentration (**Puhl's Lesion**).
   – MC hematologic finding - mild anemia and leucocytosis
   – Infraclavicular lesion is called *Assman's Focus*.

2. **Extrapulmonary TB**
   - **MC site is lymph node** (MC *cervical and supraclavicular*).
   - **Other Sites include:**
     – Pleura in the form of pleural effusion and empyema.
     – Genitourinary tract (culture negative pyuria in acidic urine).
     – Skeletal TB (**MC** site spine, hip, knee).
     – TB meningitis (paresis of cranial nerves especially *ocular*, is frequent finding).
     – GI TB (**MC** site terminal ileum and caecum).
     – Tuberculous pericarditis (**MC** cause of chronic constrictive pericarditis).

> Most common site of TB: Lung
> Most common site of extrapulmonary TB: Lymph node

Diagnosis

Specimen – sputum is best collected in the *morning* before any meal (3 sample).

i. **AFB microscopy:** smear should be prepared from thick purulent part of sputum.
   - At least **10000 AFB** should be present per ml of sputum for demonstrating in direct smears. Positive report can be given only if >2 typical bacilli have seen.
   - **Fluorescent microscopy** (stained with auramine phenol or auramine rhodamine fluorescent dye and examined under UV illumination) screen smear *rapidly* in comparison of Ziehl–Neelsen method.
   - Concentration method for microscopy can also used, e.g. Petroff's method using NaOH solution is widely used.

Slide Reporting

The number of bacilli seen in a smear reflects disease severity and patient infectivity. Therefore, it is important to record the number of bacilli seen on each smear. The standard method of reporting using 1000 × magnification is as:

Number of bacilli	Result reported
No AFB per 100 oil immersion fields	0
1–9 AFB per 100 oil immersion fields	scanty (or number AFB seen)
10–99 AFB per 100 oil immersion fields	+ (1 +)
1–10 AFB per oil immersion field	++ (2 +)
> 10 AFB per oil immersion field	+++ (3 +)

> Petroff Method: Most widely used method for sputum culture. Here sputum is mixed with 4% NaOH, neutralized with potassium dihydrogen orthophosphate and centrifuged. The deposit is then inoculated on LJ medium.

Laboratory technicians should examine both the sputum samples from each TB suspect. It is advised that the smear examined by one microscopist should not exceed 20 per day as visual fatigue leads to a deterioration of reading quality.

ii. **Culture:**
   - Very *sensitive diagnostic* technique can detect even 10 to 100 bacilli per ml.
   - LJ and Middle brook 7H10/7H11 are selective media.
   - Negative report is given, if no growth occur after 8-12 weeks.
   - Slow growing, nonpigmented niacin positive AFB is taken as *M. tuberculosis*.
   - Liquid media with radiometric growth detection (e.g. BACTEC 460) and nucleic acid probes, enables results to be given in 2-3 weeks.

- Commercial lipid culture system such as mycobacterial growth indicator tube (MGIT) are recommended by WHO as the reference standard for culture...*Harrison 20/e, p1247*

iii. **Nucleic acid technology:**
  - PCR and Ligase chain reaction are used as diagnostic technique.
  - RFLP and IS fingerprinting used for epidemiological typing of strain.
  - Xpert MTB/RIF assay: Simultaneously detect TB and rifampicin resistance in <2h and has minimal biosafety and training requirements. WHO recommends its worldwide use as initial diagnostic test in adults and children.

iv. **Immunodiagnosis:**
  a. **Tuberculin skin test**
     - Demonstration of hypersensitivity to tuberculin protein (tuberculin test/Mantoux intradermal test) is a standard procedure.
     - 1 purified protein derivative (PPD) = 50000 tuberculin units per milligram.
     - WHO advocates PPD tuberculin known as - RT 23 with Tween 80.
     - *Routinely* 1 TU used.
     - *Clinically* 5 TU used.
     - Read after 72 hours in which induration is measured in horizontal transverse diameter.
     - > 10 mm positive, < 5 mm negative.
     - < 6 and > 15 mm have more risk of developing TB.
     - Positive tuberculin test indicates exposure to bacilli *(infection, immunization)* with or without clinical disease. So persons who have never had contact with bacilli are tuberculin negative.
     - Used as aid in diagnosing active infection in infants and young children; measure prevalence of infection; to select susceptibles; as an indicator of successful vaccination.
     - Tine Multiple puncture test and heaf test is used for screening and surveys.
  b. **IFN γ Assay:**
     - Two in vitro assays that measure T cell release of IFN γ in response to stimulation with highly TB specific (IGRA) antigens ESAT-6 and CFP 10, are available by the name of **T-SPOT TB** (an enzyme linked immunospot assay) and **Quanti FERON-TB Gold** (whole blood ELISA). ...*Harrison 20/e, p1247*
     - IGRA are preferred over tuberculin test (TST) for persons above 5 years of age, in children under 5 years TST is preferred.

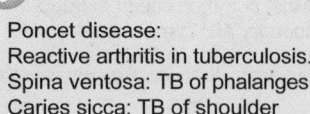

Poncet disease:
Reactive arthritis in tuberculosis.
Spina ventosa: TB of phalanges
Caries sicca: TB of shoulder

- Mantoux test: < 6 mm and > 15 mm have more risk of developing TB.
- WHO has banned use of tubercular IgM ELISA due to very high false positive rate, thus over prescription of anti-tubercular therapy.

Diagnostic test for tuberculosis	
Test	**Specimens**
Culture	Sputum, CSF
Nucleic acid amplification* (Xpert MTB/RIF assay)	Sputum, CSF, Gastric lavage, Pleural biopsy
TB LAMP assay	Sputum
AFB microscopy**	Sputum, lymph node biopsy
Mycobacterum culture***	Sputum, Endometrial biopsy
IFN-γ release assays	Blood

*WHO recommend Xpert MTB/RIF assay as the first line diagnostic test in all adults and children with sign and symptoms of active TB
**TB LED fluorescence microscopy are now recommended by WHO as the microscopy tool of choice.
***MGIT system are recommended by WHO as the reference standard for culture.

Treatment

ATT is given: First line drugs are:

- Xpert MTB/RIF based on amplification of mycobacterial nuclei acid has emerged as initial diagnostic test.
- This test has a sensitivity of 98% among AFB positive cases and 70% among AFB negative specimens.

Drugs	Daily dose	Dose in DOTS	Thrice weekly dose
H. Isoniazid	5 mg/kg	600 mg	10 mg/kg
R. Rifampein	10 mg/kg	450 mg	10 mg/kg
Z. Pyrazinamide	25 mg/kg	1500 mg	35 mg/kg
E. Ethambutol	15 mg/kg	1200 mg	30 mg/kg
S. Streptomycin	15 mg/kg	750 mg	15 mg/kg

- **MDR Strains:** Strains resistant to isoniazid and rifampicin with or without resistance to additional drugs
- **XDR Strains:** Strains resistance to at least isoniazid, rifampicin, any fluoroquinolones and any injectable agent.

Prevention

- *BCG vaccine:* Live attenuated vaccine derived from attenuated bovine strain of *tubercle bacilli.*
  - Normal saline is diluent
  - Dose of 0.05 ml for age < 4 week and 0.1 ml for > 4 weeks should be given intradermal (subcutaneous administration may lead to abscess).
- Neonate of infected mother: Give INH resistant BCG + INH prophylaxis for 6 weeks.
- *Chemoprophylaxis (preventive treatment):* INH for 1 year or INH plus ethambutol for 9 months.

Perinatal TB

..... *Nelson 17/e, 967, 971*

- MC sign and symptoms of congenital TB are respiratory distress, fever, hepatic or splenic enlargement, poor feeding, lethargy, irritability, lymphadenopathy, abdominal distension, failure to thrive, ear drainage and skin lesions.
- Symptoms most commonly begin by 2nd or 3rd week of life.
- A positive acid fast stain of an early morning gastric aspirate from newborn usually indicate TB.
- Most important clue for rapid diagnosis is maternal or family history of TB.
- Most effective way of preventing congenital TB is appropriate testing and treatment of mother and other family members.

Approach to Perinatal Tuberculosis

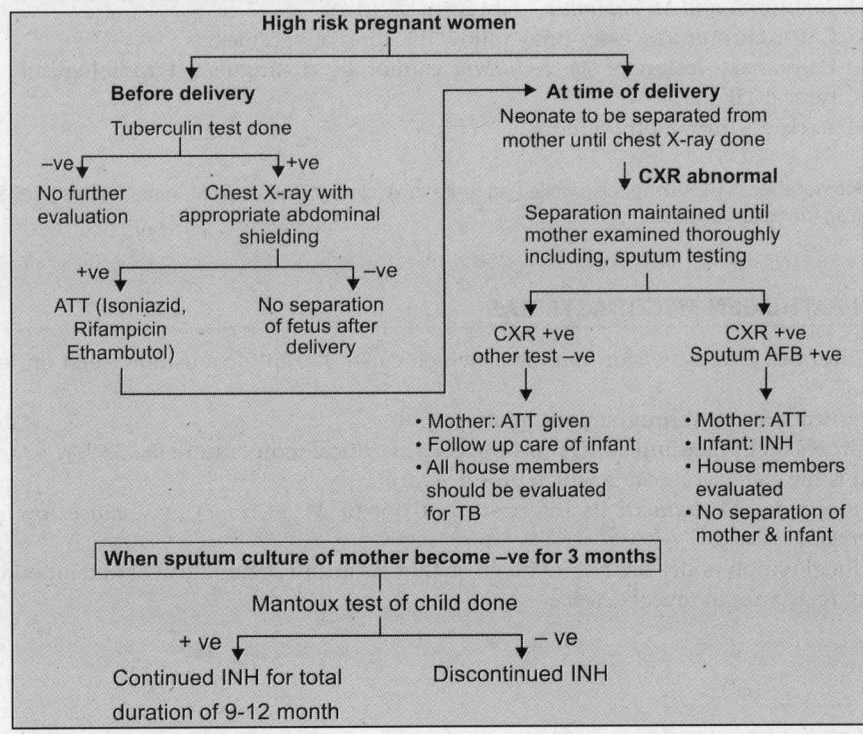

> - MDR strain (Multidrug resistant strain): Strain resistant to isoniazid and rifampicin with or without resistance to additional drugs.
> - XDR-TB (Extensively drug resistant TB): MDR Strain that is resistant to, fluoroquinolone and one of the second line injectables.
> - Mutation to drug reistance occurs at a rate of about one mutation every 10^6 cell division.

ATYPICAL MYCOBACTERIA

- Also known as Unclassified or Environmental or Opportunistic mycobacteria.
- It includes mycobacterial species other than *Mycobacterium tuberculosis* complex and *M. leprae*, hence, called as Paratubercle or tuberculoid or MOTT (mycobacteria other than tubercle) bacilli.

- It is divided into 4 groups based on colony pigmentation (Runyon's classification).
- **Group I – Photochromogens** - Produce pigment only in light.
- Slow growing though growth is faster than that of tubercle bacilli. It includes:
  a. **M. kansasii** – cause chronic pulmonary disease in old persons with pre-existing lung disease.
  b. **M. marinum** – cause warty skin lesion (*swimming pool granuloma*).
  c. M. simiae
- **Group II – Scotochromogens** - Form pigment even in dark.
  a. **M. scrofulaceum** – cause scrofula (cervical adenitis) in children.
  b. **M. gordonae** – called as *Tap water scotochromogen*.
  c. **M. szulgai** – scotochromogen and photochromogen.

Group III – non-photochromogens - Not form pigment even in light.
- Colonies may resemble those of tubercle bacilli.
  a. **M. intracellulare** – also known as *Battey bacillus*.
  b. **M. avium** – MAIS complex (i.e. avium, intracellulare, scrofulaceum) cause lymphadenopathy, pulmonary lesion and disseminated disease particularly in **AIDS** patient.
- **Other non-chromogens are:**
  – M. ulcerans, M. shinshvense, M. paratuberculosis, M. xenopi, M. malmoense, M. sylvaticum, M. lapraemurium, M. terrae, M. hemophilum, M. genevense

Group IV – Rapid growers
- Colonies appear within seven days. They can be photochromogenic, scotochromogenic, non-chromogenic. It includes:
  a. Chromogenic saprophytic rapid growers, e.g. *M. smegmatis, M. phlei*
  b. *M. fortuitum and M. chelonae* – Not form pigment.
     – Cause chronic abscesses (may follow injection of vaccines).
     – Pulmonary lesion of *M. fortuitum* cannot be distinguished radiologically from typical TB.
  c. *M. vaccae* – Immunomodulator.

> **Remember:** M. chelonei also called as turtle tubercle bacillus while M. fortuitum also called do frog tubercle bacillus.

Common site of infection
- M. kansasii: Lung
- M. marinum: Skin, swimming pool granuloma
- M. avium: AIDS patient
- M. scrofulaceum: Scrofula

SKIN PATHOGEN MYCOBACTERIAS

- **M. ulcerans:** Exclusive skin pathogen which cause *Buruli ulcer* usually seen on legs or arms.
  – Infection occur through minor injuries.
  – Grows on LJ medium slowly in 4-8 weeks at critical temperature (30-33°C).
  – It is the *only mycobacteria* which produce *toxin*.
- **M. marinum (M. balnei):** Its infection (but not of *M. ulcerans*) may cause low grade *tuberculin reaction*.
- Regional lymph nodes are not involved as they multiply optimally at skin temperature.
- Drug resistance in mycobacteria.

Buruli ulcer: Caused by M. ulcerans

Multiple Choice Questions

M. tuberculi

1. For diagnosis of tuberculosis using blood sample which of the following test is used? [NEET Pattern 2018]
   a. IFN γ assay
   b. Gene Xpert MTB/RIF
   c. BACTEC
   d. Fluorescence microscopy

2. Detection of LAM antigen in urine has been used to screen patients for infection with which of the following:
   a. Cryptococcus neoformans [AIIMS 2017]
   b. Toxoplasma gondii
   c. Mycobacterium tuberculosis
   d. Pneumocystis jiroveci

3. Basanti, 29 year aged female from Bihar present with active TB. She delivers baby. All of the following are indicated *except*: [AI 01, AIIMS 2008]
   a. Administer INH to the baby
   b. Withhold breastfeeding
   c. Give ATT to mother for 2 years
   d. Ask mother to ensure proper disposal of sputum

4. Which of the following regarding the Interferon-gamma release assays used for the diagnosis of tuberculosis is correct?: [AI 2012]
   a. 1st generation Quantiferon-TB used ESAT-6
   b. 2nd generation Quantiferon-TB (gold) used ESAT-6 and CFp-10
   c. These tests can distinguish between *M. tuberculosis* and *M. bovis*
   d. None of the non-tubercular mycobacteria give a positive reaction with this test

5. True about Mantoux test: [PGI 13]
   a. < 5 mm always +ve
   b. Usually -ve after treatment
   c. Positive reaction in children < 2 is not improtant like in adult
   d. Usually red after 48-72 hours
   e. False +ve in post measles state

6. True regarding *Mycobacterium tuberculosis* is:
   a. Produces visible colonies in 1 week time on Lowenstein Jenson media
   b. Decolorised by 20% sulphuric acid
   c. Faculatative aerobe
   d. Niacin positive [PGI 12]

7. Which of the following are acid fast positive with 20% sulphuric acid: [PGI 02, AIIMS 2012]
   a. *M. avium*
   b. *M. leprae*
   c. *M. tuberculosis*
   d. *Nocardia*

8. Selective media for TB bacilli is: [PGI 11]
   a. NNN media
   b. Dorset media
   c. LJ media
   d. Nutrient agar
   e. Mac'Conkey media

9. The picture below depicts a bacterium which is most consistent with: [AIIMS 2017]

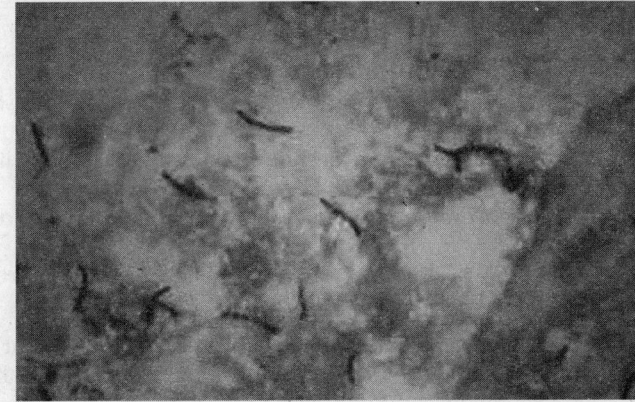

   a. Streptococcus pyogenes
   b. Mycobacterium tuberculosis
   c. Nocardia asteroides
   d. Corynebacterium diphtheriae

10. Cavitation is most often seen in: [AI 2011]
    a. Mycoplasma pneumonia
    b. Tuberculous pneumonia
    c. Streptococcal pneumonia
    d. Staphylococcal pneumonia

M. leprae

11. Leprosy affects all the following *except*: [AI 07]
    a. Testes   b. Ovaries
    c. Eyes   d. Nerves

12. In the management of leprosy, Lepromin test is most useful for: [AI 03]
    a. Herd immunity
    b. Prognosis
    c. Treatment
    d. Epidemiological investigations

13. Which of the following is true regarding globi in a patient with lepromatous leprosy: [AI 02]
    a. Consist of lipid laden macrophages
    b. Consist of macrophages filled with AFB
    c. Consist of neutrophils filled with bacteria
    d. Consist of activated lymphocytes

14. The main cytokine, involved in erythema nodosum leprosum (ENL) reaction, is: [AIIMS 06]
    a. Interleukin-2
    b. Interferon - gamma
    c. Tumor necrosis factor - alpha
    d. Macrophage colony stimulating factor

15. The following drug is not used for the treatment of type II lepra reaction: [AIIMS 06]
    a. Chloroquine   b. Thalidomide
    c. Cyclosporine   d. Corticosteroids

16. The following test is not used for diagnosis of leprosy:
    a. Lepromin test   [AIIMS 06]
    b. Slit skin smear
    c. Fine needle aspiration cytology
    d. Skin biopsy

17. Which of the following statement about lepromin test is not true: [AIIMS 07, 06]
    a. It is negative in most children in first 6 months of life
    b. It is a diagnostic test
    c. It is an important aid to classify type of leprosy disease
    d. BCG vaccination may convert lepra reaction from negative to positive

18. Under leprosy eradication program the management of single lesion is: [AIIMS 02]
    a. Single dose of Rifampicin and Dapsone
    b. Rifampicin and Dapsone for 6 months
    c. Rifampicin, Ofloxacin and Minocycline single dose
    d. Rifampicin and Monocycline for 6 months

19. The characteristic finding in a case of leprosy is:
    a. Culture test is positive in 2-3 months in LJ media
    b. Long contact with tuberculoid leprosy can transmit the disease [AIIMS 98, 2000]
    c. CMI is seen in Lepromatous leprosy
    d. Macule lesion heals spontaneously

20. Antibodies against PGL - 1 are seen in: [AIIMS 2013, AI 2011, DNB 2012]
    a. M. leprae   b. M tuberculosis
    c. Borrelia   d. Brucella

Atypical mycobacteria

21. Which one of the following statement is true regarding pathogenicity of Mycobacteria species: [AI 06]
    a. M. tuberculosis is more pathogenic than M. bovis to humans
    b. M. kansasii can cause disease indistinguishable from tuberculosis
    c. M. africanum infection is acquired from environmental source
    d. M. marinum is responsible for tubercular lymphadenopathy

22. The most common focus of Scrofuloderma is:
    a. Lung   b. Lymph node   [AI 04]
    c. Larynx   d. Skin

23. True about mycobacterium other than tuberculosis:
    a. Causes disseminated infection   [AIIMS 08]
    b. Occurs in persons with normal immunity
    c. Causes decreased efficacy of BCG due to cross immunity
    d. Person to person transmission is seen

24. Scotochromogens are: [PGI, 2008]
    a. Mycobacterium gordonae
    b. Mycobacterium marinum
    c. Mycobacterium Intracellulare
    d. Mycobacterium avium
    e. Mycobacterium kansasii

25. Which of the following are photo chromogens?
    a. M. kansasii   b. M. scrofulosorum
    c. M. marinum   d. M. TB
    e. M. leprae   [PGI 2008]

26. Which of the following is a slow grower: [AIIMS 2013]
    a. M. kansasii   b. M. chenolae
    c. M. fortuitum   d. M. abscessus

27. Rapid growing non-tuberculous mycobacteria causing lung infection are all except: [AIIMS 2013]
    a. M. kansasii   b. M. chelonae
    c. M. fortuitum   d. M. abscessus

Explanations and References with Illustrative Answers

1. **Ans. (a) IFN-γ assay** *Ref. Harrison 20/e, p 1248*

   IFN γ release Assays (IGRA)
   - In vitro assays that measure T-cell release of IFN γ in response to stimulation with the highly TB specific antigen ESAT-6 and CFP-10. Presently two such assays are available:
     (a) **T. SPOT TB:** An enzyme linked immunosorbent assay.
     (b) **Quantiferon-TB Gold:** Whole blood enzyme linked immunosorbent assay.
   - IGRA are more specific than the TST (*Mantoux test*) as they are negligibly effected by previous BCG vaccination and sensitization by non-tubercular mycobacteria.
   - IGRA require blood to be drawn from patient and delivered to lab where test is done, in contrary to tuberculin test in which PPD is injected. So, these test can be repeated without boosting response.
   - In near future IGRA are supposed to replace tuberculin skin test as preferred skin test for detection of latent tuberculin infection.
   - M. marinum, M. kansasii, M. szulgai also have ESAT 6 and CFP 10 and may cause false positive reactions.
   - Currently IGRA is preferred over TST in population above 5 years of age. In children under 5 years TST is preferred and in individuals who are at high risk of progression to active TB either test can be used.

   > **Note:** In 2013 WHO has banned IgM ELISA for tuberculosis, and described that test as one of the most misused test.

   - Though in previous reports. IGRA's found to be more specific than TST, however recent studies suggest that IGRA may not perform well in serial testing. So WHO does not recomend the replacement of TST by IGRA in low income group countries like India. *Ref. Harrison 19/e, p 1114*

2. **Ans. (c) Mycobacterium tuberculosis** *Ref. Harrison 20/e, p 1244; Internet reference*
   LAM Test based on the detection of mycobacterial lipoarabinomannan (LAM) antigen in urine have emerged as potential point-of-care tests for tuberculosis (TB).
   LAM antigen is a lipopolysaccharide present in mycobacterial cell walls, which is released from metabolically active or degenerating bacterial cells and appears to be present only in people with active TB disease.
   Urine-based testing would have advantages over sputum-based testing because urine is easy to collect and store, and lacks the infection control risks associated with sputum collection.
   As per WHO currently LF-LAM (lateral flow urine LAM testing) may be used to assist in the diagnosis of TB in HIV positive adult in-patients with signs and symptoms of TB (pulmonary and/or extrapulmonary) who have a CD4 cell count less than or equal to 100 cells/μL, or HIV positive patients who are seriously ill regardless of CD4 count or with unknown CD4 count

   > **Note:** LF-LAM should not be used for the diagnosis of TB neither it should be used as a screening test for TB.
   > LF LAM is positive in all patients of active TB irrespective of site

   Genitourinary TB
   - Accounts for 15% of all extrapulmonary cases.
   - Urinary frequency **(MC)**, dysuria, hematuria and flank pain are common presentation.

   Diagnosis:
   i. Urinalysis gives abnormal result in 90% of cases.
   ii. Culture of three morning urine specimens yields a definitve diagnosis in nearly 90% cases.
   Culture negative pyuria in acidic urine raises the suspicion of TB.
   iii. IVP – Calcification, ureteral stricture and Hydronephrosis may seen.

Genital TB	Female > male
MC site in **female** MC site in **male**	• Fallopian tube • Epididymis
Genitourinary TB respond well to chemotherapy.	

3. **Ans. (b) Withhold breastfeeding** *Ref. Nelson 17/e, p 971; Harrison 20/e, p 1256*
   If the mother is suspected of having active disease or detection of an acid fast bacilli in sputum shows evidence of current tuberculosis disease, besides giving ATT to mother certain additional steps are necessary to protect the infant:

a. **INH therapy**
   "INH therapy for newborns is so effective that separation of mother and infant is no longer considered mandatory."
   - Separation should done (until mother become non-infectious) only if:
     - Mother is so ill so as to require hospitalization.
     - She is expected to become non-adherent with her treatment.
     - There is strong suspicion that she has drug resistant tuberculosis.
   - INH treatment of infant should be continued until the mother has been shown to be sputum culture negative for at least 3 months.

b. **Appropriate treatment of mother and other family members.**
   - Though there is controversy in the question as according to 'Some books' Breastfeeding is contraindicated and isolation of infant from the mother having active TB should done.
   - But as all other three options are totally correct and as Indian child must have breastfeeding, I have to go with Nelson only.

4. **Ans (b) 2nd generation Quantiferon-TB (gold) used ESAT-6 and CFp-10**   *Ref. Harrison 20/e, p 1248*
   Already explained

5. **Ans. (d) Usually red after 48-72 hours**   *Ref. Ananthanarayan 10/e, p 360; Park 21/e, p 168; 22/e p 172*
   - Tuberculin test is the only means of estimating prevalence of infection in a population.
   - **It is of three types:**
     - Mantoux intradermal test
     - Heaf test - for testing large groups
     - Tine multiple puncture test - not recommended.
   - Standard PPD (purified protein derivative) contains 50,000 tuberculin units per milligram.
   - WHO advocates PPD tuberculin known as PPD RT-23 with Tween 80.
   - For routine testing 1 TU used, while clinically 5 TU used.

Mantoux Test

- 0.1 ml of 1 TU injected intradermally
- Examined after 72 hours and induration is measured horizontally in mm and is interpreted as:
  > 10 mm   : Positive
  < 6 mm   : Negative
  6-9 mm   : Doubtful that is the reaction may be due to M. tuberculosis or atypical mycobacteria
  > 20 mm   : Strong reactors – Greater chance of developing TB
  < 5 mm   : More risk of developing TB than those with 6-9 mm induration
- Positive reaction indicates that person has got previous exposure to M. tuberculosis but it does not prove that person is suffering from disease.
- Positive reaction is significant in younger age groups (< 2 year).
- *Negative test cannot taken as exclusion of TB* since dermal hypersensitivity to tuberculin can also be lost in immunosuppressive states which gives *false -ve result* e.g. Malignancy, Hodgkin's disease, post measles state, corticosteroid therapy.
- Repeat test may appear to be negative or exerts a booster effect.
- Positive tubercullin test may occasionally revert to negative upon INH treatment.
- *After infection patient becomes tuberculin positve in 3-6 weeks (= I.P of TB).*
- *After 8 weeks of BCG vaccination it becomes positive.*

6. **Ans. (d) Niacin positive**   *Ref. Ananthanarayan 10/e, p 354 - 355*

Mycobacteria tuberculosis is:

- Gram positive, non-motile, noncapsulated, non sporing.
- Obligate aerobic.
- Acid fast (resist decolorization by 20% H_2SO_4) and alcohol fast.
- Generation time 14-15 hours.
- Colonies appear slowly in about 2 weeks and may sometimes take up to 8 weeks.
- Niacin, Neutral red, Nitrate reduction test positive (3N is positive).
- Peroxidase and Urease test is also positive.

7. **Ans. (c) M. tuberculosis** *See below*

Features	M. tuberculosis	M. leprae
Acid fastness	Resist decolorization by 20% H_2SO_4	Resist decolorization by 5% H_2SO_4
Alcohol fastness	Present	Absent
Culture	Possible	Not possible
Niacin	Positive (also some strain of *M. microti*)	Negative
Generation time	14-15 hours	12-13 days

Remember: Nocardia resist 1-4% of sulphuric acid (weakly acid fast).

8. **Ans. (b) and (c) Dorset media and LJ media** *Ref. Ananthanarayan 10/e, p 352*

    Media for M. tuberculosis

Solid	Liquid
• Lowenstein Jensen media *(most widely used)*	• Dubos contain Tween 80
• Dorset egg media	• Middle Brook's
• Loeffler's media	• Proskauer and Beck's
• Pawlowsky media	• Sula's and Sautan

   - Selective agent inhibiting other bacteria in LJ media is Malachite green.
   - Human tubercle bacilli do not grow in presence of para-nitrobenzoic acid.
   - Traces of fatty acid is toxic for tubercle bacilli in culture media.
   - Optimum pH for M. tuberculosis: 6.4-7.0.

   Other Options:
   NNN media   – For Leishmania donovani
   Nutrient agar   – Simple media
   MacConkey media – Differential as well as indicator media for lactose and non-lactose fermenters.

9. **Ans. (b) Mycobacterium TB (See below)** *Ref. Ananthanarayan 10/e, p 358*
   Among given options both mycobacterium and nocardia are acid fast.

   Note: Nocardia are branching whereas mycobacterium are straight rods (see color plate pg xxv for related image)

10. **Ans. (b) Tuberculous pneumonia** *Ref. Harrison 20/e, p 1242*

Pneumonia pattern	Etiologic organism
Lobar distribution	Streptococcus pneumoniae
Bulging fissure	Klebsiella
Cavitation	Tuberculosis
Pneumatocele	Staphylococcus
Alveolar nodules	Varicella, Tuberculosis
Pulmonary edema	Viral/Pneumocystis pneumoniae

11. **Ans. (b) Ovaries** *Ref. Harrison 20/e, p 1262-1263; International Journal of Leprosy, Vol. 71, No. 2, p 101-105*

    Mycobacterium leprae grows best in cooler (the skin, peripheral nerves, anterior chamber of the eye, upper respiratory tract, and testes), sparing warmer areas of the skin (the axilla, groin, scalp, and midline of the back).

    Thus, ovary is the answer of exclusion.

    Complications of M. leprae
    - *Eye:*   Uveitis, cataracts, glaucoma, corneal insensitivity and lagophthalmus.
    - *Testes:*   Orchitis followed by impotence.
    - *Nerve abscesses:* Mostly seen in BT form, **ulnar nerve is most frequently involved.**
    - *Extremities:*   Plantar ulceration (most frequent complication of leprous neuropathy), footdrop, Charcot's joints.
    - *Nose:*   Epistaxis, saddle-nose deformity or anosmia.

12. **Ans. (b) Prognosis** *Ref. Ananthanarayan 10/e, p 374*

Lepromin test:
- It is intradermal test which shows delayed type IV hypersensitivity.
- It is biphasic:
  a. **Early reaction of Fernandez:** Read in 24-48 hours (analogous to tuberculin reaction)
  b. **Late reaction of Mitsuda:** –Peak in 4 weeks
  – It is more meaningful.
- It distinguishes between persons who can mount CMI against lepra bacillus antigens and those who cannot.
- So, *finally lepromin test is of little diagnostic value but has more prognostic value.*
- *It is used to:*
  - Classify the lesions of leprosy
  - To assess prognosis and response to treatment
  - To assess resistance of individual to leprosy
  - To verify the identity of candidate lepra bacilli.
- **Antigen used in lepromin test:**
  - Modern antigens contain 4×10^7 lepra bacilli per ml.
  - Standard lepromins derived from armadillo derived lepra bacilli (lepromin A) replacing human derived human lepromin H.

13. **Ans. (c) Consist of macrophages filled with AFB**   *Ref. Ananthanarayan 10/e, p 371, Robbins 7/e, p 373*
    Lepromatous lesion contain large aggregates of lipid laden macrophages (lepra cells) often filled with masses (globi) of acid fast bacilli
    ... *Robbins*

14. **Ans. (c) Tumor necrosis factor - alpha**   *Ref. Harrison 20/e, p 1262; KDT 6/e, p 756*
    TNF plays a central role in pathobiology of ENL.

Type I lepra reaction	Type II Lepra reaction
• Downgrading or reversal reaction	• Erythema nodosum leproticum
• Type IV hypersensitivity	• Type III hypersensitivity
• TNF play a central role	• IFNγ and IL-2 are main cytokines involved
• Edema is characteristic microscopic feature	• Vasculitis and panniculitis are seen
• **Treatment: DOC** – Glucocorticoid Other drugs: – Clofazimine – Chloroquine – Analgesics Thalidomide is Ineffective	• **DOC** – Thalidomide Other – Clofazimine – Chloroquine – Glucocorticoids – NSAIDs & antibiotics

15. **Ans. (c) Cyclosporine**   *Ref. Harrison 20/e, 1262; KDT 6/e, p 756*
    Cyclosporine has no role in lepra reaction.
    For more details, refer above answer.

16. **Ans. (a) Lepromin test**   *Ref. Harrison 20/e, p 1263*

    Note: PCR of the skin for M. leprae although positive MLL and BL disease negative result in 50% of tuberculoid cases.

    Lepromin test is not used for diagnosis.

17. **Ans. (b) It is a diagnostic test**   *Ref. Harrison 20/e, p 1263*
    Already explained

18. **Ans. (c) Rifampicin, Ofloxacin and Minocycline single dose**   *Ref. Harrison 20/e, p 1263*

Form of Leprosy	WHO recommended regime
i. Tuberculoid (paucibacillary)	Dapsone 100 mg/d unsupervised plus Rifampicin 600 mg/mth supervised for 6 month
ii. Single skin lesion (paucibacillary)	Single dose of **R** 600 mg **R**ifampicin **O** 400 mg **O**floxacin **M** 100 mg **M**inocycline
iii. Lepromatous (multibacillary) >6 skin lesion	Dapsone 100 mg/d plus Clofazimine 50 mg/d unsupervised; and Rifampicin 600 mg plus Clofazimine 300 mg monthly (supervised) for 1 year

19. **Ans. (b) Long contact with tuberculoid leprosy can transmit the disease** *Ref. Harrison 20/e, p 1260*

    ### Transmission of Leprosy
    - Nasal droplet infection.
    - Contact with infected soil and contact with a tuberculoid leprosy case carries a very low risk.
    - Insect vectors.
    - *Direct dermal inoculation (during tatooing).*
    - Household contact with infected lepromatous case.
    - Skin to skin contact (though can transmit infection) is *generally not considered an important route of transmission.*
    - Physicians and nurses caring for leprosy patients & the coworkers of these patients are not at risk leprosy.
    - According to *Park 18/e, p 254* "All patients with active leprosy must be considered infectious".

    > **Remember:**
    > - Cell mediated immunity (CMI) is present in tuberculoid leprosy and lepromatous leprosy patient do not exhibit CMI to leprosy bacteria Lepra bacilli cannot grow in artificial culture media.
    > - Park, Ananthanarayan, Harrison do not mention that macules of tuberculoid leprosy heals spontaneously.
    > - In India maximum leprosy patient are in Bihar > UP.

20. **Ans. (a) M. leprae** *Ref. Harrison 20/e, p 1263*

    IgM antibodies to PGL-1 are found in 95% of patients with untreated lepromatous leprosy, and 60% of patients with tuberculoid lepresy. Antibodies to PGL-1 may also be seen in exposed individual without clinical leprosy.
    Thus PGL-1 serology is of little diagnostic utility in tuberculoid leprosy.

    > **Remember:** PGL-1 stands for M. leprae specific phenolic glycolipid found in the cell wall of leprosy bacilli.

21. **Ans. (b) *M. kansasii* can cause disease indistinguishable from tuberculosis** *Ref. Jawetz 27/e, p 318*

    "Some atypical bacteria (e.g. Mycobacterium kansasii) produce human disease indistinguishable from tuberculosis."
    ..... *Jawetz, 27/e, 318*

    ### Other options:
    Option 'a': *M. tuberculosis* and *M. bovis* are equally pathogenic for humans. ......*Jawetz*

Features	M. tuberculosis	M. bovis
Shape	Curved long rod	Straighter, shorter, stouter
Staining	Less uniform	More uniform
O₂ requirement	Obligate aerobe	Microaerophilic
Colonies	Dry, rough, raised, irregular	Flat, smooth, moist, break up easily
Growth	Eugonic	Dysgonic

    Options 'c': *M. africanum* is acquired from human and cattles.

    > **Remember:**
    > - M. tuberculosis, M. bovis; M. africanum belongs to TB complex group of Runyons classification.
    > - Mycobacterium acquired from environmental source:
    >   – M. **a**vium complex
    >   – M. **m**almoense (**Mnemonic: AMU** – **A**ligarh **M**uslim **U**niversity)
    >   – M. **u**lcerans

    Option 'd': *M. marinum* causes chronic cutaneous infection when open cutaneous lesion is exposed to colonized water source.

    > **Remember:** Atypical bacteria causes lymphadenitis are: M. avium, M. intracellulare, M. malmoense, M. scrofulaceum, M. kansasii.

22. **Ans. (b) Lymph node** *Ref. Dashore Manual of Skin Disease, p 85*

    ### Scrofuloderma is a type of cutaneous tuberculosis.
    - It results from direct extension of infections from underlying tuberculous focus, i.e. infected lymph glands, muscles or bones.
    - Patient's immunity is poor or moderate.
    - Lab investigations – demonstration of bacilli in smears of biopsy material, culture.

23. **Ans. (c) Causes decreased efficacy of BCG due to cross immunity** *Ref. Park 22/e p 179*

    Exposure to some non-tuberculous environmental mycobacteria (M. vacuae, M. non-chromogenicum) may have conferred partial immunity on the population and thus masked the potential benefit of BCG vaccination. There is also evidence that exposure to other species (M. kansasii, M. scrofulososum) have an antagonistic action against BCG.

    MOTT (Mycobacteria Other Than Tuberculosis)
    - MOTT are mycobacterial species that may cause human disease but do not cause tuberculosis.
    - **Spread:** Unlike tuberculosis, which is spread from person to person, MOTT infections are not considered contagious. There is no evidence that the infection can be transmitted from one person to another. The mode of infection with MOTT is not clear.
    - **Clinical features:** – Like tuberculosis, an MOTT infection primarily affects the lungs and the symptoms are similar. Usually MOTT infections progress slowly.
        – *Symptoms include:* Fever, Weight loss, Cough, Loss of appetite, Night sweats, Blood in the sputum.
    - **Diagnosis:** MOTT infections can be more difficult to diagnose than tuberculosis. A diagnosis is generally based on the following:
        – Medical history including above symptoms
        – Chest X-ray
        – *Sputum culture:* Several sputum cultures are often necessary.
        – *Other procedures:* More complicated diagnostic procedures (BAL) may be required in certain cases.
    - *Treatment:* Many MOTT infections are benign with no need for treatment. MOTT infections are naturally resistant to conventional antibiotics and it is necessary to use several ATT at the same time in order to overcome drug resistance.

24. **Ans. (a) *Mycobacterium gordonae*** *Ref. Ananthanarayan 10/e, p 367*

    Scotochromogens:
    M. Szulgai
    M. Scrofulaceum (cause scrofula)
    M. Gordonae/M. acquae
    Mnenomic: *Sundar Sushil Girl*

25. **Ans. (a and c) *M. kansasii, M. marinum*** *Ref. Ananthanarayan 10/e, p 366*

    Photochromogens
    M. Siniae
    M. Marinum
    M. Asiaticum
    M. Kansasii

    Mnenomic: *Sridevi Marry Anil Kapoor*

26. **Ans. (a) *M. kansasii*** *Ref. Ananthanarayan 10/e, p 366*
    M. kansasii is a slow growing atypical mycobacteria belonging to photochromogens.

    Other options
    - M. fortuitum and M. chelonai belong to Group IV of atypical mycobacteria (rapid growers) and their colony usually appear within seven days.
    - ***Mycobacterium abscess*** is a rapidly growing mycobacterium that is a common water contaminant. It can cause chronic lung disease, post-traumatic wound infections, and disseminated cutaneous diseases, mostly in patients with suppressed immune systems.

    Note:
    - *M. abscessus* and *M. chelonae* can be distinguished from *M. fortuitum* by their failure to reduce nitrate and to take up iron.
    - Tolerance to 5% NaCl in Löwenstein-Jensen media, and non-utilisation of citrate as a sole carbon source are characteristics that distinguish *M. abscessus* from *M. chelonae*.

27. **Ans. (a) *M. kansasii*** *Ref. Ananthanarayan 20/e, p 367; Harrison 18/e, p 1369; 19/e, p 1129*
    M. kansasii is not a rapid grower
    M. kansasii
    - Most pathogenic nontubercular mycobacteria.
    - 2nd MC cause of lung disease due to NTM.

- Risk factors: COPD; Silicosis, Lung carcinoma, Prior tuberculosis.
- Clinical features and treatment is similar to tuberculosis with Rifampicin being the most effective drug.

Rapid Growing Mycobacteria
- Heterogeneous group to mycobacteria capable of rapid growth, colonies appearing within seven days of incubation.

Important members include:
- M. phlei : Saprophyte
- M. fortuitum : Chronic abscess, pulmonary lesions
- M. chelonae : Chronic abscess
- M. smegmatis : Round in smegma
- M. vaccae : Immunomodulator that stimulates protectine immune response in tuberculosis
- M. abscessus : Oesophageal motility disorders such as achlasia

Differentiation between tubercle bacilli and some species of atypical mycobacteria

Test	M. tuberculosis	M. bovis	M. microti	M. kansasii	M. marinum	M. scrofulaceum	M. avium-intracellulare complex	M. fortuitum	M. chelonei	M. phlei	M. smegmatis
Growth in 7 days	–	–	–	–	–	–	–	+	+	+	+
Growth at 25°C	–	–	–	+	+	+	±	+	+	+	+
Growth at 37°C	+	+	+	+	±	+	+	+	+	+	+
Growth at 45°C	–	–	–	–	–	–	±	–	–	+	+
Pigment in dark	–	–	–	–	+	–	–	–	–	+	–
Pigment in light	–	–	–	+	+	+	–	–	–	+	–
Growth in the presence of p-nitrobenzoic acid 500 µg/mL (PNB)	–	+	+	+	+	+	+	+	+	+	+
Urease	+	+	+	+	+	+	–	+	+	+	+
Niacin	+	–	±	–	–	–	–	–	–	–	–
Nitrate reduction	+	–	–	+	–	–	–	+	–	+	+

NEET Pattern Questions

1. **Which of the following is photochromogenic:**
   a. M. kansasii
   b. M. scrofulorum
   c. M. intracellulare
   d. M. avium
   [Ref. Ananthanarayan, 10/e, p 367]

2. **Which of the following is not a pathogenic mycobacteria:**
   a. M. kansasii
   b. M. scrofulorum
   c. M. cheolonei
   d. M. smegmatis
   [Ref. Ananthanarayan, 10/e, p 367]

> *Mycobacterium smegmatis* is a saprophytic mycobacteria isolated from smegma (though not regularly found in smegma). It is a frequent isolate from soft tissues lesion following trauma or surgery

> **Other saprophytic mycobacteria include:**
> - *M. butyricum* from butter
> - *M. phlei* from grass
> - *M. stercoris* from dung

3. **Buruli ulcer is caused by:**
   a. Streptococcus
   b. Spirillium minus
   c. M. ulcerans
   d. Brucella
   [Ref. Ananthanarayan, 10/e, p 368]

> **M. ulcerans**
> - A toxin producing mycobacteria producing ulcer on legs and arms called as Buruli ulcer
> - Smears from the edge of ulcer show large clumps of bacteria which are acid fast or alcohol fast

4. **Tuberculosis complex include all except:**
   a. M. tuberculosis
   b. M. bovis
   c. M. kansasii
   d. M. microti
   [Ref. Ananthanarayan, 10/e, p 350]

> Mycobacterium tuberculesis complex: Group of bacteria producing human tuberculosis include, M. bovis, M. tuberculosis, M. africanum (cause human tuberculosis in tropical Africa) and M. microti.

5. **Fish tank granuloma is seen in:**
   a. M. fortuitum
   b. M. kansasii
   c. M. marinum
   d. M. leprosy
   [Ref. Ananthanarayan, 10/e, p 369]

> Fish tank granuloma (= swimming pool granuloma) is caused by M. marinum, a natural pathogen of cold blooded animals. Normally it lives as saprophyte in salt and fresh water. Lesion begin as papule which break down to form an indolent ulcer. Usually occurs at body prominences like elbow, knee, ankle, nose, fingers or toes. Ulcer are self limiting and undergo spontaneous healing.

6. **Pigment producing atypical mycobacteria:**
   a. M. fortuitum and M. chelonae
   b. M. xenopi and MAC
   c. M. gordonae and M. szulgai
   d. M. ulcerans
   [Ref. Ananthanarayan, 10/e, p 366]

> M. scheelgai and M. gordonae are scotophoto chromogen, which produce pigment in dark

7. **ENL is seen in:**
   a. Lepromatous leprosy
   b. Tuberculoid leprosy
   c. Indeterminate leprosy
   d. Pure neuritic leprosy
   [Ref. Ananthanarayan, 10/e, p 374]

8. **Liquid medium for tuberculosis:**
   a. LJ medium
   b. Dorset medium
   c. Loeffler's medium
   d. MGIT
   [Ref. Jawetz, 27/e, p 309]

> **Culture media for M.tuberculosis**
> - **Semisynthetic agar media:** Middle brook 7H10 and 7H11 contains salt, vitamins, albumin, catalase and glycerol. Requires large inocula which makes them less sensitive for primary isolation of mycobacteria.
> - **Inspissated egg media:** Lowenstein Jensen media, small inocula can be grown on these media in 3-6 weeks. These media with antibiotics (gruft and mycobactosel) are used as selective media.
> - **Broth media:** Middle brook 7H9 and 7H12. Support small inocula. Eg MGIT system, versa TREK culture system and MB redox are other examples.
> - Use of liquid media with radiometric growth detection such as BACTEC 460 has simplified culture methods and enabled results to be given in 2-3 weeks.

9. **Live TB bacilli culture is by:**
   a. Tinsdale medium
   b. MGIT
   c. MYPA medium
   d. BYCE agar
   [Ref. Jawetz, 27/e, p 309]

10. **Radiomimetric BACTEC detect growth of M tuberculosis in how much time:**
    a. 1 week
    b. 2-3 week
    c. 4-8 week
    d. >10 weeks
    [Ref. Ananthanarayan, 10/e, p 353]

Ans.
1. a. M. kansasii
2. d. M. smegmatis
3. c. M. ulcerans
4. c. M. kansasii
5. c. M marinum
6. c. M. gordonae
7. a. Lepromatous....
8. d. MGIT
9. b. MGIT
10. b. 2-3 weeks

11. **Mycobacterium tuberculosis grows in LJ media in:**
    a. 10-14 days
    b. 2-3 weeks
    c. 4-8 weeks
    d. >10 weeks
    [Ref. Jawetz, 27/e, p 309]

12. **Which type of pulmonary TB is most likely to given sputum positive:**
    a. Fibronodular
    b. Pleural effusion
    c. Cavitary
    d. None
    [Ref. Ananthanarayan, 9/e, p 351]

13. **Fastest method for diagnosis of TB:**
    a. Genexpert
    b. LJ medium
    c. TB MGIT
    d. BACTEC
    [Ref. Jawetz, 27/e, p 315]

> **Genexpert MTB/RIF test**, a real multiplex PCR method that both identifies the MTB complex and also detects genes that encode rifampin resistance within 2 hours. Overall sensitivity is 98.2%/ for smear positive cases and 72.5% for smear negative samples. Overall specificity is 99.2%.

14. **Tuberculin test is:**
    a. Intramuscular
    b. Intradermal
    c. Subcutaneous
    d. None
    [Ref. Ananthanarayan, 10/e, p 356]

15. **Method used for acid fast staining:**
    a. Robertson's method
    b. Ziehl-Neelsen
    c. Silver imprignation method
    d. Dark ground illumination
    [Ref. Ananthanarayan, 10/e, p 352]

> **Ziehl-Neelsen Stain**
> - Described by F. Ziehl and F. Neelsen.
> - Used to identify acid fast organism.
> - Reagents used are carbol fuchsin, acid alcohol and methylene blue.
> - *Technique*: The slide is first stained with carbol fuchsin which is then heated to dry and rinsed off in tap water. The slide is then flooded with a 1% solution of hypochloric acid in ispropyl alcohol. There after the slide is stained with methylene blue.
> **Modifications:**
> - 1% sulfuric acid alcohol: Nocardia, Actinomycetes 0.5%
> - 0.5% Sulfuric acid alcohol: Oocysts of isospora, coyclospora cryptosporidium
> - 0.25–0.5% sulfuric acid alcohol for bacterial endospores.
> - *Kinyoun modification* (does not require heat): Nocardia, mycobacteria

16. **Acid fastness of tubercle bacilli is attributed to:**
    a. Presence of mycolic acid
    b. Integrity of cell wall
    c. Both of the above
    d. None of the above
    [Ref. Ananthanarayan, 10/e, p 352]

> Acid fastness is attributed to presence of mycolic acid. It is related to integrity of cell wall and appears to be the property of lipid rich waxy cell wall.

17. **XDR-TB is defined as Resistance to:**
    a. INH plus rifampicin
    b. Fluoroquinolones plus INH plus amikacin
    c. Fluoroquinolones plus rifampicin plus kanamycin
    d. Fluoroquinolones plus INH plus rifampicin plus amikacin
    [Ref. Greenwood, 18/e, p 219]

18. **Positive tuberculin test means:**
    a. Resistance to TB
    b. Susceptibility to TB
    c. Hypersensitivity
    d. None of the above
    [Ref. Park, 22/e, p 172]

> Positive reaction means person is infected with M. tuberculosis and does not necessarily means person is suffering from disease

19. **To notify a slide as AFB negative minimum how many fields should be checked?**
    a. 20
    b. 100
    c. 50
    d. 200
    [Ref. Park, 22/e, p 170]

20. **Modified Ziehl-neelsen staining is used for:**
    a. Mycobacterium tuberculosis
    b. Mycobacterium bovis
    c. Nocardia
    d. All of the above
    [Ref. Ananthanarayan, 10/e, p 352]

21. **MDR TB is defined as:**
    a. Resistance to INH and Ethambutol
    b. Resistance to Rifampicin and Ethambutol
    c. Resistance to Pyrazinamide and Rifampicin
    d. Resistance to INH and Rifampicin
    [Ref. Greenwood, 18/e, p 219]

22. **Gnexpert used for getting diagnosis of TB in:**
    a. 1–2 hrs
    b. 5 hrs
    c. 10 hrs
    d. 20 hrs
    [Ref. Jawetz, 27/e, p 315]

23. **Hansen's bacillus is cultured in:**
    a. L J medium
    b. Robertson's cooked meat medium
    c. Foot pad of mice
    d. Sabraud's agar
    [Ref. Ananthanarayan, 10/e, p 375]

24. **True about mycobacterium leprae:**
    a. Transmitted by droplet infection
    b. Phenolic glycolipid (PGL) is virulence factor
    c. Generation time 12–13 days
    d. All are true
    [Ref. Ananthanarayan, 10/e, p 375]

> - Virulence factor of M. leprae
>   – Phenolic glycolipid I (PGL-I)
>   – Lipoarabinomannan
>   – Adhesins

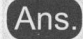

11. **c.** 4-8 weeks	12. **c.** Cavitary	13. **a.** Gene expert	14. **b.** Intradermal	15. **b.** Ziehl-Neelsen
16. **c.** Both of the above	17. **d.** Fluoroquinolones plus INH …		18. **d.** None of the above	
19. **b.** 100	20. **d.** All of the above	21. **d.** Resistance to INH and Rifampicin		
22. **a.** 1–2 hrs	23. **c.** Foot pad of mice	24. **d.** All are true		

25. **Globi in leprosy consist of:**
    a. AFB + macrophages b. Neutrophils + AFB
    c. Platelet plug   d. None of the above
    [Ref. Park, 22/e, p 172]

    > In lepromatous leprosy, the dermis is filled with rounded macrophages stuffed with bacilli which often form clumps termed Globi.

26. **Primary complex of M. bovis involves:**
    a. Tonsil and lung   b. Tonsil and intestine
    c. Tonsil and skin   d. Skin and Intestine
    [Ref. Greenwood, 18/e, p 213]

27. **Phagocytosis of mycobacterium tuberculosis by macrophages is mainly mediated by:**
    a. IL 6   b. IL 3
    c. IL 12   d. IFN Gamma
    [Ref. Greenwood, 18/e, p 214]

28. **Battey bacillus is:**
    a. Klebsiella pneumoniae
    b. Mycobacteria paratuberculosis
    c. Klebsiella ozaenae d. Mycobacteria intracellulare
    [Ref. Ananthanarayan, 10/e, p 367]

    > M. introcellulare is commonly known as Battey bacillus becused it was first identified as a human pathogen at Battey state hospital USA.

29. **Organism identified by interferons:**
    a. Staphylococcus b. Leptospira
    c. Campylobactor   d. M. tuberculosis
    [Ref. Harrison, 20/e, p 1249]

    > Two in vitro assays that measure T. cell release of IFN-α in response to stimulation with highly selective TB antigens ESAT-6 and CFP-10 are in use currently T-SPOT TB and quantiferon TB gold are example

30. **Lepra bacilli can survive outside the human body up to:**
    a. 7 days   b. 12 days
    c. Zero days d. 5 days
    [Ref. Ananthnaraya, 10/e, p 372]

    > Lepra bacilli can survive in warm humid environment for 9-16 days and in moist soil for 46 days. They survive exposure to direct sunlight for 2 hours and UV light for 30 minutes.

31. **BCG vaccine in HIV (+) newborn is:**
    a. Contraindicated   b. Double dilution
    c. Half dilution   d. Dose double
    [Ref. Ananthanarayan, 10/e, p 362]

    > BCG vaccine should not be given to infants and children with active HIV disease. Babies born to mother with AFB positive spectum should bot be given BCG at birth, but only after a course of preventive chemotherapy.

32. **Cutaneous lesions may be produced by the following mycobacteria except:**
    a. M. intracellulare
    b. M. leprae
    c. M. marinum
    d. M. tuberculosis
    e. M. ulcerans
    [See below]

    > *Mycobacterium* causing skin lesion:
    > - M. tuberculosis – M. leprae
    > - M. ulcerans   – M. marinum
    > - M. haemophilum

33. ***Mycobacterium tuberculosis* is differentiated from other atypical mycobacteria by:**
    a. Niacin test
    b. AFB staining
    c. PAS staining
    d. None
    [Ref. Ananthanarayan, 10/e, p 367]

    > Niacin test is positive in *M. tuberculosis*, *M. simiae* and few strains of *M. cheloneli*.

34. **The factor which promotes, virulence of *M. tuberculosis*:**
    a. Wax D
    b. Cord factor
    c. Muramyl dipeptide
    d. Mycolic acid
    [Ref. Jawetz, 27/e, p 312]

35. **All of the following are acid fast bacteria except:**
    a. Cryptosporidia
    b. Mycoplasma
    c. Mycobacteria
    d. Nocardia
    [Learn the list from our book]

36. **Rapid examination of Tubercle bacilli is possible with:** (2016)
    a. Ziel-neelsen stain
    b. Kinyoun stain
    c. Auramine-Rhodamine stain
    d. Giemsa stain
    [Ref. Ananthanarayan, 10/e, p 358]

    > - **Fluorescent microscopy** is preferred when several smears are to be examined daily *(rapid screening)*.
    > - In this, smears are stained with auramine phenol or auramine rhodamine fluorescent dyes and examined under UV illumination.
    > - Bacilli will appear as bright rods against dark background.

25. a. AFB + macrophages	26. b. Tonsil...	27. d. IFN gamma
28. d. Mycobacteria intracellulare	29. d. M. tuberculosis	30. b. 12 days
31. a. Contraindicated	32. a. M. intra...	33. a. Niacin ...
34. b. Cord fa ...	35. b. Mycoplasma	36. c. Auramine...

CHAPTER 15

Enterobacteriaceae

- **Enterobacteriaceae** includes large group of gram-negative rods whose natural habitat is large intestine.
- They are predominantly aerobic or facultative anaerobes, non-sporing and non-acid fast.
- They have following **common characteristics:**
  - Grow well on *MacConkey* media.
  - Catalase (+)ve; except *Shigella dysentriae* type 1.
  - Oxidase (-)ve; reduces nitrates to nitrite.
  - Urease (-)ve; except **Proteus, Klebsiella, Morganella**.
  - Motile by peritrichate flagella except *Shigella, Klebsiella* and *Salmonella gallinarum-pullorum*.
  - Ferment glucose except *Shigella*.

> - Gram (-)ve bacilli
> - Catalase positive
> - Oxidase negative
> - Classified on the basis of lactose fermentation.

Classification

- *MC* and oldest method to classify these bacteria is on *basis* of *fermentation of lactose*.

Lactose fermented rapidly = Coliforms	Lactose fermented slowly = Late lactose fermenter = Paracolons	Lactose not fermented = Mostly pathogenic
• *Escherichia* • *Klebsiella* • *Enterobacter aerogenes* They forms pink colony on Maconkey's medium and are usually part of normal flora.	• *Edwardsiella* • *Serratia* • *Citrobacter* • *Arizona* • *Providencia* • *Erwinia* • *Shigella sonnei*	• *Shigella except S. sonnei* • *Salmonella* • *Proteus*

Remember: Differential media which distinguishes lactose fermenting (colored) from non-lactose fermenting colonies (non pigmented) includes eosin methylene blue (EMB), MacConkey or deoxycholate medium.

ESCHERICHIA COLI

Morphology

Motile by peritrichate *flagella*, non-sporing. Many pathogenic isolates are *capsulated*.

Culture and Biochemical characteristics

- Grows well on ordinary media.
- *On blood agar shows hemolysis.*
- Indole and Methyl red (+)ve while VP and citrate (-)ve [IMVC ++--].
- Except certain verocytotoxin producing strain *E. Coli* are lactose fermentor.

Antigenic structure

- *Somatic antigen O* — Lipopolysaccharide in nature, heat stable. Antibodies to O-antigen are predominantly IgM.
- *Capsular antigen K* — Heat labile responsible for attachments of bacteria to epithelial cells.
  — Associated with virulence.
- *Flagellar antigen* — Important virulence factor
- Serotyping based on these three antigens is:
  - **Normal colon strains = commensal strains belong to early 'O' group (1, 2, 3, 4, etc.).** These strains generally lack specialized virulent traits. However, they may be involved in extraintestinal infection.
  - **Enteropathogenic strains: Belong to later 'O' group (25, 55, 86 etc).**

E. coli toxins
- Heat stable toxin: Rapid action.
- Heat labile toxin: Activate cAMP.
- Verocytotoxin: Phage coded inhibit protein synthesis

– **Extraintestinal pathogenic E. coli (EXPEC):** *MC* cause of extraintestinal *E. coli* infection. Like commensal *E.coli* they can be found in normal intestinal flora without causing gastroenteritis, but they have acquired diverse virulence factor that enable them to live extraintestinally.

Virulence Factors

a. Surface antigen:

- O-antigen – It has endotoxic activities and also protects bacteria from phagocytosis. These are lipopolysaccharide and are heat stable.
- K-antigen – Protect against phagocytosis.
- Fimbriae – *Plasmid coated fimbriae increase virulence,* while chromosomally determined fimbriae has no effect on virulence.
- H-antigen – Heat labile and group specific antigen. Occurs in single phase except in Salmonella where it biphasic.

b. Toxin: *E.coli* produce two kind of exotoxin:

- Hemolysins – No role in pathogenesis of diarrhea.
- Enterotoxins – Important in pathogenesis of diarrhea.

E. coli enterotoxins		
Heat stable toxin (STA)	**Heat labile toxin (LT)**	**Verocytotoxin (VT) = Shiga like toxin (SLT)**
• Plasmid mediated • Activates cGMP • Acts very rapidly	• Plasmid mediated • Consist of 2 subunit A → Activates CAMP → Diarrhea B → Binds GM_1 gangliosides	• Phage coded • Belong to ribosome inactivating protein [RIP] toxins • A subunit of SLT inhibit ribosome and ↓ protein synthesis and shows cytotoxicity

Clinical Findings

A. Diarrhea – 5 types of diarrheogenic *E. coli* are recognized:

- **Enteropathogenic = enteroadherant *E. coli***
  - Cause diarrhea in infant and children.
  - Strains that carry PEAF plasmid are termed typical EPEC while those lacking it are called atypical ...*Greenwood 18/e, p283.*
  - Non-toxigenic and non-invasive.
  - Produce diarrhea by disruption of brush border. Bacilli adhere to upper small intestine through adhesion receptor synthesized by bacteria which is then inserted in to host put wall
  - They are unable to ferment sorbitol.
  - Usually cause epidemic, but sporadic cases can also occur.

- **Enterotoxigenic *E. coli* (e.g. 06, 08, 015, 025, 027, 0167)**
  - Affect *all age group*.
  - *MC* cause of traveller's diarrhea (indistinguishable from cholera). Most cases are endemic.
  - Produce either or both LT and STa.
  - Produce diarrhea, only when it adheres to intestinal mucosa by fimbriae called colonization factor antigen and produce toxin.

- **Enteroinvasive *E. coli*** ..... *Ananthanarayan 10/e, p 285*
  - Called *atypical E. coli* as many strains do not ferment lactose or ferment it late.
  - Resemble *Shigella flexneri* except in fermenting dulcitol and forming alkali in litmus milk. They resemble 'Alkalescens–Dispar' Group
  - Cause illness resembling *shigellosis*.
  - Ability to *penetrate cells is due to* presence of plasmid which codes for outer membrane antigen called virulence marker antigen *[VMA]*.

- For *diagnosis* of EIEC - Sereny test is used. Cell penetration of Hela or HEP-2 in culture is also *diagnostic test*.
- **Enterohemorrhagic E. coli (EHEC) = Verotoxigenic E. coli (VTEC)**
  - Source of infection appears to be salad as washing only doesn't remove bacteria.
  - Produce *Verocytotoxin VT* whose major target is vascular endothelial cells.
  - VT resembles shiga toxin, genes encoding VT in E. coli are carried on a lambda like bacteriophage (in shigella they are present on chromosome). It acts by inhibiting protein synthesis, by irreversibly inhibiting ribosomal function
  - Stx2 appears to be more important than STx1 in development of HUS
    Harrison 20/e p 1152
  - Cause disease ranging from mild diarrhea to fatal hemorrhagic colitis and hemolytic uremic syndrome (HUS).
  - **HUS:** – Mainly caused by O157 H7 type which does not ferment sorbitol (Some 0157 and non 0157 strain ferment sorbitol).
    – Sorbital Mac conkey medium helps in screening of 0:157VTEC
    ..... Ananthanarayan 10/e, p 286
    – Antibiotics increase the incidence of HUS.
- **Enteroaggregative E. coli (EAEC)**
  - Cause *persistent diarrhea*.
  - Stacked brick' formation on Hep -2 cells.
  - Produce *EAST* – Enteroaggregative heat stable enterotoxin.

> Enteroadherant E. coli: Infant and Children
> ETEC: All age group.
> EIEC: Resemble *Shigella*
> EHEC: Produce verocytotoxin, causes hemorrhagic colitis and hemolytic uremic syndrome.
> Enteroaggregative E. coli: Persistent diarrhea

		Intestinal Pathogenic *E.coli*		
Pathotype	**Epidemiology**	**Clinical syndrome**[a]	**Defining Molecular trait**	**Responsible Genetic element**[b]
STEC/EHEC/ ST-EAEC	Food, water, person-to-person; all ages, industrialized countries	Hemorrhagic colitis, hemolytic uremic syndrome	Shiga toxin	Lambda-like Stx1- or Stx2-encoding bacteriophage
ETEC	Food, water; young children in and travelers to developing countries	Traveler's diarrhea	Heat-stable and labile enterotoxin, colonization factors	Virulence plasmid(s)
EPEC	Person-to-person; young children and neonates in developing countries	Watery diarrhea, persistent diarrhea	Localized adherence, attaching and effacing lesion on intestinal epithelium	EPEc adherence factor plasmid pathogenicity island (locus for enterocyte effacement (LEE)
EIEC	Food, water; children in and travelers to developing countries	Watery diarrhea, occasionally dysentery	Invasion of colonic epithelial cells, intracelluar multiplication, cell-to-cell spread	Multiple genes contained primary in a large virulence plasmid
EAEC	Food, water; children in and travelers to developing countries; all ages, industrialized countries	Traveler's diarrhea, acute diarrhea, persistent diarrhea	Aggregative/diffuse adherence, virulence factors regulated by AggR	Chromosomal or plasmid-associated adherence and toxin genes

EAEC-enteroaggregative *E. coli*; EHEC-enterohemorrhagic *E. coli*; EIEC-enteroinvaive *E. coli*; EPEC,-enteropathogenic *E. coli*; ETEC-enterotoxigenic *E. coli*.; ST-EAEC-Shiga toxin-producing enteroaggregative *E. coli*; STEC-Shiga toxin-producing *E.coli*.

B. UTI
- Urinary tract is the site most frequently infected by ExPEC.
- ***MC cause of both uncomplicated and nosocomial UTI.***
- UTI causing serotypes are those normally found in feces.
- Only one serotype is generally isolated from infected urine at a time while in diarrhea many serotypes are present in a single culture.
- Nephropathogenic *E. coli* typically produce Hemolysin.
- Pyelonephritis is associated with specific type of pilus, P. pilus.

> EHEC is the commonest cause of hemolytic uremic syndrome
> – Usually affects children < 5 years of age

- **Diagnosis**
  - UTI is said when there is:
    - Bacteriuria ≥ 10^5/mL in asymptomatic
    - Bacteriuria of ≥ 10^4/mL in symptomatic
    - Bacteriuria of ≥ 10^2/mL in catheterized sample
    - Bacteriuria of any degree in suprapubic aspirate.
- **Presumptive diagnosis of bacteriuria is made by:**
  - *Griess nitrite test*
  - *Catalase nitrite test*
  - *Triphenyl tetrazolium chloride test.*

C. Pyogenic Infection – E. coli is *MC* Cause of intra-abdominal abscess, peritonitis and cholangitis.

D. Meningitis – E. coli is *MC* cause of neonatal meningitis. 75% of meningitis causing E. coli have the K1 antigen. This antigen crossreacts with the group B capsular polysaccharide of N. Meningitidis.

E. Pneumonia – E. coli is **2nd** *MC* cause of nosocomial pneumonia (*1st being* **Staph. aureus**)

F. Bacteremia – UTI is *MC* source of E. coli bacteremia leading to septic shock
  – E. coli and S. aureus are the two most common blood isolate from patient of bacteremia.

Treatment
- **UTI –** *Fluoroquinolone* are **DOC**.
- **Diarrhea – Fluids and electrolyte correction with** *no antibiotics*.
- **Drug resistance is plasmid mediated.**

E. coli is the MC cause of:
– UTI
– Neonatal meningitis
– Intra-abdominal abscess

KLEBSIELLA

- Non motile, capsulated (capsule seen as haloes around bacilli), gas producing rod.
- **Classified into 3 species on the basis of biochemical characteristics** and into **serotypes** on basis of **K-antigen** (*capsular antigen*).

Klebsiella pneumoniae = Friedlander's bacillus
- Rarely cause disease in normal person.

Clinical manifestation
- Cause community acquired pneumonia in alcoholics, chronic bronchopulmonary disease or diabetes.
- *MC* clinical syndromes it causes are pneumonia, UTI, abdominal infections, surgical site infection, soft tissue infection and bacteremia.
- **Pneumonia :**
  – Mainly hospital acquired. Abscess are more common than in pneumococcal pneumonia.
  – Cause classic lobar infiltrate with bulging fissure.
  – Sputum is red current jelly in character.
- **UTI:** Mainly in settings of prolonged catheterization.
- **Diarrhea:** By toxin similar to ST_A of E. coli.
- Virulence is increased in iron overload conditions like thalassemia.

Capsule of type II resemble that of pneumococcus. Polysaccharide capsule is the major virulence factor

Klebsiella ozaenae
- Causative agent of ozoena characterized by foul smelling nasal discharge.

Klebsiella Granulomatis
- Only enterobacteria implicated in genital ulcers
- Cause donovanosis
- Diagnosis treatment conformed by microscopic identification of donovan bodies
- Azithromycin in the ventneto of choice
  Harrison 20/e p 1215

Klebsiella rhinoscleromatis (Frisch bacillus)
- Causative agent of rhinoscleroma (Hebra nose).

Treatment of Klebsiella
- **Carbapenem** (Imipenem) – Most active antibiotic against *klebsiella*.

Klebsiellae: Non-motile, capsulated Gram (–)ve
- **K. pneumoniae:** Pneumonia, UTI
  – One of the common cause of neonatal sepsis in India
- **K. ozaenae:** Ozone
- **K. rhinoscleromatis** Rhinoscleromatis

SHIGELLA

- Non motile, non capsulated, non lactose fermentar (except *S. sonnei* which ferments it late).
- **Classified** on the *basis of somatic O Antigen (LPS) and carbohydrate fermentation (mannitol) pattern.*
- Catalase is produced by *all except Sh. dysnteriae I.*
- Mannitol is fermented by *all except Sh. dysnteriae I.*
- MC Shigellosis worldwide – *Sh. sonnei.*
- MC Shigellosis in India – *Sh. flexneri.*
- Most clinically severe form of Shigellosis is caused by *Sh. Dysenteriae* type I while mildest form of bacillary dysentery is by *Sh. sonnei* (may occur as food poisoning).
- Only species that exist as single serotype – *Sh. sonnei.*
- **Pathogenic species of shigella are:**

Species	Group	Ornithine Decarboxylase	Mannitol Fermentation
S. dysenteriae	A	–	–
S. flexneri	B	+	–
S. boydii	C	+	–
S. sonni	D	+	+

Culture

- **Selective media:** – Xylose-lysine deoxycholate (XLD), Deoxycholate citrate agar (DCA).
  – Hektoen enteric agar or Salmonella - Shigella agar.
  ..... *Jawetz 27/e, p 238*
- *Triple sugar iron* (TSI) agar is used to differentiate salmonella and Shigella from other gram-negative rods in stool cultures.

Selective media for shigella:
– DCA Agar
– Hektoen enteric agar
– Salmonella–Shigella agar

Pathogenesis

a. **Invasiveness (main):**
   - Bacteria invade basolateral surface of colon epithelium → intracellular replication and cell to cell spread with the help of microbial protein Ics A (ATPase) and host protein cadherin L - CAM.
   - This process present in all virulent shigellae as well as in EIEC. It is responsible for late dysentery. Hence *nontoxic mutants can cause dysentery but non-invasive can't produce dysentery.*
   - Pathogenic strains carry a plasmid which is thermoregulated; such that strains become invasive when growing at 37°C but not at 30°C.

b. **Toxins:**
   i. *Endotoxin* – LPS present in all shigella causing irritation of bowel.
   ii. *Shigella Dysenteriae* – I produces a heat labile exotoxin (*Shiga bacillus exotoxin*) that affect both gut and CNS:
      - It has neurotoxicity on blood vessel of CNS and can lead to meningismus and coma.
        - *Enterotoxicity* causing fluid accumulation in ligated rabbit ileal loop.
        - *Cytotoxicity* same as Verotoxin I or Shiga like toxin produced by some strain of EHEC including 0157:H7.
      - *Toxin has two peptide subunit. A unit (N-glycosidase) of cytotoxin* hydrolyzes adenine from specific sites of 60s RNA and thus *inhibits protein synthesis.* It contributes to fatal nature of *S. dysenteriae* infection.
      - Toxins produce early, non bloody voluminous diarrhea.
      - Genes encoding shiga toxin are located on chromosome

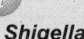

Shigella
- Non motile, non-capsulated
- Catalase (–)ve except Sh. dysenteriae
- Infective dose of bacillary dysentery is as low as 10 viable bacteria.
- Shiga toxin: Chromosome coded toxin, that inhibits protein synthesis

Clinical Features

- Most cases of bacillary dysentery occur in < 10 year children.
- Infective dose is in the order of 10^3 organisms (*while in vibrio and Salmonella 10^4-10^8*).
  ..... *Jawetz 27/e, p 238*
- Transmitted feco-orally generally direct person to person contact; *anal-oral sex* (esp. *in Sh. sonnei*).

- Majority of lesion are in *distal colon*.
- **Complications** – Toxic dilatation, Colonic perforation.
  - *Extraintestinal* (esp. with *S. dysenteriae* and *S. flexneri*) like HUS, Thrombotic thrombocytopenic purpura reactive arthritis, Reiter's syndrome.

Diagnosis

- *Specimen* – Best to use mucus flakes of stool.
- *Transport media* – Sach's buffered glycerol saline.
- *Specific diagnosis* – Culture of shigella from stool.
- Culture media – DCA agar, MacConkey agar
- Pale non-lactose fermenting colonies suggest its diagnosis.

For Shigella dysenteriae diagnosis faecal specimen is preferred over rectal swab.

Treatment

- **Mild to moderate dehydration** – Oral rehydration therapy (No antibiotics).
- **Severe cases with bloody diarrhea** – *DOC* Ampicillin or co-trimoxazole (Amoxicillin is not effective).
- *DOC* **for multiresistant:** Nalidixic acid.

SALMONELLA

- Genus consist of bacilli that parasitise small intestine leading to enteric fever, gastroenteritis, septicemia.
- They are motile with peritrichate flagella except *S. gallinarum pullorum*.
- They are non-capsulated and non-sporing.

Culture and Biochemical Characteristics

- Grows readily on simple media.
- On Wilson – Blair bismuth sulphite media S. typhi produce jet black colonies due to production of H_2S.
- *Enrichment media* – Selenite F and Tetrathionate broth.
- *Selective media* – Salmonella-shigella agar, Deoxycholate citrate agar which promotes growth of salmonella over other enterobacteria; xylose-lysine Deoxycholate agar
- Salmonella ferment sugar producing acid and gas except *S. typhi* which is anerogenic.
- *S. typhi* need *tryptophan as growth factor*.
- Boiling or chlorination of water and pasteurization of milk destroy the bacilli.

> **Note:** DCA & XLD agar are useful selective media to differentiate shigella and salmonella. Shigella do not exhibit black centre whereas salmonella appear red with black centre.

Salmonella
- Non capsulated, non-sporing, motile (except S. gallinarum pullorum).
- Enrichment media: Selenite F and tetrathionate broth
- Selective media: SS agar, DCA media

Classification

- Originally Salmonella was classified on the basis of *O, H* and *Vi antigenic* structure and biochemical reactions. But now on the *basis of DNA hybridization* studies only *7 groups have been identified*. Currently, the genus salmonella is divided into two species: Salmonella enterica (which includes five serotypes) and Salmonella bongari. ...*Jawetz 27/e p 239*
- ***Nearly all the salmonella serotypes that infect human are in DNA hybridization group 1.***

Method for Isolation of Salmonellae

- Differential culture Media: Bismuth sulfite medium permits rapid detection of salmonella (forms black colonies because of H_2S production). EMB, Mac conkey or deoxycholate medium are other differential media, but all lactose nonfermenters grow on these media.
- Selective Culture Medium: Shigella-Salmonella agar; Hektoen entire agar; XLD; deoxy cholate - citrate agar. These mediums favors growth of salmonella and shigella over other enterobacteriaceae.
- Enrichment culture: **Selenite F or tetrathionate broth**, both of them inhibit replication of bacterias other than salmonella.

Antigenic Structure

1. **Flagellar antigen (H)**
   - Heat labile protein which is strongly immunogenic. When mixed with antisera, it rapidly produce-*fluffy clumps*. Exhibit the property of diphasic variation.
2. **Somatic antigen (O)** (Biovin antigen)
   - Heat stable phospholipid polysaccharide complex identical with endotoxin. It remains unaffected by boiling. When mixed with antisera, forms chalky, granular clumps.
   - Located in outer membrane, anchored to cell wall, on the basis of difference in long chain LPS, 30 serotypes are defined.
3. **Vi antigen**
   - Heat labile surface polysaccharide antigen enveloping O antigen. Found only in *S.typhi* and *S.paratyphi*. Poorly analog to K antigen of coliforms. Heat-labile and immunogenic. *Associated with Virulence*.

> **Remember:** Order of immunogenic nature of antigen: H > O > Vi

Pathogenicity

- On reaching gut, bacilli are phagocytosed.
- Salmonella typhi *resist intracellular killing* by macrophages and polymorphs and enter mesenteric lymph node and from there via thoracic duct enter blood stream to produce bacteremia (Enteric fever).
- All the clinical manifestation begin after ileal penetration

Clinical Manifestation

I. **Enteric fever**

Systemic disease characterized by fever and abdominal pain caused by *S.typhi* (called as typhoid) and S. paratyphi. A, B and C.

S. paratyphi A is emerging as the most common cause of enteric fever specially in Asia.

- I.P. – 14 days.
- Infection is acquired through ingestion
- Infective dose: $10^3 - 10^6$
- Paratyphoid fever of S. paratyphi is generally milder.
- *Mode of transmission* – Transmitted through feco-oral; uro-oral route.
   – Making water as major vehicle
- *Typical features* – *Step ladder pyrexia with relative bradycardia*
   – *Rose spots* (located primarily on chest) usually appear at the end of 1st week and resolve after 2 - 5 days.

Carriers:
- Those who excrete bacilli for more than a year are called as Chronic carrier.
- Carrier rate is 3% (i.e. 3% of cases become chronic carrier).
- Though cases occur more in males, carriers are common in females.
- Fecal carrier are MC.
- Urinary carrier signify abnormality in urinary tract.

Diagnosis (Mnemonic: BASU)

A. *Cases*
- **Blood culture (B)**
   - Positive in 1st week (*Diagnostic gold standard*). Sensitivity is 40-80%
   - Clot culture has *higher rate of isolation*, than blood culture.
- **Bone marrow culture:** 55-90% sensitive and unlike that of blood culture, its yield is not reduced by prior antibiotic therapy.

> - Bone marrow culture is the most reliable method for diagnosis of enteric fever.
>   ...*Greenwood 18/e, p 270*
> - S. paratyphi A is now becoming a predominant cause of enteric fever specially in Asia
> - Recombinant vir EPA is the most effective vaccine.

- **Agglutination (A) = Widal reaction**
  - Detects antibodies against O and H antigen. Titer > 1:320 against O antigen and >1: 640 against H antigen is considered positive.
  - Becomes (+)ve by end of 1st week, *peaks at 3rd week*, decline afterwards.
- *Stool culture (S)* – 3rd week, particular valuable in *patient on antibiotics* in which blood culture is (-) ve Sample are plated directly on *MacConkey, DCA,* and *Wilson - Blair media (highly selective).*
- *Urine culture (U)* – (+)ve only in 2nd and 3rd weeks.

B. **Carriers**
- **Widal** – No value in detection of carrier.
- *Demonstration of Vi agglutinin has been claimed to indicate carrier state and used as screening of carrier.*

Treatment
- **Cases:**
  - First line: Ciprofloxacin, Ceftriaxone
  - Alternative: Azithromycin
  - Multidrug resistant [MDR] *S. typhi*: Ciprofloxacin is **DOC**. Multidrug resistant is due to R factor.
- **Carriers:** Amoxicillin, Co-trimoxazole, Ciprofloxacin are effective.
- **Control of typhod fever**
  - *Isolation:* The cases of typhoid should be isolated till three bacteriologically negative stools and urine reports are obtained on three separate days.
  - *Disinfection of stool and urine:* Stool and urine should be disinfected with 15% cresol for at least 2 hours, so as to kill all bacteria. All soiled cloth and linen should be soaked in a solution of 2% chlorine and steam-sterilized.
  - *Immunization:* Following vaccines are available:

Vaccine	Nature	Dose	Minimum age
Type 21a	Live attenuated	4 oral dose	6 years
Vicps	Purified Vi polysaccharide	1 Parenteral dose (subcutaneous/IM)	2 years
VirEPA	Vi bound to recombinant protein	2 parenteral dose	6 month

Vir EPA is most effective.

Salmonella carrier
- Site: Biliary tract
- Diagnosis: Culture of duodenal aspirate
- IgG Vi antibodies

II. **Gastroenteritis** = (Food poisoning)
- MC causative agent is *S. typhimurium.*
- Most frequent sources are poultry, meat, milk and milk products.
- Never caused by *S. typhi.*
- IP-6-48 hours.
- *Clinical features* – Nausea, vomiting, diarrhea, Abdominal cramps and fever.
- Blood culture is negative.
- *Treatment* – No antibiotics are given usually, except for serious invasive cases.

III. **Bacteremia and Endovascular infection**
Salmonella serotypes S. choleraesuis and S. dublin are frequently associated with sustained bacteremia.

IV. **Localized infection**
- Intra-abdominal infection: Hepatic or splenic abscess, cholecystitis.
- CNS infection: NTS meningitis most commonly develops in infants 1-4 months of age. It can cause death in up to 60% of cases.
- Pulmonary infection: Cause pneumonia and associated complications in patients with lung ca, sickle cell disease or glucocorticoid use.
- UTI and genital infection: Risk factors include malignancy, urolithiasis, structural abnormalities, HIV infection, transplant recipient.
- Bone joint and soft tissue infection: Salmonella osteomyelitis most commonly affects femur, tibia, humerus and is most often seen in conjunction with sickle cell disease, hemoglobinopathies, or pre-existing bone disease.

Proteus mirabilis
- Non lactose fermenter
- Produce enzyme phenytallanine deaminase
- Cause UTI, pneumonia.

PROTEUS BACILLI

- Non lactose fermenter, highly motile.
- *P. Mirablis* which is responsible for 90% of proteus infection is a normal commensal.
- Prominent cause of UTI in children and bacteraemia, which is attributed to its urease production
- Motility and chemotaxis have role in pathogenesis
- Proteus differs from other enterobacteria by presence of enzyme phenylalanine deaminase (responsible for PPA reaction) which convert phenyl alanine to phenyl pyruvic acid.
- Culture of proteus bacilli have characteristic fishy or seminal smell.
- *P. mirabilis* and *P. vulgaris* swarms on solid culture media.
- **Antigenic structure** – Proteus posse flagellar (H) and somatic O antigen.
- **Infectious syndromes** – UTI (20-30% of complicated UTI); Pneumonia (primarily in hospitalized patient); Intraabdominal infections; soft tissue abscess.

> **Remember:** Some strains of *P. vulgaris* called **X strains** are agglutinated by sera from typhus fever patient. This is due to sharing of carbohydrate hapten between *Rickettsiae* and proteus and forms basis of *Weil Felix reaction*.

ENTEROBACTER

- Resemble klebsiella but are readily distinguished by their motility.
  - Ent. cloacae is the most important species.
  - Important cause of bacteraemia

CRONOBACTER

- C. sakazakii is an emerging pathogen associated with powedered milk causing necrotizing enterocolitis, sepsis, and meningitis in infants.
- Ampicillin and gentamicin is the treatment.

Multiple Choice Questions

E. coli

1. With reference to infection with Escherichia coli the following are true *except*: [AI 05]
   a. Enteroaggregative E. coli is associated with persistent diarrhea
   b. Enterohemorrhagic E. coli cause hemolytic uremic syndrome
   c. Enteroinvasive E. coli produces a disease similar to salmonellosis
   d. Entero toxigenic E. coli is a common cause of traveller's diarrhea

2. A 20-year-old man presented with hemorrhagic colitis. The stool sample grow Escherichia coli in pure culture. The following serotype of E. coli is likely to be the causative agent: [AI 04]
   a. O 157:H7   b. O 159:H7
   c. O 107:H7   d. O 55:H7

3. A microbiologist wants to develop a vaccine for prevention of attachment of diarrheagenic E. coli to the specific receptors in the gastrointestinal tract. All of the following fimbrial adhesions would be appropriate vaccine candidates *except*: [AI 04]
   a. CFA-1   b. Pi-Pilli
   c. CS-2   d. K88

4. All of the following are true about HUS *except*:
   a. Infection may be transmitted by food [AI 2012]
   b. HUS is caused by serotoxin-producing *Escherichia coli*
   c. HUS is more common in children
   d. HUS is rarely associated with haemorrhagic colitis

5. All of the following are true *except*: [AI 01]
   a. E. coli is an aerobe and facultative anerobe
   b. Proteus forms uric acid stones
   c. E. coli is motile by peritrichate flagella
   d. Proteus caused deamination of phenylalanine to phenylpyrivic acid

6. Most common organism causing UTI: [PGI 10]
   a. E. coli   b. Streptococci
   c. Klebsiella   d. Staphylococci saprophyticus

7. A 20-year-old male had pain in abdomen and mild fever followed by gastroenteritis. The stool examination showed presence of pus cells and RBC's on microscopy. The most likely etiological agent is:
   a. Enteroinvasive E. coli   [AIIMS 03]
   b. Enteropathogenic E. coli
   c. Enterotoxigenic E. coli
   d. Enteroaggregative E. coli

8. Which of these are true about E. coli: [PGI 12]
   a. The L.T. (labile toxin), in ETEC acts via CAMP
   b. UTI causing E. coli attaches through pilli
   c. The ST (Stable toxin) of ETEC is responsible for causing hemolytic-uremic syndrome
   d. EIEC invasiveness is under plasmid control
   e. In EPEC, the toxin helps in invasion

9. True about Enterotoxigenic E. Coli: [AIIMS Nov 10]
   a. Causes epidemic diarrhoea in children in deve-loping countries
   b. Not a cause of traveller's diarrhoea
   c. Invasive
   d. Spread by contaminated water

10. Microbes with Et, Eh and EP strains: [AIIMS Nov 14]
    a. E. coli   b. Mycobacterium
    c. Shigella   d. Neisseria

Salmonella

11. In patient with typhoid, diagnosis after 15 days of onset of fever is best done by: [AI 12]
    a. Blood culture   b. Widal
    c. Stool culture   d. Urine culture

12. *Salmonella* typhi is the causative agent of typhoid fever. The infective dose of S. typhi is: [AIIMS 06, AI 2012]
    a. One bacillus   b. $10^8 - 10^{10}$ bacilli
    c. $10^2 - 10^5$ bacilli   d. 1 - 10 bacilli

13. There has been an outbreak of food borne *Salmonella* gastroenteritis in the community and the stool sample is received in the laboratory. Which is the enrichment medium of choice: [AIIMS 03]
    a. Cary-Blair medium   b. V - R medium
    c. Selenite F medium   d. Thioglycholate medium

14. A 24 years cook in a hostel is suffering from enteric fever 2 years back. The chronic carrier state in patient is diagnosed by: [AIIMS 02]
    a. Vi agglutination test
    b. Blood culture in brain heart infusion broth
    c. Widal test
    d. C. reactive protein

15. True about salmonella gastroenteritis is/are:
    a. Mainly diagnosed by serological tests [PGI 06]
    b. Blood and mucous are present in stool
    c. Caused by animal products
    d. Symptoms appear between 4 - 48 hours
    e. Features are mainly due to exotoxin

16. True about Salmonella typhi infection in intestine are:
    a. Affects Peyer's patches   [PGI 01]
    b. Common in mesenteric border
    c. Erythrophagocytosis is characteristic
    d. Strictures are common
    e. Typhoid ulcer always bleed very much

17. **True about maximum isolation period of enteric fever:**
    a. Till three consecutive negative urine/stool culture samples are obtained from patient. **[AIIMS 08]**
    b. After chloramphenicol treatment for 72 hours.
    c. Disappearance of fever
    d. Widal test negative

18. **About Vi polysaccharide vaccine, true is:** **[AIIMS 10]**
    a. Can be given in patients with yellow fever and hepatitis B
    b. Has many contraindications
    c. Has many serious systemic side effects
    d. Has many serious local side effects

19. **True about salmonellosis:** **[PGI 11]**
    a. ↓ed incidence in developed countries
    b. Antacid and prolonged antibiotic administration promote infection
    c. Always fatal
    d. Food born to man and animal

Others

20. **All are true about Shigella except:** **[AI 2002]**
    a. Large dose is required for infection
    b. Associated with hemolytic uremic syndrome
    c. Causes bloody diarrhea
    d. Gut pathology is due to toxin

21. **Which is/are true about Donovanosis:** **[PGI Nov 11]**
    a. Caused by Leishmania donovani
    b. Amphotericin B is drug of choice
    c. Sodium stibogluconate is drug of choice
    d. Caused by Klebsiella granulomatosis

22. **Wet mount of the scraping of genital ulcer in a sexually active female has been shown below. Identify the organism:** **[AIIMS 2017]**
    a. Klebsiella granulomatis
    b. Hemophilus ducreyi
    c. Neisseria gonorrhoeae
    d. Gardnerella vaginalis

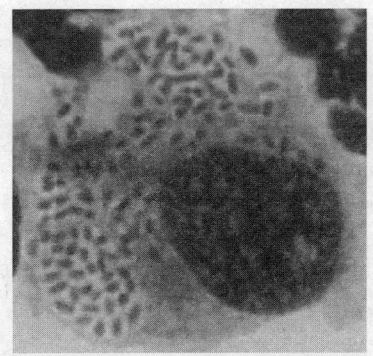

23. **HUS is caused by:** **[PGI 07]**
    a. EIEC   b. Shigella
    c. Salmonella   d. Cholera
    e. Klebsiella

24. **Which of the following is a true statement regarding Enterobacteriaceae:** **[PGI 06]**
    a. Motility is by polar flagellum
    b. Glucose is not fermented by all members of the family
    c. All members are oxidase positive
    d. Nitrate reduction negative

25. **Enterobacteriaecae includes all except:** **[PGI 06]**
    a. Pseudomonas   b. Klebsiella
    c. V. cholera   d. Proteus
    e. E. coli

26. **DT 104 strain is belongs to which of the following bacteria:** **[PGI Nov 11]**
    a. Salmonella Gallinarum   b. Salmonella Typhi
    c. Salmonella Enteritidis d. Salmonella Paratyphi A

27. **Which of the following E. coli causes diarrhoea by affecting intestinal surface villi:** **[AIIMS 2018]**
    a. EAEC   b. EHEC
    c. EAEC   d. EPEC

Explanations and References with Illustrative Answers

1. **Ans. (c) Enteroinvasive E. coli produce a disease similar to salmonellosis** *Ref. Ananthanarayan 10/e p 285*
   "Enteroinvasive E. coli produce disease similar to Shigellosis not salmonellosis."
   Enteroinvasive E. coli (EIEC):
   - Also called *atypical E. coli* as many strains don't ferment lactose or ferment it late.
   - Resemble Alkalescens-Dispar Group
   - Cause illness *similar to Shigellosis*.
   - Ability to penetrate cells is due to presence of *plasmid* which *codes for virulence marker antigen (VMA)*.
   - **Diagnosis:** – Sereny test
     – Cell penetration of Hela or HEP. 2 in culture is diagnostic.

164 Self-Assessment and Review of Microbiology and Immunology

Remember:

• Enteropathogenic *E. coli* (EPEC)	– **Diarrhea in infants and children**
• Enterotoxigenic *E. coli* (ETEC)	– **Traveller's diarrhea**
• Enteroinvasive *E. coli* (EIEC)	– Diarrhea to dysentery **similar to Shigellosis**
• Enterohemorrhagic *E. coli* (EHEC)	– **Hemolytic uremic syndrome**
• Enteroaggregative *E. coli*	– **Persistent diarrhea**

2. Ans. (a) O 157:H7 *Ref. Ananthanarayan 10/e, p 286; Harrison 20/e, p 1152*

"Typically O 157:H7 and few other such as O 26:H1 E.coli are associated with hemorrhagic colitis."
Pathogenesis of O157:H7

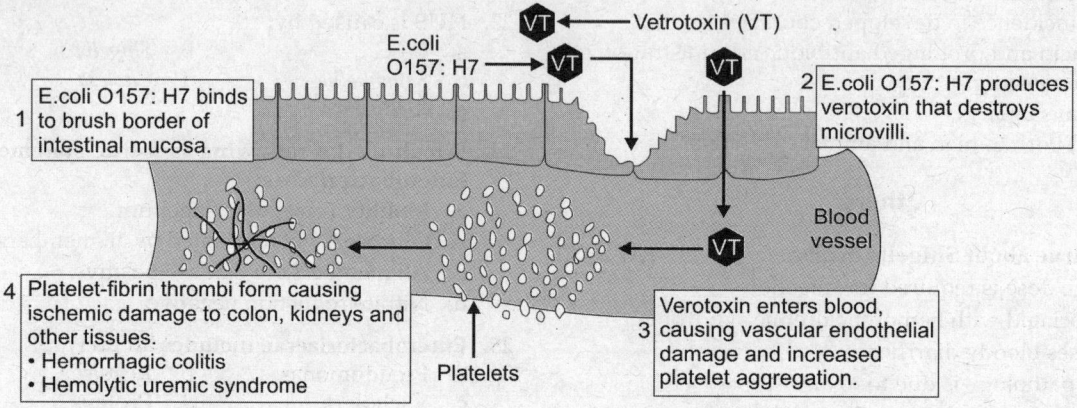

Enterohemorrhagic *E. coli* (EHEC) = Shigatoxigenic *E. coli* (STEC) = Verotoxigenic *E. coli* (VTEC):
- These strains produce verocytotoxin (VT) = Shiga like toxin (SLT).
- Cause diarrheal disease ranging in severity from mild diarrhea to *fatal hemorrhagic colitis* and *hemolytic uremic syndrome*.
- Primary *target of VT is vascular endothelial cells.*
- VT is composed of an active A subunit and five B units that mediate binding
- *'A' subunit of Shiga toxin irreversibly inhibit ribosomal function.* ... *Harrison 20/e, p 1152*
- Stx-2 mediated activation of complement may also play a role in the development of HUS.
- Typical EHEC is serotype O 157:H7 and few others such as O 26:H1.
- Diagnosis of EHEC diarrhea can be made by demonstration of bacilli or VT in feces.
- *Usually O 157:H7 serotype does not ferment sorbitol So, use of sorbitol Mac-Conkey medium helps in screening of O:157 VTEC.*

3. Ans. (b) Pi Pilli *Ref. Jawertz 25/e, p 216; Harrison 20/e, p 1152*

Correctly speaking guys we are unable to find all choices **but Pi Pilli is related in pathogenesis of pyelonephritis not GIT pathology.**
Colonizing factor (CFA1) and CS mediates attachments of E. coli, to intestinal wall.
So, most probably that would be the answer.

4. Ans. (d) HUS is rarely associated with haemorrhagic colitis *Ref. Harrison 20/e, p 1152; 19/e, p 1030*

50% of all cases of HUS and 90% of HUS cases in children are caused by STEC/EHEC.
This complication is probably mediated by the systemic translocation of shiga toxin.
Furthermore HUS is only a rare uncommon complication of hemorrhagic colitis or else it can be said that most cases of HUS are associated with EHEC, but only few cases with hemorrhagic colitis progress to HUS.
It occurs in 2-8% of cases of hemorrhagic colitis.

Pathogenesis of HUS
- There is systemic translocation of Shiga toxin, where erythrocytes serve as carrier of stx to endothelial cells located in small vessels of kidney and brain.
- Subsequently there is thrombolic microangiopathy which manifest as combination of fever, thrombocytopenia, renal failure and encephalopathy.

5. **Ans. (b) Proteus forms uric acids stone**   Ref. Harrison 19/e, p 1033, 18/e, p 1254; Ananthanarayan 10/e, p 288
   "*Proteus results in formation of struvite stone not uric acid stone.*"
   - Uric acid stone forms in acidic urine in presence of hyperuricemia.
   - All members of Enterobacteriaceae are aerobes or facultative anaerobes.
   - **Features of proteus bacilli:**
     - Non lactose fermenter
     - *Differs from other enterobacteria by presence of enzyme* phenylalanine deaminase which is responsible for deamination of phenylalanine to phenyl pyruvic acid (PPA test).
     - By producing urease it degrades urea to NH_3 and CO_2, NH_3 raises urinary pH. NH_4^+ (formed from NH_3) precipitate PO_4^{3-} Mg^{2+} to form $MgNH_4PO_4$ (Struvite.).
     - **The result is stone of struvite admixed with $CaCO_3$**
     - This precipitation of organic compounds also contribute to the formation of biofilin on catheter. As proteus resides in biofilm and stones it can be eradicated only by removal of stones and/or catheter.
     - Some strains (*X-strains*) are agglutinated by sera from *typhus fever patient* (weil felix reaction).

   P. Stuartii is a common cause of UTI and infection in burns
   P. rettgeri: Nosocomial infection of urinary tract, burns, wound and blood.

   > **Remember:**
   > - Peritrichous flagella (flagella all around the cell) seen in:
   >   - Proteus
   >   - E. coli
   >   - Listeria
   >   - Clostridia
   >   - Typhoid bacilli
   >   - Bacillus
   > - PPA test is also seen in *Morganella, Providencia.*
   > - Urine samples with unexplained alkalinity should be cultured for proteus
   > - Urease production by bacteria (in ↓ order) Proteus > Klebsiella > citrobacter

6. **Ans. (a) E. coli**   Ref. Harrison 20/e, p 1150
   "*E. coli cause 80% of acute UTI in patients with out catheterization.*"   .....Harrison 20/e, p 1150
   Strains of *E. coli* causing UTI are called extraintestinal pathogenic strains of *E. coli*.

   > **Remember:**
   > - *E. coli* is **MC** cause of catheter associate UTI too.
   > - UTI is **MC** nosocomial infection.
   > - *E. coli* is **MC** cause of neonatal meningitis.
   > - *E. coli* is **MC** cause of intraabdominal abscess.
   > - Other gram negative rods causing UTI are: Proteus, klebsiella, serratia, pseudomonas, enterobacter.

7. **Ans. (a) Enteroinvasive (E. coli)**   Ref. Ananthanarayan 10/e, p 285; Harrison 20/e, p 1153)
   EIEC cause illness resembling Shigellosis i.e. ranging from mild diarrhea to frank dysentery. However Shigella, EIEC produce disease only with a large inoculum.

Causes of bloody diarrhea	
Organism	**Incubation period**
• Shigella	>16h
• EHEC	> 16h
• EIEC	>16h
• Campylobacter jejuni	2 - 6 days

8. **Ans. (a, b) and (d) The L.T. (labile toxin), in ETEC acts via CAMP, UTI causing *E. coli* attaches through pilli, EIEC invasiveness is under plasmid control**
   Ref. Ananthanarayan 10/e, p 285-287

Enterotoxins of E. coli		
Stable Heat toxin	**Heat labile toxin**	**Verocytotoxin = Shiga like toxin**
• Acts through activation of CGMP	• Acts through activation of CAMP	• Inhibits protein synthesis

   Mnemonic: Labile Toxin cAMP
   - Fimbriae (P fimbriae) or pilli binds to epithelium of urinary tract and helps in causing UTI.
   - HUS is caused by verocytotoxin = Shiga like toxin of EHEC not by ST of ETEC.
   - Invasiveness of EIEC is due to plasmid coated outer surface antigen called virulence marker antigen.
   - EPEC or Enteroadherent E.coli causes diarrhea by disruption of brush border not by toxin or invasion.

9. **Ans. (d) Spread by contaminated water** *Ref. Harrison 20/e, p 1150*

   Enterotoxigenic E. coli (e.g. 06, 08, 015, 025, 027, 0167)
   - Affect *all age group. ETEC diarrhea is endemic in the developing countries*
   - *MC cause of traveller's diarrhea (indistinguishable from cholera).*
   - First step of pathogenesis is adherence of bacteria to intestinal mucosa which is mediated by colonisation factor antigen
   - After adhesion bacteria produce either or both LT and STa. However, toxin alone does not lead to diarrhea.
   - *Source of infection:* Contaminated water or food.

10. **Ans. (a) E. coli** *Ref. Ananthanarayan 10/e 285*
    Already explained

11. **Ans. (b) Widal test** *Ref. Ananthanarayan 10/e, p 302*
    " In 3rd week Widal test is investigation of choice."
    Diagnosis of Typhoid
    I. **Cases (BASU)**
    - ***Blood culture (B):***
      - Test of choice in first week (Diagnostic gold standard).
      - Becomes negative on treatment with antibiotics.
    - ***Widal test:***
      - Agglutinins usually appear by end of first week. Titre increase steadily till the 3rd or 4th week after which it declines gradually.
      - Maximum titre is found in 3rd week.
    - ***Stool culture (S)***
      - *Salmonella* are shed in feces throughout the course of disease, even in convalescence. A positive fecal culture occur in carriers also, so can't differentiate between case and carrier.
    - ***Urine culture:***
      - Culture is positive in 25% of cases during 2nd or 3rd week.
      - Less useful than blood culture.

    II. **Carriers**
    - *Widal* reaction – *No value* in detection of carriers.
    - Demonstration of *Vi agglutinins indicate carrier state.* This is a useful screening test which is confirmed by culture.
    - Isolation of bacillus from feces or bile. Cholagogue purgatives increase chance of isolation.
    - Tracing of carriers in cities is done by 'Sewer Swab Technique' or by filtration of sewage through millipore membrane and *culturing the membrane* on *Wilson* and *Blair* media.

    Widal reaction:
    - Test for measurement of H and O agglutinins for typhoid and paratyphoid bacilli in patient serum.
    - Agglutinins usually appear by the end of 1st week. Titre ↑ steadily till the 3rd or 4th week. Two types of tubes are generally used for the test –a narrow tube with the conical bottom (Dreyer's agglutination tube) for H agglutination and a short round bottomed tube (Felix tube) for O agglutination.
    - **O Agglutinins** – O antigen is common between S. typhi and S. paratyphi, so doesn't specify whether infection is due to S. typhi or S. paratyphi.
      - It has better diagnostic value than H.
      - O antibodies disappear after infection.
      - O agglutination is seen as disk like pattern at bottom of tube.
      - Titer > 1 : 320 is significant.
    - **H agglutinins** – H antigen are different for *S. typhi* or *S. paratyphi*, so indicates type of infection
      - May be present due to prior disease, in apparent infection, thus it does not have good diagnostic value.
      - Persist longer than O agglutinins.
      - Titer > 1: 640 is considered positive
      - Reaction to it, is rapid and leads to formation of cotton wooly clumps.
      - More immunogenic

    > **Remember:** Order of disappearance of antibody in typhoid $V_1 \rightarrow O \rightarrow H$.
    > **Widal test is false positive in case of prior infection and immunization.**

12. **Ans. (c) $10^2 - 10^5$ bacilli** *Ref. Harrison 20/e, p 1174*
    Infective dose of salmonella varies from 200 to 10^6 colony forming units and the ingested dose is an important determinant of incubation period

Organism	Infective dose
Shigella	10 - 1000
Vibrio	>10^{10} (if source of infection is water)
	$10^2 - 10^4$ (if source of infection is food)
Campylobacter jejuni	10^4
Yersinia enterocolitica	$10^8 - 10^9$
EHEC	10 - 100

13. **Ans. (c) Selenite 'F' medium**   *Ref. Ananthanarayan 10/e 306*

"*Selenite F and Tetrathionate broth are commonly employed enrichment media of salmonella.*"

Salmonella Gastroenteritis = Food poisoning
- May be caused by **any Salmonella except** *S. typhi*
- *MC* caused is *S. typhimurium*
- Human infection occurs due to ingestion of contaminated foods.
- **Most frequent source** – Poultry, meat, milk and milk products
- IP – 16 - 48 hours
- *Clinical feature* : Diarrhea, vomiting, fever
- *Diagnosis* : Isolation of salmonella from feces
- *Treatment* : No antibiotics

> **Remember:** Differential media for *Salmonella*:
> - MacConkey and Deoxycholate media: Form *colorless* colonies due to absence of lactose fermentation.
> - Wilson and Blair bismuth sulphite medium: *Jet black* colonies are formed due to production of H_2S.
> - Selective media for salmonella: SS agar, Deoxycholate citrate agar.

14. **Ans. (a) Vi. agglutination test**   *Ref. Ananthanarayan 10/e, p 299, 305*

Demonstration of antibodies to Vi. antigen has been claimed to indicate the carrier stage. Confirmation should be done by culture

Vi antigen – Polysaccharide antigen enveloping the O antigen because of which many strains of *S. typhi* fails to agglutinate with the 'O' antiserum.   *Ref. Ananthanarayan 10/e 305*

Antigens of Salmonella		
H antigen	**O antigen**	**Vi. antigen**
• Present on flagella	• Integral part of cell wall	• Envelops the 'O' antigen
• Heat labile protein	• Phospholipid - protein - polysaccharide complex	• Surface polysaccharide
• Strongly immunogenic	• Identical with endotoxin so, is less immunogenic	• Acts as virulence factor and is poorly immunogenic
• Antibody formation is rapid and in high titre	• Antibody formation is slow and titre is low	• Antibody production is slow and titres is low

Normally Vi antibody disappears early in convalescence. Its persistence indicates the development of carrier state.

> **Note:** Total absence of Vi antibody in a proven case of typhoid indicates poor prognosis.

Chronic carriers of *S. typhi*:
- Persons who excrete bacilli for more than a year after clinical attack.
- Average carrier rate is 3% (i.e. 3% cases become chronic carriers).
- Carrier state is more common in females (cases are more common in males).
- Fecal carriers are more frequent than urinary carriers but urinary carriers are more dangerous.
- Urinary carrier state is often associated with some abnormality of the urinary tract.
- Fecal carrier stage is *more common* in patients with biliary abnormality and GI malignancy.
- *Diagnosis of carriers:* – Demonstration of Vi antigen
  – Isolation of *S. typhi* by sewer swab technique.
- *Treatment:* – Ampicilin (4-6 g a day) together with probenecid for 6 week.
  – Cholecystectomy with concomitant ampicillin therapy has been regarded as the most successful approach to treatment of carriers.
  ... Park 22/e, p 215

15. **Ans. (c) and (d) Caused by animal products and symptoms appear between 4 - 48 hours** Ref. Ananthanarayan 10/e, p 306
    Already explained

16. **Ans. (a) Affects Peyer's patches** Ref. Harrison 20/e, p 1175

    Enteric manifestations of *S.typhi*:
    - *S. typhi invades peyer's* patches and form *oval ulcer* with their long axis along the length of bowel (*Tuberculosis result in transverse ulcer*).
    - Peyer's patches lie along antimesenteric border, so ulcer are common in antimesenteric border.
    - Stricture is rare but *perforation can occur* (*Stricture are common in TB ulcer*).

    > **Remember:** **Erythrophagocytosis is feature of** *E. histolytica*.

    > **Neurologic manifestations of enteric fever:**
    > - Meningitis
    > - GB syndrome
    > - Neuropsychiatric symptoms (described as muttering delirium or coma vigil)

17. **Ans. (a) Till three...** Ref. Park 22/e, p 214

    Control of Typhoid Fever
    - Control of reservoir:

      Reservoir may be case or carrier:

      A. **Cases:**
         - *Early diagnosis and treatment:* With early diagnosis and treatment, carrier stage can be prevented.
         - *Isolation:* Owing to the infectious nature of typhoid fever, cases should be isolated till three bacteriologically negative stools and urine reports are obtained on three separate days.
         - *Disinfection:* Stools and urine are sole source of infection. They should be received in closed containers and disinfected with **5% cresol** for at least 2 hours. All solid clothes and linen should be soaked in a solution of 2% chlorine and steam sterilized. All the medical and paramedical person should disinfect their hands.
         - *Follow-up:* Follow up examination of stool and urine should be done 3-4 months after discharge of patient and again after 12 months to prevent the development of carrier stage.

      B. **Carriers**
         - *Identification:* Culture of duodenal drainage establishes the presence of *Salmonella* in the biliary tract in carriers. The Vi antibody is seen in up to 80% of carriers.
         - *Treatment:* Ampicillin or amoxycillin (4-6 g a day) together with probenecid can achieve eradication of carrier stage in about 70%.
         - *Cholecystectomy with concomitant ampicillin therapy* is the **most successful** approach for treatment of carriers.
         - *Surveillance:* The carriers should be kept under surveillance and are prevented from handling food, milk for others.

    - **Control of Sanitation:**
      - The weakest link in the chain of transmission is sanitation which can be achieved easily
      - Protection and purification of drinking water supplies, improvement of basic sanitation and promotion of food hygiene are essential measures of controlling typhoid.

    - **Immunization:**
      - Immunization does not give 100% protection, but it definitely lowers both the incidence and seriousness of infection.

18. **Ans. (a) Can be given in ....** Ref. Harrison 19/e, p 1052; 18/e, 1278; Park 22/e, p 215

    Yellow fever is not a contraindication for VICPS typhoid vaccine.

    Antityphoid vaccine are:
    a. *Monovalent antityphoid vaccine* – Heat killed and phenol preserved.
    b. *Bivalent antityphoid vaccine* – Contains *S. typhi* and paratyphi A.
    c. *TAB vaccine (WHO recommended that TAB vaccine should be discontinued).*
    d. *Live oral typhoid 21a vaccine (Typhoral)*
       - Enteric coated capsule of lyophilized vaccine containing not less than 10 viable organism of attenuated *S. typhi* strain Ty 21a. *S. typhi* strain Ty21A lacks the enzyme UDP-galactose - 4 epimerase (GALE Mutant)

- It is indicated for immunization of adults and children aged more than 6 years.
- *Protection commences 2 weeks after taking last capsule and last for at least 3 years*
- **Dose** - 1 capsule on days 1, 3 and 5 one hour before meal with cold or luke warm milk or water.
- Ingestion, Ty21a strain initiates infection but self destructive after four or five cell divisions and therefore can not induce my illness.

e. **Typhin V_1 Vaccine (V_1CPS)**
- Injectable vaccine contains purified Vi polysaccharide antigen (25 µg/dose) from S.typhi strain Ty^2.
  Vaccine is injected as single subcutaneous or IM injection, which causes only minimal local reaction (Mild pain, erythema).
- Provides immunity for 2 years.
- It is contraindicated in patients with a history of hypersensitivity to any components.
- Because of T-cell independent properties, it is poorly immunogenic in children < 5 years of age.

f. **VirEPA Vaccine**
- Recently developed (not yet marketed) vaccine in which Vi is bound to a nontoxic recombinant protein that is identical to Pseudomonas aeruginosa exotoxin A. It is more immunogenic than ViCPS vaccine.

19. **Ans. (a) (b) and (d)** ↓ ed incidence in developed countries, Antacid and prolonged antibiotic administration promote infection, Food born to man and animal   *Ref. Ananthanarayan 8/e, 288-96, 9/e, 295-300; Harrison 18/e, p 1274-1276*
    Let's consider each option.

    Option 'a'
    - With improvement in food handling and water sewage treatment enteric fever has become rare in developed nations.
    - **Incidence is :**
       - *Highest* (> 100 cases per 100,000 population) in north central and southeast Asia
       - *Medium* (10-100 cases per 100,000 population) in the rest of Asia, Africa, Latin America and Oceania (including Australia and New Zealand).
       - *Low* (≥ 10 cases per 100,000 population) in the rest of world.

    Option 'b'   ...*Harrison 20/e, p1174*
    Conditions that increase susceptibility to salmonella infection
    a. *Reduced gastric acidity* : Age < 1 year, antacid ingestion, achlorhydria
    b. *Loss of intestinal integrity:* Inflammatory bowel disease, prior gastrointestinal surgery
    c. *Alteration in intestinal flora* by prior antibiotic administration

    Option 'c' Case fatality rate of enteric fever is < 1%

    Option 'd' Salmonellosis is a food borne or water borne disease resulting from ingestion of food or water contaminated by feces of case or carrier.

    Option 'e' Bacilli are killed at 55°C in one hour or at 60°C in 15 minutes. Culture may be viable for years if prevented from drying.   *Ref. Ananthanarayan 10/e, p 297*

20. **Ans. (a) Large dose is required for infection**   *Ref. Ananthanarayan 10/e, p 293*

    Correctly speaking 2 choices are wrong i.e. **option "a"** and **option "d"**.
    - *Infective dose for bacillary dysentery is just 10 to 100 bacilli as Shigella survive gastric acidity better than other enterobacteria.*

    So, option "a" is clearly wrong.
    - **Sh. dysenteraie forms enterotoxin** (acts by inhibiting protein synthesis) **which appears to be less important in pathogenesis than invasive property.** However Shiga toxins are translocated from bowel into the circulation. After binding to the cells in kidney, toxin may lead to homolytic uremic syndrome.

    Thus, **option "d"** is also wrong but not completely.
    So, Answer would be clearly wrong **option i.e. "a"**

    Remember: Small infective dose (10 - 100 bacilli) required in EHEC, *Entamoeba, Giardia*.

Differentiating features between *Shigella* and *E.coli*		
Features	**Shigella**	**E. coli**
Motility	—	+
Lactose fermentation	—	+
Glucose fermentation	+ (Produce acid)	+ (Produce acid and gas)
Lysine decarboxylase	—	+

21. **Ans. (d)** *Caused by Klebsiella granulomatosis* Ref. Harrison 20/e, p 1214

   Donovanosis (or Granuloma inguinale)
   - Veneral disease caused by Klebsiella granulomatis
   - IP: 1-12 weeks
   - Disease begins as a painless papule on genitalia which progress to auto inoculable ulcer and runs a chronic course
   - Diagnosis is confirmed by demonstration of donovan bodies in Wright-Giemsa stained smears
   - They may show bipolar condensation of chromatin, giving a closed safety pin appearance
   - Commonest site of infection are prepuce, coronal sulcus, frenum and glans in men. In women labio minora and fourchette are commonly affected
   - Lymphadenitis is uncommon
   - Treatment of choice is Azithromycin, Trimethoprim, sulfamethoxazole

22. **Ans. (a)** *Klebsiella granulomatis* Ref. Harrison 20/e, p 1214

   This is the figure showing klebsiella granulomatis along with Donovan bodies
   For details see answer no. 21

23. **Ans. (b)** *Shigella* Ref. Harrison 10/e, p 1181

   Two important complication of shigellosis are HUS and toxic megacolon.

24. **Ans. (b) Glucose is not fermented by all members of the family** Ref. Ananthanarayan 10/e p 281

   "Members of enterobacteriaceae reduce nitrates to nitrites, form catalase but not oxidase."

Enterobacteriaceae: Important features			
Features	**Escherichia**	**Salmonella**	**Shigella**
Motility by peritrichous flagella	+	+	—
Gas from glucose	+	+	—
Acid from lactose	+	—	—
Acid from sucrose	d	—	—
Growth in KCN	—	d	—
Indole	+	—	d
MR/VP	+	+	+
Citrate	—	+	—
H2S	—	+	—
Urease	—	—	—
Phenylalanine deaminase (PPA)	—	—	—
Arginine dehydrolase	d	+	—
Lysine decarboxylase	+	+	—
Ornithine decarboxylase	d	+	d

(d = result different in different species or strains)

Remember:
- Polar flagella: Vibrio, pseudomonas, legionella, spirilla, campylobacter, H. pylori, spirochetes.
- V. parahemolytic produce both polar and peritrichous flagella.

25. **Ans. (a and c)** *Pseudomonas;* **and** *V. cholerae* Ref. Ananthanarayan 10/e 279

Enterobacteriaceae			
Tribe I	**Tribe II**	**Tribe III**	**Tribe IV**
Escherichiae	Klebsiellae	Protecae	Erwinieae
Genus • *Escherichia* • *Edwardsiella* • *Citrobacter* • *Salmonella* • *Shigella*	Genus • *Klebsiella* • *Enterobacter* • *Hafnia* • *Serratia*	Genus • *Proteus* • *Morganella* • *Providencia*	Genus • *Erwinia*

26. **Ans. (b)** *Salmonella Typhi* Ref. Harrison 18/e, p 1278
    DT-104 is a multidrug resistant strain of S. typhimurium which emerged in early 1990. It is associated with increased risk of blood stream infection and hospitalization. Humans acquired infection through exposure to ill farm animals land to various meat products.

27. **Ans. (d) EPEC** Ref. Ananthanarayan 9/e, p 279
    Enteropathogenic = enteroadherent *E. coli*
    - Cause diarrhea in infant and children.
    - Strains that carry PEAF plasmid are termed typical EPEC while those lacking it are called atypical
    - Non-toxigenic and non-invasive.
    - Produce diarrhea by disruption of brush border. Bacilli adhere to upper small intestine through adhesion receptor synthesized by bacteria which is then inserted in to host put wall.

NEET Pattern Questions

1. Watery diarrhea in children is caused by:
   a. ETEC
   b. EPEC
   c. EIEC
   d. EAEC
   [Ref. Ananthanarayan, 10/e, p 285]

2. All of the following *Salmonella* are motile except:
   a. S. typhi   b. S. enteridis
   c. S. gallinarum d. S. chester
   [Ref. Ananthanarayan 10/e, p 297]

   All salmonella are motile by peritrichate flagella *except* for S. gallinarum and S. pullorum.
   [Ref. Ananthanarayan 8/e, p 289, 9/e, p 291]

3. Performed toxin is important in food poisoning due to all *except*:
   a. Staph aureus
   b. Clostridium botulism
   c. ETEC
   d. B. cereus   [Ref. Ananthanarayan, 10/e, p 285]

   ETEC first adheres with E. coli and then secretes exotoxin which causes diarrhea.

4. In E. coli true is:
   a. ETEC is invasive
   b. EPEC acts via cAMP
   c. Pilli present in uropathogenic type
   d. ETEC causes HUS
   [Ref. Ananthanarayan, 10/e, p 285]

   Strains carrying K antigens are more commonly responsible for pyelonephritis while most isolates from cystitis lacks K antigen. The P pili-positive strains are uropathogenic E. coli.

5. A child with fever with RBCs and pus in stools, causative organism is:
   a. ETEC
   b. EHEC
   c. EPEC
   d. EAEC   [Ref. Ananthanarayan, 10/e, p 286]

6. Traveller's diarrhoea, is caused by:
   a. *Shigella*   b. *E. coli*
   c. *E. histolytica* d. *Giardiasis*
   [Ref. Ananthanarayan 10/e, p 284]

Cause of Traveller's diarrhea		
Bacterial	**Viral**	**Parasitic**
ETEC (**MC**)	Rotavirus (**MC**)	Giardia (**MC**)
V. cholera	Norwalk virus	Entameba histolytica
Shigella		Cryptosporodium
Salmonella		Cyclospora
C. jejuni		

7. Recommended transport medium for stool specimen suspected to contain enteric pathogens is:
   a. Arnie's medium
   b. Buffered glycerol saline medium
   c. MacConkey medium
   d. Blood agar   [Ref. Ananthanarayan, 10/e, p 303]

   Fecal samples are plated directly on Macconkey, DCA or XLD and Wilson Blair media.

8. Phenylalanine deaminase test is positive in:
   a. Salmonella
   b. Proteus
   c. Vibrio cholerac
   d. Helicobacter   [Ref. Ananthanarayan 10/e, p 288]

9. Enteric fever is caused by:
   a. S typhi   b. S paratyphi A
   c. S paratyphi C d. All of the above
   [Ref. Harrison 19/e, p 1050; 20/e, p 1174]

10. Selective medium for shigella: [Ref. Harrison, 20/e, p 1182]
    a. Chocolate agar   b. BYCE medium
    c. Hekton agar   d. EMJH medium

11. Indicator used in MaConkey Agar:
    a. Methylene blue   b. Methyl red
    c. Neutral red   d. Bromothymol blue

    Mac Conkey's agar is a selective, indicator and differential medium. It contains peptone, agar, sodium taurocholate and neutral red. Lactose fermenters form pink colonies while non-lactose fermenters produce colourless or pale calories.

12. Shiga toxin acts by: [Ref. Ananthanarayan, 10/e, p 292]
    a. Activating adenylyl cyclase to increase cAMP
    b. activating guanylyl cyclase to increase cGMP
    c. Inhibiting protein synthesis
    d. Inhibiting DNA replication

Ans.
1. b. EPEC
2. c. S. gallinarum
3. c. ETEC
4. c. Pilli present in uropathogenic type
5. b. EHEC
6. b. E. coli
7. c. MacConkey medium
8. b. Proteus
9. d. All of the above
10. c. Hekton agar
11. c. Neutral red
12. c. Inhibiting…

13. Shigella are be divided into subgroup on the basic of ability to ferment:
    a. Lactose
    b. Maltose
    c. Fructose
    d. Mannitol [Ref. Ananthanarayan, 10/e, p 292]

> Fermentation of mannitol is of importance in classification and shigella have traditionally been divided in to mannitol fermenting and non fermenting species. S.dysenteriae being non-fermenting one.

14. True about Shiga toxin:
    a. An endotoxin
    b. Inhibit protein synthesis
    c. Activate adenylyl cyclase
    d. Increase cGMP [Ref. Ananthanarayan, 10/e, p 292]

> Exotoxin of shigella is also known as shiga token or verotoxin note. LPS of wall of shigella acts as endotoxin.

15. True about widal test:
    a. Anti-O antibody persists longer
    b. O antigen of S. paratyphi is used
    c. H-antigen is most immunogenic
    d. Felix tube is used for 'H' agglutination
    [Ref. Ananthanarayan, 10/e, p 304]

> Antigens used for widal test are the H and O antigens of S. typhi and the H. antigens of S. Paratyphi A and D
> (for details see answer no 13 in explanatory answers)

16. Salmonellae other than S. typhi and S. paratyphi cause:
    a. Typhoid fever
    b. Enteric fever
    c. Gastroenteritis
    d. All of the above [Ref. Ananthanarayan, 10/e, p 306]

> Clinical manifestations of non-typhoidal salmonellosis
> - Gastroenteritis
> - Bacteremia and endovascular infection
> - Localized infection (Intra-abdominal abscess, meningitis, pulmonary injection, UTI)
> - Bone joint and soft tissue infection

17. Chronic carrier of typhoid shed bacilli for:
    a. 1-3 weeks after cure
    b. 3 weeks to 3 months after cure
    c. 3 months -1 year after cure
    d. More than 1 year after cure [Ref. Park, 22/e, p 213]

> Convalescent carrier: Excrete bacilli for 6-8 weeks.
> Chronic carrier. Person who excrete bacilli for more than a year.

18. Culture media used for O157 : H7 enterohemorrhagic E. coli: [Ref. Ananthanarayan, 10/e, p 286]
    a. Sorbitol containing agar
    b. Mannitol containing agar
    c. Sucrose containing agar
    d. Dextrose containing agar

19. Enterobacteriaceae is classified based on:
    a. Mannitol fermentation
    b. Catalase and oxidase reaction
    c. Oxygen requirement
    d. Lactose fermentation
    [Ref. Ananthanarayan, 10/e, p 277]

20. Which of the following produces enterotoxin:
    a. Sh. dysenteriae   b. Sh. sonnei
    c. Sh. flexneri   d. Sh. boydii
    [Ref. Ananthanarayan 10/e, p 292]

> Exotoxins associated with diarrheal diseases are called as enterotoxins. They are produced by:
> - Shigella dysenteriae I   – Staph. aureus
> - B. cereus   – Cl. perfringes
> - Y. enterocolitica   – V. parahemolyticus
> - V. cholera   – ETEC
> - Klebsiella pneumonia   – Aeromonas

21. Salmonella infection is most commonly caused by:
    a. Infected water
    b. Infected vegetable
    c. Aerosol infection
    d. Through skin [Ref. Ananthanarayan, 10/e, p 301]

22. Infective dose of Salmonella typhi:
    a. 10 bacilli
    b. 1000 bacilli
    c. 10^3–10^6 bacilli
    d. 10^{10}–10^{12} bacilli
    [Ref. Ananthanarayan, 10/e, p 301]

23. Not true about Vi polysaccharide vaccine of typhoid:
    a. Single dose is given
    b. Revaccination at 3 years
    c. Given at birth
    d. Given subcutaneously
    [Ref. Ananthanarayan, 10/e, p 306]

> Vi Vaccine:
> - Contains purified Vi Polysaccharide antigen (25 ly perdose) from S typhi strain Ty2.
> - Given subcutaneous on intramuscular infection
> - Given children above 5 years of age
> - Immunity commence 2-3 weeks after and lasts for atleast 3 years

Ans.
- 13. d. Mannitol
- 14. b. Inhibit protein...
- 15. c. H-antigen...
- 16. c. Gastroenteritis
- 17. d. More than...
- 18. a. Sorbitol cont...
- 19. d. Lactose ...
- 20. a. Sh. dysenteriae
- 21. a. Infected water
- 22. c. 10^3–10^6 bacilli
- 23. c. Given ...

24. **Salmonella and shigella can be differentiated from other enterobacteriaceae member by isolation on:**
    a. MacConkey agar
    b. Mannitol salt agar
    c. BCYE medium
    d. XLD agar
    [Ref. Ananthanarayan, 10/e, p 280]

25. **Clinical significance of Vi antigen of S. typhi is:**
    a. Helps in diagnosis
    b. Highly immunogenic
    c. Most important antigen for widal test
    d. Antibody against Vi-antigen is used for diagnosis of carrier
    [Ref. Ananthanarayan, 10/e, p 299]

26. **All are important causes of UTI except:**
    a. E. coli
    b. Proteus
    c. Klebsiella
    d. Streptococcus viridans
    [Ref. Harrison, 20/e, p 969]

27. **Proteus isolated from a patient of UTI will show which biochemical reaction:**
    a. Phenylpyruvic acid reaction
    b. Bile esculin reaction
    c. Colchicine sensitivity
    d. Bacitracin sensitivity
    [Ref. Ananthanarayan, 10/e, p 288]

Proteus contain enzyme phenylalanine deaminase which converts phenylalanine to phenyl pyruvic acid (PPA reaction)

28. **Most common cause of hemolytic uremic syndrome is:**
    a. E. coli
    b. Shigella
    c. Salmonella
    d. Psedononas
    [Ref. Harrison, 10/e, p 2148]

29. *In vitro* **test for enterotoxin**
    a. Mc Conckey's culture
    b. Blood agar culture
    c. Rabbit ileal loop culture
    d. None
    [Ref. Ananthanarayan 8/e, p 274, 9/e, p 277]

In vitro test for ETEC include:
- Tissue culture tests.
- Rounding of Y_1 mouse adrenal cells
- Elongation of CHO cells
- ELISA
- Passive agglutination test
- Genetic tests (DNA probes)

30. **Most common cause of pyelonephritis in pregnancy:**
    a. Pseudomonas
    b. E. coli
    c. Proteus
    d. Klebsiella
    [Ref. Current Obt & Gyne 11/e, p 483]

UTI in pregnancy: Commonest cause *E.coli*
Diagnosis: > 10^5 organism/mL (asymptomatic bacteriuria)
> 10^2 in symptomatic

31. **Prolonged *Salmonella* septicemia is caused by:**
    a. S. enteritidis
    b. S. cholerae-suis
    c. S. typhimurium
    d. S. typhi
    [Ref. Ananthanarayan 10/e, p 307]

S. choleraesuis cause septicemic disease with focal suppurative lesions such as osteomyelitis, deep abscesses, endocarditis, pneumonia and meningitis. The case fatality may be as high as 25%.

32. **Which of the following is late lactose fermenter:**
    a. E. coli
    b. Klebsiella
    c. Salmonella
    d. Shigella sonnei
    [Ref. Ananthanarayan 10/e, p 292]

33. **The following are gas producing *Salmonella* except:**
    a. S. typhi
    b. S. enteritidis
    c. S. cholera
    d. S. typhimurium
    [Ref. Ananthanarayan 10/e, p 297]

All *Salmonella* except *S. typhi* ferment glucose, mannitol and maltose, forming acid and gas; S. typhi is anaerogenic.

Ans.
24. **d.** XLD agar
25. **d.** Antibody…
26. **d.** Streptococcus…
27. **a.** Phenylpyruvic…
28. **a.** E. coli
29. **d.** None
30. **b.** E. coli
31. **b.** S. cholerae …
32. **d.** Shigella sonnei
33. **a.** S. typhi

CHAPTER 16

Vibrio

- Gram-negative, rigid, motile curved rods. **All are halophilic except** *V. cholerae* and *V. mimicus*.
- They are *oxidase positive*, which differentiates it from gram-negative enteric bacteria.
- They are susceptible to compound *0/129* which differentiate them from *Aeromonas species*.
  ..... *Jawetz 25/e, p 236*

> **Vibrio**
> - Motile, Gr (–) ve rods that are oxidase positive and give a positive indole reaction.
> - Non sporing prefer alkalinity, require salt.
> - TCBS is the best selective media whereas alkaline peptone water is the best enrichment medium.

VIBRIO CHOLERA

- Comma shaped, isolated by Koch. (See color plate, pg xxviii for related image)
- Arranged as *fish in stream appearance.*
- Posses single polar flagella and shows *darting type motility (= swarm of gnats).*
- Natural habitate is coastal salt water and brackish estuaries where organism lives in close association with plankton.

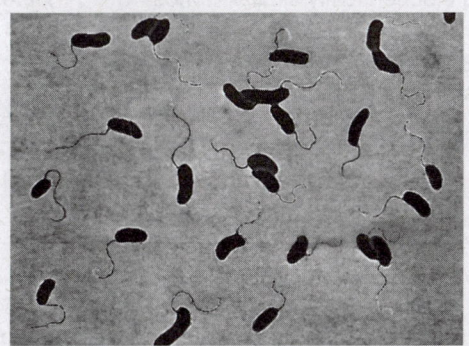

Culture Characteristics

- Grows well on ordinary media.
- Strongly aerobic, better growth in alkaline medium (pH 8.5 - 9.5) and are rapidly killed by acid.
- Ferment sucrose and mannose but not arabinose ..... *Jawetz 27/e, p 253*
- *Required NaCl* (0.5-1%) for optimal growth; however, 6% and above are inhibitory.
- *On MacConkey's agar:* Late lactose fermenters.
- *On Gelatin Stab:* Infundibuliform (funnel shaped) or napiform (turnip shaped) liquification occurs.

Special media		
Holding or transport media	**Enrichment media**	**Plating media**
- VR medium - Cary-Blair medium also for *Shigella* and *Salmonella* - Autoclaved sea water	- Alkaline peptone water at a pH of 8.6 - Monsour's taurocholate tellurite peptone water - Both used as transport media when specimen reach laboratories within few hours.	- Alkaline bile salt agar - Monsour's gelatin taurocholate trypticase tellurite agar (GTTA) - TCBS: *Best selective media*

- Colonies are identified by *string test.*
- *Vibrios are susceptible to heat drying but resist high alkalinity*

Biochemical characteristics

C : Catalase +ve
O : Oxidase +ve
I : Indole +ve
N : Nitrates reduced to nitrites
S : Sucrose fermenter

} Responsible for *cholera red* reaction

Enzymes:
- Neuraminidase [receptor destroying enzyme]
- Lipase
- Chitinase
- Elastase
- Mucinase

> Classified on the basis of lipopolysaccharide O-antigens into V.cholera O1 and Non-O1 V.cholerae.
> - Flagellar antigen is same in all V. cholerae
> - Ogawa serotype of El tor is the MC strain of vibrio, causing cholera

Classification

- *Gardner and Venkatraman's Serological Classification of vibrio:*

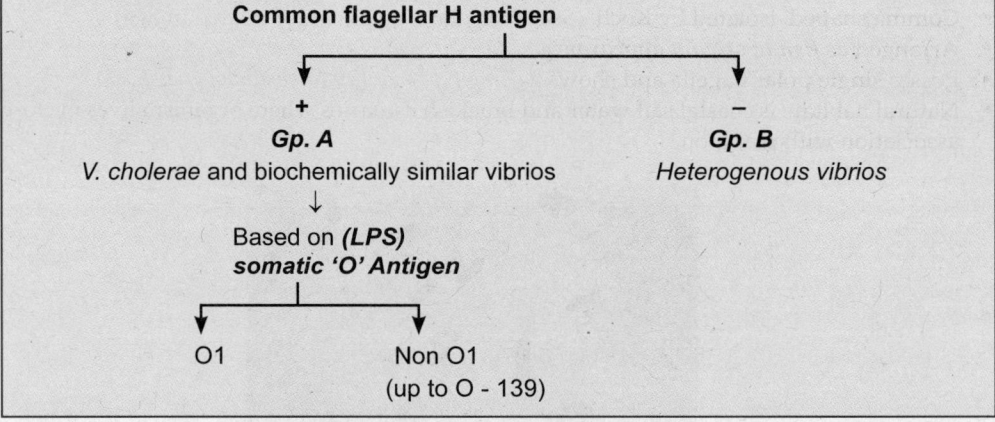

- Only O1 serogroup cause cholera till 1992, so Non O1 serogroup were known as Noncholera Vibrio (NCV) or Non-Agglutinable Vibrios (NAG vibrios).
- The latest serogroup O -139 identified in 1992 causes epidemic of cholera emphasising that they can not longer be considered as noncholera vibrios.

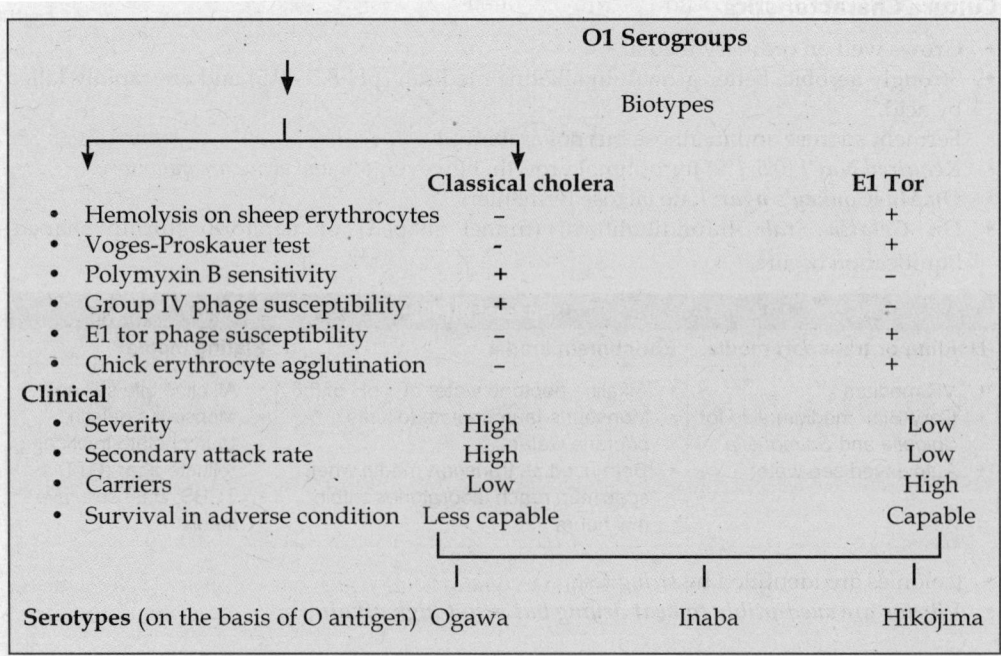

- *Ogawa serotype of E1 tor is MC* strain causing cholera [7th Pandemic].
- Ogawa and Inaba strain are agglutinated by their own antisera while hikojima is agglutinated by both Ogawa and Inaba antisera.
- *O-139 strain is called Bengal V. cholera* (arise from E1 tor by *horizontal gene transfer*) signaled begininnig of 8th pandemic. It differs from E1 tor in production of Of-139 LPS and an immunologically related O antigen polysaccharide *capsule. ..... Harrison 20/e, p 1187*

> **Remember:** *V. cholerae* belong to group I of **Heiberg grouping of vibrios**.

- V. cholerae O-139 is associated with free living aquatic amoebae and other members of zooplankton which acts as reservoir of infection.

CHOLERA

- *Incubation period* – 1-2 days.
- *Infective dose* – 10^6 bacilli. However when vehicle is food as few as 10^2–10^4 organism can cause infection.
- *Source of infection* – Water contaminated with infective feces.
- *Symptoms* – Painless rice water diarrhea.

Pathogenesis

- Individuals with *O group are most susceptible* white with blood group *AB- are least susceptible*.
- In human infection, the vibrios enter orally via contaminated water. Vibrios are highly susceptible to acids, and gastric acidity provides an effective barrier against vibrios, or else achlorhydria is a significant risk factor for cholera, so in salmonella typhi.
- Cause *non invasive toxin* mediated diarrhea.

V. Cholerae exhibit two major pathogenic mechanism:
1. Produce cholera toxin.
2. Express toxin co-regulated pilli.
Cholera toxin acts by activating adenylate cyclase.

Mechanism of Diarrhea

- Vibrio adheres to jejunal epithelial cell by special fimbria and toxin coregulated pilus [TCP].
- Then vibrio produces exotoxin called CTX = **CT (Cholera toxin)** = cholera enterotoxin = Choleragen = Permeability factor.
- The genes encoding cholera toxin (ctx AB) are part of genome of bacteriophage CTX φ.
- CT can be demonstrated by 'Skin blueing test'.
- CT *inhibits absorption of Na^+ and Cl^-* as well as, ↑ secretion of K^+ and HCO_3^-; resulting in isotonic diarrhea, acidosis with elevated anion gap (*due to increase in serum lactate, protein*). ..... *Harrison 19/e, p 1062*
- CT also ↑ intestinal secretion via prostaglandins and neural histamine receptors.
- It has no effect on any other tissue except intestinal cells.

Cholera is a local infection and organism does not reach blood stream

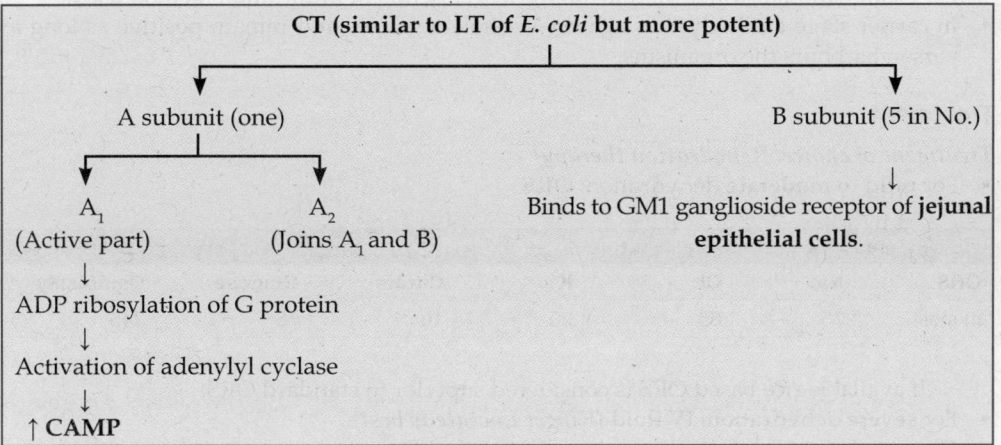

- *Vibrio cholerae* also possess LPS O Antigen (**endotoxin**) which has **no role** in pathogenesis, but *O-139 strain produce novel O-139 LPS which is responsible for its increased virulence.*
- Changes in intestine are biochemical rather than histological.

> **Virulence Factor of 01 V. cholerae are:**
> - CTx including gene encoding CTx which are part of genome of bacteriophage CTXφ.
> - TCP
> - Vibrio cholerae may express one or more of four haemolysin: Thermostable direct hemolysin, E1 Tor haemolysin, thermolabile haemolysin and thermostable hemolysin. The last three are found in pathogenic strains where they contribute to virulence.

Clinical Features

- In endemic areas, 75% of cases are asymptomatic, 20% are mild to moderate, and 2-5% are severe forms such as cholera gravis.
- Symptoms include abrupt onset of watery diarrhea (a grey and cloudy liquid), occasional vomiting, and abdominal cramps. Frequency of diarrhea can reach up to 40
- Dehydration ensues, with symptoms and signs such as thirst, dry mucous membranes, decreased skin turgor, sunken eyes, hypotension, weak or absent radial pulse, tachycardia, tachypnea, hoarse voice, oliguria, cramps, renal failure, seizures, somnolence, coma, and death.
- Death due to dehydration can occur in a few hours to days in untreated children.
- Disease is particularly dangerous in pregnant women during late pregnancy, as it may cause premature labor and fetal death.
- In cases of cholera gravis involving severe dehydration, up to 60% of patients can die; however, less than 1% of cases treated with rehydration therapy are fatal. The disease typically lasts 4–6 days.

Lab Diagnosis

- **Specimen:**
  - Rectal swabs for convalescent phase.
  - *Stool collected* by introducing a lubricating catheter into rectum is best specimen.
  - Rapid diagnosis by characteristic **darting motility** and its inhibition by antiserum under the dark field or phase contrast microscope.
  - **Culture:** Definitive, growth is rapid on peptone agar, blood agar, TCBS. Colonies can be picked in 18 hours.
- **Serological examination:**
  - Helpful in assessing prevalence of cholera in an area. Complement dependent vibriocidal antibody test is most useful. Other include antitoxin assay, indirect hemagglutination.
- For examination of water sample for vibrios, enrichment or filtration method used.
- In carrier stage antibody titer against V. cholerae raises and remain positive as long as person harbours the organisms.

..... *Park 22/e, p 209*

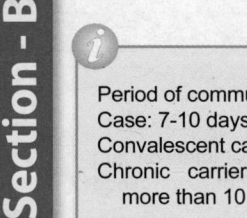

Period of communicability
Case: 7-10 days
Convalescent carries: 2-3 weeks
Chronic carriers. A month to more than 10 years

Treatment

Treatment of choice: Rehydration therapy
- For **mild to moderate** dehydration: **ORS**

Composition of WHO ORS						
ORS	Na⁺	Cl⁻	K⁺	Citrate	Glucose	Osmolality
m mol/l	75	65	20	10	75	245

..... *Harrison 20/e, p 1189*

  - If available rice based ORS is considered superior to standard ORS.
- For **severe** dehydration: IV fluid (**Ringer Lactate is best**).
- *Drug of choice for adults:* Erythromycin or Azithromycin ..... *Harrison 20/e, p 1189*
- **For children & pregnant mother :** Erythromycin or Azithromycin (10 mg/kg).
- **Control:** Water sanitation and proper excreta disposal are the most effective control measure.

VIBRIO MIMICUS

Nonhalophilic, nonsucrose fermenter causing *gastroenteritis* by eating *seafood* especially oyster.

HALOPHILIC VIBRIOS

Vibrio Parahaemolyticus

- Capsulated vibrio showing *bipolar staining* (safety pin appearance) with peritrichous flagella.
- Grows only in media containing NaCl. ***It tolerates 8% NaCl*** but not > 10%.
- String test is positive.
- *Exhibits Kanagawa Phenomenon* (ability to show hemolysis on Wagatsuma agar).
- Cause *gastroenteritis (= food poisoning)* after eating sea fish (shell fish).
  - Cause of enteritis is *invasion* not enterotoxin.

> **Note:** Bacteria with safety pin appearance
> - Yersinia pestis
> - Vibrio parahaemolyticus
> - Burkholderia mallei
> - Klebsiella granulomatis
> - Haemophilus ducreyi

Halophilic vibrios
- Vibrios, that require salt for growth
- Includes:
  - V. parahemolyticus
  - V. alginolyticus
  - V. vulnificus.

Vibrio Alginolyticus

- *Most salt tolerant* species of cholera. Can tolerate > 10% NaCl.
- Cause infection of eye, ear and wounds exposed to sea water.

Vibrio Vulnificus

VP negative lactose fermenter (but not sucrose) that has a salt tolerance of less than 8%

Cause: a. Primary sepsis in patient with underlying liver disease.
b. Primary wound infection without underlying disease.

Multiple Choice Questions

1. Gram (–) ve bacilli releasing histamine to cause scombroid poisoning are all *except*: [NEET Pattern 2018]
   a. Klebsiella　　b. E. coli
   c. Vibrio vulnificus　　d. Proteus

2. All of the following are true about *V. cholerae* O139 *except*: [AI 08]
   a. Clinical manifestations are similar to O1 E1 tor
   b. First discovered in Chennai
   c. Produces O139 lipopolysaccharide
   d. Epidemiologically indistinguishable from O1 E1 tor

3. Which of the following bacteria acts by increasing cAMP: [AI 07; AIIMS 06]
   a. *Vibrio cholerae*
   b. *Staphylococcus aureus*
   c. *E. coli* heat stable toxin
   d. *Salmonella*

4. About *V. cholerae* all statements are true *except*:
   a. Nonhalophilic　　[AI 07]
   b. Cannot grow in ordinary media
   c. Can survive outside the intestine
   d. Man is the only reservoir of cholera

5. Not true about vibrio O139: [AI 07]
   a. Can cause disease in distinguishable from E_1 or clinically
   b. First isolated in Chennai
   c. Has O polysaccharide capsule
   d. Antibody to *V. cholerae* is not protective against O139

6. All of the following *Vibrio species* are halophilic *except*: [AI 05]
   a. *V. cholerae*　　b. *V. parahemolyticus*
   c. *V. alginolyticus*　　d. *V. flovialis*

7. In the small intestine, cholera toxin acts by: [AI 05]
   a. ADP ribosylation of G regulatory protein
   b. Inhibition of adenyl cyclase
   c. Activation of GTPase
   d. Active absorption of NaCl

8. Antibiotic treatment of choice for treating cholera in an adult is a single dose of: [AI 05]
   a. Tetracycline　　b. Cotrimoxazole
   c. Doxycycline　　d. Furazolidone

9. The effect of cholera toxin is mediated via the stimulation of following second messenger: [AI 2012]
   a. cAMP　　b. cGMP
   c. Calcium-calmodulin　　d. Acetylcholine

10. Selective media for vibrio: [AIIMS 08]
    a. TCBS　　b. Stuart
    c. Skirrows　　d. MYPA

11. The endotoxin of the following gram-negative bacteria does not play any part in the pathogenesis of the natural disease: [AIIMS 06, AI 2012, AIIMS Nov 2012]
    a. *Escherichia coli*　　b. *Klebsiella sp.*
    c. *Vibrio cholerae*　　d. *Pseudomonas aeruginosa*

12. Cholera toxin: [AIIMS 06]
    a. Increases the levels of intracellular cyclic GMP
    b. Acts through the receptor for opiates
    c. Causes continued activation of adenylate cyclase
    d. Inhibits the enzyme phosphodiesterase

13. The drug of choice for treating cholera in pregnant women is: [AIIMS 05]
    a. Tetracycline　　b. Doxycycline
    c. Furazolidone　　d. Cotrimoxazole

14. Which of the following is the drug of choice for chemoprophylaxis of cholera? [AIIMS 05]
    a. Tetracycline　　b. Doxycycline
    c. Furazolidone　　d. Cotrimoxazole

15. All of the following statements about E1-Tor Vibrios are true, *except*: [AI 2010]
    a. Human are the only reservoir
    b. Can survive in ice cold water for 2-4 weeks
    c. Killed by boiling for 30 seconds
    d. Enterotoxin can have direct effects on other tissues besides intestinal epithelial cells.

16. Which toxin acts by ADP ribosylation: [PGI 07]
    a. Botulinum toxin　　b. *Shigella* toxin
    c. *V. cholerae*　　d. Diphtheria toxin
    e. Pertussis

17. *V. cholerae* able to stay in GIT because of: [PGI 06]
    a. Acid resistance　　b. Bile resistance
    c. Motility　　d. Binds to specific receptors
    e. Anaerobic potential

18. Cholera transmission by: [PGI 06]
    a. Food transmits
    b. Vaccination gives 90% efficiency
    c. Healthy carrier
    d. Chlorination is not effective

19. Cholera is caused by? [PGI June 09]
    a. *Vibrio cholerae* .01　　b. *Vibrio cholerae* 0139
    c. *V. parahemolyticus*　　d. *E. coli*
    e. NAG *vibrio*

20. A stool examination was carried out which showed organism with darting motility. Which of the following organism may be in stool: [PGI May 2013]
    a. *V. cholerae*　　b. *Shigella*
    c. *Salmonella*　　d. *Campylobacter jejuni*
    e. *E. coli*

21. True about Vibrio alginolyticus: [PGI 2013]
    a. Non-halophilic
    b. Voges Proskauer (VP) positive
    c. Swarming
    d. Cause sea borne auricular infections
    e. Does not grow in 10% NaCl

22. Cholera patient having stool output 1000–1500 mL/day is known as: [PGI 2017]
    a. Cholera mitis
    b. Cholera dumdum
    c. Cholera magna
    d. Cholera gravis
    e. Cholera intermedius

Explanations and References with Illustrative Answers

1. **Ans. (c) i.e Vibrio vulnificus** *Ref "Scombroid poisoning" CMAJ : Canadian Medical Association journal vol. 184,6 (2012): 674.*
   Scombroid poisoning
   - Scombroid poisoning (the most common causes of morbidity with fish intake) occurs after the ingestion of fresh, canned or smoked fish with high histamine levels due to improper processing or storage.
   - First described in conjunction with fish in the suborder Scombroidea (e.g., tuna and mackerel), it has since been described with other dark-fleshed fish
   - Histamine produced by the decarboxylation of histidine in the muscle of the fish is primarily responsible for the condition.
   - The decarboxylation process is induced by bacterial enzymes of enteric gram-negative bacteria (e.g., *Morganella morganii*, *Escherichia coli*, *Klebsiella* species and *Pseudomonas aeruginosa*) found in the fish's cutis and intestines
   - Symptoms
     – Resemble allergy with flushing, rash, urticaria (generally widespread erythema, usually lacking wheals), palpitations, headache, dizziness, sweating, and burning of the mouth and throat. Gastrointestinal symptoms can include abdominal cramps, nausea, vomiting and diarrhea.
     – Symptoms begin within 10 to 90 minutes after eating the implicated fish. The rash lasts 2–5 hours, and the other symptoms usually disappear within 3–36 hours.
   - Treatment involves antihistamines and supportive care

   V. vulnificus:
   - Halophillic vibrio
   - Natural habitat is sea water
   - Cause two **types of illness:**
     – In **normal host :** Wound infection following contact of open wound with sea water.
     – In **immunocompromised host** *(particularly with liver disease)* : Sepsis.

2. **Ans. (b) First discovered in Chennai** *Ref. Harrison 20/e, p 1187-1189*
   Guy's before solving this question, you must understand the epidemiology of cholera.

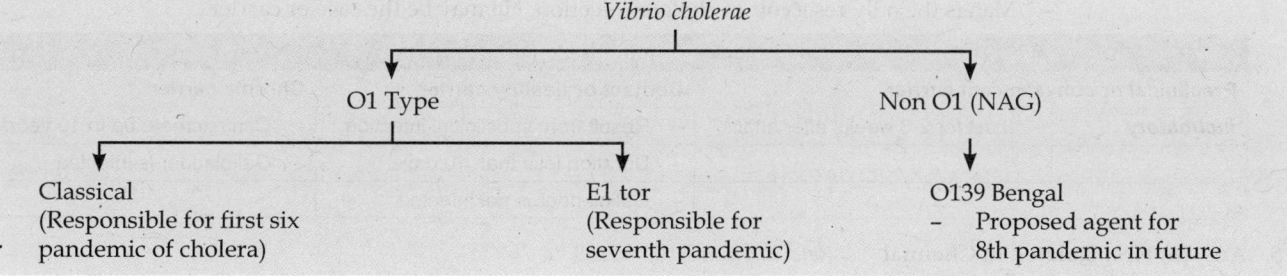

   In 1992, after its isolation O139 had initially replaced E_1 tor and become the most common causative agent of cholera in South Asia. However, by the beginning of 1994 E_1 tor had resumed its dominance in many areas and above all 0139 has not spreaded outside Asia.
   - O139 Vibrio was isolated in Bengal in 1992.
   - The clinical manifestation and epidemiological features of the disease caused by *V. cholerae* O139 are indistinguishable from those of O1 cholera.

- **O139 V. cholerae** *is identical to E_1 tor except for two important differences:*
  - Production of novel O139 Lipopolysaccharide.
  - Immunologically related O antigen polysaccharide capsule.

> **Remember:**
> - E_1 **tor biotype** was first isolated at the E_1 tor quarantine station in *Egypt* in 1905.
> - **Presently most cases of cholera are caused by E_1 tor.**

3. **Ans. (a) *Vibrio cholerae***   *Ref. Harrison 20/e, p 1188*
   Cholera toxin (CT)
   - Protein *enterotoxin*
   - Composed of 2 subunit: **A** – (Active monomeric moiety)
                              B – (Pentameric binding moiety)
   - **Mechanism of action:**

   > The B-pentamer binds to GM_1 ganglioside, a glycolipid on the surface of epithelial cells that serves as toxin receptor
   > ↓
   > The activated A subunit (A_1) irreversibly transfers ADP ribose from NAD to regulatory component of adenyl cyclase
   > ↓
   > Up regulation of adenylate cyclase
   > ↓
   > Intracellular increase in cAMP

   In intestine cAMP inhibits the absorptive sodium transport system in the villus cells and activates the secretory chloride system in the crypt cells. Thus, increased cAMP leads to leads to accumulation of sodium chloride in the intestinal lumen. To maintain osmolality water moves passively to the lumen and isotonic diarrhea starts.

   > **Note:** Though perturbation of the adenylate cylase pathway is the primary mechanism of cholera; cholera toxin also enhances the intestinal secretions via prostaglandins and/or neural histamine receptors.

   > **Remember:** *Mechanism of action* of some important bacterial toxin.
   > - Heat labile toxin of E. coli — ↑ cAMP
   > - Heat stable toxin of E. coli — Increase cGMP
   > - Botulism toxin — Inhibit release of acetylcholine from peripheral nerves.
   > - Tetanus toxin — Inhibit release of glycine and GABA at presynaptic terminals.
   > - Diphtheria toxin — Inhibit protein synthesis by inactivating EF-2.

4. **Ans. (b) Cannot grow in ordinary media** *Ref. Ananthanarayan 10/e p 310; Park 22/e, p 208*
   - Cholera grows well on ordinary media.
   - Growth is better on alkaline medium. NaCl is required for optimal growth though high concentrations are inhibitory.
   - *Option "c"* – Natural habitat of V. cholerae is coastal salt water and brackish estuaries, where the organism live in close relation to plankton.
     - Human become infected incidentally, but once infected can act as vehicle for spread.
     - Man is the only reservoir of cholera infection. He may be the case or carrier.

Carriers in cholera		
Preclinical or convalescent carrier	**Contact or healthy carrier**	**Chronic carrier**
Incubatory – Last for 2-3 weeks after attack	– Result from subclinical infection	– Can excreate up to 10 years.
	– Duration less than 10 days	– Gallbladder is infected
	– Gallbladder is not infected	

5. **Ans. (b) First isolated in Chennai**   *Ref. Harrison 20/e, p 1188*
   Already explained, refer Ans. 1

6. **Ans. (a) *V. cholerae***   *Ref. Ananthanarayan 10/e, p 317*
   Halophilic vibrios:
   - Vibrios that have high requirement of NaCl.
   - All vibrios are halophilic except *V. cholerae* and *V. mimicus*.

- Natural habitat of halophilic vibrios is sea water.

Disease caused are:

V. parahemolyticus	Gastroenteritis; wound infection
V. vulnificus	Sepsis (in immunocompromised); secondary cellulitis
V. alginolyticus (Most halophilic)	Wound infections, cellulitis

7. **Ans. (a) ADP ribosylation of G regulatory protein**   *Ref. Harrison 20/e, p 1188*
   Already explained

8. **Ans. (c) Doxycycline**   *Ref. Harrison 20/e, p 1184*
   "Doxycycline in single dose is the antibiotic of choice for adults (excepting pregnant women)." If susceptibility is confirmed
   Antibiotic treatment of Cholera
   WHO recommends administration of antibiotic to cholera patients only if they are severely dehydrated.
   - Due to increased resistances to tetracycline, erythromycin or azithromycin are agent of choice
   - Oral supplemental zinc reduce volume and severity of diarrhea

   Chemoprophylaxis – Tetracycline is *DOC* for chemoprophylaxis

9. **Ans. (a) cAMP**   *Ref. Harrison 20/e, p 1189*
   Already explained

10. **Ans. (a) TCBS**   *Ref. Ananthanarayan 10/e, p 310*
    - **TCBS** *(media containing thiosulphate, citrate, bilesalts, sucrose)* is the best **selective media** for vibrio.
    - Vibrio produces yellow convex colonies.
    - In holding or transport media, Vibrios do not multiply but remain viable.

Holding or transport media	Plating media
1. VR medium	1. Alkaline bile salt agar
2. Caryblair medium	2. GTTA
3. Alkaline peptone water*	3. TCBS (best selective media)
4. Monsur's taurocholate tellurite water*	4. Mac Conkey agar (Non-selective)
*are also enrichment media	

    Mnemonic

    Transport media – *Venkatraman carry alkaline peptone water to Maysoore* (Monsour).
    Biochemical characteristics – **[COINS]** – **C**atalase +ve; – **O**xidase +ve; – **I**ndole +ve; – **N**itrate reducer – **S**ucrose fermenter

11. **Ans. (c) *Vibrio cholerae***   *Ref. Ananthanarayan 10/e, p 314*
    Beside cholera toxin, *V. cholerae* also posses the lipopolysaccharide O antigen (LPS endotoxin) which apparently plays no role in pathogenesis of cholera but is responsible for the immunity induced by killed vaccine.

    Other options:

E. coli	–	Pathogenesis is mediated by endotoxin, adhesins, capsule present in some strain, enterotoxin.
Pseudomonas	–	Exotoxin produce tissue necrosis by blocking protein synthesis.
	–	Endotoxin plays a role in causing fever, shock, oligouria, leukocytosis, DIC, ARDS.
Klebsiella	–	Pathogenesis is mediated by endotoxin and fimbriae or other adhesin.

Remember:	–	Endotoxin levels can be assayed by 'Limulus test'.
	–	Plague toxin also has no role in natural disease.

12. **Ans. (c) Causes continued activation of adenylate cyclase**   *Ref. Harrison 20/e, p 1189*
    Already explained

13. **Ans. (c) Furazolidone** *Ref. Harrison 20/e, p 1189*
    Antibiotics used in the **treatment of cholera**.

Condition	Antibiotic
Adult	Erythromycin or Azithromycin
Chemoprophylaxis	Tetracycline 4 times a day for 3 days
Children & Pregnancy	Erythromycin or Azithromycin

    In older days furazolidone was used to treat pregnant women. As this question is old one, so the answer was furazolidone.

14. **Ans. (a) Tetracycline** *Ref. Park 22/e, p 211*
    Already explained

15. **Ans. (d) Enterotoxin can have** *Ref. Park 22/e, p 208; Ananthanarayan 10/e, p 314*

    Cholera enterotoxin does not exert extraintestinal effects.
    Resistance of vibrio to surroundings
    - Highly susceptible to heat, drying and acids. Destroyed at 55°C in 15 minutes, boiling kill, vibrio in few seconds.
    - They can remain in ice for 4-6 for weeks or longer.
    - On fruits they survive for 1-5 days at room temperature and more than a week in refrigerator.
    - E_1 tor vibrios survive longer than the classical cholera vibrios.
    - They survive in clean tap water for longer period than contaminated water.
    - They are killed in gastric juice of normal acidity but may survive for 24 hours in achlorhydria gastric juice.

16. **Ans. (c) *V. cholerae*** *Ref. Ananthanarayan 10/e, p 314*
    Already explained, refer Ans. 3

17. **Ans. (c) and (d) Motility; and Binds to specific receptors** *Ref. See below*
    - To cause cholera, *Vibrio cholerae* must reach in small intestine where it produces cholera toxin.
    - *Vibrio encounters* following barriers:

Barrier	Mechanism to invade
• Gastric acidity	– Large inoculum size (> 10^6 organism)
• Mucosal lining of small bowel	– Chemotaxis, motility and variety of protease
• Adhesion to epithelial cells	– Toxin corregulated pilus

18. **Ans. (a) and (c) Food transmits and Healthy carrier** *Ref. Ananthanarayan 10/e, p 313*
    Mode of transmission of cholera:
    - Fecally contaminated water *(MC)*
    - Contaminated food and drinks
    - Direct contact.

Cholera vaccine	
Parenteral vaccine	**Oral vaccines**
Killed	Killed *(wc/rbs)* or live *(CVD 103 HgR)*
Protective value 50%	Protective value 80% for live vaccine

    So, no vaccine of cholera provide 90% protection.

    > **Remember:**
    > - ***V. cholerae* are killed within 30 minutes by heating at 56°C or within a few seconds by boiling.** Also killed by ***chlorination***.
    > - **DOC** for chemoprophylaxis is tetracycline. Alternative is doxycycline.
    > - Carriers in cholera includes preclinical or incubatory (1-5 days), convalescent (2-3 weeks), contact or healthy (> 10 days) and chronic carrier.

Period of communicability	
Case:	7 days
Convalescent carrier:	2-3 weeks
Chronic carrier:	1 month - 10 year

19. **Ans. (a and b)** ***Vibrio cholerae* 01 and *Vibrio cholerae* O139**   *Ref. Harrison 17/e, p 969, 18/e, p 1289, 19/e, p 1062*

    Cholera now refers to disease caused by V. cholerae O1 or O139 i.e. the serogroups with epidemic potential.

    > **Note:** Causes of diarrhea with pus cells/RBCs in stool (inflammatory diarrhea or dysentery):
    > - *Shigella*
    > - EIEC, EHEC
    > - *Campylobacter*
    > - *Salmonella*
    > - *Yersinia*
    > - *Cl. difficle*
    > - *Vibrio parahemolyticus*

20. **Ans. (a and d) V. cholerae; Camplyobacter jejuni**   *Ref. Ananthanarayan 10/e, p 309*
    Bacteria showing darting type motility
    - Vibrio cholerae : Through single polar flagellum
    - Campylobacter jejuni : Through single polar flagellum. Motility can be darting or tumbling type
    - Sperillium minus

21. **Ans. (b, c, d) Voges Proskauer (VP) positive; Swarming; Cause sea borne auricular infections**
    Ref. Ananthanarayan 10/e, p 318; Greenwood 18/e, p 320
    V. alginolyticus
    - High salt tolerant, **VP positive**, sucrose fermenter halophilic vibrio that closely resembles V. parahemolyticus
    - Forms large yellow colonies on TCBS
    - It fails to grow on CLED agar but grows in presence of 10% NaCl. There is pronounced *swarming* on non selective solid media
    - It is frequently found in **sea fish**
    - It has been associated with infections of eyes, ears and wounds in human beings exposed to sea water.

22. **Ans. (d) Cholera gravis**   *Ref. Harrison 20/e, p 1188*
    Cholera gravis: Sudden onset of explosive and life threatening diarrhea.

NEET Pattern Questions

1. **Ogawa Inaba and Hikojima are the serotypes of:**
   a. Yersina
   b. Vibrio cholerae
   c. E Coli
   d. Salmonella typhi   [Ref. Ananthanarayan, 10/e, p 312]

2. **Selective plating medium for V. cholerae is:**
   a. Carry-Blair medium
   b. TCBS agar
   c. VR medium
   d. MacConkey medium
   [Ref. Ananthanarayan, 10/e, p 310]

> Carry-Blair is transport media while TCBS Alkaline bile salt agar is selective plating media

3. **True about cholerae includes all *except*:**
   a. Incubation period range from 1-5 days
   b. Produces isotonic diarrhea
   c. Cholera toxin plays principal role
   d. Antibodies 01 cholera provides protection against 0139 serotype also   [Ref. Harrison, 18/e, p 1290]

> Clinical manifestations of disease caused by 0139 V. cholerae resemble that of 01 type V. cholerae. immunity to one however is not protective against the other.

4. **Which organism grows in alkaline pH?**
   a. Vibrio   b. Klebsiella
   c. Pseudomonas   d. E. coli

> Optimum pH for vibrio is 8.2 and it an grow in pH range of 6.4–9.6

5. **Invasive infection is caused by all *except*:**
   a. V. cholerae   b. Neisseria
   c. Streptococci d. H. influenza
   [Ref. Harrison, 20/e, p 1188]

6. **Transport medium for cholera:**
   a. LJ medium
   b. Cary Blair medium
   c. MYPA medium
   d. Stewart medium   [Ref. Ananthanarayan, 10, p 310]

7. **True about cholera:**
   a. Gram negative rod
   b. Associated with fever
   c. Causes painful watery diarrhea
   d. It is an achlorhydria which renders an individual susceptible to disease
   [Ref. Ananthanarayan, 10/e, p 309-311]

> **Transportation of cholera specimen:**
> - Stool should be transported in sterilized Mc Cartney bottles containing alkaline peptone water on VR medium.
> - The specimen should be transported in alkaline peptone water on Carry blair medium if it is collected by a rectal swab.
> - It suitable plating media are available (e.g bile salt agar) at the bed side, the stools should be streaked on the media before forwarding to lab.

8. **Enrichment media for cholera:**
   a. VR medium
   b. TCBS medium
   c. Cary-Blair medium
   d. Alkaline peptone water
   [Ref. Ananthanarayan, 10/e, p 310]

9. **Optimal percentage of NaCl for V cholerae:**
   a. 1%   b. 2%
   c. 3%   d. 4%
   [Ref. Ananthanarayan, 10/e, p 310]

10. **Transmission of cholera is through:**
    a. Fecally contaminated food
    b. Fecally contaminated water
    c. Contaminated food by vomits of a case
    d. All of the above
    [Ref. Park, 22/e, p 209]

> Cases excrete around 10^7–10^{10} vibrios per ml of fecal fluid.
> Cariers excrete around 10^2–10^5 vibrios per gram of stool.

11. **True about vibrio parahemolyticus:**
    a. Polar flagella
    b. Non halophilic vibrios
    c. Non-capsulated
    d. Requires NaCl   [Ref. Ananthanarayan, 10/e, p 317]

> It has peritrichous flagella, capsule, shows bipolar staining

12. **True about vibrio vulnificus:**
    a. Causes diarrhea commonly
    b. Halophilic
    c. Drug of choice is penicillin
    d. Produces shiga toxin   [Ref. Ananthanarayan, 10/e, p 318]

13. **Most halophillic vibrio:**
    a. V. cholerae   b. V. vulnificus
    c. V. alginolyticus d. V. parahemolyticus
    [Ref. Ananthanarayan, 10/e, p 318]

> V. alginolyticus can grow in up to 10% NaCl

Ans.
1. b. Vibrio cholerae   2. b. TCBS agar   3. d Antibodies...   4. a. Vibrio   5. a. V. cholerae
6. b. Cary Blair medium 7. a. Gram negative rod   8. d. Alkaline peptone…   9. a. 1%   10. d. All of the above
11. d. Requires NaCl   12. b. Halophilic   13. c. V alginolyticus

14. **Most important step in cholera control:**
    a. Chemoprophylaxis   b. Vaccination
    c. Early treatment   d. Water sanitation
    [Ref. Park, 22/e, p 211]

15. **Non-Halophilic vibrio is:**
    a. V. cholerae   b. V. parahaemolyticus
    c. V. alginolyticus   d. V. fluvialis
    [Ref. Ananthanarayan, 10/e, p 317]

> V. cholerae is halotolerant and high NaCl concentration (6% and above) are inhibitory

16. **True about El T or vibrio:**
    a. More SAR
    b. VP reaction (+)ve
    c. Low carrier rate
    d. More severe   [Ref. Ananthanarayan, 9/e, p 312]

17. **Cholera toxin binds to which receptors in intestine:**
    a. Sphingosine through A subunit
    b. Sphingosine through B subunit
    c. GM1 gangliosides through A subunit
    d. GM1 gangliosides through B subunit
    [Ref. Ananthanarayan, 10/e, p 314]

18. **Bacteria with safety pin appearance:**
    a. H. influenzae
    b. Vibrio parahaemolyticus
    c. Vibrio vulnificus
    d. Salmonella paratyphi
    [Ref. Ananthanarayan, 10/e, p 317]

19. **7th pandemic of cholera is caused by:**
    a. E_1 tor
    b. 0139 V. cholerae
    c. Classical V. cholerae
    d. V. mimicus   [Ref. Dr Arora 3/e, p 402]

Pondemic	Year	Causative vibrio
1-6	1817-1923	Classical V. cholerae
7	1961	E_1 Tor
8	Not yet	0139 (proposed)

20. **Peritrichous flagella is seen in all except:**
    a. E. coli   b. Salmonella
    c. Bacillus   d. Vibrio cholerae
    [Ref. Ananthanarayan 10/e, p 309]

21. **All of the following statements about cholera are true except:**
    a. O and H antigens measure carrier state
    b. Culture medium is TCBS agar
    c. Produces indole and reduces nitrate
    d. Synthesize neuraminidase   [Ref. Park 22/e, 209]

> • **Enzymes produced by Vibrio cholerae:**
>   – **N**euraminidase   – **E**lastase
>   – **L**ipase   – **M**ucinase
>   – **C**hintinase.
>   **Mnemonic** - Cute NELaM

22. **True about cholera vibrios is:**
    a. Can tolerate wide range of alkaline pH
    b. Nonmotile bacilli
    c. Cannot be grown in media
    d. NaCl stimulates growth   [Ref. Ananthanarayan 10/e, 309]

> • Vibrio cholerae can grow in pH range 6.4-9.6 (Optimum - 8.2).
> • NaCl (0.5-1%) is required for optimal growth though high concentration (6% and above) is inhibitory.

23. **A patient with acute onset of diarrhea comes to emergency. After culture on enriched media, colonies as shown below were visualized. Identify the causative organism:**

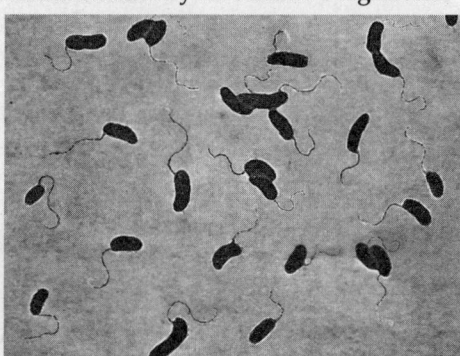

    a. Vibrio cholera
    b. Salmonella typhi
    c. Campylobacter jejuni
    d. E. coli   [Ref. Ananthanarayan, 10/e, p 309]

> Comma shaped bacteria with single sheathed polar flagellum can be none other than V. cholera

---

Ans.
14. **d.** Water sanitation   15. **a.** V. cholerae   16. **b.** VP reaction (+)ve   18. **b.** Vibrio Parahaemolyticus   19. **a.** E_1 tor
17. **d.** GM1 gangliosides through B subunit
20. **d.** Vibrio ...   21. **a.** O and H ....   22. **a, d.** Can tolerate.... and NaCl stimulates...   23. **a.** Vibrio cholera

Pseudomonas and Yersinia

CHAPTER 17

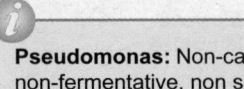

Pseudomonas: Non-capsulate, non-fermentative, non sporing, Aerobic Gr (–)ve, pigment producing, motile (two flagella) bacteria
Selective media: Cetrimide agar

PSEUDOMONAS

Gram (–)ve aerobic motile bacilli with polar flagella.
Pseudomonas aeruginosa is the *MC* human pathogen in this group.

P. AERUGINOSA = P. PYOCYANEA

- *Non-sporing, obligate aerobic bacilli* which is differentiated from enteric gram (–)ve bacilli by its *ability to oxidise indophenol and inability to ferment lactose.*
- *Noncapsulated* but many strains have mucoid slime layer of alginate particularly in patient of cystic fibrosis.
- Part of normal intestinal flora.   ...*Jawetz 27/e, p 245*

Note: Can grow anaerobically if nitrate is available as a terminal electron acceptor.

Culture and Growth characteristic

- Grows well at 37-42°C on ordinary media.
- *Growth at 42°C helps differentiate it from other Pseudomonas species.*
- *Selective media* – Cetrimide agar
- Pigment
  a. *Pyocyanin*   –   Bluish green pigment produce *only by P. aeruginsoa*. It inhibits growth of many other bacteria.
  b. *Fluorescein*   –   Greenish yellow. Produce by all species of *Pseudomonas*.
  c. *Pyorubin*
  d. *Pyomelanin*] – Some strains of P. aeroginosa

Fluorescent pigment: pyoverdin
Red pigment: Pyorubin
Black pigment: Pyomelanin

Classification

- *On the basis of difference of lipopolysaccharide.*
- Restriction endonuclease typing with pulsed gel electrophoresis is most reliable method.
- Used for epidemiological purpose.

Pathogenicity and Resistance

- *P. aeruginosa* is pathogenic only when inoculated into areas devoid of normal defences's e.g. when mucous membrane is disrupted, patient is catheterized, neutropenia is there.
- Broad spectrum antibiotic use is the another important risk factor.
- *MC* and *most serious* cause to infection in burns.
- *MC infection* outside hospital is suppurative otitis media.
- Can infect all body sites but shows strong predilection for lungs   *Ref.: Harristion 20/e p 1168*
- Pseudomonas bacteria has mortality rate > 50%
- Causative agent of Shanghai fever.
- MC infection inside hospital in pneumonia
- *Produce Blue pus* with characteristic fruity odour.
- *Pathognomonic* skin lesion are called as *ecthyma gangrenosum*, which occur singly or in small number on the perineum, buttocks and extremities (*lesions are due to vascular invasion and contains bacteria*).
- Resistant to common antiseptic and disinfectant such as dettol. Contrary it may grow profusely in bottle of these antiseptic. Resistant to quaternary ammonium compounds, chloroxylenol.

Virulence Factors

Motility and colonization:
a. **Pilli:** Demonstrate adhesive property to variety of cells, and adheres best to injured cell surface.
b. **Flagellin:** Flagellin molecule binds to cells and the flagellar cap attaches to mucins through the recognition of glycan chains.
c. Lipopolysaccharide (LPS) molecule: Binds to cFTR and aids in internalization of organism in cystic fibrosis patient.

Evasion of host defenses: Attached bacteria inject four known toxins (EXOS or EXOU, EXOT and EXOY) via type III secretion which evade phagocytic cell either directly or by inhibition of phagocytosis.

Multiple protease secreted by type II secretion system degrade cytokines and chemokines.

- **Tissue injury:** Exotoxin A, four different protease, phospholipase induce host injury. Pyocyanin and hydrocyanic acid also injured tissue.
- **Inflammatory components:** Flagellin; LPS.
- *Exotoxin A* – As, ↓ protein synthesis via ADP ribosylation and thereby inactivation of EF-2.
- *Exotoxin S* – Ribosylation of GTP binding protein, disruption of cellular actin cytoskeleton.
- Exoenzyme U is a phospholipase.
- Exoenzyme Y is an adenylyl cyclase.

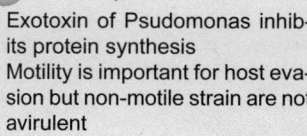
Exotoxin of Psudomonas inhibits protein synthesis
Motility is important for host evasion but non-motile strain are not avirulent

> **Remember:** Extracellular virulence factors exhibits Quorum Sensing (= cell to cell signaling system). P. aeruginosa can be typed by lipopolysaccharide immunophenotype and by pyocin (bacteriocin susceptibility) ... *Jawetz 27/e, p 247*

Sterilization –Killed at 55°C in 1 hour; Sensitive to acids, β glutaraldehyde, silver salts and strong phenolic disinfectants

Treatment

Antimicrobials effective against Pseudomonas are:

Penicillin	Cephalosporins	Aminoglycoside	Quinolones
Piperacillin/tazobactam	Ceftazidime	Tobramycin	Ciprofloxacin
Tazobactam	Cefoperazone	Gentamicin	Levofloxacin
Ticarcillin/Clavulanate	Cefepime	Amikacin	Trovafloxacin
Mezlocillin			

- **Other Agent:** Polymyxin B. Colistin, *Monobactams* - Aztreonam
- **Drug of Choices: Aminoglycoside + Penicillin** except:
  a. **In UTI** – Ciprofloxacin
  b. **In CNS infection** – Ceftozidime ± Aminoglycoside.
  c. **In Malignant external otitis** – Cephalosporin or carbapenem or ciprofloxacin.

BURKHOLDERIA PSEUDOMALLEI [PSEUDOMONAS PSEUDOMALLEI]

- *Causative agent of* 'Melioidosis'.
- Resembles *Ps. mallei* but differs in being motile.
- Organism is oxidase positive and motile but does not produce diffusible pigments.
- Among all pseudomonas, P. pseudomallei is most virulent   ... *Harrison, 20/e, 1172*
- *MC* manifestation of melioidosis: Acute pulmonary infection.
- May cause hemoptysis resembling TB.
- Another common manifestation is acutely localizead skin infection with ulceration or abscess that is associated with nodular lymphangitis and regional lymphadenitis.
- Latency and reactivation may occur as bacillus can survive intracellulary in reticuloendothelial system.
- Human infection occurs commonly through skin abrasion or by inhalation.

B. pseudomallei
- Causative agent of meliodesis
- Motile, oxidase (+)ve.
- Bipolar safety pin appearance

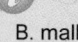
B. mallei
- Causative agent of glanders
- Non-motile
- Both mallei and pseudomallei are potential bioterrorism agent.

- **Diagnosis:** – *Typical bipolar safety pin appearance* of bacillus in exudates on microscopy.
  – Confirmed by culture or ≥ 4 fold rise in antibody.
- **Treatment:** – *Ceftazidime or carbapenems* is **DOC**.

BURKHOLDERIA MALLEI (PSEUDOMONAS MALLEI)

- *Causative agent of* 'Glanders', a disease of equine.
- Non-motile with bipolar staining imparting safety pin appearance.
- *On potato:* characteristic amber, honey like growth appears, becoming greenish yellow resembling Ps. aeruginosa
- It is agent of biological Warfare and terrorism, classified as 'category B biological agent'.
- In human, it cause acute localized suppurative infection, acute pulmonary infection; acute septicemic infection and chronic suppurative infection.
- It induces **'Straus reaction'**.
- Human infection is usually *occupational*.
- **Diagnosis:** – *Mallein test* which is analogous to tuberculin test.
  – Molecular methods for rapid identificatiion – 16s rRNA gene sequencing. Also distinguish it from B. pseudomallei.
- **Treatment:** – Same as **melioidosis**.

Burkholderia Cepacia

- Gained popularity as the cause of rapidly fatal syndrome of respiratory distress and septicaemia in cystic fibrosis patients.
- Patients with chronic granulomatous disease are also predisposed to B. cepacia lungs disease.
- Organism binds to lung mucous and secret toxins like P. aeruginosa.
- Treatment: Due to intrinsic resistance to antibiotics, trimethoprim sulfamethoxazole, meropenem and doxycycline are most affective agent.

PASTEURELLAE

- Group consists of gram-negative, short, pleomorphic bacilli that are primary pathogen of rodents.
- It is divided into 3 genus:
  a **Yersinia:** – Includes plague bacillus (Y.pestis); Y. pseudotuberculosis (primary pathogen of rodents); Y. enterocolitica.
  – It is assigned in the family Enterobacteriaceae.
  b. **Pasteurella:** – Includes P. multocida (non-motile, oxidase positive).
  c. **Francisella:** – Includes F. tularensis.

YERSINIA PESTIS = PLAGUE BACILLUS

Morphology

- Nonmotile, nonsporing, microaerophilic, biochemically unreactive, pleomorphic bacilli/coccobacillus.
- Characteristic bipolar (safety pin) appearance, with Wayson's stain/Giemsa/methylene.
- It is noncapsulated but at ≥ 30°C it produces envelop (= **F1 antigen**) – a virulence factor that serves as the principal immunodiagnostic marker of infection.
- *Serotypes do not exist.*
- Central Asia or Himalayas is believed to be the original home of plague.
- The last pandemic was started in Hong Kong in 1894 and was caused by Y. pestis var orientalis.

Cultural Characteristics

- *Optimum* growth occurs at **27°C and pH 7.2** (unlike most pathogens which usually grow at 37°C).
- Shows 'Stalactite growth' in ghee broth.

Yersinia
- Non-motile
- Non-sporing
- Microaerophillic
- Safety pin appearance on Wayson's stain
- Cause plague

Non-capsulated but at ≥ 30°C it produces envelop

> **Remember:** Growth is *fastest* at 30°C and envelops develop best at 37°C. It produce coagulase at 28°C but not at 35°C.
> ..... *Jawetz 25/e, p 257*
> **Resistance:** Killed at 55°C in 5 min and by 0.5% phenol in 15 min.

Biochemical Reactions

- Based on fermentation of glycerol and reduction of nitrate, it is divided into 3 varieties.
- Catalase and aesculin positive; Urease and oxidase negative.

Pathogenesis

- From the site of flea bite *(xenopsylla cheopis)* it is carried to regional lymph nodes (=bubo) via lymphatic channel.
- Mononuclear phagocytes play role in dissemination of infection to distant sites (secondary pneumonia and septicemia).
- **Primary pneumonia** results by droplet infection of plague patient.
- **Primary septicemic plague** consist of sepsis in absence of bubo while secondary septicemic plague is complication of bubonic or pneumonic plague.
- Heat stable somatic antigen complex of Y. pestis has endotoxic activity which contribute to terminal toxemia. Heat labile portion resist phagocytosis.

> Y. pestis fits the profile of potential agent of bioterrorism

Clinical Features

- Characterized by rapid onset of fever and other systemic manifestations of Gram −ve bacterial infections.
- It is of 3 types:

  a. **Bubonic Plague:**
  - I.P 2 - 7 days
  - MC type of plague and is almost always caused by *bite of infected flea.*
  - MC site of bubo, inguinal region >axillary, cervical.
  ... *Harrison 20/e, p 1202*
  - Distinguished from lymphadenitis by its rapid onset, extreme tenderness, accompanying signs of toxemia and absence of cellulitis or obvious ascending lymphadenitis.
  - DIC is common and may lead to gangrene.
  - *Y. pestis can also be cultured from blood of most bubonic plague patient.*

  b. **Septicemic plague:** (black death)
  - Most fatal, often present with GI symptoms, DIC, multiorgan failure.
  - I P 2 - 7 days

  c. **Pneumonic plague:**
  - *Most infectious,* type of plague with I P of 1-3 days. Can cause:
    (i) Primary pneumonia: Cyanosis is very prominent, with bloody mucoid sputum.
    (ii) Secondary pneumonia: Diffuse *interstitial* pneumonia, less infectious.

> MC site of bubo: Axillary node

Diagnosis:
- Demonstrating the bacilli in fluid from buboes or local skin lesion
- Blood culture
- PCR is rapid & less hazardous.

> - Bubonic plague is the most common type of plague
> - Pneunonic plague is the most fatal type
> - Plague can be transmitted from rat to rat, rat to human, human to human.

Treatment:
- Streptomycin is drug of choice

Prevention:
- *Prophylaxis of choice* – Tetracycline.
- Recombinant vaccine that use F_1 and V antigen is available.

FRANCISELLA OR PASTEURELLA OR BRUCELLA TULARENSIS

- Capsulated, nonmotile, intracellular parasite which grows in special media such as Francis blood dextrose cystine agar.
- It resembles *Mycoplasma*.
- It cause **tularemia**, a disease of rabbits and other rodents which is transmitted by ticks.
- In human it presents as local ulceration with lymphadenitis, typhoid like fever with glandular enlargement or influenza like respiratory infection.
- **Treatment:** Streptomycin is *DOC* for adults and children.

YERSINOSIS

- *It denotes infection with Yersiniae other than Y. pestis* (i.e. by enterocolitica and pseudotuberculosis).
- They are motile at 25°C but non-motile at 37°C.
- They show antigenic cross-reaction with Y. pestis, *Vibrio, Salmonella, Brucella*.
- For culture *'cold enrichment'* is done.

Y. pseudotuberculosis
- Most human infection occur by serotype 01.
- ***Commonest presentation is abdominal pain & fever***
- Associated with Far-Eastern scarlet like fever (a childhood illness with rash, arthralgia and toxic shock) similar illness is called as Izumi fever in Japan.

Y. enterocolitica
- Most human infections occur by serotypes 03, 08, 09.
- It causes gastroenteritis or enterocolitis; Mesenteric adenitis or terminal ileitis; system disease with bacteremia; erythema nodosum, reactive arthritis (in HLA - B 27).

Multiple Choice Questions

1. Burkolderia cepacia is resistant to: [NEET Pattern 2018]
   a. Polymyxin B
   b. Trimethoprim-sulfamethoxazole
   c. Amoxicillin-clavulanic acid
   d. 3rd generation cephalosporins

2. The mode of infection of *Pasteurella multocida*? [AI 09]
   a. Endogenous infection
   b. Animal bites or scratches
   c. Human beings
   d. Aerosols and dust

3. A young boy had a flea bite while working in a wheat grain godown. After 5 days he developed fever and had axillary lymphadenopathy. A smear was sent to the laboratory to perform a specific staining. Which one of the following staining method would help in the identification of the suspected pathogen? [AI 06]
   a. Albert staining
   b. Ziehl-Neelsen staining
   c. McFadyean's staining
   d. Wayson staining

4. Which one of the following drugs is an antipseudomonal penicillin? [AI 06]
   a. Cephalexin   b. Cloxacillin
   c. Piperacillin   d. Dicloxacillin

5. The following statements are true regarding melioidosis except: [AI 05]
   a. It is caused by *Burkholderia mallei*
   b. The agent is a gram-negative aerobic bacteria
   c. Bipolar staining of etiological agent is seen with methylene blue
   d. The most common form of meliodosis is pulmonary infection

6. An organism grown on agar shows green colored colonies; likely organism is: [AI 01]
   a. *Staphylococcus*   b. *E. coli*
   c. *Pseudomonas*   d. *Peptostreptococcus*

7. A girl from Shimla presented with fever, malaise and axillary/inguinal lymphadenopathy and organism shows stalactite growth on culture. Which of the following is the causative organism? [AIIMS 08]
   a. *Yersinia pestis*
   b. *Francisella*
   c. *Burkholderia pseudomallei*
   d. *Pasteurella*

8. Which species of *Pseudomonas* is the most common cause of intravenous catheter related infection? [AIIMS 08]
   a. *Pseudomonas cepacia*   b. *P. aeruginosa*
   c. *P. maltophilia*   d. *Burkholderia pseudomallei*

9. A 50-year-old chronic alcoholic male agriculture worker presented with high grade fever of one week with spells of chills and rigor. Examination of the respiratory system reveals bilateral crepitation with scattered rhonchi. Multiple subcutaneous nodules were found on extensor surface of left forearm and left leg. Direct microscopy of the pus aspirate from the nodules reveals plenty of grams (–)ve bacilli with bipolar staining. Culture reveals distinct rough corrugated grey white colonies on blood agar. The organisms were motile and oxidase-positive. The most likely diagnosis is: [AIIMS 03]
   a. Plague   b. Melioidosis
   c. Bartonellosis   d. Actinomycosis

10. True about *Y. pestis*: [PGI 06, 03]
    a. Gram +ve   b. Gram –ve
    c. Motile   d. Non-motile
    e. It is coccobacilli

11. A farmer from Himachal Pradesh present with inguinal lymphadenopathy. On examination multiple small ulcers are seen in leg. Which of the following stain would you prefer for bipolar staining of etiologic agents of this case? [AIIMS 2010]
    a. KOH   b. Gram stain
    c. Wayson's   d. Nigrosin

12. A farmer presents to the emergency department with painful inguinal lymphadenopathy and history of fever and flu like symptoms. Clinical examination reveals on ulcer in the leg. Which of the following stain should be used to detect suspected bipolar stained organism. [AI 2011, AIIMS 2012]
    a. Alberts stain   b. Ziehl Neelsen stain
    c. Wayson's stain   d. McFayden's stain

Explanations and References with Illustrative Answers

1. **Ans (a) Polymyxin B** *Ref. 20/e p 1172; Katjung 13/e p 1035*
   Burkholderia species is usually resistant to aminoglycosides cosides and Polymyxin B'

Antibiotic sensitivity of B. cepacia	
Resistant	**Sensitive**
• Aminoglycoside • Penicillin • Polymyxin B • Macrolides • Rifamycins • Colistin	• Trimethoprim sulfamethoxazole • Carbapenem • Doxycycline • Amoxicillin Clavulanic acid • Ureidopenicillin • Advance cephalosporin • Fluoroquinolones

2. **Ans (b) Animal bites or scratches** *Ref. Ananthanarayan 10/e, p 331*
   Pasteurella multocida
   - Group of bacteria similar to *Yersinia* often carried in the upper respiratory tract of variety of animals such as dogs, cats, cattle. It may cause hemorrhagic septicemia in these animals.
   - *P. multocida* is **nonmotile**, Gram-negative bacilus, resembling *Yersinia*, but differing in being oxidase-positive, ***producing indole*** and *failing to grow on MacConkey agar.*
   - Human infection is rare but may occur following animal bites or scratches.
   - Clinical manifestation includes local suppuration, meningitis (following bite in head) respiratory tract infection.
   - Tetracycline and streptomycin are drug of choice.

3. **Ans. (d) Wayson staining** *Ref. Park 22/e, p 267-268; Ananthanarayan 10/e, p 329*
   "It is typical clinical presentation of bubonic plague."
   PLAGUE:
   - It is a zoonosis.
   - Causative agent is Yersinia pestis which is:
     - Gram-negative, non-motile, coccobacilli
     - Exhibits bipolar staining with ***Wayson's stain/giemsa stain/methylene blue, Wright Stain***
     - Plague bacilli can survive and indeed multiply in the soil of rodent burrows where microclimate and other conditions are favourable.
   - Reservoir:
     - ***Wild rodents*** (e.g. field mice) *are natural reservoirs* of plague.
     - In India wild rodent, **Tatera indica** *has been incriminated as main reservoir,* not the domestic rat.
   - Source of infection:
     - ***Infected rodents*** and ***fleas*** and ***case of pneumonic plague (not bubonic plague).***
   - Immunity:
     - After recovery there is relative immunity.
   - Vector:
     - Commonest vector is rat flea, (X-cheopis). Infected flea may live upto 4 year.
     - Human **infection** is *most frequently* contracted from bite of infected flea.
     - **Basic cycle** in epidemic bubonic plague is: Commensal rats → rat fleas → man
   - **Incubation period:**   – Bubonic plague   - 2 to 7 days
                              – Septicaemic plague - 2 to 7 days
                              – Pneumonic plague   - 1 to 3 days
   - Clinical Presentation:
     - **MC type** of human *plague* is **bubonic plague** characterized by enlarged tender lymph nodes (Bubos).
     - MC site of bubo is inguinal, axillary and cervical nodes.
     - **Pneumonic plague** – Rare variety but most infectious variety of plague.
     - **Septicaemic plague** – Rare variety.
   - Diagnosis:
     - *Specimens* - Blood for culture.
                   - Aspirates of enlarged lymph nodes for smear and culture.
     - *Smears* - Stain with Giemsa and specific immunofluorescent stains.
                - Prime face diagnosis is by examination of smears which show characteristic ***bipolar appearance with Wayson's stain.***

- *Culture* - Blood culture are often positive in 24 hours. Show stalactite growth
  - Definite identification of culture is best done by immunofluorescence.
- *Serology* - Antibodies to F. 1 antigen may be detected by passive hemagglutination.
- **Treatment:** – **DOC** – Streptomycin (Alternative tetracycline, chloramphenicol)
- **Chemoprophylaxis:** – **DOC** – Tetracycline (Alternative sulfonamide)

> **Remember:** Flea borne disease — Endemic typhus — Chiggerosis
> — Hymenoplepis diminata

Other Options

Stain	Organism
Albert's	C. diphtheria
Ziehl-Neelsen	Acid fast organism
Mc Fadyean's	B. anthrax

4. **Ans. (c) Piperacillin** *Ref. Harrison 20/e p 1168; 16/e, p 894*

Antimicrobial agents active against Pseudomonas aeruginosa		
Antipseudomonal penicillins	**Antipseudomonal cephalosporins**	**Carbapenems/Other agents**
• Piperacillin	• Ceftazidime	• Imipenem/cilastatin
• Mezlocillin	• Cefoperazone	• Meropenem
• Ticarcillin	• Cefepime	• Polymyxin B
• Ticarcillin/clavulanate		• Colistin
Monobactams	**Aminoglycosides**	**Fluoroquinolones**
• Aztreonam	• Tobramycin	• Ciprofloxacin
	• Gentamicin	• Levofloxacin
	• Amikacin	

5. **Ans. (a) It is caused by *Burkholderia mallei*** *Ref. Harrison 20/e, p 1172; Jawetz 27/e, p 248*
   Meliodoisis
   - Caused by *Burkhoderia pseudomallei (Pseudomonas pseudomallei)*.
   - It is free living small, motile (differentiating feature from pseudo. mallei) *aerobic gram-negative* bacillary saprophyte normally found in soily ponds and rice paddies.
   - It grows at 42°C and oxidise glucose, lactose and is *oxidase positive*.
   - It forms colonies that vary from mucoid and smooth to rough and wrinkled and in colour from cream to orange.
   - *MC* form of melioidosis is *Acute pulmonary* infection.
   - Acute pulmonary infection vary from mild bronchitis to extensive necrotizing pneumonia.
   - Chronic pulmonary infection mimics TB.
   - It also cause acute, localized skin infection with ulceration or abscess that is associated with nodular lymphangitis and regional lymphadenitis.
   - Also cause suppurative parotitis particularly in children.
   - Progression of disease is more common in chronic debilitated patient (DM, chronic renal disease, alcoholics).

   Diagnosis
   - Considered in patient present with acute lower respiratory tract illness, parotitis, lymphadenitis or unusual skin or subcutaneous lesion or chest X-ray suggest TB (upper lobe infiltrate) in absence of tubercle bacilli in sputum.
   - Gram's stain of appropriate specimen will show small Gram-negative bacilli; **bipolar regularly staining** (safety pin appearance) is seen by Wright's stain or methylene blue stain.
   - **Positive culture is diagnostic.**
   - Positive serologic test is evidence of past infection.
   - X-ray - upper lobe infiltrate occasionally with thin walled cavities.

   Treatment:
   - Ceftazidime or carbepenems are DOC.

6. **Ans. (c) Pseudomonas** *Ref. Ananthanarayan 10/e, p 321*
   Pseudomonas
   Aerobic, nonsporing gram-negative, motile bacilli, forms many pigments:
   a. **Pyocyanin:** – Bluish green pigment, produced **only by** Ps. aeruginosa
   b. **Fluorescin (Pyoverdin):** – Greenish yellow pigment which oxidise in old culture to yellowish brown pigment
   c. **Pyrubin:** – Red
   d. **Pyomelanin:** – Brown

Other Pigment forming bacteria	
• S. aureus	– Golden yellow pigment
• B. melanogenicus	– Black pigment
• Rhodococcus	– Red pigment
• Nocardia	– Yellow to red pigment
• Peptostreptococcus	
• Photo and Scotochromogen	– Yellow orange pigment

7. **Ans. (a) *Yersenia pestis***   Ref. Ananthonarayan 10/e, p 327
   In India presently there are four foci of plague
   1. Near kolar in Tamil Nadu
   2. Beed Latur belt of Maharashtra
   3. Rhoru near Shimla in Himachal Pradesh
   4. Small pocket in Uttaranchal
   So, in a girl of Shimla with clinical features of plague and organism showing stalactite growth can be none other than Y. pestis.

8. **Ans. (b) *P. aeruginosa***   See below

Etiology of bacteremia associated with IV catheters	
• Staph. epidermidis	85%
• S. aureus	7%
• Candida albicans	3%
• Enterococcus	2%

• Others
  – E. coli
  – Klebsiella
  – P. aeruginosa
  – Viridans streptococci
	3%

9. **Ans. (b) Melioidosis**   Ref. Harrison 20/e, p 1172
   - Actinomycosis is ruled out as it is gram-positive bacilli.
   - Plague is ruled out as it is gram-negative nonmotile coccobacilli.
   - Bartonellosis is ruled out as it does not exhibits bipolar staining.
   - Bacteria showing bipolar staining = safety pin appearance are:
     - Calymmatobactcrium granulomatis   – Yersinia and Pasteurella   – H. ducreyi
     - V. parahemolyticus   – Ps. pseudomallei

10. **Ans. (b, d) and (e) Gram –ve, Non-motile; and It is coccobacilli**   Ref. Ananthanarayan 10/e, p 325
    Yersinia is gram –ve, nonmotile cocobacilli.

11. **Ans. (c) Wayson's**   Ref. Jawetz 27/e 276; Ananthanarayan 10/e 327, 329
    This is a case of bubonic plague
    Why?
    - The geographical Area - Himachal Pradesh which is one of the foci of plague in India
      Other are: • Kolar at the trijunction of AP, TN, Karnataka
                       • Beed - Latur belt in Maharashtra
                       • Small pocket in Uttaranchal

    Clinical Presentation of Patient
    - Enlarged tender inguinal lymphnodes is commonest manifestation of bubonic plague.
    - Multiple small ulcer, represent flea bites

    Now coming to question
    - Plague is caused by Yersina pestis a gram-negative short bacilli
    - In smear stained with Wayson, Giemsa or methylene blue, it shows bipolar staining (*safety pin appearance*) with the two ends densely stained and the central area clear.
    - The bacilli characteristically show pleomorphism which gets enhanced in media containing 3% NaCl. It is non- motile, non-sporing and non-acid fast.

12. **Ans. (c) Wayson's stains**   Ref. Ananthanarayan 10/e, p 329; Jawetz 27/e, p 276
    Aready explained

NEET Pattern Questions

1. Pseudomonas toxin acts by:
   a. ↑cAMP
   b. ↓cAMP
   c. ↓Protein synthesis
   d. ↓cGMP
   [Ref. Ananthanarayan, 10/e, p 372]

2. A diabetic person presents with multiple abscess in leg. Microscopic examination of pus shows gram (–)ve bacilli. On staining with methylene blue bacteria shows bipolar staining. The most likely causative agent is:
   a. B. pseudomallei
   b. Y. Pestis
   c. Pseudomonas mallei
   d. Botromycosis [Ref. Ananthanarayan, 10/e, p 323]

3. Pseudomonal infection, not cleaned by:
   a. Dettol
   b. Hypochloritic
   c. Chlorine
   d. Betadine [Ref. Ananthanarayan, 10/e, p 371]

> Pseudomonas is resistant to common antiseptics and disinfectants such as quaternary ammonium compounds, chloroxylenol and hexachlorophane. Indeed P. aeroginosa can grow in dettol or cetrimide selective medium.

4. Ecthyma gangrenosum is caused by:
   a. Pseudomonas
   b. Streptococcus
   c. Staphylcoccus
   d. H. influenza
   [Ref. Harrison, 20/e, p 1168]

> **Ecthyma gangrenosum**
> - Occurs exclusively in markedly neutropenic patient or AIDS patient.
> - The disease is characterized by small or large, painful, — maculopopular lesions, which are initially pink then darken to purple and finally to black.
> - These lesions are due to vascular invasion and are teeming with bacteria.

5. Selective media for Pseudomonas:
   a. EMJH medium
   b. PALCAM agar
   c. PLET medium
   d. Cetrimide agar [Ref. Ananthanarayan, 10/e, p 371]

> Cetrimide prevents the growth of alternate flora and also entrances the production of Pseudomonas pigments such as pyocyanin and fluorescein.

6. An organism grown on agar shows green coloured colonies, likely organism is:
   a. Staphylococcus
   b. Streptococcus
   c. Pseudomonas
   d. E. coli [Ref. Ananthanarayan, 10/e, p 370]

7. Pseudomonas exotoxin inhibits protein synthesisly by:
   a. RNA polymerase
   b. EF-2
   c. Transpeptidase
   d. Reverse transcriptase [Ref. Internet]

> Exotoxin A, the main virulence factor of betadomonas exerts its pathogenic effect by inhibition of protein synthesis via ADP-ribosylation and there by inactivation of elongation factor 2.

8. Bacteria that can grow even in the presence of antiseptic:
   a. Staphylococcus
   b. Streptococcus
   c. E. coli
   d. Pseudomonas [Ref. Ananthanarayan, 10/e; p 371]

9. Which of the following is non-motile:
   a. Pseudomonas aeruginosa
   b. Burkholderia mallei
   c. Burkholderia pseudomallei
   d. None of the above [Ref. Ananthanarayan, 10/e, p 323]

10. A patient in ICU and on ventilator develops cough with fever. The gram-staining on microscopy will show:
    a. Gram negative cocci
    b. Gram negative bacilli
    c. Gram positive bacilli
    d. Gram variable organism [Ref. Harrison, 20/e, p 1168]

11. Pyocyanin is formed by:
    a. *Yersinia*
    b. *Pseudomonas*
    c. *Burkholderia*
    d. *Pasteurella*
    [Ref. Ananthanarayan 10/e, 322]

12. Glanders is caused by:
    a. *Protozoa*
    b. *Virus*
    c. *Fungi*
    d. *Bacteria*
    [Ref. Greenwood 18/e, 303]

Ans.
1. c. ↓ Protein synthesis
2. a. B. pseudomallei
3. a. Dettol
4. a. Pseudomonas
5. d. Cetrimide agar
6. c. Pseudomonas
7. b. EF-2
8. d. Pseudomonas
9. b. Burkholderia mallei
10. b. Gram negative bacilli
11. b. *Pseudomonas*
12. d. *Bacteria*

13. In India last outbreak of plague occurred in which state:
    a. Gujarat
    b. Maharashtra
    c. Himachal Pradesh
    d. MP   [Ref. Ananthanarayan, 10/e, p 328]

    Last outbreak occurred in February 2002 near Shimla

14. What is not true about yersiniosis:
    a. Zoonosis
    b. Caused by Y. pestis
    c. By Yersinia enterocolitica
    d. By Yersinia pseudotuberculosis
    [Ref. Ananthanarayan, 10/e, p 330]

15. Pneumonic plague is spread by:
    a. Bite of infected flae
    b. Direct contact with infected tissue
    c. Ingestion of contaminated food
    d. Droplet infection   [Ref. Ananthanarayan, 10/e, p 328]

16. Izumi fever is caused by:
    a. Pseudomonas aeruginosa
    b. Burkholderia mallei
    c. Yersinia pseudotuberculosis
    d. Pasteurella multocida   [Ref. Harrison, 20/e, p 1207]

    Izumi fever (Japanese name) is characterized by abdominal pain and fever. Y. pseudotuberculosis mitogen (YPM) is implicated as causative factor

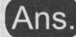
13. c. Himachal Pradesh   14. b. Caused by Y. pestis
15. d. Droplet infection   16. c. Yersinia pseudotuberculosis

Hemophilus, Bordetella and Brucella

CHAPTER 18

HEMOPHILUS

- Genus comprised of nonmotile, nonsporing, oxidase positive gram-negative bacilli, characterized by requirement of one or both of two accessory growth factors (X and V) in blood. These requirement are used to identify the bacteria.
- Important species are *H. influenza*, *H. aegypticus* and *H. ducreyi*.
- Both *H. influenzae* and *H. haemolyticus* have identical growth (factors X and V) requirement. So *H. hemolyticus* is distinguished from *H. influenzae* by hemolysis on horse blood agar.

Hemophilus:
- Non motile, Gram (–)ve bacilli
- *H. influenzae* and *H. hemolyticus* require factors X and V for growth
- Flides agar is best for isolation of *H. influenzae*
- *H. influenzae* shows satellitism cause meningitis, epiglottitis, cellulitis

H. INFLUENZAE = PFEIFFER'S BACILLUS

Morphology

- Capsulated Coccobacilli shows pleomorphism.
- Stained by **Loeffler's methylene blue** or Dilute carbol fuchsin.
- On the basis of indole production, urease and ornithine decarboxylase activity, it is divided into eight biotypes.

Culture

- *Flides agar* is *best for* primary isolation.
- On **Levinthal's medium** — capsulated strain shows distinctive iridescence.
- Require **both X factor** (heat stable hemin) and V factor (heat labile coenzyme present in RBC) so heated or boiled blood agar (Chocolate agar) is superior to plain agar. X factor is not required for anaerobic growth.
- Shows 'Satellitism' (dependence on V factor) when *S. aureus* is streaked across blood agar. Staphylococus on sheep blood agar cause the release of NAD which favours the growth of *H. influenzae*.

Antigenic Properties

- **There are three major surface antigen** - the capsular polysaccharide; the outer membrane protein (OMP) and Lipo-oligosaccharide.
- Major antigenic determinant is **capsular polysaccharide** based on which, it is typed into six capsular types **a to f** while noncapsulated strains are nontypable.
- Most isolates from **acute invasive** infections belong **to 'b'**.
- Type b capsule has unique structure containing pentose sugar (ribose and ribitol) in the form of Polyribosyl ribitol phosphate (PRP) instead of hexoses and hexosamines as in other 5 serotypes. The capsule of type b *H. influenzae* is the major virulence factor.
- Hib PRP is used in vaccine.
- *H. influenza* is first free living organism whose *complete genome is sequenced*.

Invasive disease is more common.

Feature	Type b Strains	Nontypable Strains
Capsule	Ribosyl-ribitol phosphate	Noncapsulated
Pathogenesis	Invasive infections due to hematogenous spread	Mucosal infections due to contiguous spread
Age	2 months–3 years	Adults
Clinical manifestations	Meningitis and invasive infections in incompletely immunized infants and children	Otitis media in infants and children; lower respiratory tract infections in adults with chronic bronchitis and pneumonia, puerperal sepsis
Vaccine	Highly effective conjugate vaccines	None available; under development

- **Serotyping of *H. influenzae*** is done by agglutination or quelling reaction

Many non-encapsulated H influenzae are the part of normal microbiota of the upper respiratory tract.

H. egyptius – Conjunctivitis
– Brazilian purpuric fever
H. ducreyi : Chancroid

Non typable H. influenzae is the most common bacterial cause of exacerbation of COPD.

Resistant to ampicillin d/t production of ß lactamase and altered penicillin binding protein

Clinical Features

Meningitis: **Most** frequently by **biotype - I** of type **b** strain
- Occur in children (<2 years of age) due to absence of PRP antibodies.
- **MC Complication** of its meningitis - *Subdural effusion*

Epiglottitis: – Particularly affects 2-7 years age group.
Cellulitis: – Seen in young children. The most common location is on the head or neck.
Pneumonia: – Particularly in infants.
– Hib is more likely to involve pleura   ...Harrison 20/e, 1130

Diagnosis:

Viability of H. influenzae declines with time particularly at 4°C. So they should be transported rapidly.
Meningitis: – CSF Gram's stain and culture on IsoVitale X-enriched chocolate agar
... Jawetz 27/e, 265
– If culture negative - **Detection of PRP**.
Respiratory tract infection: – Suggested by predominance of gram-negative coccobacilli among abundant polymorphonucelar leukocytes in sputum.
Treatment : *DOC* ceftriaxone or cefotaxime (also in other invasive infection).
Administration of glucocorticoids reduces neurologic sequelae
... Harrison 20/e, 1130
Vaccination : Hib conjugate vaccine: – 1st dose : 2 months
– Rest of primary series : 2-6 months
– Booster dose : 12-15 months.

Remember: No vaccine is available for nontypable *H. influenzae*.

HAEMOPHILUS DUCREYI

- Bipolar stained *(safety pin)* bacilli arranged in group or whorls or parallel chains (school of fish or rail-road track appearance).
- Causative agent of *Chancroid or soft sore*—STD characterized *by tender*, non-indurated irregular genital ulceration and inguinal adenitis, i.e painful penile ulcer with inguinal lymphadenopathy.
- Primary isolation is difficult. It can be grown on fresh clotted rabbit blood. Smears made after 24–48 hours of incubation show tangled chains of bacilli.
  Treatment: – Single oral dose of azithromycin.
  – Alternative ciprofloxacin or erythromycin.

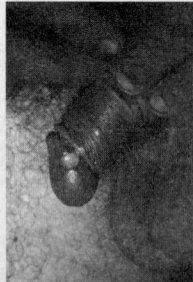 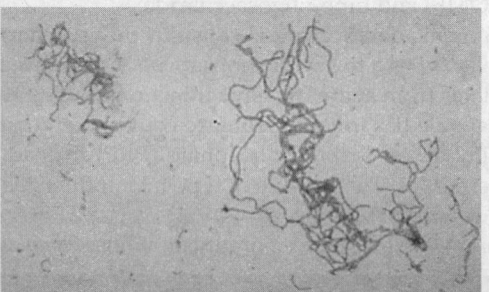

Note: An unrelated Gram negative rod calymmatobacterium Klebsiella granulomatis cause similar STD called as granuloma inguinale or donovanosis

HAEMOPHILUS AEGYPTIUS

Identical to non-capsulated *H. influenzae*, therefore now named as *H. influenzae* biotype aegypticus. Cause highly contagious form of conjunctivitis *(PINK EYE)* and Brazilian purpuric fever *(BPF)*.

BPF: Conjunctivitis proceed to fulminant septicemia in infants and children with high fatality.

Hemophilus, Bordetella and Brucella

Clinical Features of penile ulcer

Feature	Syphilis	Herpes	Chancroid	Lymphogranuloma venereum	Donovanosis
Incubation period	9–90 days	2–7 days	1–14 days	3 days–6 weeks	1–4 weeks (up to 6 months)
Early primary lesions	Papule	Vesicle	Pustule	Papule, pustule, or vesicle	Papule
No. of lesions	Usually one	Multiple	Usually multiple, may coalesce	Usually one; often not detected, despite lymphadenopathy	Variable
Diameter	5–15 mm	1–2 mm	Variable	2–10 mm	Variable
Edges	Sharply demarcated, elevated, round, or oval	Erythematous	Undermined, ragged, irregular	Elevated, round, or oval	Elevated, irregular
Depth	Superficial or deep	Superficial	Excavated	Superficial or deep	Elevated
Induration	Firm	None	Soft	Occasionally firm	Firm
Pain	Uncommon	Tender	Very tender	Variable	Uncommon
Lymphadenopathy	Firm, nontender, bilateral	Firm, tender, often bilateral	Tender, may suppurate, usually unilateral	Tender, may suppurate, loculated, usually unilateral	None; pseudobulboes

BORDETELLA

- Genus consist of gram-negative, strict aerobic coccobacilli which grows only on complex media.
- Its two important members:
  a. *B. pertussis* – Causative agent of pertussis (whooping cough = 100 day fever).
  b. *B. parapertussis* – Silent copy of pertussis toxin gene causing milder form of pertussis.

Morphology

- *B. Pertussis* is pleomorphic, nonmotile, nonsporing, *capsulated, fimbriated* coccobacilli, which show Bipolar metachromatic granules on staining with toluidine blue. Most fastidious of all bordetellae
- Obligate human parasite

Culture

- Grows on enriched media like *Regan Towe or Bordet-Gengou glycerine potato blood agar*, forming colonies with bisected pearls or Mercury drops or Aluminium paint appearance.
- Culture films has **Thumb print** appearance.
- Charcoal containing media (as for legionella) is preferred.
- Blood is required to neutralize the inhibitory materials formed during bacterial growth.

Virulent Factors

- **Pertussis toxin**
  - Most important virulence factor
  - *PT is a exotoxin* protein consist of B - (binding unit) and A (active unit) having ADP ribosylating activity of G protein *(like of cholera toxin)*
  - B parapertussis do not express the gene coding for pertussis toxin.
  - Pertusis toxin also serves as adhesin, lymphocytosis producting factor, histamine sensitizer and islet activating protein.
- *Filamentous hemagglutinin (FHA) secreted protein.*
  - Both PT and FHA hemagglutinin promotes secondary infection by coating *H. influenza* and pneumococci so that they bind. This is known as 'Piracy of Adhesins'.
- **Tracheal cytotoxin**
  - It is responsible for destruction of the ciliated respiratory epithelial cells. Tracheal cytotoxin inhibits DNA synthesis in ciliated cells
- Surface adhesins (pertactin, Fimbriae), Adenylate cyclase, hemolysin, heat labile toxin LPS endotoxin, pertactin agglutinogens are other virulence factor.
- Impairment of host defence by B pertussis is mediated by pertusis toxin and adenylate cyclase toxin.

... Harrison 20/e 1143

Bordetella
- Gr (–)ve, aerobic coccobacilli
- **Enriched media:**
  - Regan Towe
  - Bordet-Gengou glycerine potato
- B. pertussis is the most fastideus bordetella
- Pertussis toxin acts by activating G protein
- Acellular vaccine, containing PT and filamentous hemaglutinin is the preferred vaccine

Whooping cough is non-invasive infection of respiratory mucosa.

Purpose of antibiotic therapy is to eradicate the infecting bacteria from the nasopharynx. Therapy doesn't alter the clinical course unless given early in catarrhal phase.

Pathogenesis

- Infection is initiated by attachment of the organism to the ciliated epithelial cells of the nasopharynx, attachment is mediated by surface adhesions.
- Infection is limited to respiratory mucosa only, local cellular invasion with intracellular persistence (systemic dissemination not occurs). Systemic manifestation is due to toxin.
- Both cellular and humoral immunity are important.
- First defence is by antibody which prevents attachments of bacteria.
- Neurological manifestations are due to hypoxia.

Clinical Features

- *Incubation period:* 7–14 days.
- It has 3 stages:
  a. *Catarrhal stage:* Maximum infectivity
  b. *Paroxysmal stage:* – Post-tussive vomiting is frequent with mucus plug occassionally at end of episode.
     – Vomiting with cough is the best predictor of diagnosis of pertussis.
     – Episodes are often worsening at night and interfere with sleep.
     – Most complications occur during paroxysmal stage.
     – Paroxysm is precipitated by noise, eating and physical contact
  c. *Convalescent stage*

Complications

Subconjunctival hemorrhages, abdominal and inguinal hernia, pneumothorax, petechiae, weight loss, apnea, pneumonia, seizures, encephalopathy.

Diagnosis

i. *Best specimen* is obtained by **nasopharyngeal aspiration** ..... *Harrison 20/e, p 1144*
ii. Gold standard – Culture of nasopharyngeal secretion
iii. Absolute lymphocytosis without ↑ in ESR
iv. *Most sensitive is PCR*
v. Serology — If symptoms > 4 weeks.

Treatment

- *DOC* – Macrolide (Erythromycin, Clarithromycin, Azithromycin)
- Alternative – Cotrimoxazole
- β agonist, Glucocorticoids and cough suppressants are *not effective*.

Prevention

- *Chemoprophylaxis* – For household contact of cases.
  – Erythromycin is *DOC*.
- *Immunization — main stay* of preventions is active immunization.
  Two types of vaccine are available:
  a. *Whole cell vaccine:*
     - Associated with many adverse effects and may also cause — encephalopathy, sudden infant death syndrome, and autism.
     - It is contraindicated in individual ≥ 7 year age.
  b. *Acellular vaccine:*
     - Less reactogenic and is recommended for routine immunization.
     - All variety of acellular vaccine contain pertussis toxoid and filamentous hemagglutinin.
     - It contains pertussis toxoid.
     - Two component vaccine are more effective than monocomponent, since addition of pertactin increase efficacy.
     - Protection against pertussis by vaccine correlated best with the production of antibody to pertactin, fimbriae, and pertussis toxin.

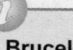

Brucella
- Gr (–)ve, intracellular coccobacilli that grows on strict aerobic condition
- B. abortis requires 5-10% CO_2
- B. melitensis is the most common and most virulent cause of brucellosis
- Diagnosis requires castaneda method of blood culture.

BRUCELLA

- Gram-negative, nonmotile, noncapsulated, non-sporing, strict aerobic, intracellular coccobacilli.
- Major virulence factor: LPS which possess endotoxin activity.
- Brucella is agent of biological warfare.
- Form both caseating and non-caseating granuloma.
- Resist intracellular killing by suppression of myeloperoxidase—hydrogen peroxide-halide system and production of superoxide dismutase.
- Organism are sensitive to sunlight, heat, ionizing radiation but are resistant to freezing and drying.

> **Source of infection:** Sheep, goats, camel
> **Mode of infection:** Usually occupational.
> **Most serious manifestation:** Pancarditis.

Culture

- B. abortus require 5-10% CO_2 for growth, where as other three species can grow in air.
- Fresh specimens from animal or human source are usually inoculated on trypticase soy agar or blood culture media: Optimum temperature is 37°C. Erythritol has a stimulating effect on the growth of brucellae.
- In vivo brucellae behave as facultative intracellular parasite. ... *Harrison 18/e, p 1296*

Classification

- On the basis of CO_2 requirements, H_2S production, sensitivity to dyes, phage lysis, oxidative metabolic tests four species are identified–B. melitensis, B. abortus are major species.

> MC and most virulent cause of Brucellosis: B. melitensis

Clinical Features

- It cause Brucellosis, a zoonotic diseases, also known as mediterranean fever or Malta or undulant fever.
- *Source:* Sheep, goats, camels.
- *Route of transmission:* Occupational exposure, ingestion of untreated milk or milk products, raw meat (blood); inhalation; transplacental; during breastfeeding and during sexual activity.
- MC and *most virulent* cause of brucellosis: B. melitensis.
- MC symptoms are fever, chills, diaphoresis, headaches.
- Pancarditis, Sleep disturbances, lymphadenopathy, Hepatosplenomegaly, GBS syndrome, abortion or IUD during pregnancy are other important findings.
- MC focal feature is musculoskeletal pain.
- **Death is** usually a consequence of *cardiac involvement*.
- Immunity is mainly cell-mediated.

Diagnosis

1. Most definitive method—Blood culture
   - **Castaneda** method of blood culture is employed.
   - Preferred media are serum dextrose agar; trypticase soy agar.
2. *PCR: More sensitive* and more quicker than blood culture.
3. *Serological test:*
   a. Acute infection — Standard agglutination (SAT) test done
      - Shows prozone phenomenon
      - SAT also +ve in cholera, tularemia, yersinia, and immunization.
   b. Chronic infection — Complement fixation test.
   c. For diagnosing animal infection – Rapid *plate agglutination, rose Bengal card* and *milk ring test done.*

Treatment

- TB must always be excluded.
- *Gold standard* treatment in adults: **IM Streptomycin + doxycycline.**

   ... *Harrison 20/e, p 1195*

- Alternative rifampin + doxycycline.
- In children, pregnant women or who cannot tolerate tetracycline—Cotrimoxazole given.

Multiple Choice Questions

Hemophilus

1. In a child admitted with H. Influenza meningitis, Cefotaxime was started instead of ampicillin. Which of these is the likely reason for this? **[AIIMS 15]**
   a. H. influenzae stains known to produce Beta lactamase
   b. H. influenzae stains known to have altered penicillin binding protein
   c. More easier to give
   d. It is cheap

2. A 2-year-old child is brought to the emergency with history of fever and vomiting. On examination he has neck rigidity. CSF examination shows polymorphs more than 200/mL; protein 100 mg/dL and glucose 10 mg/dL. the Gram's stain shows the presence of Gram-negative coccobacilli. The culture shows of bacteria only on chocolate. Agar and not on blood agar. The causative agent is:
   a. *Neisseria meningitidis* **[AIIMS 02]**
   b. *Haemophilus influenzae*
   c. *Branhamella catarrhalis*
   d. *Legionella pneumophila*

3. Disease caused by *Hemophilus* species: **[PGI June 09]**
   a. Chancroid   b. Influenza
   c. Acute epiglottitis   d. Brain abscess
   e. Brazilian purpuric fever

4. False about H. influenzae: **[AIIMS Nov 10]**
   a. It needs X and V factor for growth
   b. Protein capsule plays an important role in pathogenecity
   c. It is a rare cause of meningitis in the first 2 months of life
   d. Most common invasive manifestation is meningitis

5. Non-typable H. influenzae can cause all *except*: **[NEET Pattern 2018]**
   a. Meningitis   b. Otitis media
   c. Puerperal infection   d. Pneumonia

Bordetella

6. The usual incubation period of pertussis is: **[AIIMS 05]**
   a. 7-14 days   b. 3-5 days
   c. 21-25 days   d. Less than 3 days

7. True regarding pertussis vaccine is: **[AIIMS 10]**
   a. 95% of vaccinated are protected
   b. Erythromycin should be given to contacts
   c. Neuroparalytic complication is seen in 1 in 15000
   d. Leukocytosis is diagnostic

8. Mechanism of action of pertussis toxin is all *except*:
   a. Act by ADP ribosylation of GI subunit **[AIIMS 08]**
   b. Increase in calcium
   c. Act by decreasing GTP

9. In which of the following organism does the capsule does not act as a virulence factor? **[AI 2011]**
   a. H. influenzae   b. Strep pneumoniae
   c. N. meningitidis   d. Bordetella pertusis

10. A 7-month-old, partially immunized child presented with cough ending in characteristic whoop. Which of the following is considered the best type of specimen to isolate the organism and confirm the diagnosis?
    a. Nasopharyngeal swab **[AI 11, AIIMS May 11]**
    b. Cough plate culture
    c. Tracheal-aspirates
    d. Sputum

11. Acellular pertussis vaccine contains: **[AIIMS 2011]**
    a. Pertactin, flagillary hemagglutinin, cytotoxin, endotoxin
    b. Pertactin, flagillary hemagglutinin, fimbriae, endotoxin
    c. Pertactin cytotoxin, fimbriae
    d. Flagillary hemagglutinin, pertussis toxin, pertactin

12. All are true statement regarding pertussis, *except*:
    a. Secondary attack rate averages 90% in unimmunized contacts **[PGI 2012]**
    b. Incubation period is around 14 days
    c. Erythromycin is the drug of choice
    d. Can affect people of any age
    e. Main source of infection is chronic carriers

Brucella

13. A veterinary doctor had pyrexia of unknown origin. His blood culture in special laboratory media was positive for gram-negative short bacilli which was oxidase positive. Which one of the following is the likely organism grown in culture? **[AI 06]**
    a. *Pasturella spp.*   b. *Francisella spp.*
    c. *Bartonella spp.*   d. *Brucella spp.*

14. A farmer presenting with fever off and on for the past 4 years was diagnosed to be suffering from chronic Brucellosis. All of the following serological tests would be helpful in the diagnosis at this state *except*: **[AI 04]**
    a. Standard agglutination test
    b. 2-mercapto-ethanol test
    c. Complement fixation test
    d. Coomb's test

15. Malta fever is caused by: **[AIIMS 08]**
    a. *Legionella*   b. *Borrelia burgdorferi*
    c. *Brucella melitensis*   d. *Pseudomonas*

16. Brucellosis can be transmitted by all of the following modes, *except*: **[AIIMS 07, 06]**
    a. Contact with infected placenta
    b. Ingestion of raw vegetables from infected farms
    c. Person to person transmission
    d. Inhalation of infected dust or aerosol

Hemophilus, Bordetella and Brucella

17. All are true about brucella *except*: [AIIMS May 11]
    a. B. abortus is capnophilic
    b. Transmitted by aerosol can occur occasionally
    c. Paesturisation destroys it
    d. 2 ME is used to detect IgA

18. Brucella melitensis is commonly found in (animal): [PGI 2011]
    a. Pig
    b. Camel
    c. Sheep
    d. Goat
    e. Reindeer

Explanations and References with Illustrative Answers

1. **Ans. (a) H. influenzae stains known to produce Beta lactamase** Ref. Harrison 20/e, p 1131
   Approximately 20-35% of nontypable strains of hemophilus produce β-lactamase. In addition to β-lactamase alteration of penicillin binding proteins is a second mechanism of ampicillin resistance has been detected in isolates of H. influenzae.
   ..... Harrison
   Treatment of H. influenzae infection:
   - Invasive infections: Antibiotics e.g. third-generation cephalosporin (ceftriaxone) should be started as soon as appropriate specimens have been collected for culture.
   - Sinusitis, otitis media, and other upper RTI: Trimethoprim–Sulfamethoxazole or amoxicillin clavulanate combination.

2. **Ans. (b) H. influenzae** Ref. Ananthanarayan 10/e, p 333
   See the morphology of asked bacteria, you will know the answer.

H. influenzae	– Gram-negative coccobacilli
N. meningitidis	– Gram-negative cocci
Legionella	– Gram-negative coccobacilli
B. catarrhalis	– Gram-negative cocci

3. **Ans. (a), (c) and (e) Chancroid, Acute epiglottitis, Brazilian purpuric fever** Ref. Harrison 20/e, p 1130

Disease Caused by *Haemophilus*	
Species	**Disease**
H. influenzae	– Meningites – Epiglottitis – Pneumonia – Bronchitis, arthritis, pericarditis, – Endocarditis
H. aegypticus	– Brazilian purpuric fever – Conjuctivitis
H. ducreyi	– Chancroid or soft sore

   Note: Influenza is a viral disease.

4. **Ans. (b) Protein capsule plays an important....** Ref. Ananthanarayan 10/e, p 334
   Capsule is made up of polysaccharide (not protein)

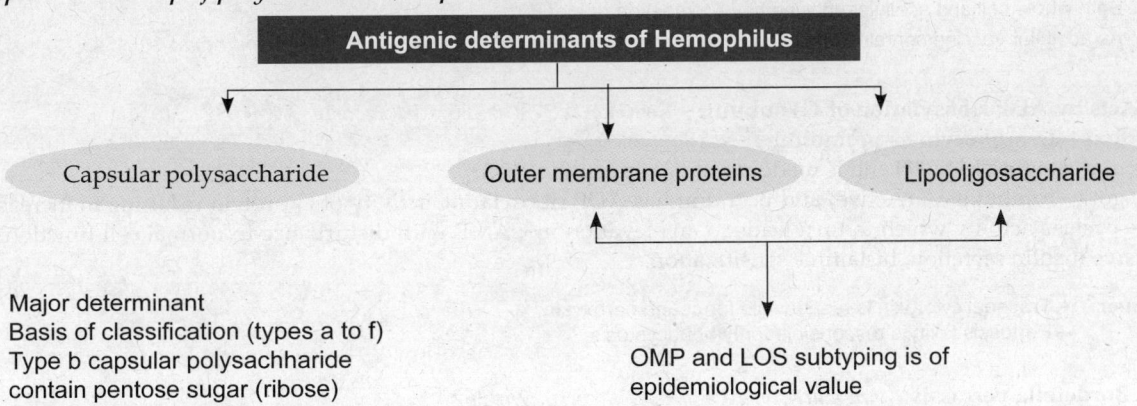

- Major determinant
- Basis of classification (types a to f)
- Type b capsular polysachharide contain pentose sugar (ribose) other types have hexose sugar

OMP and LOS subtyping is of epidemiological value

5. **Ans. (a) Meningitis**   *Ref. Harrison 20/e, p 1130*
   Strains of Hemophilus which lacks polysaccharide capsule are referred as Non-typable Strains
   - Non-typable H. influenza is the commonest bacterial cause of exacerbations of COPD.
   - They also cause community acquired pneumonia, otitis media (3rd most common cause after pneumococci, and Moraxella catarrhalis), puerperal sepsis, neonatal bacteraemia, sinusitis.

   | \multicolumn{3}{c}{Characteristics of Type b and Nontypable Strains of Haemophilus influenzae} |||
Feature	Type b Strains	Nontypable strains
Capsule	Ribosyl-ribitol phosphate	Unencapsulated
Pathogenesis	Invasive infections due to haematogenous spread	Mucosal infections due to contiguous spread
Clinical manifestations	Meningitis and invasive infections in incompletely immunized infants and children	Otitis media in infants and children; lower respiratory tract infections in adults with chronic bronchitis
Evolutionary history	Basically clonal	Genetically diverse
Vaccine	High effective conjugate vaccines	Under development

6. **Ans. (a) 7-14 days**   *Ref. Park 22/e, p 154*
   Incubation period of pertussis is usually 7 to 14 days, but never exceed 3 weeks.
   Important points about pertussis:
   - Caused by *Pertussis*
   - Source of infection is case, there is no evidence of subclinical infection
   - Pertussis is most infectious in catarrhal stage
   - Infective period extends from a week after exposure to about 3 weeks after the onset of paroxysmal stage
   - Secondary attack rate is about 90% in unimmunized contacts.

7. **Ans. (b) Erythromycin should be given to contacts**   *Ref. Harrison 20/e, p 1145*
   Those known to have in contact with whooping cough should be given prophylactic erythromycin or ampicillin for 10 days.
   Pertussis vaccine
   1. **Killed whole cell vaccine:**
      - Given in the form of DPT
      - Protection 70-90%

      Adverse reaction:
      - Neurologic complication 1:170000
      - Convulsions
      - Prolonged screaming
      - Hyporesponsible state.

      Contraindication: — Epilepsy, convulsion or other CNS disorder.
   2. **Acellular vaccine:**
      - Contain pertussis toxoid and filamentous hemagglutinin.
      - Same efficacy but less reactogenic
      - Two component (which contain pertactin and pertussis toxoid. are more effective than monocomponent acellular vaccine. The further addition of fimbriae appears to enhance protective efficacy.   ..... *Harrison 20/e, p 1146*

   > **Note:** In pertussis lymphocytosis (not leukocytosis) is diagnostic. Whole cell and acellular vaccine have protection rate of 90%
   > - Both whole cell and acellular vaccine have protection rate of 80%
   > - As acellular vaccine contains toxid, they only prevent infection not disease.   *Ref. Ananthanarayan 10/e 343*

8. **Ans (a) Acts by ADP ribosylation of GI subunit**   *Ref. Jawetz 27/e, p 266; Chakraborty 2/e, p 387*
   Pertusis toxin (Lymphocytosis promoting factor)
   - Molecular weight of 117000 and is made-up of 6 polypeptide chain
   - It has got two subunits A (Active) and B. A unit has ADP ribosylating activity of G protein resulting in increased adenylate cyclase activity which in turn leads to an elevation in CAMP with disturbance to normal cell function such as excessive insulin secretion, histamine sensitization.

   > **Remember:** — Tracheal cytotoxin is responsible for cough paroxysm.
   > — Pertussis toxin is responsible for lymphocystosis

9. **Ans. (d) Bordetella pertussis**   *Ref. Harrison 20/e, p 1142; Jawetz 27/e, 267*

Antigenic constituents and Virulence factor of Bordetella
- Pertussis toxin (most important)
- Dermonecrotic toxin
- Adenylate cyclase toxin (impair host defence)
- Filamentous hemagglutinin (a component of cell wall)
- Tracheal cytotoxin
- Lipo oligosoccharide
- Fimbriae
- Pertactin (an outer membrane protein)

Note: All virulance factors of Bordetella are regulated by a single locus on chromosome. This locus has two Bordetella virulence genes bvg A and bvg S. 'bvg' S responds to environmental signal whereas bvg A is a transcriptional activator of virulence gene.

10. **Ans. (a) Nasopharyngeal swab** *Ref. Harrison 20/e, p 1144*

    Culture of nasopharyngeal secretion is the gold standard for diagnosis. The best specimen is collected by nasopharyngeal aspirations. An alternative to the aspirate is a dacron or rayon nasopharyngeal swab.

    Note: PCR, due to its quick result, is replacing culture in many laboratories.

11. **Ans. (d) Flagillary ...** *Ref. Harrison 20/e 1146*
    All acellular pertussis vaccines contain pertussis toxoid and filamentous hemagglutinin. One acellular vaccine also contain pertactin and another contains pertactin plus two types of fimbriae.
    Phase III studies suggest that addition of pertactin and fimbriae increase the efficacy of vaccine.

12. **Ans. (e) Main source of infection.....** *Ref. Ananthanarayan 10/e 341*
    "Source of pertussis infection is always a case, a chronic carrier state does not exists and there is no evidence that infection is ever subclinical."
    For full details see previous answers.

13. **Ans. (d) Brucella spp.** *Ref. Ananthanarayan 10/e, p 345*
    Oxidase positive gram-negative organism producing pyrexia of unknown origin in veterinary doctor is pointing towards Brucella (coccobacilli or short rods).
    - **Brucella is the causative agent of Brucellosis** (*Malta fever, undulant fever*).
    - Other options:
      Pasturella spp. (P. multocida)
      – It is also short bacilli and oxidase positive, but it can grow over normal media and does not present with pyrexia of unknown origin. It is nonmotile and produces indole.
      – Manifestation of pasturella: Local suppuration, Meningitis, Respiratory tract infection.
      Francisella (Casuative agent of Tularemia):
      – It is also short bacilli with fastidious growth requirement. But it is oxidase negative.

    Remember:
    – Brucella is oxidase and catalase positive except *B. neotomae* and *B. ovis*.
    – **Risk factors for Brucellosis** (Zoonotic disease).
        - *Occupational*—Farmers, shepherds, Veterinarians, Goats herds, Slaughter-house workers.
        - *Domestic*—family members of individual in animal husbandry.
        - *Laboratory workers*—involved in handing cultures.
        - Travellers and Urban dwellers.
    – Brucella can grow over normal media but growth is improved by addition of serum or liver extract.

14. **Ans. (a) Standard agglutination test** *Ref. Ananthanarayan 10/e, p348; Harrison 17/e p 972, 18/e, p1299; Jawetz 27/e, p270*
    Diagnosis of Brucellosis
    1. Culture:
       - Blood culture is the most definitive method.
       - *Castaneda method* of blood culture is recommended.
    2. Serology
        a. *Standard agglutination (tube agglutination) test (SAT)* is performed most often. It identifies mainly the IgM antibody.
        – *Titre tends to decline after acute phase of the illness* so not helpful in chronic brucellosis.
        – Positive agglutination test may be produced by cholera, Tularemia or Yersinia infection or immunization.
        – Cholera induced agglutinins may be differentiated by agglutination absorption test and also as they are removed by treatment with 2-mercapto ethanol.

b. ***Blocking or nonagglutinating antibodies***—Most reliable method for obviating the blocking effect and detecting the incomplete antibodies is antiglobulin (Coomb's) test.
c. ***Complement fixation test***—Detects both IgG and IgM so it is more useful in chronic cases.
d. ***ELISA***—Sesitive, specific and can detect IgM and IgG antibody separately so useful for differentiating acute and chronic infections.
e. ***PCR***—To detect bacteremia, to predict relapse and to exclude chronic brucellosis. More sensitive and quicker than blood culture.
f. ***Brucellacapt***: Rapid immunocapture agglutination method based on the combs test that detects non agglutinating IgG and IgA antibodies. It has a high sensitivity and specificity.
3. **Hypersensitivity test** – **Not useful** in diagnosing acute infections.

15. Ans. (c) *Brucella melitensis*   *Ref. Ananthanarayana 10/e, p 347*

Clinical features of Brucellosis
- Fever with profuse sweats, especially at night. If untreated fever follows undulating pattern, i.e. fever → afebrile period → fever. (Malta Fever)
- Fever is associated with musculoskeletal symptoms, i.e. pain.
- Osteomyelitis commonly in lumbar and low thoracic vertebrae.
- Septic arthritis *(MC knee)*
- Neurologic involvement with depression and lethargy
- Endocarditis *(MC in aortic valve)*

16. Ans. (c) Person to person transmission   *Ref. Park 22/e, p 265*

Brucellosis is transmitted from infected animal to man and ***there is no evidence of transmission from man to man.***

Mode of Transmission of Brucella		
Contact infection (MC)	**Food-borne infection**	**Airborne infection**
– Direct contact with infected tissue, blood, urine, etc.	– Ingestion of raw milk or dairy products	– From aerosols in cowshed and slaughter house
– Mostly occupational	– Water contaminated with excreta of infected animal	

17. Ans. (d) 2 ME is used to detect IgA   *Ref. Ananthanarayan 10/e, p 349*

2ME (2-Mercaptoethonol test) detect IgM and IgG

Serological tests for Brucellosis
- Standard Agglutination test
- Rose Bengal test
- Enzyme Immune Assay (detects IgM, IgG, IgA)

Culture Characteristics of Brucella
- Strict aerobs, B. abortus is capnophillic
- Optimum temperature 37°C
- Can grow on normal media, growth is improved by the addition of serum or liver extract. Erythritol has a specific stimulating effect on the growth of brucellae.

Resistance
- They survive in soil and manure for several weeks; remain viable for 10 days in refrigerated milk, 1 month in ice cream and for > 4 months in butter
- They are sensitive to 1%, destroyed by heat at 60°C in 10 minutes. They are killed by pasteurisation. They are sensitive to sunlight and acid.

18. Ans. (b, c and d) i.e. Camel, Sheep, Goat   *Ref. Park 22/e, p 265*

- Animals that commonly acts as source of human brucellosis are: Goats, sheep, cattle, buffaloes, and swine
- In some part of world infection may also come from dogs, reindeer caribou, camels and yalks
- Most important vehicle of infection is raw milk. Milk products, meat from infected animal and raw vegetables or water supply contaminated by feces or urine of infected animal may also be responsible.

NEET Pattern Questions

1. **True about H. influenza:**
   a. Grown on sheep blood agar and CO_2
   b. It is not capsulated
   c. Invasive strain is most common
   d. Gram positive
   [Ref. Harrison, 20/e, p 1129; Ananthanarayan, 10/e p 334]

   > Hib strains cause systemic disease by invasion and hematogenous spread from the respiratory tract to distant site such as meninges, bones and joints. The type b polysaccharide capsule is an important virulence factor and imparts bacterium the ability to avoid opsonisation and cause systemic disease.
   > Type b and non typable strains are most common.
   > Grows on blood agar if source of Vth factor is also provided.

2. **Chancroid is caused by:**
   a. H. ducreyi   b. T. pallidum
   c. Gonococcus   d. HSV
   [Ref. Ananthanarayan, 10/e p 337]

3. **Agar media used for Haemophilus influenza:**
   a. Blood agar   b. Chocolate agar
   c. Tryptose agar   d. BYCE agar
   [Ref. Ananthanarayan, 10/e p 336]

4. **Satellitism is seen in cultures of:**
   a. Hemophilus   b. Streptococcus
   c. Klebsiella   d. Proteus
   [Ref. Ananthanarayan, 10/e p 334]

5. **Causative organism of which STD has safety pin appearance:**
   a. LGV   b. Chancroid
   c. Syphilis   d. Herpes genitalis
   [Ref. Ananthanarayan, 10/e p 337]

6. **School of fish appearance is characteristic of:**
   a. Bordetella pertussis   b. Yersinia enterocolitica
   c. Haemophillus ducreyi   d. Legionella
   [Ref. Ananthanarayan, 10/e p 337]

   > H. ducreyi is a short Gr(-)ne ovoid bacillus with a tendency to occur in end to end pairs or short-chain. Bacilli often shows bipolar staining. The bacilli may be arranged in small group on whorls or in parallel chain, giving a school of fish or rail road track appearance.

7. **Brazilian purpuric fever is caused by:**
   a. Bordetella pertussis   b. Haemophilus aegypticus
   c. Haemophilus duceryi
   d. Haemophilus parinfluenzae
   [Ref. Ananthanarayan, 10/e p 336]

> Brazilian purpuric fever: Conjunctivitis proceeding to fulminant septicemia in infants and children with high fatality.

8. **Painful vaginal ulcer with inguinal lymphadenopathy and school of fish appearance of microorganism or microscopy are characteristic of:**
   a. Syphilis   b. LGV
   c. Granuloma inguinale   d. Chancroid
   [Ref. Ananthanarayan, 10/e p 336]

9. **Hemophilus influenzae requires:**
   a. Factor V   b. Factor X
   c. Factor V & X   d. Factor VII
   [Ref. Greenwood, 18/e p 325]

10. **Penile ulcer is painful in:**
    a. Syphilis
    b. LGV
    c. Donovanosis
    d. Chancroid
    [Ref. AA, 10/e p 337]

11. **Safety pin appearance is seen in:**
    a. Vibrio vululfieus
    b. Vibrio cholera
    c. Pseudomonas aeuroginosa
    d. H. ducreyi

    > **Safety pin Appearance**
    > • Yersinia pestis.
    > • Vibrio parahemolyticus
    > • Burkholderia mallei
    > • Klebsiella granulomatis
    > • Haemophilus ducreyi

12. **Whooping cough is caused by:**
    a. B. pertussis
    b. H. influenzae
    c. Pneumococcus
    d. Meningococcus   [Ref. Ananthanarayan, 10/e, p 341]

13. **All are true statement regarding pertussis except:**
    a. Secondary attack rate averages 90% in unimmunized contacts
    b. Incubation period is around 14 days
    c. Can affect people of any age
    d. Main source of infection is chronic carriers
    [Ref. Ananthanarayan 10/e p 341]

Ans.
1. c. Invasive strain...   2. a. H. ducreyi   3. b. Chocolate agar   4. a. Hemophilus
5. b. Chancroid   6. c. Haemophillus ducreyi   7. b. Haemophilus...
8. d. Chancroid   9. c. Factor V & X   10. d. Chancroid
11. d. H. ducreyi   12. a. B. pertussis   13. d. Main source of infection...

14. All of the following are virulence factors of pertussis, *except*:
    a. Tracheal cytotoxin
    b. Pertussis toxin
    c. Capsule
    d. Pertactin
    [Ref. Harrison 20/e, p 1142]

15. Which does not has a known animal reservoir?
    a. Brucella melitensis
    b. Bordettela pertussis
    c. Pasturella multocida
    d. Francisella tularensis
    [Ref. Ananthanarayan, 10/e p 341]

> Bordetella pertussis infect only human. A related species B. bronchiseplica had been isolated from dogs with bronchopneumonia.

16. Milk ring test is for: [MP 2009]
    a. Brucellosis
    b. Bacteroides
    c. Tuberculosis
    d. Salmonellosis
    [Ref. Ananthanarayan 10/e, p 349]

> Milk ring test is used to detect brucella infection in cattle. In this test a sample of whole milk is mixed with a drop of stained brucella antigen and incubated in water bath at 70°C for 40-50 min. If antibodies are present, bacilli are agglutinated and form a blue ring at the top; leaving the milk unstained.

Other tests are:
- Rapid plate agglutination test
- Rose Bengal card test

Ans. 14. c. Capsule   15. b. Bordettela pertussis   16. a. Brucellosis

Campylobacter and Helicobacter

CHAPTER 19

CAMPYLOBACTER

- Motile, curved rods; non-sporing (comma shaped on S shaped) shows *darting motility*. with single polar flagellum.
- Important pathogenic organisms are C. jejuni and C. fetus.

CAMPYLOBACTER JEJUNI

Comma's or gull-wing shaped bacteria motile with single polar flagellum at one or both ends
...*Greenwood 18/e 305*

- Very common cause of diarrhea, especially in west.
- Readily take surrounding naked DNA and gets incorporated into genome making them genetically diverse.

Culture

- Growth occurs under microaerophilic condition 5% O_2 optimal with added CO2 [10%]. Although *C. jejuni* grows well at 36-37° C, but incubation at 42°C prevents most of other fecal bacteria thus helps in selective growth.
- *Selective media* – Skirrow's medium; Butzler's media; Campy BAP (*selective media*)

Pathogenesis and Clinical Feature

- Infection is acquired by oral route. *Source of infection is raw or under cooked food products from poultry, cattle sheep, swine.* **Most common being raw milk.** Though organism is susceptible to gastric acid as few as **500–800** organism can produce infection when ingested with bolus of food, which protects them from acid.
...*Greenwood 18/e 306*
- Organism multiply in small intestine, invade the epithelium and cause inflammation.
- Usually present: within 2-4 days.
- *Clinically* present as acute onset of crampy abdominal pain, profuse bloody diarrhoea.

Diagnosis

- Faeces show polymorphonuclear leucocytes.
- Gram stained smear may show **typical 'S' shaped** bacteria.
- Dark field or phase contrast microscopy may show *darting motility*.
- Culture on selective media at 42°C is **definitive diagnostic test.**
- In cases of delay, specimen should be transported in Carry Blair transport media
- In patient with campylobacter enteritis peripheral leucocyte count reflects severety.

Treatment

- *Erythromycin is DOC.*

CAMPYLOBACTER FETUS

- Oppurtunistic pathogen that cause systemic infection in immunocompromised.
- Cause diarrhoeal illness in normal host.
- Cause abortion in cattle

Campylobacter:
- Gr (–)ve, non-sporing bacilli that are motile with a single flagellum
- Show darting motility
- Grows best at 37–42°C under microaerophilic condition
- Infective dose of *C. jejuni*: 500-800 viable bacilli

Helicobacter pylori:
- Gram (–)ve, rod that is motile with lopotrichous flagella.
- Vacuolating cytotoxin is the major virulence factor.
- Associated with 80% of duodenal ulcer and 60% of gastric ulcer.

Helicobacter cinaedi and H. fennelliae are intestinal rather than gastric organism.

HELICOBACTER PYLORI

- Discovered by Warren & Marshall in 1982 for which they were awarded with Noble prize in 2005.
- Spiral shaped gram (–)ve microaerophilic rod associated with gastritis and peptic ulcer.
- Motile with *lopotrichous flagella*. (3-7 sheathed flagella at one end)
- The sole source is human gastric mucosa.

  Culture:
  - Grows well when incubated at 37°C in microaerophilic condition.
  - Media used include skirrow's medium, chocolate medium.

  Biochemical reaction: Catalase (+)ve, Oxidase +ve, Urease +ve

Pathogenesis

- Grows optimally at pH 6.0-7.0 and are likely to be killed at gastric pH.
- But it survives as it is found deep in mucus layer near epithelial surface, without invading mucosa where physiologic pH is present. Produces potent urease which provides ammonia to buffer acid.
- Major disease associated *H.pylori virulence factor* are vacuolating cytotoxin *(Vac A)* and group of genes termed CagPaI.
  - *H pylori* colonization decrease somatostatin producing cells → ↑ Gastrin → ↑ Acid → Gastric metaplasia in duodenum → Inflammation → Ulceration.
  - *Best characterized host determinant* of disease is enhanced *H. pylori* stimulated secretion of IL - 1 β in some people due to genetic polymorphism are at risk for gestric adenocarcinoma. ..... *Harrison 20/e, p 1163*
- Colonization induce chronic superficial gastritis which includes both mononuclear and polymorphonuclear cell infiltration. **Gastric antrum is MC site of** colonization.

> **Note:** H. pylori appears to be associated with idiopathic thrombocytopenic purpura, ischemic heart disease, cerebrovascular disease.   ..... *Harrison 19/e, p 1040*

Clinical Manifestation

- *H. pylori* colonizes the stomach in 50% of world population ..... *Harrison 20/e, p 1162*
- Though all patients have histologic gastritis only 10 to 15% of patient develop clinical illness.
- *80% of duodenal* ulcer and *60% of gastric* ulcer are related to *H. pylori.*
- *Increase risk of gastric adenocarcinoma, Gastric MALT lymphoma, autoimmune gastritis*
- Extragastrointestinal pathologies that are linked include ischemic heart disease and cerebrovascular disease, but association is not confirmed.

Diagnosis

Invasive test	Non-invasive tests
Requires upper GI endoscopic biopsy	Most consistently accurate test is urea breath test
Most convenient biopsy based test is biopsy urease test or rapid urease test	Stool antigen test is less expensive and more conveniente
Microbiologic culture is **most specific** but insensitive	Simplest tests are serologic assays measuring IgG levels in serum by ELISA or immunoblot

Urea breath test, the stool antigen test, and biopsy based tests can all be used to assess the success of treatment. However for accurate results these test should be performed only after 4 weeks of uninterrupted treatment.

> **Note:** With improvement in immunochromatography, currently stool antigen test is the most sensitive (94%) and specific (98%) test for detection of H. pylori.

Treatment

Symptomatic cases		
First line:		
Regimen 1 -	14 days	PPI BD, Clarithromycin 500 mg BD, Amoxicillin 1g BD (or Metronidazole 500 mg BD in penicillin allergic)
Regimen 2 -	10 days	PPI BD, Amoxicillin 1g BD (days 1-5), days 6-10 Clarithromycin 500 mg + Metronidazole 500 mg both BD
Second line:	14 days	**O**meprazole, **B**ismuth, **T**etracycline, **M**etronidazole (OBTM)

*PPI - Proton pump inhibitor
No treatment is given **for asymptomatic cases**.

Remember: *H. pylori* and *H. influenzae* are bacteria whose complete genome has been mapped.

Multiple Choice Questions

Campylobacter

1. A child was diagnosed to be suffering from diarrhea due to *Campylobacter jejuni*. Which of the following will be the correct environmental conditions of incubation of culture plates of the stool sample: [AI 05]
   a. Temperature of 42°C and microaerophilic
   b. Temperature of 42°C and 10% CO_2
   c. Temperature of 37°C and microaerophilic
   d. Temperature of 37°C and 10% CO_2

2. Darting motility occur in *V. cholerae*, also found in: [PGI Dec 2008]
   a. Shigella
   b. Campylobacter jejuni
   c. Pneumococcus
   d. Bacillus anthrax
   e. Aeronomas

3. *Campylobacter* culture media are: [PGI Dec 2008]
   a. Schaedler's agar
   b. CVA medium
   c. Regan-Lowe medium
   d. Skirrow medium
   e. Compylobacter blood agar

4. All are true statement about *Campylobacter jejuni*, except: [AIIMS Nov 09, May 11]
   a. Human is the only reservoir
   b. Can cause GB syndrome
   c. Poultry is the source of infection
   d. Common cause of campylobacteriosis

5(a). A 35-year-old patient complaints of abdominal cramps along with profuse diarrhea. Treating physician wants to process the stool specimen for isolation of *Campylobacter jejuni*. Which of the following is method of choice for culture of stool: [AIIMS 04]
   a. Culture on TCBS media incubated at 37°C on aerobic condition
   b. Culture on Skirrow's medium incubated at 42°C under microaerophilic condition
   c. Culture on MacConkey medium incubated at 42°C under anaerobic condition
   d. Culture on Wilson and Blairs medium at 37°C under microaerophilic condition

5(b). Microaerophilic bacteria: [AIIMS 09]
   a. Campylobacter
   b. Vibrio cholera
   c. Pseudomonas
   d. Salmonella

6. Urea breath test is used for diagnosis of: [NEET Pattern 18]
   a. H. pylori
   b. E. coli
   c. C. jejuni
   d. Proteus

7. Gram (–) bacillus which can grow in acidic pH: [NEET Pattern 18]
   a. Salmonella
   b. E. coli
   c. H. pylori
   d. Campylobacter

Helicobacter

8. *Helicobacter pylori* is not associated with:
   a. Gastrointestinal lymphoma [AIIMS 03]
   b. Gastric cancer
   c. Gastric leiomyoma
   d. Peptic ulcer

9. Which of following is false regarding *H. pylori*:
   a. With chronic infection urease breath test become negative
   b. *H. pylori* infection remains lifelong if untreated
   c. Endoscopy is diagnostic
   d. Toxigenic strains usually cause ulcer

10. Which of the following correctly describe *H. pylori*:
    a. Gram-negative cocci curved [PGI 05]
    b. Gram-positive cocci straight
    c. Gram-positive bacilli curved
    d. Gram-negative bacilli straight
    e. Gram-negative bacilli curved rod

11. True about *H. pylori*: [PGI 12]
    a. Seen in 85 to 90% cases of gastric ulcer
    b. Seen in 20 to 25% cases of duodenal ulcer
    c. Transmitted from man to man, feco-orally and by oro-gastric route
    d. Common in adults of developing countries

12. True statement about *H. pylori*: [PGI 09]
    a. 75% of ulcers are a/w *H. pylori*
    b. Medical therapy is Tx of choice
    c. 90% cases of duodenal ulcer a/w *H. pylori*
    d. 60% of *H. pyulori* colonization develop ulcer

13. Gastric ulcers of *H. pylori*, True: [PGI 09]
    a. Gm+ve aerobes
    b. Invade mucosa and muscularis layers
    c. Rapid urease test on endoscopy is diagnostic
    d. Culture confirm eradication
    e. Causes MALT of stomach

Explanations and References with Illustrative Answers

1. **Ans. (a) Temprature of 42°C and microaerophilic** *Ref. Jawetz; 27/e, p 257; Ananthnarayan 10/e, p 406*
   Diagnosis of *C. jejuni* diarrhoea:
   - Specimen: Stool
   - Direct microscopy: Dark field or phase contrast microscope shows *gull-wing shaped C. jejuni* with characterstic *darting motility*.
   - Culture: Growth occurs under microaerophilic conditions 5% O_2 and 85% N_2 with added CO_2 (10%). Though *C. jejuni* grows well at 36-37°C but incubation at 42°C prevents growth of other faecal bacteria and thus helps in selective growth.

Culture Media for Campylobacter
Selective Media 1. **CVA medium** (*Cefoperazone – Vancomycin – amphotericin B*) 2. Skirrow medium 3. Charcoal cefoperazone deoxycholate agar (CCDA) medium 4. Charcoal based selective medium (CSM) 5. Charcoal based medium containing cefoperazone, amphotericin & teicoplan (CAT) medium 6. Campy BAP selective media
Enrichment Culture 1. Preston enrichment medium 2. Compy-thio medium 3. Campylobacter enrichment broth

   - Fecal specimens are the preferred sample for isolating campylobacter species from patients with gastrointestinal infections.
   - Campylobacter species primarily *C. fetus, C. jejuni* have also been isolated from blood.

   Remember: *C. jejuni* cause inflammatory diarrhoea (i.e. presence of WBC in stool).

2. **Ans (b) *Campylobacter jejuni*** *Ref. DR Arora 3/e, p 411, 415*

Bacteria Showing Darting motility
• Spirillum minus (causative agent of rat bite fever)
• ***Campylobacter jejuni***
• *Vibrio cholerae*
Mnemonic: Spicavi

3. **Ans (b), (d) and (e) CVA medium, Skirrow medium, Campylobacter blood agar**
   Already explained

4. **Ans. (a) Human is the only reservoir** *Ref. Harrison 20/e p 1184; Ananthnarayan 10/e p 406*
   "*Campylobacter jejuni is part of normal intestinal flora of domestic animals and birds including poultry, cattle, sheep and swine. Human infection is acquired through raw or under cooked meat or other food products.*"
   - *Campylobacter jejuni* is the most common cause of *Campylobacter* infection (campylobacteriosis).
   - *Campylobacter* fetus infection is common in immunocompromised patients.

   Complications of Campylobacter infection
   - **Generalised:** Bacteremia - (Common with C. fetus)
   - **Local suppurative:** Cholecystitis; pancreatitis, cystitis
   - **Distant:** Meningitis, endocarditis, arthritis, peritonitis, cellulitis, septic abortion; hepatitis; interstitial nephritis.
   - **Immunologic:**
     – Reactive arthritis
     – GB syndrome (specially after C. 019 subtype)
     – Immunoproliferative small intestinal disease (α chain disease)

Infectious causes of GB syndrome	
Bacterial	**Viral**
Campylobacter jejuni	CMV
Mycoplasma pneumoniae	Epstein-Barr virus

5(a). Ans. (b) Culture on Skirrow's medium incubated at 42°C under microaerophilic condition *Ref. Jawetz 27/e, p 257*
Already explained

> **Note:** Skirrow's medium contains vancomycin, polymycin B and trimethoprin to inhibit growth of other bacteria.

5(b). Ans. (a) *Campylobacter*
Microaerophilic organism are organisms that require oxygen to survive, but in concentration less than that present in atmosphere, i.e. less than 21%.
Example include:
- Treponema pallidum
- Helicobacter pylori
- Borrelia burgdorferi
- Campylobacter

Mnemonic: Temp. Helicopter bording camp.

6. Ans. (a) H. pylori *Ref. Harrison 20/e p 1164*

Urea breath test is simple, best established and very accurate test for *H. pylori*. In this test patient drinks a solution of urea labelled with non-radioactive isotope ^{13}C and then blows into a tube. If *H. pylori* urease is present, the urea in hydrolyzed, and labelled CO_2 is detected in breath samples. This test becomes (-)ve after treatment. Thus used for followup too.

Diagnosis of H. Pylori		
Test	**Advantages**	**Disadvantages**
Invasive (based on endoscopic biopsy)		
Biopsy urease test	Quick, simple	Not fully sensitive before 24h
Histology	May give additional histologic information	Sensitivity dependent on experience & use of special stains
Culture	Permits determination of antibiotic susceptibility	Sensitivity dependent on experience
Noninvasive		
Serology	Inexpensive and convenient	Cannot be used for early follow-up;
^{13}C or ^{14}C urea breath test	Inexpensive and simpler than endoscopy; useful for follow-up after treatment	Radiation exposure in ^{14}C test
Stool antigen test	Inexpensive & convenient; useful for follow-up after treatment; may be useful in children	New test; appears less accurate than urea breath test

7. Ans. (c) H. pylori

Optimum pH for growth for some microorganisms (Jay. 1992. Bourgeois et.al., 1988)			
Moulds	4.5–6.8	E.coli	6–7
Yeasts	5–6.5	Clostridium botulinum	–
Bacillus	6.8–7.5	Clostridium perfringens	6.0–7.6
Lactic acid bacteria	5.5–6.5	Clostridium sporogenes	6.0–7.6
Lactobacillus acidophilus	5.8–6.6	Staphylococcus aureus	7.0–7.5
Thiobacillus thiooxidans	2.0–2.8	Pseudomonas aeruginosa	6.6–7.0
Enterobacteria	6.5–7.5	Streptococcus pneumoniae	7.8
Salmonella	6.5–7.5		

8. Ans. (c) Gastric leiomyoma *Ref. Harrison 20/e, p 1163-64*
Important features of *H. pylori*:
- Gram (–)ve cocobacilli motile with lophotrichous flagella.
- 80% of *duodenal ulcer* and 60% of *gastric ulcer* are related to *H. pylori*.
- *Increase the risk of:*
  - Gastric adenocarcinoma
  - Gatric MALT lymphoma
  - Reflux esophagitis
  - Autoimmune gastritis
  - Oesophageal adenocarcinoma
- Also increase the risk of non-gasric pathlogies like iron deficiency anemia, idiopathic thrombocytopenic purpura.
- Urea breath test is most consistently accurate test for diagnosis.
- Microbiologic culture is most specific but insensitive.

9. **Ans. (a) With chronic infection urease breath test becomes negative**
   Urease breath test is most consistently accurate test for diagnosis of H. pylori.
   It becomes negative only after treatment and is used to assess outcome of treatment. Ref. Harrison 20/e, p 1164

   > **Remember:**
   > - Most specific test is microbiologic culture of specimen obtaining by upper GI endoscopic biopsy.
   > - Major virulence factor of *H. pylori* are vacuolating cytotoxin (VaCA) and group of genes called *CagPal*.
   > - Urea breath test, stool antigen test, and biopsy based tests can all be used to assess the success of treatment.

10. **Ans. (e) Gram-negative bacilli curved rod** Ref. Ananthnarayan 10/e, p 407
    "H.pylori is a gram-negative curved spiral rod motile by unipolar tuft of lopnotrichous flagella."
    Correctly speaking *H. pylori* is a coccobacilli.

    > **Remember:**
    >
    > | Other Gram (–)ve coccobacilli | |
    > | --- | --- |
    > | – Hemophilus | – Bordetella |
    > | – Brucella | – Campylobacter |
    > | – Helicobacter | – Legionella |
    > | – Rickettsiaceae | – Chlamydiae |
    >
    > | All important bacilli are gram negative except | |
    > | --- | --- |
    > | – **A**ctinomycetes | – **B**acillus |
    > | – **C**lostridium | – **C**orynebacterium |
    > | – **M**ycobacteria | – **L**isteria |
    > | **Mnemonic:** ABC CML | |

11. **Ans. (c) and (d) Transmitted from man to man, feco-orally and by orogastric route; Common in adults of developing countries** Ref. Harrison 20/e, p 1162
    Mechanism of transmission is likely to be oral-oral or fecal-oral.
    - 70% of **duodenal** ulcer and 50% of gastric ulcer are associated with *H. pylori*.
    - Prevalance of *H. pylori* in developing countries is 80%.
    - *H. pylori* is virtually always associated with chronic active gastritis but only 10-15% of infected individual develop frank ulceration.

12. **Ans. (a) and (b) 75% of ulcers are a/w *H. pylori*, Medical therapy is Tx of choice** Ref. Harrison 20/e, p 1163
    - *H. pylori* is associated with 70% of duodenal ulcer and 50% of gastric ulcer or it can be said that 75% (Mean of 80% and 60%) of peptic ulcers are a/w *H. pylori*.
    - It is also worth to mention that only 10-15% of individual infected with *H. pylori* develop peptic ulcer.
    - Treatment is medical with OCA (omeprazole, clarithromycin, amoxicillin) being treatment of choice.
    - Indications for treatment
      - Duodenal or gastric ulceration
      - Low grade gastric B-cell lymphoma
      - Functional dyspepsia
      - ITP
      - Iron deficiency anemia
      - Vit B_{12} deficiency anemia

13. **Ans. (c) and (e) Rapid urease test on endoscopy is diagnostic, Causes MALT of stomach**
    Ref. Harrison 19/e p 1039, 18/e, p 1263
    - Under normal circumstances *H. pylori* do not invade gastric mucosa. It is found deep is the mucous layer near the epithelial surface where physiologic pH is present.

NEET Pattern Questions

1. **True about *H. pylori* includes all *except*:**
   a. Gram positive bacillus
   b. Urease positive bacillus
   c. Highly associated with deodenal ulcer
   d. Urease breath test can be performed only in specialized labs
   [Ref. Ananthanarayan, 10/e, p 407]

   > The main limitation of urea breath test is its availability and lost
   > ... Harrison 20/e p 1165

2. **The most sensitive test for *H. pylori* is:**
   a. Breath test
   b. Stool antigen test
   c. Culture of biopsy
   d. Microscopy of biopsy   [Ref. Harrison 20/e, p 1184]

   > **Senstivity of H. pylori tests:** Stool antigen test > Urea breath test > H. pylori serology > Histology Journals

3. **Seven sheathed flagella is seen in:**
   a. V cholera   b. H pylori
   c. Ps aeroginosa   d. Spirochetes
   [Ref. Ananthanarayan, 10/e, p 407]

   > H. pylori has five to seven sheathed polar flagella

4. **Which of the following is microaerophilic:**
   a. *E. coli*   b. *Bacteroides*
   c. *Clostridium*   d. *Helicobacter pylori*
   [Ref. Ananthanarayan 10/e, p 407]

   > **Psychrophilic bacteria:** Bacteria that grow at low temperature (< 15°C) of e.g. listeria moncytogenes

5. **True about Campylobacter jejuni:**
   a. Exclusively found in jejunum only
   b. Shows darting motility by peritracheal flagella
   c. Can grow at temperature around 42°C
   d. Common cause of diarrhea in India
   [Ref. Ananthanarayan, 9/e, p 399]

   > Darting motility is due to single polar flagellum

6. **Culture medium for Campylobacter jejuni:**
   a. BYCE medium
   b. Skirrow's medium
   c. Thayer-Martin medium
   d. TCBS medium   [Ref. Jawetz, 27/e, p 257]

7. **True about Campylobacter jejuni:**
   a. Obligate aerobe
   b. Oxidase negative
   c. Grows at 42°C
   d. Non-motile   [Ref. Jawetz, 27/e, p 257]

8. **True about campylobacter:**
   a. Polar flagella
   b. Grows at 25°C
   c. Strict aerobe
   d. Psychrophilic   [Ref. Ananthanarayan 10/e, p 405]

   > Campylobacter are thermophilic, as they grow best at 37–42°C

9. **Temperature required for isolation of compylobacter:**
   a. 20°C   b. 25°C
   c. 37°C   d. 42°C
   [Ref. Ananthanarayan 10/e, p 407]

Ans.
1. a. Gram positive...   2. b. Stool antigen test   3. b. H pylori   4. d. *Helicobacter pylori*
5. c. Can grow at...   6. b. Skirrow's medium   7. c. Grows at 42°C   8. a. Polar flagella
9. d. 42°C

CHAPTER 20
Legionella

- Gram-negative non-capsulated, intracellular cocobacilli.
- They are motile (with polar or subpolar Flagella), aerobic, catalase and oxidase positive.

Culture
- Not grow on ordinary media.
- Buffered charcoal yeast extract *'BCYE'* is selective medium used to grow *Legionella*. It grows best at pH - 6.9, temperature 35°C and 90% humidity, 5% CO_2
- Colonies have a 'cut glass' appearance and exhibit blue white autofluorescence
  ...*Greenwood 18/e, p 340*
- **MC** species associated with human infection *is L. pneumophilia*, (**MC** with **serogroup 1**).
- Other important species is *L. micdadei* (Pittsburgh pneumonia agent). It is partial acid fast (AFB).
- *Natural habitat* is *aquatic bodies including lakes and streams*. Shows symbiotic relations with algae, amebas, ciliated protozoa.
- Factors enhancing colonization are warm temperature, stagnation and sediments. It can form *microcolonies within biofilms*. Its eradication require disinfectants that can penetrate the biofilm.

- Gram (–)ve, non motile aerobic intracellular coccobacilli
- Buffered charcoal yeast agar is selective medium
- BCYE contains iron and cysteine

Mode of Transmission
- *Aspiration* is predominant mode of transmission. Other modes include aerosolization, direct instillation into lungs.
- *No man-to-man transmission occurs.*
- Aerosolization by AC, nebulizer, humidifier, overhead showers and direct installation into lung are other modes.

Risk Factors and Pathogenesis
- Conditions that impair mucociliary clearance predispose to legionnaires disease, most commonly being cigarette smoking.
- *Hairy cell leukemia* (not other leukemia) and immunocompromised state are other risk-factors.
- Legionella enters the lung through aspiration or direct inhalation. Attachment to host cells is mediated by bacterial type IV pilli, heat shock proteins, and the major outer membrane protein. *Legionella* then binds complement CR1 and CR3 integrin receptors of phagocytic cells. Entry into the cell is by phagocytic process. Alveolar macrophages readily phagocytose *Legionella* but bacteria actively multiply with in macrophages, when cells are destroyed the bacteria are released and infect other macrophages.
- The presence of iron is essential for intracellular growth of the bacteria.
- *Cell mediated immunity is primary mechanism of host defense* (Role of neutrophil appears to be minimal).
- Humoral immunity plays no role.

- *L. pneumophila* is the most common *Legionella* species associated with human infection
- Aspiration is predominant mode of transmission.

- *L. pneumophila* is oxidase positive (others are variable)
- *L. pneumophila* hydrolyzes hippurate whereas others do not.

LEGIONELLOSIS

Legionella causes 2 clinical syndromes:
A. **Pontiac fever:**
   - Acute febrile self-limited illness. Airbone transmission with high attack rate.
   - Pneumonia does not develop. **MC symptom**—malaise, fatigue and myalgia.
B. **Legionnaires' disease:** Designation for pneumonia.
   - **4th MC** cause of community acquired pneumonia (**MC**—*S.pneumoniae* **2nd MC**—*H. influenzae* **3rd MC** *Chlamydia pneumoniae*). ..... *Harrison 20/e, p 1138*

Legionella cause atypical pneumonia and legionnaires disease
- Heart is the most common site for extrapulmonary legionellosis
- Diarrhea with pneumonia suggest *Legionella* pneumonia.

- Cause atypical pneumonia which is more serious than atypical pneumonia of other agents.
- *Clinical features suggestive of* **L. pneumonia:**
  - Diarrhea   – High fever
  - Hyponatremia   – Proteinuria
  - Onset of symptom if occur within 10 days after discharge from hospital, suggest nosocomial legionnaires disease.
- Mostly caused by serotype 1 but serotype 6 is associated more commonly with hospital acquired and has poor prognosis.
- Relative bradycardia is useful diagnostic finding.

Extrapulmonary Legionellosis

- Results from blood-borne dissemination from lung.
- *MC* extrapulmonary site is **heart (myocarditis, pericarditis)**.
- Most cases are hospital acquired.
- *MC* neurological **abnormality** are **confusion** or changed mental status.

Diagnosis

Transplant recipients appears to be at unusually high risk of legionella pneumonia.

Specimen	Sensitivity of bronchoscopy specimens is approximately the same as that of sputum. Bronchoalveolar lavage fluid gives higher yield than bronchial wash specimen.
Staining	Gram-staining usually show numerous leukocytes but no organisms.
	DFA test is rapid and highly specific but less sensitive.
Culture	*Definitive* method of diagnosis.
	Requires 3-5 days to become grossly visible.
	B'CYE media is used.
Antibody detection	Requires 12 weeks, so used for retrospective diagnosis or epidemiologic studies.
Urinary antigen	Cheap, rapid, second in sensitivity (70–90%) and highly specific (95–100%).
	Detectable within 3 days.
	The test is not affected by antibiotic administration.
	Reliable only for L pneumophilia serogroup I which causes 80% of legionella infection.
Radiographic abnormalities	Pleural effusion
	In immunosuppressed distinct round nodular opacity may be seen.
	Nucleic acid based detection methods (PCR) are highly sensitive, fast and specific.

Treatment

- Azithromycin and respiratory tract quinolones (Levofloxacin, gemifloxacin, moxifloxacin) are *DOC*.
- Quinolones are preferred antibiotic in transplant recipients.

Prevention

- Disinfection of water by:
  - Superheat and flush method—*Ideal* for *emergency* situation
  - Copper and silver ionization method
  - Tap water filters particularly in transplant units.

Note: **Superchlorination** is *not* effective against legionella.

Multiple Choice Questions

1. BCYE. medium is used to culture: [New Pattern 2019]
   a. *Mycoplasma*
   b. *T pallidum*
   c. *H. pylori*
   d. *Legionella*

2. A 70-year-old patient presents with high grade fever, dry cough and abdominal pain. Sputum sample collected from patient, shows gram negative organisms that are able to grow only on charcoal yeast extract medium. The most likely organism is: [AI 07; AIIMS 06]
   a. *H. influenza*
   b. *Legionella*
   c. *Lesteria monocytogenes*
   d. *M. catarrhalis*

3. A 60-year-old man is diagnosed to be suffering from Legionnaires disease after he returns home from attending a convention. He could have acquired it: [AIIMS 16]
   a. From a person suffering from the infection while traveling in the aeroplane
   b. From a chronic carrier in the convention center
   c. From inhalation of the aerosol in the air conditioned room at convention center
   d. By sharing an infected towel with a fellow delegate at the convention

4. Anju, a 28-years-female, has diarrhea, confusion, high grade fever with bilateral pneumonitis. Organism causing this: [AI 12]
   a. *Legionella*
   b. *Neisseria meningitidis*
   c. *Streptococcus pneumoniae*
   d. *H. influenzae*

5. Pontiac fever is caused by: [PGI Dec. 07]
   a. *Legionella*   b. *Listeria*
   c. *Scrub typhus*   d. *Leptospira*
   e. *Rickettsia*

6. Aerosol spread leading to epidemics is seen in infection with: [AIIMS 2012]
   a. *Legionella*
   b. *Hemophilus*
   c. *Influenza virus*
   d. *Mycoplasma*

7. Method of transmission of legionella includes all, except: [AIIMS 2013]
   a. Patients suffering from legionella to contacts
   b. Aerosol from air cooling systems
   c. From contaminated food
   d. Through contaminated tracheal tubes

Explanations and References with Illustrative Answers

1. **Ans. (d) *Legionella*** *Ref. Harrison 20/e, p 1140*
   - **BCYE agar** is the medium used to grow *Legionella*.
   - This highly enhanced medium contains the **amino acid L-cysteine** which is an **absolute growth requirement** for *Legionella*.
   - Addition of vancomycin, polymyxin B and an antifungal agent increases the selectivity.
   - Best specimen is respiratory secretions.
   - Culture takes 3–5 days sometime upto 2 weeks
   - Pretreatment of specimen with acid or heat markedly improves the yield.

2. **Ans. (b) *Legionella*** *Ref. Harrison 20/e, p 1138, 1140; Jawetz 27/e, p 301*
   Dry cough, high grade fever and growth on charcoal yeast medium suggest legionella.
   Legionella have fastidious requirements and grow on complex media such as buffered charcoal, yeast extract (BCYE) agar with L. cysteine and antibiotic supplements with 5% CO_2 at pH 6.9, 35°C and 90% humidity.

3. **Ans. (c) From inhalation of the aerosol in the air conditioned room at convention center** *Ref. Harrison 20/e, p 1137–1138*
   Important features of *Legionella*
   - Aerobic, Gram-negative motile, nonencapsulated bacilli
   - Natural habitat are aquatic bodies such as stagnant water, mud, hot springs.
   - Outbreaks are associated with contaminated water source such as air conditioning cooling towers.
   - Multiple modes of transmission—**Aspiration (MC)**, aerosolization, direct instillation.

- *No man-to-man transmission,* no animal reservoir.
- It causes:

Manifestations	
Pneumonia	***Pontiac fever***
Atypical pneumonia	Acute febrile self-limiting illness
Presents with high fever, diarrhea, pneumonia	
MC extrapulmonary site of Legionella is heart.	

- **Selective media** – Buffered charcoal yeast extract **(BCYE) agar.**

Treatment: – Macrolides and quinolones.
– β-lactams are not effective.

4. **Ans. (a) Legionella**   *Ref. Harrison 20/e, p 1138*

Clinical features suggestive of Legionnaire's disease
- Diarrhea
- High fever (>40°C or >104°F).
- Numerous neutrophils but no organisms revealed by Gram's staining of respiratory secretions.
- Hyponatremia (serum sodium level of < 131 mEq/L).
- Failure to respond to β-lactam drugs (penicillins or cephalosporins) and aminoglycoside antibiotics.
- Occurrence of illness in an environment in which the potable water supply is known to be contaminated with Legionella.
- Onset of symptoms within 10 days after discharge from the hospital.

Risk factors for Legionnaires disease
- **Cigarette** *smoking and other condition that impair mucociliary clearance*
- Chronic lung disease
- Advances age
- Immunosuppression
- Surgery is predisposing factor in nosocomial infection with transplant recipient at highest risk.

Remember: MC extrapulmonary site in heart in which it causes myocarditis, pericarditis.

5. **Ans. (a) Legionella**   *Ref. Harrison 20/e, p 1138*
Pontiac fever is a mild nonfatal influenza like illness caused by Legionella pneumophila.

Pontiac fever
- An acute self limiting flue like illness with IP of 24-48 hours
- Malaise, fatigue and myalgia are the most frequent presenting symptoms
- Pneumonia doesn't develop.
- Complete recovery takes place, without antibiotic therapy.
- Diagnosis is established by antibody detection.

6. **Ans. (a) Legionella**   *Ref. Harrison 20/e 1138*
- *Aerosolization of Legionella by devices filled with tap water including whirlpools, nebulizers and humidifiers has been implicated"*
- *Pontaic fever has been linked to Legionella containing aerosols from water using machinery, a cooling tower, AC and whirlpools.*

Other Options:
- **Hemophilus:** Transmitted by airborne droplets or by direct contact with secretions or fomites.
- **Influenzae virus:** Same as hemophilus
- **Mycoplasma:** Person to person by respiratory droplets expectorated during coughing.

7. **Ans. (a) Patients suffering from**   *Ref. Ananthanarayan 10/e, p 408; Harrison 20/e, 1138*
Human to human transmission does not occur in legionella

Mode of Infection of Legionella:
- **Source:**
  - Natural habitat for L. pneumophila are aquatic bodies including lakes and streams. However, their number is very low in aquatic bodies
  - When the contaminated water from these aquatic bodies is stored in human constructed water reservoirs (water cooler), legionella grow and proliferate.
  - Warm temperature and sediment enhances the proliferation
  - L. pneumophila can form microcolonies within biofilms in water coolers, its eradication requires disinfectants that can penetrate the biofilm
  - Ameboe, alga, ciliated protozoans are symbiotic to L. pneumophila and promotes the growth
- **Mode of transmission:**
  - **Aspiration:** Predominant mode. Aspiration can occur either from oropharyngeal colonization, or through contaminated water
  - **Aerosolization:** Air conditioners, whirlpools, nebulizers aerosolize the legionella which then gets inhaled.
  - **Direct instillation into the lungs:** Either through contaminated instruments (endotracheal tube) or through respiratory tract manipulation which mobilizes the oropharyngeal colonies to respiratory tract.

NEET Pattern Questions

1. **Buffered charcoal yeast agar is the selective medium for:**
   a. Listeria monocytogenes
   b. Legionella pneumophila
   c. Pseudomonas aeroginosa
   d. T. pallidum
   [Ref. Ananthanarayan, 10/e, p 408]

2. **Which of the following pneumonia is caused by contaminated air conditioner:**
   a. Pneumococci
   b. Staphylococci
   c. E. coli
   d. Legionella
   [Ref. Harrison, 20/e, p 1138]

3. **Legionnaire disease is caused by:**
   a. Motile gram positive
   b. Motile gram negative
   c. Non-motile gram positive
   d. Non-motile gram negative
   [Ref. Ananthanarayan, 10/e, p 408]

4. **In pontiac fever, which antigen is seen in urine:**
   a. Group specific antigen of Legionella serogroup 1 (LP 1)
   b. Group specific antigen of Legionella serogroup 2 (LP 2)
   c. Group specific antigen of Legionella serogroup 4 (LP 4)
   d. Group specific antigen of Legionella serogroup 6 (LP 6)
   [Ref. Harrison, 20/e, p 1141]

5. **Legionella causes:**
   a. Pontiac fever
   b. Myocarditis
   c. Diarrhea
   d. All of the above
   [Ref. Harrison, 20/e, p 1138]

Ans.
1. b. Legionella...
2. d. Legionella
3. b. Motile gram...
4. a. Group specific...
5. d. All of the above

Rickettsiae and Chlamydiae

CHAPTER 21

CHLAMYDIAE [PLT AGENT]

- **Obligate intracellular** bacteria, so *unable to grow in cell free media*.
- Lacks enzymes of electron transport chain and require ATP from host cell, so they are often called as *energy parasites*.
- Cell wall resemble that of Gr(-)ve bacteria
- ***Peptidoglycan and N-acetylmuramic acid is absent*** from its cell wall. Its cell wall contain tetrapeptide linked matrix and relatively high lipid content.
- Show tropism for squamous epithelial cells and lymph nodes.
- Genome of chlamydiae is 1.04 megabases in length encodes 900 genes, and is one of the smallest bacterial genomes.

Chlamydia
- Obligate intracellular bacilli, also called as energy parasites
- Cell wall lacks peptidoglycan and N-acetylmuramic acid

Growth Cycle

Replicate by *binary fission* without an eclipse phase.
Chlamydiae occur in 2 forms:

Elementary Body (EB)	Reticular Body (RB)
Extracellular metabolically inactive infective form	Intracellular growing, metabolically active and replicative form
Contain rigid trilaminar cell wall	Friable cell wall lacking peptidoglycan
Contain electron dense nucleoid	No electron dense nucleoid
DNA = RNA	RNA > DNA about 4 times

Chlamydia
- Elementary body usually attach near the base of microvilli

Reticular body undergoes binary fission resulting in chlamydial microcolony called *inclusion body*. This whole cycle takes about 24 - 48 hours.

Effect on Host Cell

- *C. trachoma* leave host cell with scar while *C. psittacosis* leaves host cell severely damaged which is usually followed by lysis.

Classification

Chlamydiae are divided into four species:
i. *C. trachomatis*
ii. *C. pneumoniae* } (Affect humans)
iii. *C. psittaci.*
iv. *C. pecourum*   (Affect ruminants)

Features	C. trachoma	C. pneumoniae	C. psittaci
Serovars	15	1	≥ 4
Inclusion body	Round vacuolar called *HP bodies	Round dense	Large dense called *LCL bodies
Glycogen in inclusions	+	–	–
Susceptibility to sulfonamide	+	–	–
Plasmid	+	–	+
Natural host	Humans	Humans	Birds
Transmission	Person-to-person Mother to infant	Airborne person-to person	Airborne bird excreta to humans
Elementary body morphology	Round	Pear-shaped, round	Round

*HP = Halberstaedter Prowazek
*LCL = Levinthal - cole - lillie

Chlamydia
- Elementary body: Infective entity
- Reticular body: Metabolically active entity.

- C. pneumoniae grows well on HL and Hep-2 cells.
- C. trachomatis grows well on McCoy cells.

Antigen

- **Heat stable LPS** — Genus (Group) specific
- (Lipopolysaccharide) — Common to all chlamydia
  - Responsible for complement fixation test (CFT).
  - Species specific protein antigen, present at envelope surface, so classify chlamydiae into trachomatis, psittaci, pneumoniae and pecorum.
- **Major outer membrane protein (MOMP)** — Used for intraspecies typing, i.e. for serovar or serotypes.
  - Demonstrated by microimmuno-fluorescence.

Lab Diagnosis

- *Microscopy*
  a. Staining — By Giemsa or castaneda or Machiavello particularly in neonatal inclusion conjunctivitis. As C. trachomatis inclusions contain glycogen matrix they can be stained with Lugol's iodine
    - *Iodine staining* of conjunctival scrapping is a *rapid and simple screening method for trachoma*
  b. Immunofluorescence — Using monoclonal antibody
    - More sensitive and specific.
- *Isolation* — *Cell culture* is the preferred mode.
  - Can also be done by inoculation into embryonated eggs or experimental animals.
  - McCoy & HeLa All lines are commonly used   ...*Ananthanarayan 9/e, p 418*
- *Demonstration of antigen*
  a. Microimmunofluorescence – Commonly used method.
  b. ELISA – Preferred for screening.
  c. DNA probes and amplification techniques (PCR and LCR) – More sensitive and specific.
- *Detection of antibody* — CFT: Cannot distinguish species as it is Group = Genus specific.
  - Micro IF: More useful for TRIC (inclusion conjunctivitis).

Remember:
- High titre antibody are seen only in:
  - Infant pneumonia — Salpingitis — LGV.
- *C. pneumoniae*, grows better in HL and HEp - 2 cells than in HeLa 22q or McCoy cells.
- McCoy cells are widely used to culture C. trachomatis.
- Skin hypersensitivity in LGV can be demonstrated by Frie's test.

CHLAMYDIA TRACHOMATIS

- *MC* cause of STD worldwide.
- *MC* cause of ophthalmia neonatorum.
- 15 serotypes [A to K and L1, L2, L3] are known:
  - A, B, Ba, C - Endemic blinding trachoma.
  - D to K - Inclusion conjunctivitis, genital infection, infant pneumonia.
  - L_1, L_2, L_3 Lymphogranuloma venereum.

Serovars can be distinguished by serologic typing with monoclonal antibodies or by molecular gene typing.
- *C. trachomatis* is *MC* cause of non-gonococcal urethritis, post-gonococcal urethritis.
- *MC* cause of epididymitis.
- **Inclusion conjunctivitis** of *neonate* is called *inclusion blenorrhea* while *adult* form is called as "Swimming pool disease."

Clinical Manifestations

- **IP:** 5–10 days.
1. **Trachoma**
   - Chronic keratoconjunctivitis characterized by follicular hypertrophy, papillary hyperplasia, pannus formation and in late stage, cicatrisation

- C. trachomatis is the most common STD worldwide, and is the most common cause of non-gonococcal urethritis
  - Associated with ophthalmia neonatorum, lymphogranuloma venereum.

- **Stages include**
  - Trachoma dubium (earliest), when disease is just suspicion
  - Protrachoma (stage of conjunctival lesion).
  - Established trachoma (Stages I-IV)
  - Inclusion bodies are not demonstrable in trachoma dubium and protrachoma

2. **Genital Infection**
   - Chlamydia serovars D-K and L causes two types of genital infection viz. LGV and miscellaneous urogenital syndrome, Collectivity referred as genital chlamydiasis.

   a. **LGV - Lymphogranuloma venereum**
      - Most cases occur due to **L2** serovar–LGV serovars are more invasive than other serotypes.
      - **MC presentation** in heterosexual man and women is painful lymphadenopathy called inguinal syndrome/Tropical bubo.
      - LGV strains are **more invasive** than the other serovars.
      - **MC** LN involved in woman - *Intrapelvic and pararectal*.
      - In women it causes rectal stricture and elephantiasis of vulva (esthiomene).
      - Elementary bodies are known as *Miyagawa's corpuscles*.

> - L_1–L_3 serovar are more invasive and replicates in macrophages
> - Trachoma serovars are more common and replicates in eye (A–C) on genital tract (D–K)

Lymphogranuloma venereum

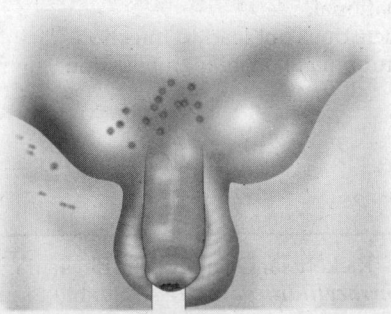

Lymphogranuloma venereum

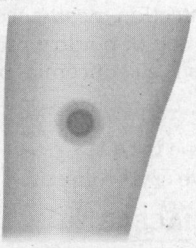

Positive Frei test

Lymphogranuloma Venereum		
Primary stage	**Secondary stage**	**Tertiary stage**
• 3 – 30 days of IP	• 2 – 6 weeks after primary lesion	• After several years
• Painless small papule which may ulcerate at the site of lesion	• Characterized by inguinal lymphadenopathy which is painful	• Elephantiasis of genitalia
	• Proctitis	• Esthiomene syndrome
	• Cervical adenopathy after oral intercourse	

> • **LCR and PCR are most sensitive** chlamydial diagnostic test available

Note: Sign of groove: Extensive enlargement of chain of inguinal nodes above and below the inguinal ligament (the sign of the groove). Present only in minority of cases of LGV.

b. **Genital chlamydiasis:**
   - MC form of STD worldwide (caused by serotype D-K)
   - In *men* they cause urethritis (nongonococcal urethritis), epididymitis, prostitis, conjunctivitis and urethritis.
   - In *women* bartholinitis, mucopurulent cerviticis, endometritis, salpingitis are seen.
   - Reiter syndrome and Fitz-Hugh -Curtis syndrome can be seen in both sexes.

3. **Reiter's syndrome**
   - Conjunctivitis, urethritis, arthritis and characteristic mucocutaneous lesions
   - Associated with HLA B - 27.

   Diagnosis:
   - Cell culture once considered to be the gold standard has been replaced by NAAT.
   - LCR and PCR are most sensitive chlamydial diagnostic test available.
     ..... *Harrison 19/e, p 1071, 18/e, p 1426*
   - *Specimen*: Urine and vaginal swabs have replaced urethral and cervical swabs in males and females respectively.

> C. pneumoniae: Atypical pneumoniae.
> C. psittaci: Psitticosis.

Rickettsiae
- Gr (−)ve obligate intracellular parasite.
- Only louse borne typhus is the primary human disease, in other rickettsial disease, human are incidental host.
- Rocky mountain spotted fever is the most severe rickettsial disease.
- Rickettsia pox is the mildest rickettsial disease.

- **Treatment:**
- Azithromycin is the DOC for STD.
- Tetracycline, erythromycin, rifampicin are effective in trachoma

CHLAMYDIA PNEUMONIAE (TWAR STRAIN)

- Distinguished from other 2 species on the basis of DNA morphology.
- Only one serovar identified.
- Associated with increased risk of atherosclerosis, asthma, sarcoidosis.
- **HL and HEP-2 cells** - Most effective cell line for isolation.
- Causes atypical pneumonia, similar to M pneumoniae, 5-20% of community acquired pneumonia are thought to be caused by C. pneumoniae
- Pharyngitis, otitis, sinusitis, bronchitis are other manifestation

Treatment: Erythromycin/Tetracycline.

CHLAMYDIA PSITTACI

- Primarily disease of parrots.
- Acquired in humans by inhalation of dropping or nasal discharge.
- Human infection mostly occupational.
- Consumption of poultry products does not lead to infection.
- Psittacosis is a septicemia, pneumonia is usual manifestation.

Treatment:
- Tetracycline is *DOC*
- Alternative erythromycin.

RICKETTSIACEAE

Rickettsial disease with Eschar
- Scrub typhus.
- Indian tick typhus.
- Siberian tick typhus.
- Rickettsial pox.

- This family consist of 3 genera - Rickettsia, Orientia and Ehrlichia.
- These are *Gram −ve obligate intracellular parasite* so unable to grow in cell free media, except Rochalimaea quintana.
- Transmitted by arthropod vectors.
- In humans they infect vascular and reticuloendothelial cells.
- *Except for louse-borne typhus, humans are incidental hosts.*
- *Coxiella burnetii* is notorious for its ability to survive outside reservoir or vector and for its extreme infectiousness. *(Non arthropod air-borne rickettsial disease).*
- Severity of rickettsial disease are enhanced by sulphonamide. Penicillin is also ineffective in rickettsial disease.
- Rickettsia are stained by Giemsa, Castaneda, Machiavello and Gimenez stains.
- Rickettsia grow best in cells that are not metabolizing actively.
- Rickettsia are non-motile non-capsulated, pleomorphic coccobacilli.

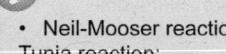

- Neil-Mooser reaction.
  Tunia reaction:
  - Used to differentiate R.typhi and R.prowazekii (−ve reaction)

Classification of Rickettsial Cell Disease

Diseases	Rickettsial agent	Insect vectors	Mammalian reservoirs	Incubation period	Clinical features	Lymph-adenopathy	Diagnosis
Typhus group							
Epidemic typhus	Rickettsia prowazekii	Louse	Humans	7–12 days	No eschar, petechial rash, suffused conjunctiva, epistaxis	–	W-F: ≥1:160 OX-19
Murine typhus/ Endemic typhus	Rickettsia typhi	Flea	Rodents	1–2 weeks	Rash-maculopapular, petechial	–	W-F ≥1:160 OX-19
Scrub typhus	Orientia tutsugamushi	Mite	Rodents	1–3 weeks	Eschar, rash-maculopapular, retiform purpura	+++	W-F: ≥1:160 OX-K
Spotted fever group							
Indian tick typhus (Mediterranean spotted fever)	Rickettsia conorii	Tick	Rodents, dogs	3–7 days	Eschar: Rare, retiform, purpura	+	W-F: ≥1:160 OX-2
Rocky Mountain spotted fever	Rickettsia rickettsii	Tick	Rodents, dogs	2–14 days	Rash around wrist and ankle	+	W-F: ≥1:160 OX-19

Contd...

Contd...

Diseases	Rickettsial agent	Insect vectors	Mammalian reservoirs	Incubation period	Clinical features	Lymph-adenopathy	Diagnosis
Rickettsialpox	*Rickettsia akari*	Mite	Mice	6–15 days	Eschar present, rash-maculopapular, vesicular, photophobia	+++	W-F: Negative
Others							
Q fever	*Coxiella burnetti*	Nil	Cattle sheep, goats	2–6 weeks	Rash is absent	–	W-F: Negative
Trench fever	*Rochalimaea quintana*	Louse	Human	15–25 days	Rash (maculopapular)	–	W-F: Negative IIF: IgG titers ≥ 1:50

(W-F: Weil-Felix; IIF: Indirect immunofluorescence)
- Don't go into DETAILS of Individual disease as they are asked very rarely.

Mnemonic to Learn this Confusing Table

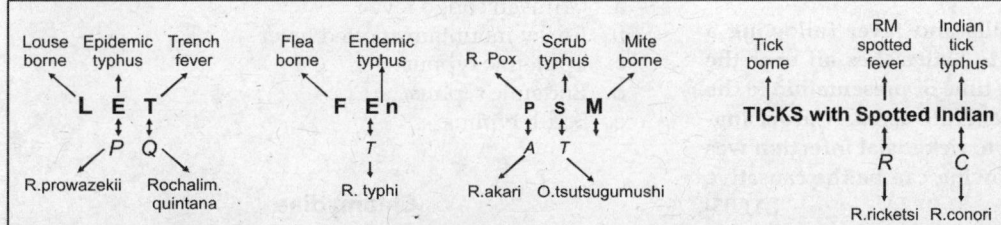

Important Points About Rickettsial Diseases

- **Most severe** rickettsial disease is Rocky mountain spotted fever.
- **Most mild** rickettsial disease—Rickettsia pox.
- Rickettsial infections are characterized by fever, headache, malaise, prostration, skin, rash (except in Q fever) and hepatosplenomegaly.
- Neil—Mooser or tunica reaction positive in *R. typhi* (*R.mooseri*), *R. conori*, *R.akari* and negative for *R. prowazekii*.
- **Weil Felix reaction** - It is heterophile agglutination test. Based on sharing of alkali stable polysaccharide between typhus rickettsia and some strain of *Proteus* bacilli. (OX 19, OX - 2, OX K)
  - OX 19: (+++): In epidemic and endemic typhus, Tick born spotted fever.
  - OX - 2: (++): In rocky mountain spotted fever.
  - OXK: (+++): In scrub typhus.
  - *No value in*: Q fever, trench fever, rickettsial pox.
  - *False positive in:* Typhoid, liver disease, *Proteus* infection, *Pseudomonas*, *Borrelia*, *S.typhi*.
- Diagnosis of most disease is made by serology, the most common serologic test is indirect immunofluorescence. However serologic test may be negative at the time of presentation. The only diagnostic test that has proven useful during the acute illness in case of Rocky mountain spotted fever is immunohistologic examination of cutaneous biopsy sample.

Bartonella

- Tiny Gram(-)ve bacilli usually transmitted by arthropods
- Human pathogenic strains are *B. bacillifornis, B. Quintana* and *B. henselae*
- Identification and classification depends upon 16 SRNA analysis
- Cat scratch disease: Transmitted by B. hemelae
- Oraya fever: Caused by Bartonella bacilliformis
- Causative agent of Trench fever i.e. Rochalimaea quintana is also classified as Bartonella quintana as unlike other rickettsiae. It can grow in cell free media.
- **Note:** B. henselae has been linked with bacillary angiomatosis and bacillary peliosis.

Multiple Choice Questions

Rickettsiae

1. Lice are not the vectors of: [AI 07; AIMS 06]
   a. Relapsing fever 4
   b. Q fever
   c. Trench fever
   d. Epidemic typhus

2. All are true about scrub typhus, *except*: [AI 2010]
   a. Causative organism is R.TSUTSUGAMOSHI
   b. Vector is trombiculide mite
   c. Adult female feeds on vertebrate hosts
   d. Tetracycline is the drug of choice

3. A patient complained of chills and fever following a louse bite 2 weeks before. He had rashes all over the body and was delirious at the time of presentation to the hospital and subsequently went into coma. A provisional diagnosis of vasculitis due to rickettsial infection was made. Which one of the following can be the causative agent? [AI 05]
   a. *Rickettsia typhi*
   b. *Rickettsia rickettsiae*
   c. *Rickettsia prowazekii*
   d. *Rickettsia akari*

4. True about scrub typhus: [PGI Nov 11]
   a. Zoonotic disease
   b. Positive Weil-Felix reaction
   c. Spread by adult mite
   d. Eschar indicates the location of mite bite
   e. Spread by infected chigger

5. Scrub typhus is transmitted by: [AIIMS 07]
   a. Reduvid bug
   b. Trombiculid mite
   c. Enteric pathogens
   d. Cyclops

6. It is true regarding endemic typhus that: [AIIMS 06]
   a. Man is the only reservoir of infection
   b. Flea is a vector of the disease
   c. The rash developing into eschar is a characteristic presentation
   d. Culture of the etiological agent in tissue culture is a diagnostic

7. Following is the etiological agent of Rocky Mountain spotted fever: [AIIMS 05]
   a. *R. rickettsii*
   b. *Rochalimae quintana*
   c. *R. tsutsugamushi*
   d. *Coxiella burnetii*

8. Mode of transmission of Q-fever is: [AIIMS 09]
   a. Bite of infected louse
   b. Bite of infected tick
   c. Inhalation of aerosol
   d. Bite of infected mice

9. Disease caused by both *Rickettsia* and *Orientia* is transmitted by: [PGI 2011]
   a. Rat flea
   b. Tick
   c. Louse
   d. Trombiculid mite
   e. Gamaxid mite

10. Which is caused by *Rickettsia*? [PGI 07]
    a. Weil's disease
    b. Rocky mountain spotted fever
    c. Scrub typhus
    d. Lymes disease

11. Tick is vector for: [PGI 2012]
    a. Crimean congo fever
    b. Rocky mountain spotted fever
    c. Epidemic typhus
    d. Endemic typhus
    e. Scrub typhus

Chlamydiae

12. A 14-year-old infant presented with conjunctivitis following which 5 days later, the patient developed pneumonitis. Which is the most likely causative agent? [AIIMS 2017]
    a. Chlamydia trachomatis
    b. Streptococcus agalactiae
    c. Gonococcus
    d. Haemophilus influenzae

13. Regarding *Chlamydia* infection of the eyes, true statement include the following *except*: [AI 09]
    a. Mostly asymptomatic
    b. Can be cultured
    c. Inclusion conjunctivitis is an acute ocular infection caused by sexually transmitted *C. trachomatis* strains (usually serovars D through K)
    d. Penicillin is the treatment

14. In a patient with UTI; on smear, no bacteria are found on Gram stain with abundant pus cells, to demonstrate organism, which of the following is useful? [AI 07; AIIMS May 2012, 11, 06]
    a. McCoy cell line
    b. Thayer Martin medium
    c. L J medium
    d. Acid fast staining

15. Which of the following is not true regarding *Chlamydia*? [AI 07; AIIMS 06]
    a. Has biphasic life
    b. Elementary body is metabolically active
    c. Reticulate body undergoes binary fission
    d. Once it invades into cell it abates phagolysosomal fusion

16. *Chlamydia trachomatis* is associated with the following except: [AI 05]
    a. Endemic trachoma
    b. Inclusion conjunctivitis
    c. LGV
    d. Community acquired pneumonia

17. Which one of the following statements is true regarding *Chlamydia pneumoniae*? [AI 05]
    a. Fifteen serovars have been identified as human pathogen
    b. Mode of transmission is by the air-borne bird excreta
    c. The cytoplasmic inclusions presents in the sputum specimen are rich in glycogen
    d. The group specific antigen is responsible for the production of complement fixing antibodies

18. All are true regarding *Chlamydia psittaci except*:
    a. Endemic in birds [AIMS 06]
    b. Cause non-gonococcal urethritis
    c. Grow in a specified laboratory
    d. Tetracycline is treatment of choice

19. A 45-year female complains of lower abdominal pain and vaginal discharge. On examination there is cervicitis along with a mucopurulent cervical discharge. The gram smear of the discharge shows presence of abundant pus cells but no bacteria. The best approach to isolate the possible causative agent would be: [AIIMS 05]
    a. Culture on chocolate agar supplemented with Haemin
    b. Culture on McCoy cells
    c. Culture on a bilayer human blood agar
    d. Culture on vero cell lines

20. The following is not a method of isolation of *Chlamydia* from clinical specimens: [AIIMS 05]
    a. Yolk inoculation
    b. Enzyme immunoassay
    c. Tissue culture using irradiated McCoy
    d. Tissue culture using irradiated BHK cells

21. The following statements are true regarding *Chlamydia except*: [AIIMS 05]
    a. Erythromycin is effective for therapy of Chlamydial infections
    b. Their cell wall lacks a peptidoglycan layer
    c. They can grow in cell free culture media
    d. They are obligate intracellular bacteria

22. A man presents to STD clinic with urethritis and urethral discharge. Gram stain shows numerous pus cells but no microorganism. Culture is negative on routine laboratory media. The most likely agent is: [AIIMS 02]
    a. *Chlamydia trachomatis*   b. *H. ducreyi*
    c. *T. pallidum*   d. *N. Gonorrhoeae*

23. *Chlamydia trachomatis* serovars D-K cause:
    a. Arteriosclerosis [AIIMS 02]
    b. Trachoma
    c. *Lymphogranuloma venereum*
    d. Urethritis

24. Triad of Reiter's syndrome: [PGI 07]
    a. Conjunctivitis   b. Uveitis
    c. Polyarthritis   d. Mucosal lesions
    e. Glaucoma

25. Most sensitive test for diagnosing asymptomatic chlamydia infection is: [AIIMS 09]
    a. Tissue culture   b. Nucleic acid amplification
    c. Serology   d. Serum electrophoresis

26. Isolation of Chlamydia from tissue specimen can be done by: [AI 10]
    a. ELISA (Enzyme Linked Immune Assay)
    b. Yolk sac inoculation
    c. Direct Immunofluorescence Antibody test (DFA)
    d. Polymerase Chain Reaction (PCR)

27. Which of the following statement is not true regarding *Chlamydia Trachomatis*? [AI 2012]
    a. Elementary body is metabolically active
    b. It is biphasic
    c. Reticulate body divides by binary fission
    d. Inside the cell it evades phagolysosome

28. A male patient with symptoms of urethritis. Examination reveals only pus cells without any organism. Most likely cause is: [AI 08; AIIMS 07]
    a. *Chlamydia trachomatis*   b. *H. ducreyi*
    c. *Treponema pallidum*   d. *M. tuberculi*

29. Most sensitive test for diagnosing chlamydia:
    a. Gram's staining [AI 09; AIIMS 17]
    b. Nucleic acid amplification testing
    c. ELIS A
    d. Fluorecent microscopy

Explanations and References with Illustrative Answers

1. **Ans. (b) Q fever** *Ref. Ananthnarayan 10/e, p 413*
   "Q fever is air-borne disease."
   Lice act as vector in following diseases:

Disease	Causative agent
Epidemic typhus	R. prowazekii
Relapsing fever	Borrelia recurrentis
Trench fever	Rochalimaea quintana
Dermatitis	
Pediculosis	

   Note: Relapsing fever can be tick-borne also.

2. **Ans. (c) Adult female feeds on vertebrate hosts** *Ref. Ananthnarayan 10/e 415; Harrison 18/e, p 1413, 19/e, p 1159*
   "Mite feeds on serum of warm blood animals only during there larval stage (chiggers) and adult mites feed only on plants"
   Scrub typhus
   - Caused by *O. tsutsugamushi*
   - **Transmitted** by *trombiculid mite* which also shows transovarian spread. It must be noted that disease is transmitted by chiggers (larva), not by adult mite
   - **Clinical features:** – Fever, headache, myalgia, cough and GI symptoms.
     – Classic case present with an eschar, regional lymphadenopathy and a maculopapular rash.
   - **Diagnosis:** Serologic assays (IFA, indirect immunoperoxidase and enzyme immunoassays) are main stay of diagnosis.

   Treatment – Rifampin
   – Azithromycin and clarithromycin
   Truely speaking doxycycline is not drug of choice but it can be used for all rickettsial infections.

3. **Ans. (c) Rickettsia prowazekii** *Ref. Ananthnarayan 10/e, p 414; Park; 22/e, p 276*
   Most important point in the given question is "louse-borne rickettsial infection" which is only one i.e., Epidemic typhus which is caused by *R. prowazekii*.
   Epidemic Typhus
   - Also called as louse-borne typhus or classical typhus or Gaol fever.
   - Usually seen among military and refugee populations and famine areas.
   - Humans are only natural vertebrate host.
   - **Vector:** Body or head louse (*Pediculus humanus*) not pubic louse.
   - **Causative agent:** *R. prowazekii*
   - **Route of transmission:** Louse feces is rubbed over abraded skin. So, infection is transmitted from man-to-man by infected louse.
   - **Incubation period:** 5 to 15 days
   - **Clinical feature:** Fever, chills, rash (starts on trunk and spread over limbs sparing face, palms and soles), stupor and delirium.
   - Rickettsia may become latent in lymphoid tissue causing recrudescent typhus or Brill-Zinsser disease.

   Remember: Trench fever is also transmitted by louse but causative agent is Rochalimaea or Bartonella quintana which is excluded from Rickettsiaea, because it can grow in cell free media.

4. **Ans. (a) (b) (d) (e) Zoonotic…, Positive…, Eschar…, Spread…** *Ref. Ananthnarayan 10/e, p 417, 9/e, p 407, 410*

Disease	Agglutination pattern		
	OX 19	OX 2	OX K
Epidemic typhus	+++	+	–
Brill-Zinsser disease	– –/+		–
Endemic typhus	+++	±	–
Tickborne spotted fever	++	++	–
Scrub typhus	–	–	+++

5. **Ans. (b) Trombiculid mite** *Ref. Ananthnarayan 10/e, p 1413*
   Already explained

6. **Ans. (b) Flea is a vector of the disease** *Ref. Ananthnarayan 10/e, p 414*
   Endemic typhus or Murine or fleaborne typhus
   - Caused by *R. typhi* or *R. mooseri*. It is zoonotic disease.
   - No direct man-to-man transmission occur.
   - Human acquire infection usually when saliva or feces of infected flea is rubbed over skin.
   - Clinical features is similar to epidemic typhus in milder form.
   - Its mammalian reservoir is rodents.
   - Serology is *diagnostic test.*
   - Human infection is dead end infection.

   Remember: Rickettsia cannot grow in artificial culture media.
   Bacterial Zoonotic diseases:
   – Q fever
   – Anthrax
   – Brucellosis
   – Leptospirosis
   – TB
   – Plague

   Rashes are seen in:
   - Epidemic typhus (no eschar)
   - Endemic typhus (no eschar)
   - Scrub typhus (50% have eschar)
   - RMSF (no eschar)
   - Rickettsial pox (eschar)
   - Fever boutonneuse (tache noire eschar).

7. **Ans. (a) R. rickettsii** *Ref. Ananthnarayan 10/e, p 413*
   Already explained

8. **Ans. (c) Inhalation of aerosol** *Ref. Harrison 20/e, p 1131; Jawetz 27/e, p 347*
   "Q fever is transmitted by inhalation of dust contaminated with rickettsia from placenta, dried feces, urine or milk or aerosols in slaughter houses."
   Q fever:
   - Caused by *Coxiella burnetii*
   - A *zoonotic* disease
   - Primary source of human infection are cattle, sheep and goats
   - **Mode of transmission:**

   In infected female animal, *C. burnetii* localizes uterus
   ↓
   Infection reactivates during pregnancy
   ↓
   High concentration of *Coxiella* in placenta
   ↓
   Soil gets contaminated during parturation
   ↓
   Coxiella aerosols generates during storms
   ↓
   Human infection

- **Diagnosis:**
  - Mainly serological through microagglutination, compliment fixation.
  - Isolation is possible but is not recommended due to hazard of laboratory infection.

> **Remember:** Q fever: – Gives negative Weil-Felix reaction.
> – Also transmitted by infected milk.

9. **Ans. (d) Trombiculid mite** Ref. Ananthnarayan 10/e, p 413; Park 22/e p 712
   Trombiculid mite transmit both rickettsia disease (Rickettsial pox) and orientea disease (scrub typhus)

Arthropod-borne diseases	
Arthropod	*Disease transmitted*
Mosquito	Malaria, filaria, viral encephalitis (e.g. Japanese encephalitis), viral fevers (e.g. dengue, West Nile, viral haemorrhagic fevers (e.g. yellow fever, dengue haemorrhagic fever)
Housefly	Typhoid and paratyphoid fever, diarrhoea, dysentery, cholera, gastroenteritis, amoebiasis, helminthic infestations, poliomyelitis, conjunctivitis, trachomas, anthrax, yaws, etc.
Sandfly	**Kala-azar**, oriental sore sandfly fever, oraya fever
Tsetse fly	Sleeping sickness
Louse	Epidemic typhus, relapsing fever, trench fever, pediculosis
Rat flea	Bubonic plague, endemic typhus, chiggerosis, hymenolepis diminuata
Blackfly	Onchocerciasis
Reduviid bug	Chagas disease
Hard tick	Tick typhus, viral encephalitis, viral fevers, viral haemorrhagic fever, (e.g. Kyasanur forest disease), tularemia, tick paralysis, human babesiosis
Soft tick	Q fever, relapsing fever Mnemonic: **QRST**
Trombiculid mite	Scrub typhus, Rickettsial-pox
Itch mite	Scabies
Cyclops	Guinea-worm disease, fish tapeworm (D. latus)
Cockroaches	Enteric pathogens

10. **Ans. (b) Rocky mountain ...** Ref. Ananthnarayan 10/e, p 413

    Family rickettsiae includes six genera:

    - *Rickettsia*   - *Ehrlichia*
    - *Orientia*   - *Anaplasma*
    - *Neorickettsia*   - *Coxiella*

    As question is about disease by rickettsia answer is RMSF (which is caused by *Rickettsia rickettsii*) only as scrub typhus is caused by *Orientia tsutsugamushi*.

11. **Ans (a) crimean... and (b) Rock...** Ref. Park 22/e p 712

    Crimean congo is a viral illness, caused by flavi virus and is transmitted by ticks
    For full details see previous answers

12. **Ans (a) Chlamydia trachomatis** Ref. Ananthnarayan 10/e, p 427
    "Conjuctivitis followed by pneumonia suggest *C. trachomatis*"
    C. trachomatis is also of the commest cause of pneumonia in infant particularly around 2–12 weeks of age.

Clinical manifestations	
Conjunctivitis	**Pneumonia**
• Most frequent clinical manifestation of C. trachomatis infection in the new born. • Sometimes referred to as **inclusion conjunctivitis** of the newborn (ICN) or inclusion blennorrhoea. • **The incubation period for C. Trachomatis conjunctivitis is 5 to 14 days after delivery.** – Presentation before five days is unusual. **Clinical findings of trachoma conjunctivitis range from:** **Mild swelling:** • Watery eye discharge which becomes mucopurulent, • Marked swelling of the eyelids with red and thickened conjunctivae (chemosis). • A pseudo membrane may form as the exudate adheres to conjunctiva. • Blood-stained eye discharge was found to have high specificity and positive predictive value for chlamydial conjunctivitis. • A membrane of granulation tissue (micropannus) may form, especially if the patient is untreated for more than two weeks.	• **Among infants born to mothers with cervical C. trachomatis infection, 5 to 30 percept develop pneumonia.** • Approximately one-half of these have a history of conjunctivitis. • Pneumonia due to C. trachomatis is recognized in most affected infants between **12 weeks** of age, although essentially all are symptomatic before **8 weeks**. • Cough and nasal congestion without significant discharge are common, although occasional infants may have thick nasal secretions. • Otitis media may be present. • Patients usually are afebrile or have minimal fever. • Rales are often present on auscultation of the lungs; • Wheezing is uncommon. • The liver and spleen may be easily palpable because of the hyper inflated lungs. • Preterm infants may have apneic spells associated with the infection.

13. **Ans (d) Penicillin is the treatment**   *Ref. Parson 20/e, p 1070, 1074*

    Penicillin is not effective against Chlamydia

    Drugs effective against *Chlamydia* include

    - Tetracycline
    - Erythromycin
    - Azithromycin
    - Sulfonamides
    - Rifampicin

    • *Chlamydia* can be cultured, but not in cell free media.
    • In most cases trachoma inflammation undergoes spontaneous resolution and only few cases progress to conjunctival scarring.

14. **Ans. (a) McCoy cell line**   *Ref. Ananthnarayan 10/e, p 425, 426; Jawetz 27/e, p 354*

    "Complaint of urethritis with no result on gram staining signifies nongonococcal urethritis."

    MC cause of NGU is *Chlamydia trachomatis* and urethritis is one of the commonest manifestation of genital chlamydiasis.

    Diagnosis of genital chlamydiasis (D-K serovars)

    I. **Culture:**
        – Scarpe epithelial cells from 1-2 cm deep into endocervix.
        – Dacron, cotton, rayon or calcium alginate on plastic shaft should be used to collect specimen.
        – Inoculum is centrifuged onto the monolayer of cyclohexinide treated McCoy cells.
        – This is incubated at 35-37°C for 48-72 hours.
        – Monolayers can be increased.
        – Examine monolayers by direct IF to see inclusion bodies.
        – This method is 80% sensitive but 100% specific.

        Remember: Cell lines for Chlamydia: McCoy, HeLA, HEP-2, HL.

    II. **Direct cytologic examination** (direct fluorescent antibody) and enzyme-linked immunoassay.
    III. **Nucleic acid detection** by PCR and LCR are test of choice to diagnose genital *C. trachomatis* infections.
    IV. **Serology**–Serum antibodies are more common than trachoma because of more antigenicity in genital tract.

        Remember: LJ medium is for *Mycobacteria tuberculosis*. Thayer Martin medium is for *Neiersia*.

15. **Ans. (b) Elementary body is metabolically active**   *Ref. Ananthnarayan 10/e, p 423; Jawetz 27/e, p 351*

Reproductive Cycle of Chlamydiae

Elementary body (EB)
- Stable spherical form, metabolically inactive
- Extracellular phase
- Infectious form
- 200 - 300 nm diameter
- Rigid trilaminar cell wall
- Electron dense nucleoid (contains DNA)
- DNA = RNA

↓

Attach to surface of susceptible epithelial cell near base of microvilli by adhesins (e.g. major outer membrane protein); receptors (heparin sulfate like proteoglycans in case of *C. trachomatis*)

↓

Engulfment of EB into host cell either by endocytosis into clathrin-coated pits or pinocytosis into non-coated pits. Lysosomal fusion is inhibited by unknown mechanism, so EB form of chlamydiae is protected under membrane bound environment.

↓

Reorganisation of EB by spheroplast-like transformation/loss of cross-linking of EB membrane proteins.

↓

Reticulate body (Initial body form)
- Pleomorphic stage
- Intracellular form
- Growing and replicative form
- 500-1000 nm size
- No electron dense nucleoid
- RNA > DNA

Within membrane bound vacuole RB divides by binary fission repeatedly to form EB.

↓

Cytoplasmic inclusion bodies form (EB filled vacuole)

↓

This EB liberate from host cell to infect new cells.

---

16. Ans. (d) Community acquired pneumonia *Ref. Harrison 18/e, p 1422-1425, 19/e, p 1172; Ananthnarayan 10/e, p 426*

Human disease caused by Chlamydiae		
Species	**Serotype**	**Disease**
C. trachomatis	A, B, Ba, C	Endemic blinding trachoma
C. trachomatis	D - K	Inclusion conjunctivitis, genital chlamydiasis, infant pneumonia
C. trachomatis	L1, L2, L3	Lymphogranuloma venereum
C. psittaci	Many serotype	Psittacosis
C. pneumoniae	Only one serotype	Acute respiratory disease

Remember: Inclusion conjunctivitis include inclusion blenorrhea or ophthalmia—neonatorum and swimming pool conjunctivitis. C.pneumoniae is associated with 10% of cases of community acquired pneumonia

Remember: *Four most common cause of community acquired pneumonia are:*
- S. pneumoniae
- Chlamydia pneumoniae
- H. influenzae
- Legionella.

17. Ans. (d) The group specific antigen is responsible for the production of complement fixing antibodies *Ref. Jawetz 27/e, p 355; Ananthnarayan 10/e, p 425*

"*Genus or Group specific heat stable LPS antigen is responsible for CFT while serovar specific major membrane protein is responsible for microimmunofluorescence.*"

Note: Species specific protein antigen helps in classifying chlamydia into chlamydial species.
Serotype specific antigen: Intraspecies typing and demonstrated by microimmunofluorescence.

Characteristic of Chlamydiae			
Feature	**C. trachomatis**	**C. pneumoniae**	**C psittaci**
Inclusion morphology	Round, vacuolar	Round, dense	Large, variable shape, dense
Glycogen in inclusions	Yes	No	No
Elementary body morphology	Round	Pear-shaped, round	Round
Susceptible to sulfonamides	Yes	No	No
DNA homology to C pneumoniae	<10%	100%	<10%

Contd...

Contd...

Characteristic of Chlamydiae

Feature	C. trachomatis	C. pneumoniae	C psittaci
Plasmid	Yes	No	Yes
Serovars	15	1	> 4
Natural host	Humans	Humans	Birds
Mode of transmission	Person-to-person, mother-to-infant	Airborne person-to-person	Airborne bird excreta to humans
Major diseases	Trachoma, STDs, infants pneumonia, LGV	Pneumonia, bronchitis, sinusitis	Psittacosis, pneumonia, fever of unexplained origin

Nucleic Acid Amplification "*Amplification assays such as ligase chain reaction and polymerase chain reaction are the most sensitive chlamydial diagnostic method available.*"

Diagnostic methods for Chlamydia	Accuracy
Cell culture technique	Low sensitivity (60 to 80%)
Direct immunofluorescent antibody test	70-80% sensitive and quite specific
ELISA	60-80% sensitive
LCR and PCR	Most sensitive method available

Note: For occular disease nucleic acid amplification test (NAAT) are not approved by FDA.
For genital chlamydiasis NAAT specimen can be:
– Urine in males
– Cervical/vaginal swabs in females

18. **Ans. (b) Cause non-gonococcal urethritis** *Ref. Ananthnarayan 10/e, p 428; Jawetz 27/e, p 358*
    C. Psittaci
    - Causes psittacoses in humans/birds, ornithosis in birds, meningopneumonitis, feline pneumonitis and other animal diseases.
    - Form *diffuse intracytoplasmic inclusions* that lack glycogen, not stained by I_2 and not inhibited by sulphadiazine or cycloserine. Heat stable group reactive. CF antigen resist proteolytic enzymes so seems to be lipopolysaccharide.
    - Psittacosis is disease of human acquired from contact with birds and also includes infection of psittacine birds.
    - Ornithosis is infection in all types of domestic birds.
    - Infection in birds is usually subclinical (carriers).
    - *Human infection* is usually **occupational** as in poultry workers, pigeon farmers, pet-shop owners, bird fencers and veterinarian. Usually occur by inhalation of infected dried feces.
    - *Incubation period* is about **10 days.**
    - Manifest as influenza/atypical pneumonia/sepsis.
    - Antibodies to species specific antigen can neutralize toxicity and infectivity.
    - **Diagnosis:** – Culture is dangerous and if done; then isolation should be attempted only in special laboratories as laboratory infection is serious hazard.
        – *Detection of antigen by direct fluorescent antibody staining or by immunoassay or PCR is preferred*, serology (confirmatory) by CFT or MIF.
    - **Treatment:** – DOC is tetracycline.
        – Should be continued for 10 days after defervescence to prevent relapse.

19. **Ans. (b) Culture on McCoy cells** *Ref. Ananthnarayan, 10/e, p 425*
    "*Genital chlamydiasis is suspected if Gram stained smear of urogenital exudates show significant number of neutrophils (> 4/oil immersion field in urethritis, > 30 in cervicitis) in absence of gonococcal bacteria.*"
    McCoy and HeLa cell lines are the most common cell lines to cultivate chlamydia

20. **Ans. (b) Enzyme immunoassay** *Ref. Ananthnarayan 10/e, p 425*
    Isolation of Chlamydiae can be done by:
    a. Inoculation into yolk sac of embryonated eggs of 6 - 8 day old chick embryo which may be pretreated by streptomycin or polymyxin B.
    b. Inoculation into experimental animals (mice): Intranasal; intraperitoneal or intracerebral inoculation
    c. Tissue/cell culture:
        – *Preferred mode*
        – Commonly used cell lines are McCoy and HeLa cells.
        – Cell cultures are pretreated by irradiation or chemicals such as 5-iodo-2 deoxyuridic or cycloheximide to enhance replication and detection of inclusion bodies.
        – Pretreatment with DEAE dextrax or centrifugation after inoculation promotes contact between chlamydiae particles and cell monolayer.

21. **Ans. (c) They can grow in cell free culture media** *Ref. Ananthnarayan 10/e, p 425*
    - *Chlamydia* are obligate intracellular parasite so, they cannot be grown in cell free media.
    - McCoy and HeLa cell lines are *MC cell lines* used to culture chlamydiae.
    - Chlamydia are Gram-negative coccobacilli.
    - Chlamydia do not have peptidoglycan cell wall.
    - They lack enzymes of electron transport chain. So require ATP from host cells and are called energy parasites.
    - *Drugs effective against chlamydiae:* Doxycycline azithromycin, erythromycin.

    Remember: Other obligate parasite: Rickettsiaceae, M. laprae, pathogenic treponemas and Coxiella burnetii.

22. **Ans. (a) *Chlamydia trachomatis*** *Ref. Harrison 19/e, p 1167, 20/e 1318; Ananthnarayan 10/e, p 427*
    "Complaint of urethritis with no result on Gram staining signifies Non-gonoccocal urethritis."
    Chlamydia is the commonest cause of non-gonococcal and post gonococcal urethritis

23. **Ans. (d) Urethritis** *Ref. Ananthnarayan 10/e, p 427*
    - Urethritis is one of the presentation of serovar D-K
    - Genital chlamydiasis, caused by serotype D-K of *C. trachomatis*.
    - *C. pneumonia* increase the risk of arthrosclerosis, asthma, sarcoidosis.

24. **Ans. (a), (c) and (d) Conjunctivitis, Polyarthritis, Mucosal lesions** *Ref. Harrison 19/e, p 1168, 20/e, p 1368*
    Reiter's syndrome consists of *conjunctivitis, urethritis, (or in female patient cervicitis) arthritis and characteristic mucocutaneous lesion.*
    - Pathogenesis is unknown. However more than 80% affected patient belong **to HLA-B-27.**
    - It may develop in 1-2% cases of non-gonococcal urethritis and is thought to be the *most common type of peripheral inflammatory arthritis in young men.*
    - Other implicated bacteria includes Salmonella, Shigella, Yersinia or Campylobacter
    - Arthritis usually begin 4 weeks after the onset of urethritis
    - *Knees followed by ankle are the most frequently involved joint*

25. **Ans. (b) Nucleic acid amplification test** *Ref. Harrison, 20/e p 1318*
    "At least 1/3 of males with C. trachomatis urethral infection have no symptoms. Use of NAAT (Nucleic acid amplification test) using PCR, LCR, TMA on first void urine specimen is highly sensitive in detecting these infections".
    Among all test for detection of chlamydia these NAAT tests are most sensitive. They can be applied for all infection sites viz conjunctiva (on conjunctival scrapings); pneumonia (on sputum); proctitis (rectal secretions) etc.

    Types of NAAT for Chlamydia
    - PCR (Polymerase chain reaction)
    - LCR (Ligase chain reaction)
    - TMA (Transcription mediated assay)
    - Gene probe optima CT assay

    - In all NAAT the *Gen Probe optima CT assay* which utilises target capture and RNA amplification is *most sensitive and specific.*
    - The main limitation of these tests is their cost and availability

26. **Ans. (b) Yolk Sac inoculation** ...*Ref. Ananthnarayan 10/e, p 425*
    Already explained

27. **Ans. (a) Elimentary body is** ...*Ref. Ananthnarayan 10/e, p 423*
    Already explained

28. **Ans. (a) *Chlamydia trachomatis*** ...*Ref. Harrison 20/e, p 1318*
    The patient is suffering from non-gonoccocal urethritis and *C. trachomatis* is the most common cause of non gonococcal urethritis.

Cause of non-gonococcal urethritis	
Chlamydia trachomatis (MC)	**Ureaplasma urealyticum**
Trichomonas vaginalis	Herpes simplex virus
Mycoplasma hominis	CMV
Gardnerella vaginalis	Acinetobacter iwoffii, Ac calcoaceticus
Candida albicans	

29. **Ans. (b) Nucleic acid amplification testing** *Ref. Harisson 18/e, p1426*
    Already explained

NEET Pattern Questions

1. **Inclusion body is seen in:**
   a. Rickettsiae   b. Chlamydia
   c. Mycoplasma   d. H. Pylori
   [Ref. Ananthanarayan, 10/e, p 423]

2. **All of the following are true about Chlamydia except:**
   a. Gram positive   b. Causes trachoma
   c. Causative organism of psittacosis
   d. Are also called tasophilic viruses
   [Ref. Ananthanarayan, 10/e, p 423]

3. **True about chlamydia are all except:**
   a. Obligate intracellular organism
   b. Gram positive
   c. Reticulate body is metabolically active
   d. Replicate by binary fission
   [Ref. Ananthanarayan 10/e p 423]

- Cell wall of chlamydia resemble Gr (−)ve bacteria.

4. **Obligatory intracellular organism is:**
   a. Mycoplasma   b. Chlamydia
   c. Cryptococcus   d. H. pylori
   [Ref. Ananthanarayan, 10/e, p422]

5. **Chlamydia pneumoniae causes:**
   a. LGV   b. Atherosclerosis
   c. Inclusion conjunctivitis
   d. Trachoma   [Ref. Ananthanarayan, 10/e, p 423]

6. **True about chlamydia is:**
   a. Replicative form is elementary body
   b. Infective form to host cell is elementary body
   c. Cell wall contains N-acetylmuramic acid and peptidoglycan
   d. All of the above are correct   [Ref. AA, 10/e, p 423]

7. **LGV (lymphogranuloma venereum) is caused by:**
   a. Treponema pallidum   b. Chlamydia trachomatis
   c. Calymmatobacter granulomatosis
   d. H.ducreyi   [Ref. Harrison, 20/e, p 1320]

8. **How does chlamydia differ from other usual bacteria?**
   a. Lack cell wall
   b. Cannot grow in cell free culture media
   c. Contains inclusion body
   d. None of the above   [Ref. Ananthanarayan, 10/e, p 423]

- Cell wall of chlamydia resemble that of Gr(-)ve bacteria.

9. **Frie's test is useful for diagnosis of:**
   a. Mycoplasma   b. Rickettsia
   c. Sarcoidosis   d. Chlamydia
   [Ref. Ananthanarayan, 10/e, p 428]

- **Frie test:** Demonstration of hypersensitivity by skin testing was widely used for diagnosis of LGV. But due to high false positivity it has been given up.

10. **True about chlamydia:**
    a. Extracellular bacteria   b. HeLa cells for isolation
    c. Gram positive   d. Penicillin is drug of choice
    [Ref. Ananthanarayan, 10/e, p 425]

11. **"Genital elephantiasis" is seen in:**
    a. Rickettsia
    b. Chancroid
    c. Lymphogranuloma venereum
    d. Syphilis   [Ref. Anantharayan 10/e, p 428]

In tertiary stage of LGV elephantiasis of vulva is there

12. **Trachoma is caused by which serotype of chlamydia trachomatis?**
    a. D to K   b. A, B, C
    c. $L_1 L_2 L_3$ d. All of the above
    [Ref. Ananthanarayan, 10/e, p 423]

13. **Bubus form is which stage of LGV?**
    a. Prmary   b. Secondary
    c. Tertiary   d. Latent
    [Ref. Harrison 19/e, p 1170, Greenwood 18/e, p 385]

14. **Weil Felix reaction for Scrub typhus shows positivity for:**
    a. OXK   b. OXK + OX19
    c. OX-2   d. OX-19
    [Ref. Ananthanarayan, 10/e, p417]

15. **Which of the following is used for Rickettsia?**
    a. Weil-Felix reaction   b. Rose-Waler test
    c. Paul-Bunnell test   d. VDRL   [Ref. AA, 10/e, p417]

16. **Tunica reaction is positive in:**
    a. R prowazekii   b. R typhi
    c. R tsutsugamushi   d. R akari
    [Ref. Ananthanarayan, 10/e, p 414]

- **Neil-Mooser = Tunica reaction:** When male guinea pigs are inoculated intraperitoneally with blood from a case of endemic typhus or with culture of *R. typhi*, they develop fever and a characteristic scrotal inflammation. The testes can not be pushed back into scrotum because of inflammatory adhesions between the layers of tunica vaginalis. The reaction is negative with *R. prowazakaii*.

1. b. Chlamydia	2. a. Gram positive	3. b. Gram positive	4. b. Chlamydiae	5. b. Atherosclerosis
6. b. Infective form…	7. b. Chlamydia…	8. b. Cannot grow…	9. d. Chlamydia	10. b. HeLa cells…
11. c. Lympho…	12. b. A, B, C	13. b. Secondary	14. a. OXK	
15. a. Weil-Felix reaction	16. b. *R typhi*			

17. Rickettsial infections cause 30% mortality due to:
    a. Endothelial injury
    b. Hemodynamic instability
    c. Endocarditis
    d. Renal failure   [Ref. Ananthanarayan, 10/e, p 413–14]

18. Vector for scrub typhus:
    a. Reduvid bug
    b. Trombiculid mite
    c. Enteric pathogens
    d. Cyclops
                              [Ref. Ananthanarayan, 10/e, p 413]

19. Endemic typhus is caused by:
    a. R prowazekii   b. R typhi
    c. R tsutsugamushi   d. R akari
                              [Ref. Ananthanarayan, 10/e, p 413]

20. Brill-Zinsser disease is:
    a. Recrudescent of R prowazekii infection
    b. Recrudescent of R typhi infection
    c. Recrudescent of R conorii infection
                              [Ref. Ananthanarayan, 10/e, p 414]

> In some patients who recover from epidemic typhus, (caused by R. Prowazekii) the rickettsiae may remain latent in lymphoid tissue. Such latent injection may at times get reactivated leading to recuredescent typhus.

21. Eschar is seen in all the Rickettsial diseases *except*:
    a. Scrub typhus
    b. Rickettsial pox
    c. Indian tick typhus
    d. Endemic typhus   [Ref. Jawetz 27/e, p 343]

22. The primary site of multiplication of rickettsial organisms is in the:
    a. Parenchymal cells of the liver
    b. Endothelial cells of small vessels
    c. Media of arteries
    d. Adventitia of all blood vessels
                              [Ref. Ananthanarayan 10/e, p 413]

> On entry into the human body, the rickettsiae multiply locally and enter the blood. They become localized in vascular endothelial cells which gets enlarged, degenerate and cause thrombus formation with partial or complete occlusion of vascular lumen.

23. Bartonella henselae causes all *except*:
    a. Oraya fever
    b. Cat scratch disease
    c. Bacillary angiomatosis
    d. SABE
                              [Ref. Ananthanarayan 10/e, p 420]

- Bartonella are tiny gram negative bacteria, usually transmitted by arthropods which invades mammalian endothelial cells and blood cells. Human pathogenic strains are:
- B. Baciliformis, B. quintana and B. henslae

Organism	Disease
B. Henslae	Cat scratch disease, bacillary angiomatosis bacillary peliosis, bacterial endocarditis.
B. quintana	Trench fever or five day fever
B. bacilliformis	Oraya fever, Verruga peruana (carrions disease)

24. Cat scratch disease is caused by:
    a. Streptobacillus moniliformis
    b. Spirillum minus
    c. B. Henselae
    d. R. tsutsugamushi   [Ref. Ananthanarayan, 10/e, p 420]

Disease caused by bartonella henselae
- Cat scratch desease
- Bacillary angiomatosis
- Bacillary peliosis

25. Bartonella quintana causes:
    a. Trench fever   b. Scrub typhus
    c. Endemic typhus   d. Epidemic typhus
                              [Ref. Ananthanarayan, 10/e, p 419]

Trench fever or five day fever is an exclusive human disease seen in European soldiers fighting in trenches.
- Transmitted by body louse. Body louse remain infective for whole life
- Etiologic agent is Rochalimae quintana also called as B. quintana

26. Which of the following infection is mainly diagnosed by serological tests?
    a. Actinomycosis   b. Q Fever
    c. TB   d. Leprosy
                              [Ref. Ananthanarayan, 10/e, p 418]

Q fever is caused by pleomorphic coccobacilli Coxiella burnetti which is an obligate intracellular pathogen primarily infecting monocyte-macrophage cellls.
Diagnosis is made by serology: Compliment fixation-list or indirect immunofluorescence assay.

27. Anthropozoonosis are all *except*:
    a. Guinea worm infection
    b. Rabies
    c. Plague
    d. Hydatid cyst   [Ref. Park 22/e, p 90]

- Anthropozoonoses: Infections transmitted to non from vertebrate animal e.g. Rabies, plague
- Zoonthroposis: Infections transmitted from non to vertebrate animal e.g. human tuberculosis in cattle.

17. a. Endothelial injury	18. b. Trombiculid...	19. b. *R typhi*	20. a. Recrudescent...	
21. d. Endemic typhus	22. b. Endothelial ...	23. a. Oraya fever	24. c. B. Henselae	
25. a. Trench fever	26. b. Q Fever	27. a. Guinea worm ...		

CHAPTER 22

Spirochetes

Group comprising: Elongated, motile, flexible bacteria.
Characteristic feature of spirochetes is *presence of varying number of endoflagella* which are polar flagella situated between outer membrane and cell wall (periplasmic space). Unlike flagella of other bacteria they *don't protrude outside*.
Pathogenic spirochetes belong to genera:
1. *Treponema*
2. *Borrelia*
3. *Leptospira*

> **Treponema**
> - Spiral bacteria actively motile (by endoflagella)
> - Don't stain by Gram's method
> - Possess fine cytoplasmic filaments which are absent in Borrelia
> - Pathogenic treponemes cannot be cultivated.

TREPONEMA

- Relatively short slender spirochetes with fine spiral and **pointed or rounded ends.**
- Pathogenic treponemes **have not been successfully cultivated in** cell free media while the non-pathogenic [which are commensals] can be cultivated.
- **Pathogenic treponemes include:**
  - *T. pallidum* (causative agent of endemic and venereal syphilis)
  - *T. partenue* (causative agent of yaws)
  - *T. carateum* (causative agent of pinta)

  They are identical in their morphology, antigenic structure and other biochemical features, differs only in clinical feature of disease they produce. But recently molecular signatures have been identified that can differentiate the three subspecies of *T. pallidum* by PCR based methods.
  ... *Harrison 20/e, p 1280*

> - *T. pallidum:* Syphilis
> - *T. partenue:* Yaws
> - *T. carateum:* Pinta

TREPONEMA PALLIDUM

Morphology
- A thin spiral organism which is actively motile through endoflagella.
- *Seen* by **immunofluorescence staining** or dark field illumination or phase contrast microscope.
- *Stained* by **silver impregnation methods.** Fontana method useful for staining films and Levaditi method for tissue sections.

Cultures and Growth
- **Pathogenic treponemes** have **never been cultured** continuously on artificial media, in fertile eggs or in tissue culture as pathogenic treponemes lack genes required for de novo synthesis of amino acids, nucleotides and lipids. They also lacks the genes encoding for the enzymes of Krebs cycle and oxidative phosphorylation
- *Reiter strain (T. phagedenis)* - Non-pathogenic. treponeme; shows morphological and antigenic similarities with *T. pallidum*; can grow in artificial culture.
- As such *T. pallidum* is *microaerophilic* organism and survives best in 1-4% O_2.
- Virulent *T. pallidum* strains can be maintained by serial testicular passage in rabbits. One such strains called **Nichol strain** was isolated in 1912 and is still being propagated.
- In whole blood or plasma stored at 4°C, organisms remain viable for at least 24 hours, which is of potential importance in blood transfusions.

T-pallidum
- Microaerophilic
- Enters tissue by penetrating intact mucosa or abraded skin
- Primary syphilis: Chancre
- Secondary syphilis: Macular or pustular lesion on the trunk and extremities
- Tertiary: Neurosyphilis, cardiovascular syphilis, gummatous syphilis.
- Lesions of secondary syphilis are most infectious.

Antigenic Structure

- Treponemal infection induce 3 antibodies:
  - **Reagin antibody:** It is responsible for *Wasermann reaction, Kahn test* and **VDRL**. In these reactions a hapten called cardiolipin *[extracted from beef heart]* is used as antigen. Chemically cardiolipin is diphosphatidylglycerol.
  - *Antibody to group antigen* which is found in both pathogenic and non-pathogenic treponemes.
  - **Antibody to species specific** antigen which is polysaccharide in nature and is positive only with sera of patients infected with pathogenic treponemes.

Clinical Manifestations

Natural infection with *T. pallidum* occurs *only in* human beings. It causes:

1. **Venereal Syphilis** (See color plate, pg xxxi for related image)
   - Acquired by sexual contact. **Infectivity** of patient to its sexual partner is maximum during *1st two years of disease.*
   - *In 1905, Schaudinn and Hoffmann discovered Treponema pallidum in tissue of patients with syphilis. One year later, the first effective test for syphilis, the Wassermann test, was developed*
   - Treponema rapidly penetrates intact mucous membrane or microscopic abrasions in skin and within few hours enters the lymphatics and blood to produce systematic infection.
   - Blood from the patient with incubating or early syphilis is infectious.
   - Natural history fall into *3 stages:*

Location of chancre:
- Heterosexual male: penis
- Female: Cervix, Labia

Primary syphilis	Primary lesion of syphilis *is painless hard chancre* at the site of entry of spirochete which heal without scar in 10 - 40 days.
	Cases in which syphilis is acquired non-venerally [as occupationally in doctors] primary chancre is *extragenital usually on fingers*.
	Cases in which syphilis is transmitted by blood transfusion chancre don't occur.
	Persistent or multiple chancres may be seen in HIV infected or other immunodeficient patient.
Secondary syphilis	3 months after primary lesion.
	Reseolar or papular skin rashes, mucous patches in oropharynx and condylomata at mucocutaneous junction are characteristic lesions. Spirochetes are abundant in the lesions. These condylomata lata are highly infectious and are *most common* in groin or inner thigh.
	Patient *is most infectious* during this stage.
Tertiary syphilis	Consist of *cardiovascular lesions; chronic granuloma (gummata) & meningovascular manifestations such as tabes dorsalis.*

Remember: Latent syphilis: – Period of quiescence between secondary and tertiary stage.
– During this period diagnosis is only possible by serological test.

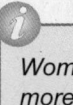

Woman with early syphilis is more infective to her child

2. **Congenital syphilis**
   - *Woman with early syphilis is more infective* to her child.
   - Transmission across placenta can take place at any time, but lesions of congenital syphilis have their onset after 4th month of gestation. So, adequate treatment of mother before 4th month of pregnancy prevents fetal damage.
   - **Earliest sign** of congenital syphilis is rhinitis or snuffles (23%), mucocutaneous Lesions (35–41%). ....Harrison 20/e, p 1283
   - MC early **manifestation** are bone changes, hepatosplenomegaly, lymphadenopathy.
   - *Clutton's joint (Bilateral knee effusion), interstitial keratitis* are late manifestation.
   - Residual stigmata of congenital syphilis are:

Hutchinson's teeth	:	Centrally notched, widely placed upper central incisor.
Mulberry molars	:	Sixth year molars with poorly developed cusps.
Rhagades	:	Linear scars at angle of mouth.

Spirochetes

3. **Neurosyphilis**
- Traditionally neurosyphilis is considered a late manifestation of syphilis which is now proved to be wrong.
- Asymptomatic neurosyphilis: Patient who lack neurologic symptoms and signs but have CSF abnormalities like mononuclear pleocytosis.
- Asymptomatic infection is seen in 40% of primary and secondary syphilis and in 25% of cases of latent syphilis.
- Symptomatic neurosyphilis:

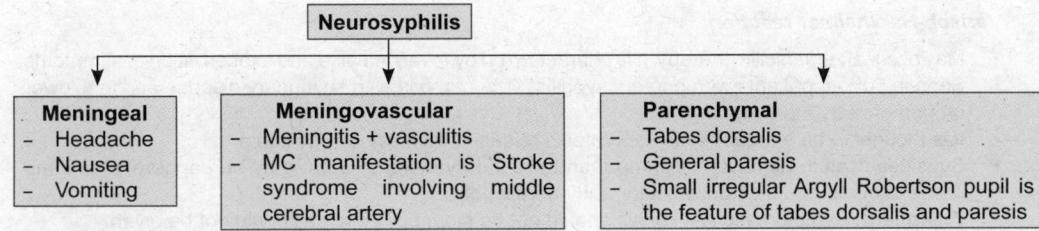

Meningeal	Meningovascular	Parenchymal
- Headache - Nausea - Vomiting	- Meningitis + vasculitis - MC manifestation is Stroke syndrome involving middle cerebral artery	- Tabes dorsalis - General paresis - Small irregular Argyll Robertson pupil is the feature of tabes dorsalis and paresis

4. **Cardiovascular syphilis:**
   - Aortitis, Aortic regurgitation, saccular aneurysm.

Diagnosis

1. *Demonstration of Organism*
   - **Darkfield microscopic examination of lesion** exudate such as chancre of primary syphilis or more reliably by immunofluorescence or immunohistochemical method.

2. *Serological test for syphilis*

Nontreponemal test	Treponemal test
Detect IgG or IgM against cardiolipin antigen	Detect specific antibody against T. pallidum
1. RPR (Rapid plasma reagin) *[test of choice for rapid diagnosis]*	Includes: Fluorescent treponemal antibody absorption test **[F-TAABS]**
2. VDRL *[test of choice for response to therapy and for examining CSF]*	- Agglutination assays **(MHATP, TPHA, TPPA)**
VDRL is type of slide flocculation test while Kahn flocculation is tube test	- TPI (Treponemal pallidum immobilisation) test
Group specific treponemal tests: • These tests used the Reiter treponemes to avoid biological false positive • Reiter protein complement fixation (RPCF) test is the most commonly employed group specific treponemal test. • RPCF uses a lipopolysaccharide - protein complex antibody using a lipopolysaccharide - protein complex	

> *FTA-ABS is the most sensitive test for syphilis TPI is the most specific test.*

> *RPR test of choice for rapid clinical diagnosis.*

Remember:
- FTA-ABS, TPPA are most sensitive test. FTA - ABS is (+) ve in approx. 80%, 100% & 95% of primary, secondary and late syphilis respectively [Greenwood 18/e p 370]
- TPI is most specific serological test.
- TPPA has supplanted the FTA-ABS test as diagnostic test. ... CMDT' 2014, p 1419
- RPR is the test of choice for rapid diagnosis in clinically setting
  ...Harrison 20/e p 1284

3. **EIA and CIA (chemiluminescence)**
   - These test are simple sensitive specific and yield rapid result so they are now the initial test for screening. ...CMDT 2014, p 1419

4. **Diagnosis of neurosyphilis**
   - Examination of CSF for pleocytosis, increase protein concentration, VDRL reactivity.

5. **Diagnosis of congenital syphilis**
   - If both test i.e. **VDRL** and **FTA- ABS IgM** (specific) test are positive in the infant then congenital syphilis should be strongly suspected and the child should be treated.

Diagnosis of congenital syphilis: FTA-ABS IgM

Treatment

Stage of syphilis	DOC	Patient with penicillin allergy
Primary secondary or early latent	Penicillin benzathine	Tetracycline or Doxycycline
Late latent	Penicillin G	Tetracycline
Neurosyphilis	Aqueous penicillin G	Desensitization and treatment with penicillin
Syphilis in pregnancy	Penicillin	Desensitization and treatment with penicillin

Jarisch-Herxheimer reaction:

- May occur after penicillin therapy. It is characterized by fever, malaise and exacerbation of symptoms
- Seen in 50% of patients with primary syphilis, 90% of those with secondary disease and in a lower proportion with late stage disease
- It is thought to be a response to lipoproteins released from dying T. pallidum
- Subsides itself in all cases of primary and secondary syphilis. But it may be dangerous in some cases of gummatous cardiovascular and neurosyphilis
- *Treatment:* Symptomatic - Antibiotic should not be stopped. Steroids should not be given.

JH reaction
Mediated by release of lipoproteins, cytokines and immune complexes.

Evaluation of response to therapy:
- Response to treatment is determined by monitoring VDRL or RPR titer.
- Activity *of neurosyphilis is* best correlated with CSF pleocytosis.

Remember: Continued susceptibility of treponema to penicillin is due to its highly conserved genome.

NON-VENEREAL TREPONEMATOSIS

Infection usually transmitted by body to body contact. It includes:

A. Endemic syphilis: (Bejel)
 - Caused by *T. pallidum* subspecies endemicum
 - Disease is common in young children, primary chancre is not usually seen.
 - *Treatment:* Same as venereal syphilis.

B. Yaws:
 - Caused *by T. pallidum* subspecies *T. pertenue* which is morphologically and Immunologically identical to T. pallidum. *(Mnemonic Py)*
 - Primary lesion is extragenital papule which enlarges and ulcerate to form an ulcerating granuloma.

C. Pinta:
 - *Causative agent T.carateum (Mnemonic Cap).*
 - It is not identical but closely related to T. pallidum.
 - *Primary lesion* is extragenital papule which doesn't ulcerate but develop into lichenoid or psoriatic patch.

Remember: In non-venereal treponematosis, yaws (*always*) and pinta (*usually*) **serological test of syphilis are positive**.

LEPTOSPIRA

Leptospira
- Zoonosis with widest geographical distribution.
- Rodents are the most important reservoir
- Mainly affects liver and kidney where it damages endothelial cells to produce vasculitis.

Actively motile spirochetes possessing a large number of closely wound spirals and characteristic *hooked ends.*

Genus contains two species **L. interoorgans** being **pathogenic** and **L. biflexo** which is **saprophytic**

- **Culture:** Grow *best* under **aerobic condition at 28-32°C**. Leptospirae derive energy from oxidation of long chain fatty acid and cannot use amino acid or carbohydrate as major energy source. So, for isolation **EMJH** media is used.
- **Fletcher medium** is another selective media.

Pathogenesis and clinical manifestation:

- Leptospirosis is a **zoonosis** with **rodents** being most important reservoir.

- **Transmission** results from ingestion or contact with urine, blood or tissue from infected animal but not from bite. Since leptospires are excreted in urine of infected rat, *water is important vehicle*. Human to human transmission is rare.
- **Vasculitis is responsible for most clinical manifestation.**
- It mainly infects: – Liver *(centrilobular necrosis is found)*
  – Kidney *(cause interstitial nephritis, tubular necrosis)*
- After formation of antibody, leptospires are eliminated from all sites except *the eye, proximal renal tubules and brain.*
- More than 40% of symptomatic person have mild and anti-icteric form of leptospirosis.
- Severe leptospirosis is characterized by **profound jaundice, renal dysfunction, hemorrhagic diathesis called as** Weil's syndrome or Icterohemorrhagic fever.

Compared with serology, **PCR** offers a great advantage, particularly early diagnosis within first 5 days of illness
Harrison, 18/e, p 1145

Diagnosis

1. Direct demonstration	– PCR, dark field examination of centrifuged urine
2. Isolation of organism	– From blood or CSF during 1st 10 days
	– From urine after 1 week
	– For *isolation EMJH medium is useful*
3. Serology Type specific (indicates serovar)	– **Microscopic agglutination test [MAT] (Gold Standard)**
	– **Macroscopic agglutination test**
Gene specific (Identity infection without indicating serovar)	– **ELISA**
	– Sensitized erythrocyte lysis
	– CFT
	– Indirect immunofluorescence

– ....*Harrison 20/e, p 1283*

Treatment
– *Mild* - Doxycycline or Ampicillin.
– *Moderate/severe* - Penicillin or Erythromycin.
Chemoprophylaxis: Doxycycline

BORRELIA

- Large, refractile spirochetes which can be *stained by ordinary method* and are Gram (–) ve.
- Pathogenic species are:

B. burgdorferi	-	Causes Lyme's disease
B. recurrentis	-	Causes Relapsing fever
B. vincenti	-	Causes Vincent angina

Borrelia
Causative agent of:
- **Relapsing fever:** Borrelia recurrentis
- **Lyme disease:** B. burgdorferi. The most common vector borne (Ixodid tick) infection in Europe.

LYMES' DISEASE (LYME BORRELIOSIS)

- Causative agent *B.burgdorferi.*
- **MC** vector born infection in **Europe. Transmitted by bite of Ixodid ticks.**
  .... *Harrison 19/e, p 1149, 18/e, p 1401*
- **Clinical features**
  a. **Stage I. (Localized infection)**
    - After incubation period of 3 to 32 days EM occurs at the site of bite. EM (Erythema migrans) is not painful.
    - Erythema migrans usually begin as red macule or papule at the site of the tick bite that expands slowly to form a large annular lesion.
  b. **Stage II. Disseminated infection**
    - Disseminate hematogenously to produce secondary annular skin lesion, meningitis, carditis (*MC* cardiac finding is fluctuating degree of Atrioventricular heart block).
  c. **Stage III. Persistent infection**
    - Usually present as oligoarticular arthritis (*MC* knee), encephalopathy, polyneuropathy. Acrodermatitis chronica atrophicans is late skin manifestation.

For diagnosis of Lyme's disease serological tests are preferred.
Harrison 19/e p 1151

- **Diagnosis**
  - ELISA followed by western blot is *best investigation*.
  - VIsEC$_6$ peptide IgG ELISA is the most promising second generation serological test.
  - Culture in BSK medium gives definitive diagnosis but not useful clinically.
  - PCR particularly in persistent infection.
- **Treatment**
  - For **nervous manifestation** and 3° heart block – *Ceftriaxone* is *DOC*.
    ..... Harrison 19/e, p 1153, 18/e, p 1405
  - For **skin manifestation, arthritis 1° and 2° AV block** – *Doxycycline* is *DOC*.

RELAPSING FEVER

- Causative agent *B. recurrentis*.
- It is of 2 types:
  - *Louse borne* and *Tick borne*, *Borrelia* causing them are indistinguishable.
  - *Louse borne* relapsing fever occur as *epidemic*.
  - *B. recurrentis* is an *exclusive human pathogen* transmitted from person to person through body lice (Pediculus humanus corporis)
  - *Tick borne* occur as *sporadic/endemic* cases.
- **Treatment:** Erythromycin is *DOC*.

VINCENT ANGINA

- Causative agent *B. vincenti*
- Normal mouth commensal, but when associated with fusiform bacilli (Fusobacterium fusiform) causes ulcerative gingivostomatitis or oropharyngitis called vincent angina.
- **Treatment:** Penicillin and Metronidazole.

Multiple Choice Questions

Syphilis

1. Diagnosis of neurosyphilis is made by: [NEET Pattern 2019]
   a. FTa Abs
   b. RPR
   c. VDRL
   d. TPI

2. Congenital syphilis can be diagnosed by: [AI 11]
   a. IgM FTA BS
   b. IgG FTA ABS
   c. VDRL
   d. TPI

3. False +ve VDRL is/are seen in: [PGI 2011]
   a. Leprosy
   b. Malaria
   c. Relapsing fever
   d. IV drug user
   e. HIV infection

4. All are true about FTA-ABS Syphilis, except: [AI 00]
   a. FTA-ABS becomes negative after treatment
   b. Present in secondary syphilis
   c. It is a sensitive test
   d. May be positive in Lyme's disease

5. 'Chancre redux' is a clinical feature of: [AIIMS 06]
   a. Early relapsing syphilis
   b. Late syphilis
   c. Chancroid
   d. Recurrent herpes simplex infection

6. A 23-year-old male had unprotected sexual intercourse with a commercial sex worker. Two weeks later he developed a painless, indurated ulcer on the glans that exudated clear serum on pressure. Inguinal lymph nodes in both groins were enlarged and non-tender. Most appropriate diagnostic test is: [AIIMS 18]
   a. Gram's stain of ulcer discharge
   b. Dark field microscopy of ulcer discharge
   c. Giemsa stain of lymph node aspirate
   d. ELISA for HIV infection

7. Spirochetes among following are: [PGI 06]
   a. Syphilis
   b. Leptospira
   c. Mycoplasma
   d. Brucella
   e. Borrelia

8. True about primary chancre: [PGI Dec 2008]
   a. Painless ulcer
   b. Painless lymphadenopathy
   c. Covered with exudate
   d. Indurated lesion
   e. Organism can be cultured from exudative fluid

9. False positive Nontreponemal serological test for syphilis are seen in: [PGI Dec 2008]
   a. HIV Infection
   b. Collagen disorders
   c. Paediatric age group
   d. Tuberculosis

10. Most sensitive test for Treponema: [AIIMS 10]
    a. VDRL
    b. RPR
    c. FTA-ABS
    d. Kahn

11. A 25-year-old labourer presented 3 years back with penile ulcer which remain untreated. Later he presented with neurological symptoms for which he has taken appropriate treatment. Test to monitor response to treatment is: [AIIMS 09]
    a. VDRL
    b. TPI
    c. FTA Abs
    d. ELISA

12. A male patient presented with agitation, restlessness and neck stiffness. He had undergone treatment for penile ulcer - 3 years back. Lab investigation used for prognosis of treatment: [AIIMS 10]
    a. TPI
    b. VDRL
    c. FTA-ABS
    d. Dark field microscopy

13. Which is true about syphilis? [PGI 2017]
    a. VDRL test detects antibodies
    b. Jarisch herxheimer reaction-IgE mediated
    c. Penicillin is preferred treatment for primary and secondary stage
    d. RPR can be done for CSF

Non-venereal Treponemas

14. Which is not true about Yaws? [AI 08]
    a. Spread by sexual transmission
    b. Caused by T. pertenue
    c. Has cross immunity with syphilis
    d. Cannot be differentiated serologically from T. pallidum

15. Non-venereal treponemas is/are: [PGI 14]
    a. T. pertenue
    b. T. carateum
    c. T. pallidum
    d. T. cuniculi

16. About yaws all are true except: [AI 11]
    a. Caused by T. pertenue
    b. Transmitted non-venereally
    c. Secondary yaw can involve bones
    d. Later stages involves heart and nerves

17. True about Yaws: [PGI May 2013]
    a. Sexually transmitted disease
    b. Transmitted by fomites
    c. Mother-child transmission
    d. Periostitis occurs
    e. Caused by T. pallidum subspecies endemicum

Leptospira

18. Conjunctival hyperemia is the manifestation of:
    [NEET Pattern 2019]
    a. Viral hepatitis   b. Leptospirosis
    c. Malaria   d. Meningitis

19. Serological test for leptospirosis
    [NEET Pattern 2019; AIIMS 2016]
    a. Cold agglatination
    b. Hemagglutination
    c. Microscopic agglutination
    d. None of the above

20. A bacterial disease with 3 'R's i.e. rats, rice fields and rainfall is: [AI 05]
    a. Leptospirosis   b. Plague
    c. Melioidosis   d. Rodent bite fever

21. A sweeper involved with repair-work of sewers was admitted with fever, jaundice and renal failure. The most appropriate test to diagnose infection of this patients:
    a. Weill-Felix test   [AI 18]
    b. Paul-Bunnell test
    c. Microscopic agglutination test
    d. Microimmunofluorescence test

22. Which bacterium best exemplifies the information provided in the image? [AIIMS 2017]

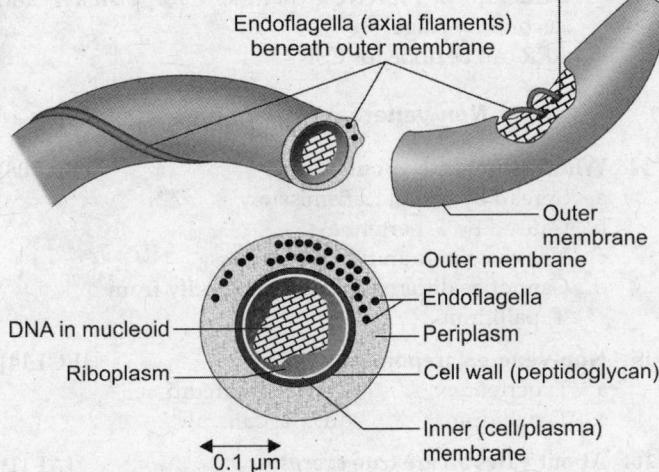

    a. Helicobacter pylori
    b. Leptospira icterohaemorrhagiae
    c. Mycobacterium tuberculosis
    d. Vibrio cholerae

23. The following statements are true regarding leptospirosis, except: [AIIMS 06]
    a. It is a zoonosis
    b. Man is the dead end host
    c. Man is an accidental host
    d. Lice acts as reservoir of infection

24. True regarding leptospirosis is: [AI 11]
    a. Rats are the only reservoirs
    b. Fluoroquinolones are the DOC
    c. Person to person transmission rare
    d. Hepatorenal syndrome occurs in 50% cases

Borrelia

25. The following are true regarding Lyme's Disease, except: [PGI 13]
    a. It is transmitted by Ixodes tick
    b. Erythema chronicum migraines may be a clinical feature
    c. Borrelia recurrentis is the etiologic agent
    d. Rodents act as natural hosts

26. A 25-year-old farmer presented with history of high grade fever for 7 days and altered sensorium for 2 day. On examination, he was comatosed and had conjunctival hemorrhage. Urgent investigations showed a hemoglobin of 11 gm/dl. Peripheral blood smear was negative for malarial parasite. What is the most likely diagnosis? [AIIMS 05]
    a. Brucellosis   b. Weil's disease
    c. Acute viral hepatitis d. Q fever

27. Which one of the following microorganisms uses antigenic variation as a major means of invading host defenses? [AIIMS 04]
    a. Streptococcus pneumonia
    b. Borrelia recurrentis
    c. Mycobacterium tuberculosis
    d. Listeria monocytogenes

28. Which of the following species of borrelia cause relapsing fever? [AI 09]
    a. Borrelia recurrentis b. Borrelia hermsii
    c. Borrelia turicatae   d. Borrelia duttonii

29. Tick born relapsing fever is/are caused by: [PGI 14]
    a. Borrelia recurrentis b. Borrelia duttonii
    c. Borrelia burgdorferi d. Borrelia hermsii
    e. None of above

30. Lymes disease all are true except:
    [AIIMS 10, 11]
    a. Borrelia burgdorferi replicates locally and invades locally
    b. Infection progresses in spite of good humoral immunity
    c. Polymorphonuclear leukocytoses in CSF suggest meningeal involvement
    d. Intrathecal IgA confirms meningitis.

Spirochetes

Explanations and References with Illustrative Answers

1. **Ans. (c) VDRL**   *Ref. Harrison 20/e, p1284*
   Evaluation of Neurosyphilis
   - Involvement of CNS is detected by examination of CSF for mono-nuclear pleocytosis (>5 WBc/μl), increased protein concentration (> 45 mg/dl) or CSF VDRL reactivity.
   - CSF WBC counts ≥20 cell/μl is diagnostic of neurosyphilis in HIV injected patient with syphilis
   - CSF VDRl test is highly specific when reactive and is considered diagnostic of neurosyphilis. However the sensitivity of VDRL is poor and it may be negative even in patient with symptomatic neurosyphilis
   - FTA-ABS test on CSF is more sensitive but less specific and may reflect passive transfer of serum antibody into the CSF.
   - Measuring CXCL13 is CSF can distinguish between neurosyphilis and HIV related CSF abnormalities.

2. **Ans. (a) IgM FTABS**   *Ref. Ananthanarayan 10/e, p382; Harrison 20/e, p 1284*
   "Newborn infant of mother with reactive VDRL or FTA-ABS shows (+) ve test irrespective of infection because of transplacental transfer of maternal IgG antibody."
   As IgM antibody don't cross placenta, neonatal IgM antibody can be detected in cord or neonatal serum with the syphilis capita M or 19S IgM FTA-ABS test. ..... *Harrison 16/e, p 984*

   Important points about Congenital syphilis:
   - Transmission across placenta can take place any time, but lesion appear after 4 month of gestation.
   - *Earliest sign* of congenital syphilis — Rhinitis, snuffles
   - *Residual stigmata* of congenital syphilis — Hutchinson's teeth, Mulberry molars, Rhagades
   - *DOC* of congenital syphilis — Penicillin G.

   Adequate treatment of the woman before the 6th week of pregnancy should prevent fetal damage.

   Among infants born alive only fulminant congenital syphilis is clinically apparent at birth.

3. **Ans. (b, c, d and e) Malaria, relapsing fever, IV drug user, HIV infection**   *Ref. Harrison 20/e, p 1284; CMDT 2014, p 1419*

Causes of False-positive VDRL	
Acute false-positive reaction <6 months	**Chronic false-positive reaction > 6 month**
Recent viral illness or immunization	– Aging
Genital herpes	Autoimmune disorders
HIV infection	– SLE
Malaria	– Rheumatoid arthritis
Parenteral drug used	– Parenteral drug used
Other	
Infective endocarditis	– Hepatitis infection
Pregnancy	– Infectious mononucleosis

4. **Ans. (a) FTA-ABS becomes negative after treatment**   *Ref. Harrison 20/e, p 1286*
   - Only **VDRL** and **RPR** for syphilis becomes negative after treatment and are recommended for evaluation of therapy. VDRL or RPR titer progressively declines, becomes (–ve) by 12 months in 40-75% of primary cases and in 20-40% of secondary cases.
   - **FTA-ABS** and agglutination test remains positive after treatment, so these test are not useful in evaluating the response to therapy. HIV coinfected patients are less likely to become nonreactive.

Follow-up Evaluation after Therapy for Syphilis		
Stage of Syphilis	**Tests to Perform**	**When to Perform**
Primary or Secondary	Quantitative RPR or VDRL[b]	HIV-uninfected: 6 and 12 months HIV-infected: 3, 6, 9, 12 and 24 months
Latent or late	Quantitative RPR or VDRL[b]	HIV-uninfected: 6, 12, 24 months HIV-infected: 6, 12, 18 and 24 months
Neurosyphilis (Asymptomatic or symptomatic)	1. If CSF pleocytosis was documented initially, repeat CSF exam. 2. Monitor decline in CSF protein and CSF-VDRL. (Note: Rate of decline may be slow). 3. Quantitative serum RPR or VDRL[b]	1. Every 6 months until CSF cell count is normal 2. Until normal 3. 6, 12, 18 and 24 months

   [b]Try to distinguish between reinfection and treatment failure. If no clear evidence of reinfection exists, perform CSF examination. If CSF is normal, treat as for late latent syphilis.

5. **Ans. is (a) Early relapsing syphilis** *Ref. Br J Clin Prac 1978:32 206-207*
Chancre redux or chancre monoredive is thought to be due to insufficient treatment of a syphilitic chancre, which after disappearance may relapse and accompanied by enlarged lymph nodes and the presence of numerous treponemes at the site of recurrence.

6. **Ans. (b) Dark field microscopy of ulcer discharge** *Ref. Ananthanarayan 10/e, p 380; Harrison 20/e, p 1283*
Painless indurated ulcer (Hard chancre) with non-tender inguinal lymphadenopathy signifies diagnosis of syphilis.

   Organism examine under dark ground microscope are:
   – Leptospira   – Treponema   – Vibrio cholera   – Campylobacter jejuni.
   Mnemonic: Local Train Via Chandigarh

   ### Diagnosis of Syphilis
   a. Demonstration of organism:
   - *Dark field microscopic examination* of lesion exudate is useful in moist cutaneous lesion such *as chancre* of primary syphilis; *condylomata* of secondary syphilis.
   - A treponemal concentration of $>10^4$/ml in exudate is required for visibility under dark field microscope
   - *Direct fluorescent antibody T. pallidum (DFA-TP) test* – Use fluorescent conjugated antibody for detection of T. pallidum in fixed culture.
   b. Serological test for Syphilis

Non-treponemal test	Treponemal test
– Detect antibody against cardiolipin	– Detect specific antibody against T. pallidum antigen
Includes	**Includes**
• VDRL (test of choice for response to therapy); RPR (test of choice for rapid diagnosis)	• FTA-ABS **(most sensitive test)**
• RPR (Rapid Plasma Reagin)	• Agglutination assays (MHA-TP; TPHA; TPPA)
• TRUS (Toluidine red unheated serum test)	• TPPA has supplanted the FTA-ABS test as diagnostic test.
	• TPI - **most specific serological test**. (not used now)

7. **Ans. (a), (b) and (e) Syphilis, *Leptospira* and *Borrelia*** *Ref. See below*

Spirochete	Species	Diseases
Treponema	T. pallidum T. endemicum T. pertenue T. carateum	– Syphilis – Bejel/Endemic syphilis – Yaws – Pinta
Borrelia	B. burgdorferi B. recurrentis B. vincenti	– Lyme disease – Relapsing fever – Vincent's angina
Leptospira	L. interrogans L. canicola	– Weil's disease – Canicola fever

8. **Ans (a,b,c,d) Painless ulcer, Painless lymphadenopathy, Covered with exudate, Indurated lesion**
   Ref. Harrison 20/e, p 1281; Textbook of Microbiology by DR Arora 3/e p 330, 331
   Primary chancre (Hunterian chancre) (See color plate, pg xxxi for related image)
   - The primary lesion of syphilis is the chancre which usually begins as a single painless papule that rapidly become eroded and usually gets indurated.
   - It is relatively avascular and has characteristic cartilaginous consistency.
   - **Site:** It is located at the entry site of spirochete i.e. penis in heterosexual male, anal canal or rectum in homosexual; cervix and labia in females.
   - The regional lymph node are swollen, discrete, rubbery and non-tender.
   - Large number of treponemes are present in primary lesion and in the serum that exudes from it.
   - *T. pallidum* do not grow in artificial media and so they cannot be cultured.

9. **Ans (a, b) HIV infection, Collagen disorders** *Ref. Harrison 20/e, p 1284; Ananthanarayan 10/e, p 381*
   Non-treponemal test
   Serological test in which cardiolipin or lipoidal antigen is used. Includes:
   – Wasermann reaction   – Kahn test
   – VDRL   – RPR
   - As cardiolipin antigen is present in both *T. pallidum* and mammalian tissue, reagent antibody may be induced which accounts for biological false positive (BFP).

10. **Ans. (c) FTA-ABS** *Ref. Harisson 20/e, p 1284*

    Most sensitive test for syphilis: FTA-ABS
    Most specific test for syphilis: TPI

    > **Note:** Treponemal test are likely to remain reactive even after adequate treatment and cannot differentiate past from current treponemal infection.

11. **Ans. (a) VDRL** *Ref. Harrison 20/e 1284*
    - This is a case of neurosyphilis. The efficiency of treatment of neurosyphilis is assessed by monitoring of quantitative VDRL or RPR Titer.
    - FTA Abs agglutination test remain positive in most patients treated for seropositive syphilis, so these tests are not useful for monitoring the response.
    - VDRL test can be performed on both serum and CSF, while RPR can not be performed on CSF, this makes VDRL test of choice for monitoring response particularly in neurosyphilis.
    - CSF VDRL is highly specific and when reactive is considered diagnostic of neurosyphilis.

    > **Remember:** The activity of neurosyphilis is correlated best with CSF pleocytosis and this measure provides the most sensitive index of response to treatment.

12. **Ans. (b) VDRL** *Ref. Harisson 20/e, p 1284*
    Already explained

13. **Ans. (a and c) VDRL test detects antibodies, Penicillin is preferred treatment for primary and secondary stage**
    Ref. Harrison 20/e, p 1284-1286

    Jarisch: Herxheimer reaction is mediated by release of lipoproteins, cytokines and immune complex.

    Evaluation for neurosyphilis:
    - Pleocytosis, increased protein concentration
    - CSF VDRL is highly specific and when reactive is considered diagnostic of neurosyphilis
    - Patient with RPR titre ≥ 1:32 are at higher risk for developing neurosyphilis.

14. **Ans. (a) Spread by sexual transmission** *Ref. Harrison 20/e, p 1287 Table*
    Yaws is caused by *T. pallidum* subspecies pertenue.
    - *T. pertenue* is antigenically identical to T. Pallidum.

    Mode of transmission : Infection is transmitted by direct contact with infectious lesions, often during play or group sleeping. Fly acts as mechanical vector.

    Clinical features : After 3-4 weeks the initial lesion begins as a papule usually on extremity which enlarges and breaks down to form an ulcerating granuloma (mother yaw). It is followed by appearance of multiple skin lesion.
    As in syphilis secondary and tertiary manifestations follows but cardiovascular or neurological involvement is rare. Destructive lesions of bones are common.

    Treatment of choice : Benzathine penicillin.

15. **Ans. (a) and (b) T. pertenue and T. carateum** *Ref. Ananthanarayan 10/e, p 384*

Non-venereal Treponematosis	
Endemic syphilis	– Caused by *T. pallidum* subspecies endemicum. – Transmitted by body to body contact. – Mainly seen in young children. – Primary chancre is not formed. – **Treatment** - penicillin is **DOC**.
Yaws (=pian = Parangi)	– Caused by *T. pallidum* subspecies *T. pertenue*. – Primary lesion is extragenital papule which ulcerate to form an ulcerating granuloma.
Pinta	– Caused by *T. carateum* – Not identical but closely related to *T. pallidum* – Primary lesion is extragenital papule which does not ulcerate but develop into lichenoid or psoriatic patch.

> **Remember:** *T. pallidum* subspecies *endemicum* and *T. pertenue* are morphologically and immunologically identical to *T. pallidum* subspecies *pallidum* (causative agent of syphilis), So VDRL is positive.

16. **Ans. (d) Later stages involves heart and nerves** Ref. Harrison 20/e, p 1287

Feature	Yaw (pian, framboesia)	Pinta (carate, azul)
Organism	T. pallidum subspecies pertenue	T. carateum
Mode of transmission	Skin to skin	Skin to skin
Usual age	Early childhood	Late childhood
Primary lesion	Ulcerative Papilloma (Mother yaw)	Non ulcerative papule with satellite
Site	Extremities	Extremities, face
Secondary lesion	Cutaneous papulosquamous lesion, osteoperiostitis	Pintides, pigmented, pruritic
Relapses	Common	Rare
Late complication	Destructive gummas of skin, bone, cartilage	Nondestructive macules
Treatment	Benzathine penicillin	Benzathine penicillin

17. **Ans. (b, d) Transmitted by fomites, Periostitis occurs** Ref. Ananthanarayan 10/e, p 384; Harrison 20/e, p 1287
    Painful papillomatous lesions on the soles of the feet, periostitis, polydactilitis are the secondary manifestations of yaws.
    Late yaws also manifest as *gummas* of skin and long bones, hyperkeratosis of palm and soles, osteitis and periostitis and hydrarthrosis.

18. **Ans. (b) Leptospirosis** Ref. Harrison 20/e 1291; Ananthanarayan 10/e, p 387
    Conjuctival suffusion is one of the characteristic manifestation of Leptospirosis

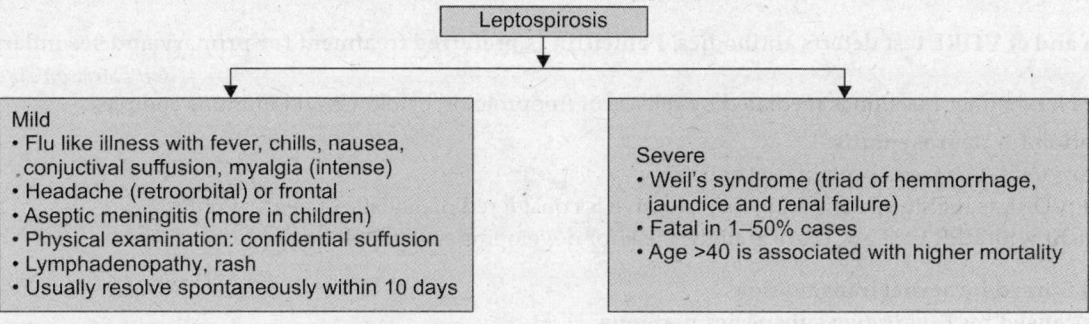

19. **Ans. (c) Microscopic ...** Ref. Ananthanarayan 10/e, p 399
    Diagnosis of Leptospirosis
    - Specimen: Blood, Urine, or by inoculation of guinea pigs.
    - Microscopy: Dark field examination of blood: Effective only in 1st week
        Dark field examination of urine: Appear in 2nd week
    - Culture: 3 or 4 drops of blood in EMJH media for 2 days at 37°C and thereafter at room temperature for 2 weeks.
    - Direct culture of urine in seldom successful.
    - Animal inoculation: Blood from patient is inoculated intraperitoneally into young guinea pigs. Virulent serotype produce human like illness in 7–10 days
    - Serological tests: Antibodies appear towards the end of the 1st week and increase till 4th week serological tests include:
        (a) **Broadly reactive or genus specific test:** Identify leptospiral injection without indicating the exact infecting serovar. Tests employed include sensitised erythrocyte lysis, complement fixation, agglutination and indirect immunofluorescence. The antigen for these test are prepared from non-pathogenic L.biflexa.
        (b) **Type specific test:** Identify the infective serovar. Include microscopic and microscopic agglutination tests. Microscopic agglutination test is more specific. MAT however is available only in reference laboratory.

Diagnosis of leptospirosis	
Isolation of organism	**Serology**
EMJH medium is useful	Raise in antibody titre (>: 100) in *microscopic agglutination test (MAT)*.
Dark field examination of patient blood	*Macroscopic agglutination test* is useful for screening but is *not specific*.
	IgM enzyme-linked immunosorbent assay (EIA) - particularly useful in making an *early* diagnosis.

20. **Ans. (a) Leptospirosis** Ref. Ananthanarayan 10/e, p 387; Harrison 20/e, p 1291
    Leptospirosis
    - *Dead end infection* of leptospira characterized by clinical manifestations ranging from inapparent infection to fulminant icterohemorrhagic fever *(Weil's syndrome).*

Modes of transmission:
- **Rodents** are most important reservoir.
- Transmission occur by direct contact with urine, blood or tissue from an infected animal.
- Indirect contact: Contact of broken skin or ingestion of soil, water or vegetation contaminated by urine of infected animal.
- Direct man to man transmission is rare
- **Water is** an important vehicle of transmission.
- Out breaks mostly occur as a result of heavy rainfall and consequent flooding.

So, guys Leptospirosis is associated with:
- Rats
- Rainfall
- Rice - Rats usually live in rice farms.

Other options
- **Heavy rainfall** tends *to protect against plague and Rodent bite fever* by damaging rodent burrows.
- Melioidosis is not associated with Rat.

21. **Ans. (c) Microscopic agglutination test** Ref. Harrison 20/e, p 1294; Ananthanarayan 10/e, p 390
    - The patient is a case of *Weil's syndrome* or *icterohemorrhagic fever* which is caused by **Leptospira** and manifest as:
        - *Fever*
        - *Jaundice*
        - *Renal failure (Hematuria)*
    - Human infections are usually due to occupational exposure to urine of infected animal e.g.,
        - Farmers
        - Workers in rice field and sugarcane field
        - Workers in underground Sewers
        - Meat and animal handlers
        - Veterinarians

    > **Remember:**
    > - Leptospirosis is most widespread zoonotic disease in world.
    > - Vasculitis is responsible for most manifestation of Leptospirosis
    > - Penicillin G is **DOC** for Leptospirosis.
    > - Fletcher medium and Korthof medium can also be used for isolation of leptospira.

22. **Ans. (b) Leptospira...**
    The clue is endoflagella which are the characteristic of spirochetes. Among given options Leptospira is the only spirochetes. See colour palette for details.

23. **Ans. (d) Lice acts as reservoir...** Ref. Park 22/e, p 266; Harrison 20/e p 1291
    "Reservoir of leptospirosis are rats not lice." Other wild mammals as well as farm animals may also harbor leptospires.
    - Most important source of infection are rats, dogs, cattle and pig.
    - Human infection is *mostly accidental.*
    - *Transmission occur through direct contact Leptospira enter the body through:*
        - Skin abrasions or through intact mucous membrane.
        - Ingestion of food and water contaminated with urine of rat (minor important).
        - Inhalation of droplets of urine of infected animal.
    - Direct man to man infection is rare.

24. **Ans. (c) Person to person transmission rare** Ref. Park 21/e p 267; Harrison 20/e, p 1292
    Already explained

    > **Note:**
    > - Weil syndrome develops in 5-10% of infected individual
    > - Treatment of choice for leptospirosis is Ampicillin
    > - Doxycycline is the drug of choice for chemoprophylaxis.

25. **Ans. (c) Borrelia recurrentis is the etiologic agent** Ref. Ananthanarayan 10/e, p 387; Harrison 19/e, p 1149, 20/e, p 1299
    "Lyme's disease is caused by Borrelia burgdorferi not B. recurrentis."
    Lyme's disease
    - *Causative agent* — Borrelia burgdorferi
    - *Vector* — Ixodes tick
    - Natural reservoir host — Rodents, deer and other mammals.

    Clinical Manifestation
    - *Stage 1* – After I.P of 3-32 days
        - Erythema migrans occur at the site of tick bite.
        - *MC site* - Thigh, groin, axilla

- **Stage 2** – Disseminate hematogenously to produce: – *Secondary annular skin lesion*
  – *Meningitis*
  – *Carditis*
- **Stage 3 (Persistent infection)** – Intermittent attacks of oligoarticular arthritis (*MC* - Knee).
  Acrodermatitis atrophicans – Late skin manifestation.

Diagnosis
- *Serology* – ELISA followed by western blot can't distinguish active and inactive infection.
- *Isolation of organism* – B. burgdorferi may be cultured from skin lesions of patient.
  – Grows best in BSK medium at 33°C.
- Detection of DNA by PCR, particularly in joint fluid.
- Later in infection PCR is greatly superior to culture.

Remember: *B. recurrentis* is etiological agent of Relapsing fever.

26. **Ans. (b) Weil's disease** *Ref. Harrison 20/e, p 1299*
    This is **classic** case of **Weil disease** with: – Fever
    – Jaundice
    – Renal failure (increase urea).

27. **Ans. (b) Borrelia recurrentis** *Ref. Ananthanarayan 10/e, p 385*
    "Borrelia readily undergoes antigenic variations in vivo and this is believed to be the reason for relapsing in the disease."
    .... *Ananthanarayan 10/e, p 385*

    Borrelia recurrentis
    - Causative agent of epidemic or lice born relapsing fever
    - Antigenic variation occur due to DNA rearrangement in linear plasmids present in Borrelia.

    Remember: Other bacteria exhibiting antigenic variation are:
    - Neisseria
    - Group A streptococci

28. **Ans (a) Borrelia recurrentis** *Ref. Ananthanarayan 10/e, p 385*
    Already Explained

29. **Ans (b) and (d) Borrelia duttonii, Borrelia hermsii** *Ref. Ananthanarayan 10/e, p 385*

Relapsing Fever	
Louse born (Epidemic)	Tick born (Endemic)
– Borrelia recurrentis	– B. duttonii
	– B. hermsii
	– B. Parkeri

30. **Ans. (c) Polymorphonuclear leucocytosis in CSF suggest meningeal involvement**
    Spread of Infection in Lyme Disease *Ref. Ananthanarayan 10/e 387; Harrison 20/e p 1299*
    - In lyme disease B. burgdorferi in inoculated in skin by the bite of ixodes tick
    - Bacteria replicates locally and migrate outward into the dermis.
    - Days to week after the tick bite, hematogenous dissemination to secondary sites takes place. If untreated bacteria persist in the body for month or even years, despite the production of antibodies.
    - **Following mechanism have been described for the resistance of B. burgdorferi:**
      – Tick saliva contains substance that disrupt immune response at the site of bite
      – Once inside the body, Borrelia changes shape. In the tick, bacterium has a thick cell wall and spiral shape. However, in the human body, Borrelia can shed its cell wall and can take a different shape. When under attack from immune system, it simply changes shape to remain unrecognized.
      – Borrelia burgdorferi produces antigenic variation in a "cell surface lipo protein VIsE", during the course of infection. by using this type of antigenic variation, B. burgdorferi can escape the adaptive immune system.

    CSF Findings of Lyme Meningitis
    - Pleocytosis with predominantly lymphocytosis (not polymorphonuclear leukocytosis)
    - Increased protein
    - Glucose content is usually normal, but it falls below the serum concentration in 20% of patients
    - Immunoglobulin abnormalities are common in the CSF of patients with lyme meningitis.
      – Specific IgM, IgG or IgA antibody against B. Burgdorferi appears in CSF and indicates intrathecal antibody synthesis.

NEET Pattern Questions

1. Incubation period of syphilis:
   a. 1 hour - 5 hour
   b. 24 hour - 48 hour
   c. 1 day - 10 days
   d. 10 days - 90 days [Ref. Ananthanarayan, 10/e, p 379]

2. Stain for treponema:
   a. Fontana's
   b. Acid-facid
   c. Methenamine-silver
   d. PAS [Ref. Ananthanarayan, 10/e, p 378]

> Treponema Pallidum is stained by silver impregnation methods. Fontana's method is useful for staining films and Levaditi's method for tissue section.

3. Painless genital ulcer in male with everted margin is seen in:
   a. Syphilis   b. Chancroid
   c. Herpes   d. LGV
   [Ref. Ananthanarayan, 10/e, p 379]

4. Dark field microscopy used in:
   a. Vibrio   b. Syphilis
   c. TB   d. Brucellosis
   [Ref. Ananthanarayan, 10/e, p 380]

5. In a syphilis patient, site which does not help in isolation of organism:
   a. Gumma
   b. Chancre
   c. Mucosal patch
   d. Maculopapular rash [Ref. Ananthanarayan, 10/e, p 380]

> Gumma represent tertiary tension which are due to delayed hypersensitivity and contains few if any spirochetes

6. Confirmatory test for syphilis:
   a. VDRL   b. FTA-ABS
   c. RPO   d. None
   [Ref. Ananthanarayan, 10/e, p 382]

7. True about B. recurrentis:
   a. Causes leptospirosis   b. Water borne disease
   c. Vector borne disease   d. Transmitted by tick
   [Ref. Ananthanarayan, 9/e, p 380]

8. Tabes dorsalis is manifestation of:
   a. Primary syphilis   b. Secondary syphilis
   c. Tertiary syphilis   d. Latent syphilis
   [Ref. Ananthanarayan, 10/e, p380]

> Tabes dorsalis is a late manifestation of syphilis that presents with symptoms and signs of demyelination of the posterior columns, dorsal root and dorsal root ganglia.

9. Syphilis was first identified by:
   a. Fraenkel
   b. Nicolaricu
   c. Schaudinn and Hoffman
   d. Ogston
   [Ref. AA 10/e, p 378]

> Remember: Name pallidum refers to its pale staining

10. Dark ground microscopy is used for:
    a. TPI
    b. FTA-ABS
    c. Kahn's test
    d. VDRL
    [Ref. Ananthanarayan 10/e, p 382]

- **TPI** is *most specific* test for syphilis, but not performed now, as it requires Treponoma in Tissue culture.
  - In TPI treponema is combined with antibody and complement of patient sample, if it results in immobilization (which is seen in dark ground) infection is confirmed.

11. Painless ulcer along with painless lymphadenopathy is characteristic of which STD?
    a. Syphilis   b. Chancroid
    c. LGV   d. Donovanosis
    [Ref. Harrison, 20/e, p 1281]

12. The following is not true of syphilis: [NEET 2016]
    a. TPI is most specific
    b. VDRL is not specific
    c. VDRL is negative in secondary syphilis
    d. IgM test is specific for congenital syphilis
    [Ref. Harrison 20/e, p 1283–84]

13. RPR is done for diagnosis of: [NEET 2016]
    a. Malaria   b. Syphilis
    c. Leishmaniasis
    d. None   [Ref. Ananthanarayan 10/e, p 381]

Ans.
1. d. 10 days - 90 days
2. a. Fontana's
3. a. Syphilis
4. b. Syphilis
5. a. Gumma
6. b. FTA-ABS
7. c. Vector borne disease
8. c. Tertiary syphilis
9. c. Schaudinn...
10. a. TPI
11. a. Syphilis
12. c. VDRL ...
13. b. Syphilis

14. Leptospirosis is transmitted by:
    a. Rat
    b. Cat
    c. Dog
    d. Fish
    [Ref. Ananthanarayan, 10/e, p 387]

15. Culture medium used for leptospira for laboratory diagnosis:
    a. Skirrows medium
    b. EMJH medium
    c. BYCE agar
    d. Pike's medium
    [Ref. Ananthanarayan, 10/e, p 388]

16. Fletcher's medium containing Rabbit serum is used for:
    a. Streptococcus
    b. Bacillus anthracis
    c. Leptospira
    d. Borrelia
    [Ref. Ananthanarayan 10/e, p 388]

Leptospira require media enriched with robbit serum e.g. Korthofis, Stuart, Flutcher. GMJH is a semisynthetic media which is used nowadays.

17. Most common form of leptospirosis:
    a. Weil's disease
    b. Icteric form
    c. Hepatorenal form
    d. Anicteric form
    [Ref. AA, 10/e, p 388]

18. Borrelia undergoes antigenic variation due to:
    a. Plasmids
    b. Transposons
    c. Intrinsic mutation
    d. All of the above
    [Ref. Ananthanarayan, 10/e, p 385]

Antigenic variation of Borelia are due to DNA rearrangements in linear plasmids.

19. Vincent's angina is caused by Borrelia vincentii along with:
    a. Lactobacillus
    b. Peptostreptococcus
    c. Fusobacterium
    d. Bacteroides
    [Ref. Ananthanarayan, 10/e, p 386]

This symbiotic infection of B. Vincentii with Fusobacterium fusiforme is known as fusospirochetosis

Ans.
14. a. Rat
15. b. EMJH medium
16. c. Leptospira
17. d. Anicteric form
18. a. Plasmids
19. c. Fusobacterium

CHAPTER 23

Mycoplasma

- *Smallest free living bacteria, that lacks cell wall and is* bounded by sterols containing soft trilaminar membrane, so are highly pleomorphic.
- **Lack cell wall** so are resistant to cell wall active antimicrobial agent such as penicillin, cephalosporin and lysozyme.
- Also called as *PPLO = Stable L forms.*
- Even cell precursors like *muramic acid or diaminopimelic acid are absent.*
- Do not possess spores flagella or fimbria. Some species exhibit *gliding motility.*

Morphology

- Gram negative but better stained *by Giemsa.*
- Can be grown on cell free media, that contain lipoprotein and sterol.
- Colony is typically biphasic with **"Fried egg appearance" best studied** after staining *by Dienes* method. Most mycoplasma colonies are hemolytic.
- Pathogenic mycoplasma grows best at 35-37°C. Media are enriched with 20% horse or human serum and yeast extract. Penicillin and thallium acetate are added as selective agents.
- Some species shows bulbous enlargement with a differentiated tip structure which aids in attachment of organism to host cell carrying neuraminic acid receptor.

Mechanism of Pathogenicity

- Adherence to host cell
- H_2O_2 production (as in *M. pneumonia*)
- Ammonia production (as in *M. hominis*).
- Urease activity to produce ammonia (as in *U. urealyticum*).
- IgM autoantibodies that agglutinate human group O erythrocyte at 4°C. This *cold agglutinin* produces anemia.

Classification

- *M. pneumoniae* — Upper and lower respiratory tract infection.
- *M. genitalium* and *Ureaplasma urealyticum* — Urethritis and other genital condition.
- *M. hominis* and *U. urealyticum* — *Part of flora of bacterial vaginosis.*

Smallest free living bacteria
- Smallest organism capable of independent replication
- Lacks cells wall
- Exhibit biphasic colony with fried egg appearance
- Grows best at 35 to 37°C
- Causative agent of walking pneumonia.
- Smallest organism capable of independent replication.

MYCOPLASMA PNEUMONIA = PRIMARY ATYPICAL PNEUMONIA = WALKING PNEUMONIA

- Caused by *M. pneumonia* (= Eaton agent) in which pneumonia is classic presentation but **non-pneumonic** infection is more common with prolonged incubation period.
- Interstitial type of pneumonia characterized by paucity of respiratory signs on auscultation with striking radiological abnormality.
- **Extrapulmonary manifestations** (e.g. Erythema multiforme, anemia, pancreatitis, coagulopathies) is due to autoantibodies against brain, heart and muscle.

Diagnosis

i. *Isolation*: Throat swab/respiratory secretions are inoculated into medium containing glucose and phenol.
ii. *Serological diagnosis*:
   a. **Specific test** - Immunofluorescence hemagglutination inhibition and metabolic inhibition are most sensitive test.
   b. **Non-specific serological test** are Streptococcus MG (group F) and cold agglutination test.

- Non-gonococcal Urethritis: U. urealyticum and M. genitalium are the most common non-chlamydial cause of NGU.
- Cell wall deficient form of Gr(+) bacteria: Protoplast
- Cell wall deficient form of Gr(−) bacteria: Spheroplast.

GENITAL MYCOPLASMAS

- Non-gonococcal Urethritis (NGU) - *U. urealyticum* and *M. genitalium* cause most of non-chlamydial cases of NGU.
- *U. urealyticum* called as **T. strain/T. form of mycoplasma** use urea as a source of energy. Hence, **Urea and cholesterol are essential growth factor**.

> **Treatment:** Tetracycline [Doxycycline] is DOC for treatment of mycoplasma infection.

CELL WALL DEFECTIVE BACTERIA

L phase variants (L. forms)

- Wall defective microbial forms that can replicate serially as non-rigid cells and produce colonies on solid media.
- *Protoplasts* are such forms usually derived from Gram +ve organisms. They are osmotically fragile.
- *Spheroplasts* are cell wall defective form usually derived from Gram –ve bacteria. They retain outer membrane.
- These L forms results from spontaneous mutation or by the effect of chemicals.
- ***Reversion of L-form to the parental bacterial form is enhanced by growth in the presence of 15-30% gelatin or 2-5% agar.***

Multiple Choice Questions

1. **Mycoplasma is resistant to which antibiotic:** [NEET Pattern 2018]
   a. Aminoglycosides   b. Chloramphenicol
   c. Beta-lactams   d. Erythromycin

2. **Atypical pneumonia can be caused by the following microbial agents** *except*: [AI 05]
   a. *Mycoplasma*
   b. *Legionella pneumophila*
   c. Human corona virus
   d. *Klebsiella pneumoniae*

3. **All are features of** *ureaplasma urealyticum except*:
   a. Non-gongococcal urethritis   [AI 11]
   b. Salpingitis
   c. Epididymitis
   d. Bacterial vaginosis

4. **The following statements are true with references to Mycoplasma** *except* : [AIIMS 05]
   a. They are the smallest prokaryotic organisms that can grow in cell free culture media
   b. They are obligate intracellular organisms
   c. They lack a cell wall
   d. They are resistant to Beta-lactam drugs

5. **In reference to Mycoplasma, the following are true** *except*: [AIIMS 05]
   a. They are inhibited by penicillins
   b. They can reproduce in cell free media
   c. They have an affinity for mammalian cell membranes
   d. They can pass through fiters of 450 nm pore size

6. *Mycoplasma pneumonia* **is characterized by all** *except* : [AIIMS 18]
   a. Diagnosed by serum cold antibody
   b. Treatment is erythromycin
   c. Cannot be cultured from sputum
   d. Resistant to β lactams

Explanations and References with Illustrative Answers

1. **Ans. (c) Beta-lactams**   Ref. Ananthanarayan 10/e, p 394
   - Mycoplasmas are **devoid of cell walls** (but bound by soft trilaminar unit membrane of sterols) and so **they are resistant to** β. lactams (penicillin, cephalosporins, vancomycin, bacitracin) and lysozymes that act on cell wall.
   - Due to lack of cell wall they are highly pleomorphic and pass through bacterial filters of 450 nm since size varies from 50-300 nm in diameter.
   - Parasitic mycoplasma requires cholesterol or other sterols as an essential growth factor.
   - They have affinity for mammalian cell membrane.   .....*Jawertz 27/e, p 335*
   - It typically colonizes mucosal surfaces of respiratory, gastrointestinal and genitourinary tracts.
   - Mycoplasmas occur as granules and filaments (shows *true branching*).
   - They multiply by asynchronous binary fission producing budding forms and chains of beads.
   - Some species get attached to suitable host cells carrying neuraminic acid receptors by bulbous enlargement.
   - *Mycoplasmas can grow in cell free media.*
   - **Media** of *Mycoplasma* are **enriched with 20% horse** or **human serum** and **yeast extract**
     - Penicillin and thallium are *selective agents*.
     - Colonies is typically biphasic with a *fried egg appearance* and are best studied after staining by Dienes method.
     - Growth of mycoplasma is inhibited by specific antibody.

   Note: Doxycycline is drug of choice for mycoplasma.

2. **Ans. (d)** *Klebsiella pneumoniae*   [Ref. Robbin's 7/e, p 751]
   Atypical pneumonia is characterized by patchy inflammatory changes in the lung, largely confined to alveolar septa and pulmonary interstitium.

Causes of atypical pneumonia	
Mycoplasma (MC)	Coxiella burnettii (Q fever)
Legionella pneumonia	Pneumocystis carinii
Francisella tularensis	Histoplasma capsulatum
Chlamydia psittacosis, Chlamydia pneumoniae	Coccidiodis immitis.
Viruses (influenzae A and B, RSV, Adeno, rhino, rubeola, varicella, etc).	

Klebsiella is associated with community acquired pneumonia classically in alcoholics (also in diabetics and chronic lung disease). It usually affects upper lobes producing expansion of lobes (bulging fissure) and Red current jelly sputum.

Note: Causes of community acquired pneumoniae in decreasing frequency **Strep. pneumoniae > H. influenza > Chlamydia > Legionella**.

3. **Ans. (b) Salpingitis** [Ref. Harrison 20/e, p 1163; Ananthanarayan 10/e, p 396; CGDT 9/e, p 654]

   ***Ureaplasma urealyticum* are T. form mycoplasmas which are urease positive.**

   It causes:
   - Nongonococcal urethritis (**MC** cause is *Chlamydia trachomatis* also caused by *U. urealyticum* and *M. genitalium.*)
   - Epididymitis **(no role of M. homins).**
   - Chorioamnionitis
   - Postpartum fever
   - Proctitis
   - Reiter's syndrome
   - Acute salpingitis
   - Infertility in both men and women
   - Late abortion
   - Low birth weight infant
   - Balanoposthitis
   - Cervicitis and vaginitis

   ... *Not given in Harrison and CGDT*
   - Pneumonia and chronic lung disease in very low birth weight infants
   - PID and bacterial vaginosis : by *M. hominis* and *U. urealyticum*

   Bacterial vaginosis (Altered vaginal normal microbial flora) is associated with *Gardenrella* and *Hemophilus vaginitis*, in which **clue cells** are present and **Amide test** is positive.

   If 'none' is given as option then it is more appropriate than 'Salpingitis' as salpingitis is given in few books.

4. **Ans. (b) They are obligate intracellular organisms** [Ref. See below]
   - Mycoplasma is not obligate intracellular bacteria.
   - ***Obligate intracellular bacteria:***
     - M. leprae
     - Chlamydia
     - Rickettsiae and Coxiella burnettii
     - Pathogenic treponemes.
   - Obligate intracellular bacteria cannot grow in cell free media.

5. **Ans. (a) They are inhibited by penicillins** [Ref. Ananthanarayan 8/e, p 387-89, 9/e, p 387]

   Already explained

6. **Ans. (c) Cannot be cultured from sputum** Ref. Ananthanarayan 8/e, p 389, 9/e, p 387; Harrison 19/e, p 1163, 18/e, p 1418
   - *Mycoplasma pneumoniae* is **MC** cause of Atypical pneumonia which is characterized by reticulonodular or interstitial infiltration of lower lobes on X-ray with paucity of signs on auscultation.
   - Diagnosis is mainly clinical. Lab test are of secondary value.

   Lab Diagnosis
   - *Specimen:* – Throat swabs, sputum or respiratory secretions.
   - *Microscopy:* – It cannot be detected on Gram's stain as it lacks cell wall.
     – Gram's stain of sputum shows leukocytes without predominance of any bacteria morphologic type.
   - *Culture:* It can be grown on artificial media but process is difficult as it requires special media and takes more than 2 weeks so cultures do not provide timely information.

- **Serology:**
  a. *Specific*   :   Antibodies are detected by enzyme linked immunoassays, indirect immunofluorescence, or complement fixation test.
  b. *Nonspecific* :   Cold agglutinin aids in diagnosis since they develops within 7-10 days of infection and can be easily detected.
     - They are IgM autoantibodies which agglutinate human erythrocytes at 4°C,
     - Cold agglutinin titer > 1:32 supports diagnosis of *M. pneumoniae*.
     - It can also be performed at the bedside.
- *Antigen Detection test:* Includes antigen capture, indirect enzyme immunoassays, DNA probing and multiplex nucleic acid amplification test.

Note: EIA which detect IgG and IgM antibody is highly sensitive and specific.

Treatment

Ambulatory patients with community acquired pneumonia	Hospitalized patients with community acquired pneumonia
Oral doxycycline Oral erythromycin Oral clarithromycin, azithromycin; Levofloxacin, Moxifloxacin; ciprofloxacin	IV ceftriaxone or IV cefotaxime

Remember: Media for cultivating mycoplasma are enriched with 20% horse or human serum and yeast extract. Penicillin and thallium acetate are added as selective agent.

NEET Pattern Questions

1. **Diene's method is used for:**
   a. Mycoplasma
   b. Chlamydiae
   c. Plague
   d. Diphtheria
   [Ref. Ananthanarayan, 10/e, p394]

   > In Dienes method a block of agar containing the colony is cut and placed on a slide. It is covered with a cover slip on which on alcohol solution of methylena blue and azure has been dried.

2. **Ureaplasma is naturally resistant to:**
   a. Erythromycin   b. Tetracycline
   c. Chloramphenicol   d. Cephalosporins
   [Ref. Ananthanarayan, 10/e, p396]

3. **True about mycoplasma:**
   a. L-form   b. Multidrug resistant
   c. Cause NGU   d. Penicillin effective
   [Ref. Ananthanarayan, 10/e, p394]

4. **True about ureaplasma:**
   a. Obligate intracellular organism
   b. Penicillin is effective treatment
   c. Require cholesterol for growth
   d. Have thick cell wall
   [Ref. Ananthanarayan, 10/e, p347]

   > Urea and cholesterol are essential growth factors in addition to cholesterol.

Ans.
1. a. Mycoplasma
2. d. Cephalosporins
3. a. L-form, c. Cause NGU
4. c. Require cholesterol for growth

SECTION B

UNIT II

Virology

- DNA Virus
- RNA Virus
- Slow Virus Disease
- Hepatitis Virus
- HIV and Other Retrovirus

CHAPTER 24

DNA Virus

HERPES VIRUSES

- *Enveloped* virus with linear double stranded genome.
- Characterised by their ability to establish life long persistent infection in their host and to undergo periodic reactivation.
- Replicate in host cell **nucleus** forming **cowdry type A intranuclear** (*Lipshutz*) inclusion bodies.
- Virus are relatively thermolabile and readily inactivated by lipid solvents like ether.

> **Herpes Virus**
> - Enveloped virus
> - Forms cowdry type A intra-nuclear inclusion bodies

Classification of human herpes viruses

	Species			
Official name	Common name	Sub-family	Cytopathology	Site of latent infection
Human herpesvirus type 1	Herpes simplex virus type 1	Alpha	Cytolytic	Neurons/gasserian or Trigeminal ganglia
Human herpesvirus type 2	Herpes simplex virus type 2	Alpha	Cytolytic	Neurons/sacral ganglia
Human herpesvirus type 3	Varicella zoster virus	alpha	Cytolytic	Neurons/T3 - L3 (**MC**).
Human herpesvirus type 4	Epstein–Barr virus	Gamma	Lymphoproliferative	Lymphoid tissue (B cells)
Human herpesvirus type 5	Cytomegalovirus	Beta	Cytomegalic	Secretory glands Kidneys, (salivary glands and bowel)
Human herpesvirus type 6	Human B cell lymphotropic virus	Beta	Lymphoproliferative	Lymphoid tissues
Human herpesvirus type 7	R K virus	Beta	Lymphoproliferative	Lymphoid tissues
Human herpesvirus type 8		Gamma		

> - Neurotropic herpes virus: HSV and VZV
> - Lymphotropic herpes virus: EBV, HHV-6 &7

- **HHV – 6** cause exanthem subitum/roseola infantum or *sixth disease*.
- Different Herpes virus species don't show any antigenic cross reaction except Herpes simplex types 1 and 2.
- HHV-8 is associated with AIDS/Non-AIDS **Kaposi sarcoma.**

HERPES SIMPLEX VIRUS (HSV)

- HSV includes HSV-1 and HSV-2, both of them are associated with variety of infections affecting both immunocompromised and immunocompetent individuals.
- The genomic structure of both HSV are similar (~50% similarity). Proteome homology is >80%.

HSV Type 1	HSV Type 2
Cause lesion in and around mouth	Cause lesion around genital area
Transmitted by direct contact or droplet spread	Usually transmitted sexually
Replicate poorly in chick embryofibroblast cell	Replicate well
Relatively sensitive to antiviral agents	Resistant
Less neurovirulent	More neurovirulent
Infectivity is less temperature sensitive	More temperature sensitive
Site of latency-trigeminal ganglia	Sacral ganglia
On chick embryo CAM, form smaller pock	Form larger pock

> **Site of latency:**
> 1. HSV-1: Trigeminal ganglia, vagus ganglia, adrenal tissue and brain
> 2. HSV-1: Sacral ganglia
> ... *Greenwood, 18/e, p422*

Herpes simplex virus
Type I Fragile, less neuro-virulent, cause lesion around mouth.
Type II Resistant, neurovirulent cause lesion around genital area.
- Genital herpes most frequently involves cervix and urethra in females and penis in males.
- In viscera oesophagus is the MC site.
- HSV-1 is the most common cause of sporadic encephalitis
- HSV is the MC cause of Mollaret's meningitis.

- Genomes of HSV-1 and HSV-2 are similar and both cross react serologically. They can be distinguished by sequence analysis or by restriction enzyme analysis of viral DNA.
...Jawetz 27/e, p 460

Pathogenesis

- Humans are only natural host.
- *Source of infection* Saliva, skin lesion or respiratory secretion.
- On exposure mucosal surfaces or abraded skin permits entry of virus and initiates its replication in epidermis and dermis.
- On entry into neuronal cells the virus is transported intra-axonally (centripetally) to nerve cell bodies in ganglia.
- During initial phase of infection virus replication occur in ganglia, virus then spread to other mucosal surfaces through centrifugal migration of infectious virions via peripheral sensory nerves.
- Both antibody mediated and cell mediated immunity are important.
- *CD8 + T cell* responses are critical for clearance of virus from lesion.
- Typical lesion produced by HSV is the vesicle, a ballooning degeneration of intra-epithelial cells.

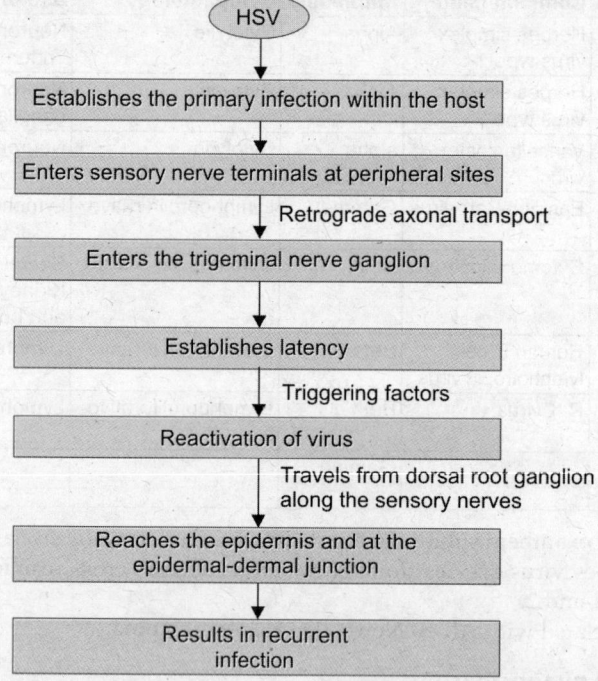

Gingivitis and pharyngitis are most frequent clinical manifestation of primary infections

Clinical Features

- **Orofacial Infection**
  - Gingivitis and pharyngitis are most frequent clinical manifestation of first episode of HSV-1 infection **(primary infection)**.
  - Recurrent herpes *labialis* is *MC* manifestation of *reactivation* (occur by stress stimulus).
  - *Erythema multiforme may* be associated with HSV infection.
  - HSV-1, varicella zoster virus (VZV) may cause Bell's palsy.

- **Genital Infection (HSV-2)**
  - Widely placed bilateral lesion (vesicles, pustules, or *painful* erythematous ulcer) are characteristic of primary infection.
  - *Cervix* and *urethra* are most commonly involved *in* women with primary infection and penis in males.

Typical lesion of HSV: Vesicle
- Base of vesicle contains Tzank cells

- Primary infection in patient who has prior HSV-1 infection are associated with *less* frequent systemic manifestation and there is faster healing of lesion.
- A clear mucoid discharge and dysuria are characteristic of symptomatic HSV urethritis.

- **Herpetic Whitlow**
  - HSV infection of finger may occur as a complication of primary oral or genital herpes by inoculation of virus through abraded skin. Seen in doctors, dentists.
- **Eczema Herpeticum (Usually with HSV-1)**
  - Generalized eruption caused by herpes infection in children suffering from eczema.
- **Herpes Gladiatorum**
  - Mucocutaneous HSV infection of thorax, ears, face and hands.
  - Seen in wrestlers due to recurrent trauma.
- **Eye Infection (HSV-1)**
  - *MC* cause of corneal blindness in USA
  - Cause keratitis, stromal keratitis, necrotizing retinitis, chorioretinitis (in neonates and HIV patients)
- Central and peripheral nervous system manifestation

  A. Encephalitis
  - HSV-1 is *MC* cause of *sporadic encephalitis*.
  - Present as acute onset of fever, focal neurologic signs especially of *temporal lobe*.
  - *Most sensitive non-invasive* method for early diagnosis of HSV encephalitis is demonstration of HSV DNA in CSF by PCR **(Investigation of choice)**.
  - Demonstration in **brain tissue by biopsy** is over all most sensitive but **invasive** method.

  B. Meningitis
  - HSV is *MC* cause of recurrent Lymphocytic meningitis (*Mollaret's meningitis*).
  - HSV-2 is the usual cause
  - Diagnosed by demonstration of HSV DNA or HSV antibodies in CSF.
- **Visceral infection**
  - **Oesophagitis**, *MC* site is **distal oesophagus.**
  - Endoscopically obtained secretion for cytology and culture provide most useful material for diagnosis.
  - Pneumonia in immunocompromised.
  - Hepatitis – may lead to disseminated intravascular coagulation.
- **Neonatal HSV infection**
  - Infection is usually acquired perinatally at the time of delivery.
  - Of all age group, neonates have highest frequency of visceral or CNS infection.
  - 70% are due to HSV-2 and 30% due to HSV-1
  - Skin lesion are the most commonly recognized feature but may not be seen in all cases.

Neonates have highest propensity to visceral or CNS infection

Diagnosis

- Both clinical and laboratory. Multiple vesicular lesion on an erythematous base suggest its diagnosis.
- Scrapings from base of characteristic lesion is taken and stained with Wright's, Giemsa (Tzanck preparations) to detect giant cell or intranuclear inclusions. Sensitivity is low and this can't differentiate between VZV and HSV.
- HSV infection is best confirmed (specific test) by *isolation* of virus in tissue culture. Human diploid fibroblast is the preferred tissue.
- *PCR* for detection of HSV DNA is most sensitive.   ... Harrison 20/e, p 1351
- **Serology:** Type specific antibodies are useful to diagnose primary infection and asymptomatic carriers.
- Serologic assays that identify antibodies to glycoprotein G of HSV-1 and HSV-2 can reliably differentiate between two types.

Varicella Zoster:
- Human are the only reservoir
- Cause chicken pox and shingles
- CNS is the MC extracutaneous site of involvement in chicken-pox

- Herpes zoster most frequently involves T_3-L_3
- Herpes zoster is the reactivation of latent infection of VZV

Treatment

- Acyclovir is most frequently used drug. Other are valacyclovir and vidarabine.

HERPES VIRUS SIMAE: B VIRUS

- Infect old world monkeys in a manner similar to the herpes simplex infection of human.
- Human cases may occur after bite of monkey or in some cases through handling of monkey tissue. Human disease is usually fatal.
- Properties are similar to H. simplex, but antibody against H. simplex are not protective.

VARICELLA - ZOSTER

- Causative agents of:
  - Varicella = Chickenpox (Primary infection)
  - Herpes zoster = Shingles (Reactivation of latent infection).

Pathogenesis

- Humans are *only* known reservoir of VZV.
- **Primary infection** *(Chickenpox)* – Transmitted by respiratory route or through conjunctiva.
- **Recurrent infection** – (Herpes zoster)- During primary infection virus infect dorsal root ganglia, where it remains latent. When immunity wanes, virus reactivates and travel along sensory nerve to produce zoster lesion on mucosa, or skin supplied by it.

Clinical Manifestation

I. Chickenpox

- Highly contagious disease (secondary attack rate 90%) affecting 5-9 year children most commonly.
- IP – 10 to 21 days
- Patient **is infectious** *48 hours prior to onset of vesicular rash to until all vesicles are crusted.*
- Skin lesions – The hallmark of infection includes maculopapules, vesicles and scabs in various stage of evolution.
- Immunocompromised have severe (often hemorrhagic) and long lasting lesion with higher rate of visceral complication and fatality.
- Most common infectious complication is secondary bacterial superinfection of skin usually by S. pyogenes or S. aureus. ... *Harrison 20/e, p 1355*
- The *MC site of extracutaneous* involvement in children **is CNS**.
- Varicella pneumonia is the most serious complication occurring mostly in adults.
- *Perinatal varicella* is associated with high mortality when maternal disease develop **with in 5 days before delivery or** within 48 hr **thereafter.**

II. Herpes zoster (Shingles)

- Reactivation of latent infection from dorsal root ganglia.
- *Age group* – 60 and beyond.
- Characterized by **unilateral** lesion within a dermatome associated with severe pain. The dermatome from T3 to L3 is most frequently affected.
- Patient with herpes zoster can transmit infection to seronegative individual which will develop chickenpox.
- **Zoster sine herpetica:** Zoster without skin lesion, characterized by pain in specific dermatome with seropositivity.
- **Zoster Ophthalmicus** – Due to reactivation in ophthalmic branch of trigeminal (gasserian) ganglia.
- **Ramsay Hunt syndrome** – Due to reactivation in geniculate ganglion of facial nerve.
- Most debiliating complication of Shingles is pain associated with acute neuritis and post-herpetic neuralgia.
- Patient with Hodgkin's disease and NHL are at greatest risk for progressive Herpes zoster.

Diagnosis

- Diagnosis is usually clinical. Tzank smear shows multinucleated giant cells.
- Confirmation can be done by isolation of VZV from vesicles in tissue culture cell lines or detection of DNA by PCR.

Zoster Ophthalmicus: Reactivation of VZV infection in ophthalmic branch of trigeminal (gasserian) ganglia.

CMV
- Largest virus of herpes family
- MC pathogen complicating organ transplant
- Heterophile antibody (-ve) infectious mononucleosis is the MC manifestation
- PCR is the most sensitive technique of diagnosis.

- Serology: Most frequently used are:
  - FAMA (fluorescent antibody to membrane antigen) test
  - ELISA
  - Immunoadherent hemagglutination.
- *FAMA Test and ELISA are most sensitive.*

Treatment
- No antiviral for immunocompetent child.
- *Aspirin should be* **avoided** during episode of chickenpox as it increases risk of development of Reye's syndrome.
- **Acyclovir** therapy is recommended for adolescent and adults with chickenpox of < 24 hours duration. However it does not appear to prevent postherpetic neuralgia.
- Herpes zoster – Famciclovir and valacyclovir are more effective than acyclovir.
- **Postherpetic neuralgia** and acute neuritis:
  - Analgesics
  - Amitryptyline
  - Gabapentin
  - Lidocaine patch
  - Glucocorticoid (with concomitant antiviral therapy).
- In immunocompromised patient IV acyclovir should be given.

Prevention
Vaccine: A live varicella vaccine developed by Takahashi in Japan by attenuation a strain of varicella virus (oka strain) through various passage in tissue culture
- Administered subcutaneously
- Recommended for all children at 12-15 months of age and all sero negative adults
- Contraindicated in pregnancy

Varicella zoster immunoglobulin
- Susceptible high risk individual who have significant exposure
- Product should be given within 46 hours (preferably) within 72 hours

CMV = SALIVARY GLAND VIRUS

- Characterised by enlargement of infected cell and prominent intranuclear inclusion (Owl's eye appearance).
- *Largest virus* of herpes family.
- *MC* organism causing intrauterine infection.
- *MC* pathogen complicating organ transplantation.

Pathogenesis
- Transmitted by sexual route, transplacental, blood transfusion, organ transplant.
- Once infected, individual carry CMV for whole life.
- Infection usually remains latent, reactivation may occur when cell mediated immunity is compromised.

Clinical Features
I. **Congenital infection**
   - CMV infection is the most common congenital infection.
   - Characterized by involvement of CNS and reticuloendothelial system.
   - IUGR, Petechiae, Hepatosplenomegaly, Jaundice are *MC* manifestation.
   - Intracerebral calcification (usually periventricular) and chorioretinitis, deafness are other important findings.
II. **Perinatal infection**
   - Infection is acquired through birth canal at the time of delivery or through breast milk.
   - Mostly asymptomatic, but may lead to interstitial pneumonia in preterm infant.
III. **Beyond neonatal period in immunocompetent host**
   - Heterophile antibody (-)ve infectious mononucleosis is *MC* manifestation.
   - Clinically present with malaise, protracted fever, myalgia, liver function abnormality and lymphocytosis.
   - Salivary gland involvement is common and is probably chronic.
   - Associated with restenosis following coronary angioplasty.

EBV
- Cause heterophile antibody positive infectious mononucleosis
- Salivary secretions are the predominant mode of infection
- Diagnosed by heterophile antibody test (Paul Bunnel test)

B-lymphocytes are the principal and essential cell infected through attachment of the major viral envelope glycoprotein gp 350/220 to C-BV receptors (CD-21)
...Ref. Greenwood, 18/e, p434

IV. Immunocompromised host
a. Organ transplant patient:
 – Period of maximal risk of infection – Between 1 and 4 months after transplantation.
 – Retinitis is late complication.
 – Transplanted organ is particularly vulnerable as a target for CMV infection, e.g. CMV hepatitis in liver transplant holder.
b. AIDS patient: – Cause retinitis (cottage and cheese appearance/pizza pie retinopathy) or disseminated disease particularly when $CD4+ < 50 - 100/\mu l$.

Remember: Prolong CMV infection of the Kidney does not seen to be deleterious in normal person

Diagnosis
- *Most sensitive* method to detect CMV in blood is **PCR**.
- Congenital infection is diagnosed by culture *(best specimen saliva and urine)*; PCR. Human fibroblast are used for virus isolation. Usually 2-3 weeks are needed for culture.

Treatment
- Ganciclovir or Valganciclovir is **DOC**. Foscarnet is recommended for CMV retinitis.

EPSTEIN - BARR VIRUS

- **Causative agent of Heterophile (+)ve infectious mononucleosis** (Kissing disease) = Glandular fever.
- **Associated with:**
 – Nasopharyngeal Ca
 – Burkitt's lymphoma
 – Hodgkin's disease (mixed cellularity type)
 – B cell lymphoma in patients with immunodeficiency
 – Fatal lymphoproliferative disorder in patient of Duncon disease
 – CNS lymphoma in AIDS patient and transplant recipient
 – Increase risk of thymoma, tonsillar and gastric carcinoma.
 – Oral hairy leukoplakia
 – Chronic fatigue syndrome

Pathogenesis
- Source of infection is usually salivary secretions, so *kissing* is predominate mode of transmission.
- The virus infect epithelium of oropharynx and the salivary gland; tonsillar crypts can also be infected directly. Virus then spreads through the bloodstream.
- EBV receptor CR_2/CD21 present on B cell is also receptor for C_3 component of complement; So EBV infection immortalise B cell, at least in vitro.
- Memory B cell are reservoir of EBV in body.
- Cellular immunity is more important than humoral immunity in controlling EBV infection.
- If *T cell immunity decreased, infected B cells begins to proliferate hence producing lymphoma.*

Clinical Features
- Most EBV infection in infant and young children are asymptomatic; Second peak occurs in adults
- In adolescent, most infection present as **infectious mononucleosis**.
 – IP: 4-8 weeks
 – *MC symptom* sore throat
 – *MC sign* - Lymphadenopathy *(mostly of posterior cervical nodes)*
 – Erythema nodosum, erythema multiforme may also occur.

Diagnosis
- During initial phase there is leucopenia, which is followed by increase in TLC; Lymphocytosis with *> 10%* atypical lymphocytes.
 – Atypical lymphocytes are *mainly CD8+ cells* which have undergone blast transformation.

- Thrombocytopenia
- Serological testing
  - Heterophile agglutination test *(Paul Bunnell test)* is used for diagnosis of IM in children and adults. Titer of 40-fold or greater is diagnostic in patient having symptoms. Titer remains positive for 3 months. Commercially available monospot test is more sensitive.
  - False positive monospot test are seen in patient with connective tissue disorder, lymphoma, viral hepatitis, malaria.
  - EBV specific antibody test: *IgM antibody to VCA* is most useful for diagnosis of IM. Used in patients with atypical presentation or in those who lack heterophile antibody.
  - Nucleic acid hybridization is *the most sensitive* means of detecting EBV in patient materials.

Serology in EBV infection						
		Anti-VCA			Anti-EA	
Condition	Heterophile	IgM	IgG		EA-D	EA-R
Acute infectious mononucleosis	+	+	++		+	–
Convalescence	±	–	+		–	±
Past infection	–	–	+		–	–
Reactivation with immunodeficiency	–	–	++		+	+
Burkitt's lymphoma	–	–	+++		±	++
Nasopharyngeal carcinoma	–	–	+++		++	±

VCA viral capsid antigen; EA, early antigen; EA-D antibody, antibody to early antigen in locally diffuse pattern in nucleus and cytoplasm of infected cells; EA-R antibody, antibody to early antigen restricted to the cytoplasm.

> **Pox Virus**
> - Include
>   Variola: small Pox
>   Vaccinia: Small pox vaccine
>   Molluscum contagiosum

Complication
- Most cases are self limited.
- *Most deaths* which occur very rarely are due to *CNS complications.*
- Coombs (+)ve autoimmune hemolytic *anemia*.
- Acute EBV may be associated with *Guillain-Barre' syndrome, CN palsy (MC-facial nerve).*

Herpes Virus Type 6
- Also called as human *B-lymphotropic* virus. Infect *CD4 + T cells*
- Cause common childhood illness exanthem subitum (sixth disease)
- In older age groups it has been associated with infectious mononucleosis syndrome, focal encephalitis.

HHV 7
- Isolated from some cases of exanthem subitum.

HHV 8
- Classified in rhadinovirus genius
- Infects dividing B cells   ...Ref. Greenwood, 18/e, p443
- Associated with Kaposi sarcoma, Body cavity-associated B-lymphoma/multicentric Castleman's disease.

POX VIRUS

Largest pathogenic virus of vertebrates
Important pox virus are: – Variola (causative agent of smallpox)
               – Vaccinia (Artificial virus which was used as smallpox vaccine)
               – Molluscum contagiosum.

VARIOLA

- *Brick shaped* enveloped ds DNA virus
- Elementary bodies are called Paschen bodies.

Adenovirus
- Ds DNA containing enveloped virus
- Potential candidate for gene therapy
- Upper respiratory tract infection is MC Manifestation.

VACCINIA

- It is an artificial virus whose genome can accommodate about 25000 foreign base pairs.
- Eosinophillic inclusion bodies called Guarnieri bodies can be demonstrated in stained preparation.
- But it is not suitable as a vector for human use due to its pathogenic effects.
- Properties are similar to variola.

Smallpox

- On 8th May 1980 WHO announced global eradication of smallpox.
- In India last case was found in 1975.
  Note: *Disease had been eradicated, so clinical features etc are rarely going to be asked.*

Cultivation of Poxvirus

- Both Variola and Vaccinia grow on **CAM** producing pocks.
  - Variola pocks are small, shiny, white convex, non-necrotic, non-hemorrhagic lesions with *ceiling temperature* (highest temperature above which pocks are not produced) of *38°C*.
  - Vaccinia pocks are larger, irregular, flat, greyish, hemorrhagic and Necrotic with ceiling temperature of *41°C*.
- *On tissue culture*
  - Cytopathic effect are produced by Vaccinia in 24 - 48 hours and more slowly by Variola.
  - *Inclusion bodies* called **Guarnieri bodies** can be seen.

MOLLUSCUM CONTAGIOSUM

- *Most common human disease resulting from pox virus.* ...Harrison 20/e, 1366
- Out of the four types (MCV 1 to MCV 4), type 1 is most prevalent
- Molluscum contagiosum virus is an obligate human pathogen.
- Usually seen in children and young adults.
- Characterised by *pink or pearly white nodules* on skin which show large *inclusion bodies* called **Molluscum bodies**.
- Virus *cannot be grown in* eggs, tissues culture or animals.

ADENOVIRUS

- Space vehicle (Hexagonal shape) shaped, non-enveloped virus containing *ds DNA*.
- They have capacity to carry DNA up to 7 kb so, are potential vectors of gene therapy.

Classification

- There are about 50 serotype. Type 1-7 illness account for most disease casually respiratory illness. ......Ananthanarayan, 8/e, p 479
- Types 1, 2, 5 and 6 are more commonly associated with endemic infections.
- Types 3, 4 and 7 are more in epidemic.
- Human adenovirus have been divided into 6 subgenera on the basis of DNA homology.

Clinical Manifestation

- *MC is upper respiratory tract infection* with rhinitis in pediatric age group
- In adults MC is acute respiratory disease caused by types 4, 7

Syndromes	Principal serotypes
Respiratory disease in children	1, 2, 5, 6
Sore throat, febrile cold, pneumonia	3, 4, 7, 14, 21
ARD in military recruits	4, 7, 21
Follicular (swimming pool) conjunctivitis	3, 7
Epidemic keratoconjunctivitis (ship-yard eye)	8, 19, 37
Diarrhea	40, 41
Hemorrhagic cystitis	11, 21
Pharyngoconjunctival fever	3,7,14

Generalized exanthem, mesenteric adenitis and intussusception are other manifestation.

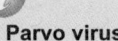

Parvo virus
- Non-enveloped SS DNA-virus
- B-19 is one of the few parvo virus which are pathogenic to humans
- B-19 causes
  - Fifth disease
  - Transient aplastic crisis

Lab Diagnosis

- Isolation of virus from throat, eye, urine or feces.
- It grows only in tissue cultures of human origin, e.g. human embryonic kidney, Hela or HEP-3.
- All mammalian adenovirus share a common complement fixing antigen which is detected by immunofluorescence or ELISA.

ADENO ASSOCIATED VIRUS – (DEPENDOVIRUS)

- These are virus which can multiply only in cells infected with adenovirus as they lack enough DNA.
- It is classified under family parvoviridae.

PARVO VIRUS

Human papilloma virus
- Member of papova virus family
- Non-enveloped DNA virus
- Selectively infects the epithelium of skin and mucous membranes where it immortalize the keratinocytes

- Non enveloped *SS DNA* virus
- Most parvo virus are pathogenic to animals. Human pathogen is **B-19**, the causative agent of **fifth disease**.

Pathogenesis and Clinical Manifestation

- Most of the severe manifestation of B-19 viremia are due *to its ability to lyse erythroid precursor*.
- **Erythema Infectiosum (fifth disease)**
  - *MC* manifestation of B-19 infection.
  - Child present with facial rash (slapped cheek appearance) which is preceded by low grade fever.
- **Arthropathy**
  - In *adults* B-19 infection *most commonly* present as acute arthralgia and arthritis which is symmetrical and *involves wrist (most often), knee*.
- **Transient aplastic crisis**
  - B-19 infection is the *MC cause of transient aplastic crisis in patient* with chronic hemolytic disease.
  - Unlike patient with erythema infectiosum or arthropathy, these patients can readily transmit B-19 infection to other people.
- **Immunodeficient patient**
  - *MC* manifestation is chronic anemia with reticulocytopenia (Pure red cell aplasia)
- **Fetal and congenital infection**
  - Maternal B-19 infection usually does not adversely affect fetus but can rarely cause nonimmunohydrops fetalis if infection occur in first 20 weeks of pregnancy.

HPV-16 is the commonest HPV associated with Ca cervix

Diagnosis

- Most commonly relies on B-19 specific IgM and IgG antibodies.

PAPOVA VIRUS

- Nonenveloped, Icosahedral double stranded DNA, tumor viruses
- Family contains 2 genera:
  1. *Polyoma virus* – which contains SV 40, polyoma viruses.
  2. *Papilloma virus* – which contain human and animal papilloma virus.

HUMAN PAPILLOMA VIRUS (HPV)

- HPV *selectively infects* the epithelium of skin and mucous membrane and may immortalize the keratinocyte leading either asymptomatic infection or warts or neoplasia.
- Genome consists of:
  - Early (E) region
  - Late (L) region
  - Upstream regulatory region (URR).
- Products of E genes **(E6; E7)** are related to immortalization or malignant transformation of keratinocytes by interfering with **P53, Rb gene** respectively.
- HPV *infects only* human skin and *grows only* in organ cultures of human skin.

Clinical Features
- Replication of HPV begins with the infection of **basal cells**.
- **Koilocytes** appear in granular cells.

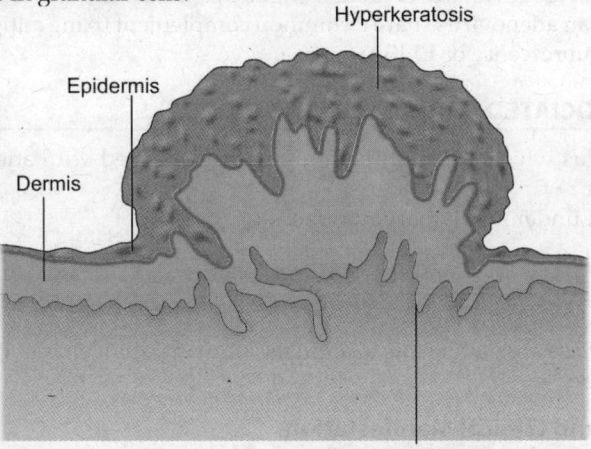

Clinical Presentation
a. **Cutaneous Warts**
   - Common Warts (verruca vulgaris) — Type 1, 2, 3, 4
   - Plantar warts (verruca plantaris)
   - Flat warts (verruca plana) – *MC* among children – Type 3, 10
   - Also associated with Sq cell carcinoma and dysplasia of penis, anus, vagina and vulva; epidermodysplasia verruciformis (type 5, 8).
   - HPV-7 is particularly seen in Butchers and Fishmongers
b. **Anogenital warts (condyloma acuminatum)**
   - Caused by type 6 and 11
   - In women vulva & vgina are commonest site.
   - In male, the most common site of lesion are: Shaft of penis, peri-anal skin and the anal canal.
c. **Orolaryngeal lesion**
   - Recurrent respiratory papillomatosis: Caused by HPV type 6 & 11. Child acquire infection while passage through birth canal
   - Adult acquire infection from orogenital contact with an infected sexual partner
   - Disease is characterized by presence of benign squamous papillomata on the mucosa of the respiratory tract, most commonly on the larynx.
   - Surgery is the only treatment and recurrence is common Oral papillomatosis is the other disease caused by variety of HPV infections.
d. **Neoplastic lesion**
   - CIN-1: – Type 6, 11 (low risk)
   - Cervical cancer – 16, 18, 31, 33, 45 (high risk types)
   - Squamous cell Ca – HPV types 5 or 8 in patients of epiderm
     - odysplasia verruciformis
   - Oropharyngeal squamous cell Ca

Diagnosis
- The *most sensitive* and *specific* method of diagnosis is PCR or hybrid capture assay to detect HPV nucleic acids and to identify specific virus type.

Treatment
- *Cryosurgery* is initial *treatment of choice* for condyloma accuminatum.
- Topically – Podophyllum, podofilox
  - Interferon (IFN)

Prevention
- **Two vaccines are available:** Quadrivalent (Gardasil, Merck) and bivalent (Cervarix) vaccines.

Multiple Choice Questions

Herpes Virus

1a. Vaccine contraindicated in pregnancy: [NEET Pattern 2019]
   a. Typhoid
   b. Varicella
   c. Measles
   d. Rubella

1b. The most common cause of sporadic viral encephalitis is:
   a. Japanese B encephalitis [AIIMS 07]
   b. Herpes simplex encephalitis
   c. HIV encephalitis
   d. Rubeola encephalitis

2. A 29-year-old person comes with focal seizures. MRI shows frontal and temporal enhancement. What is the most probable diagnosis? [AI 10]
   a. Meningococcal meningitis
   b. Herpes simplex encephalitis
   c. Japanese encephalitis
   d. Enterovirus encephalitis

3. Disseminated unilateral lesion of 5 day duration: [NEET Pattern 2019]

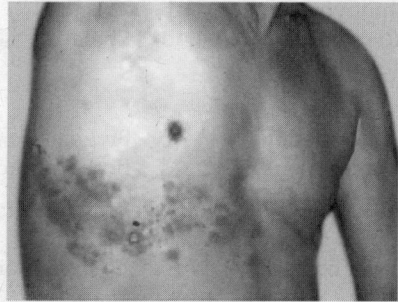

   a. Disseminated HSV
   b. Varicella zoster virus
   c. Herpes simplex
   d. Vaccinia

4. A 6-year-old girl presented to OPD with complaint of painful vesicular lesion on her lower extremity for the past 4 days. What is the most likely etiologic virus. [NEET Pattern 2019]

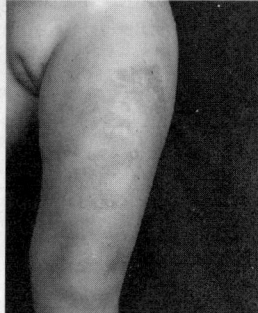

   a. Cox sackie virus
   b. HPV
   c. HHV 6
   d. Varicella Zoster

5. Herpes Zoster virus remain latent in:
   a. Dorsal root ganglion [NEET Pattern 2018]
   b. Ventral horn cells
   c. Pain receptors in skin
   d. Spinal cord

6. Shingles is caused by: [NEET Pattern 2018]
   a. Human herpes virus 1
   b. Human herpes virus 2
   c. Human herpes virus 3
   d. Human herpes virus 4

Varicella Zoster Virus

7. Infectivity of chickenpox lasts for:
   a. Till the last scab falls off [AI 02, AIIMS 00]
   b. 6 days after onset of rash
   c. 3 days after onset of rash
   d. Till the fever subsides

8. Which of the following pair is correct? [PGI 05]
   a. RSV – Bronchiolitis
   b. HHV5 – Infectious mononucleosis
   c. Parvovirus exanthem subitum
   d. HHV-6 – Kaposi sarcoma
   e. VZV – Chickenpox

9. Varicella Zoster remains latent in: [NEET Pattern 2018]
   a. Trigeminal Ganglion
   b. Macrophages
   c. T-cells
   d. B-cells

CMV

10. Which of the following does not establish a diagnosis of congenital CMV infection in a neonate? [AI 09]
    a. Urine culture of CMV
    b. IgG CMV antibodies in blood
    c. Intra-nuclear inclusion bodies in hepatocytes
    d. CMV viral DNA in blood by polymerase chain reaction

11. A 7 days old neonate with microcephaly and periventricular calcification was suspected to have CMV. Which is the best sample that should be collected for DNA-PCR?
    a. Liver biopsy
    b. CSF [AIIMS 2017]
    c. Blood
    d. Urine

12. All of the following statement are true regarding CNS infection *except*: [AIIMS 16]
    a. Measles virus is causative agent of subacute sclerosing panencephalitis
    b. Cytomegalovirus causes bilateral temporal lobe hemorrhagic infarction
    c. Prion infection cause spongiform encephalopathy
    d. JC virus is causative agent of progressive multifocal leucoencephalopathy

13. A 40-year-old man underwent kidney transplantation. Two month after transplantation, he developed fever and feature suggestive of bilateral diffuse interstitial pneumonia. Which of the following is most likely etiologic agent? [AIIMS 13]
    a. Herpes simplex virus b. Cytomegalovirus
    c. Epstein-Barr virus   d. Varicella - zoster virus

14. In a patient with a vesicle on shin. Microscopy on Tzank smear showed giant cells. Causative agents is: [AIIMS 15]
    a. Vaccinia virus   b. Varicella zoster
    c. Tuberculous   d. Molluscum contagiosum

15. Infection with which virus resemble megaloblastic anemia? [NEET Pattern 2019]
    a. EBV   b. VZV
    c. HSV   d. CMV

16. Which virus is most likely to be transmitted by organ transplantation? [NEET Pattern 2018]
    a. EBV   b. CMV
    c. HSV-1   d. VZV

EBV

17. The following diseases are associated with Epstein-Barr virus infection, *except*: [AI 06]
    a. Infectious mononucleosis
    b. Epidermodysplasia verruciformis
    c. Nasopharyngeal carcinoma
    d. Oral hairy leukoplakia

18. A patient with sore throat has a positive Paul Bunnell test. The causative organism is: [AI 10]
    a. EBV   b. Herpes virus
    c. Adenovirus   d. Cytomegalovirus

19. A 20-year-old male with history of fever and enlarged lymph nodes and sore throat, suspected to have infections mononucleosis and was ordered a Paul Bunnell test. What is the principle of the test? [AIIMS 2016, 2017]
    a. Heterophile agglutination test
    b. Neutralization test
    c. Complement fixation test
    d. Agglutination reaction

20. Epstein-Barr virus causes autoimmunity by:
    a. Molecular mimicry [AI 2012]
    b. Inducing inappropriate expression of class II MHC
    c. Release of sequestered antigens
    d. Polyclonal B cell activation

Others

21. Hypoplasia of limb and scarring is caused by: [AIIMS May 2011]
    a. Varicella   b. Herpes simplex
    c. Rubella   d. Toxoplasma

22. Viral enterotoxin is detected as a possible mechanism of pathogenesis in: [PGI 13]
    a. Adenovirus   b. Rotavirus
    c. Calcivirus   d. Astrovirus

23. Parvovirus B-19 does not cause: [AIIMS 08]
    a. Roseola infantum
    b. Aplastic anemia in sickle cell
    c. Fetal hydrops
    d. Collapsing FSGS

24. Parvo virus causes: [PGI 07]
    a. Aplastic anemia   b. Erythema infectiosum
    c. Roseola infantum   d. Arthritis

25. In parvovirus infection what is common in adult? [PGI 07]
    a. Bone marrow   b. PRCA
    c. Erythema infectiosum d. Arthropathy

26. True about parvovirus is: [NEET Pattern 2018]
    a. Proliferates in T-cells
    b. Proliferates in erythroid progenitor cells
    c. Proliferates in megakaryocytes
    d. Proliferates in B-cells

27. Which of the following statement is correct? [PGI 05]
    a. Viral warts usually resolve spontaneously
    b. Plantar warts should not be excised
    c. Callosity are formed occupationally
    d. Corns are viral in etiology
    e. Plantar warts are painless

28. Vaccine preparation requires which virus as vector?
    a. Rhinovirus   b. Vaccinia   [AIIMS 17]
    c. Adenovirus   d. Ebola
    e. Hepatitis B

29. HPV vaccine is: [AIIMS 09]
    a. Monovalent   b. Bivalent
    c. Quadrivalent d. Both b and c

30. About parvovirus B19 all are true *except*: [AI 2011]
    a. Spread by respiratory route
    b. Has affinity for erythrocyte progenitor cells
    c. Causes transient aplastic crisis
    d. Transplacental transfer occurs in only 10% of cases

31. Virus causing head and neck cancer: [PGI Nov. 11]
    a. EBV   b. HSV
    c. HPV   d. HBV
    e. HCV

32. Not a cause of epidemic encephalitis: [PGI May 2013]
    a. Herpes simplex virus   b. Rabies
    c. West Nile virus   d. Nipah virus
    e. Japanese encephalitis virus

33. Post-transplant nephropathy after 1 month is most likely be due to: [AIIMS May 2014]
    a. Hepatitis C   b. HHV-6
    c. Polyoma BK virus d. Herpes simplex viruses

34. Not associated with HHV8: [AIIMS 2018]
    a. Castleman's disease
    b. Kaposi sarcoma
    c. Body cavity lymphoma
    d. Adult T cell lymphoma

Explanations and References with Illustrative Answers

1a. Ans. (b) Varicella *Internet Resource*

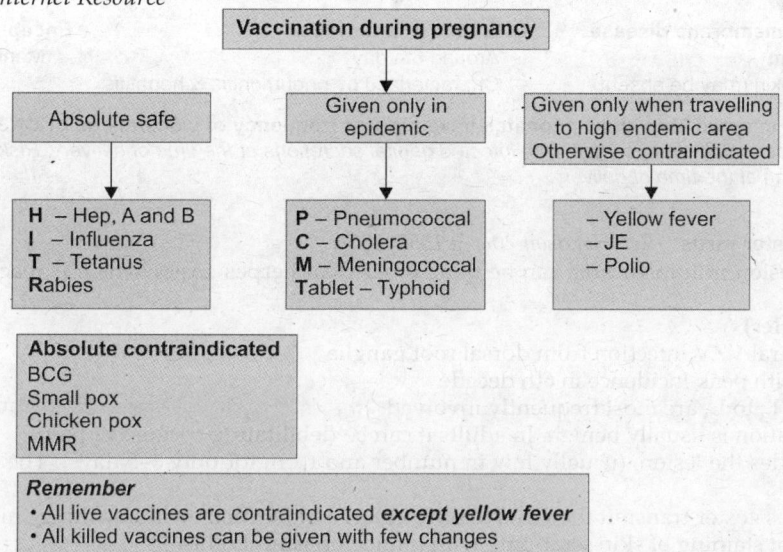

1b. Ans. (b) Herpes simplex encephalitis *Ref. Harrison 19/e, p 891, 20/e, p 1349*

"The most common virus causing sporadic cases of encephalitis in immunocompetent adult are HSV-1, VZV, EBV and less commonly enterovirus." HSV accounts for 10–20% of all cases of sporadic viral encephalitis.

Remember: Epidemic of encephalitis are caused by Arbovirus: **1. Alphaviruses, 2. Toga viruses, 3. Bunyaviruses**

Virus causing encephalitis			
• Common:	– Arbovirus – HSV-1	– Enterovirus – Mumps	– EBV – VZV
• Less common:	– CMV, HIV, measles		
• Rare:	– Adenovirus, influenza virus, parainfluenza virus, rabies, rubella		

Neurological manifestation of Herpes			
CNS manifestation		**ANS manifestation**	**PNS manifestation**
Encephalitis (HSV-1 > HSV-2) Meningitis (HSV-2 > HSV-1)	Involving temporal lobe especially HSV is *MC* cause of recurrent lymphocytic meningitis **(Mollaret's meningitis)**	• ANS dysfunction especially of sacral region leading to numbness, tingling of the buttocks or perineal areas. • Urinary retention, constipation, impotence. • **Guillain-Barre' syndrome**	• Bell's palsy • Cranial polyneuritis

2. Ans. (b) Herpes simplex encephalitis *Ref. Harrison 20/e, p 1349, 19/e p 1178*

Herpes simplex encephalitis

- In children and young adults primary HSV infection can led to encephalitis, by neurotropic spread of virus from periphery via olfactory bulb.
- Reactivation of latent CNS infection is another mechanism for the development of HSV encephalitis.
- In other majority of cases, there is prior mucocutaneous HSV-1 infection which gets reactivated.
- **Clinical hallmark** of HSV infection include acute onset of fever, and *focal neurological symptoms and signs, especially of temporal lobe.*

Diagnosis	– CSF protein and CSF lymphocytosis – Brain biopsy is gold standard – HSV DNA detection in CSF by PCR has largely replaced biopsy
Treatment	– IV acyclovir

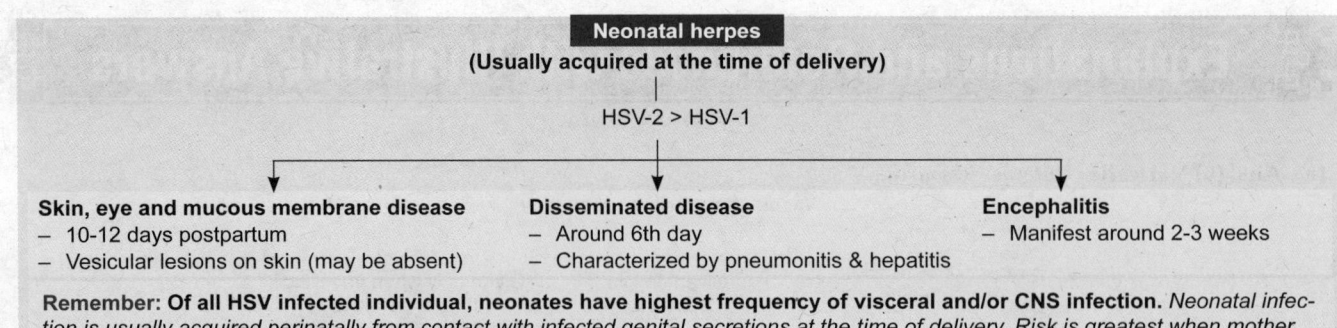

3. **Ans. (b) Varicella Zoster virus** *Ref. Harrison 20/e, p 1355, 1356*
   Unilateral vesicular lesion in lumbar area can be none other than herpes zoster which is reactivation of varicella zoster virus infection.
   Herpes Zoster (Shingles)
   - Reactivation of lateral VZV infection from dorsal root ganglia
   - Occurs at all age with peak incidence in 6th decade
   - Dermatomes from T_3 to L_3 are most frequently involved
   - In children reactivation is usually benign. In adults it can be debilitating because of pain
   - Pain usually precedes the lesion, (usually few in number and form for only 3–5 days). The total duration of disease is 7–10 days
   - Patients with herpes zoster transmit the virus to seronegative individuals with resulting chickenpox
   Diagnosis: Fluorescent staining of skin scrapping with monoclonal antibodies
   - Treatment Acyclovir

4. **Ans. (d) Varicella Zoster** *Ref. Harrison 20/e, p 1355*
   Though herpes zoster usually occur in 6th decade. It can affect child group too
   Other options:
   - Coxsackie virus: Cause vesicular lesion in and around oral cavity
   - HPV: Produce warts (not vesicular lesion)
   - HHV-6: Cause roseola infantum. In older age group HHV-6 is associated with mononucleosis syndromes

5. **Ans. (a) Dorsal root ganglion** *Ref. Harrison 20/e, p 1355*
   Allready explained.

6. **Ans. (c) Human herpes virus 3** *Ref. Harrison 20/e, p 1355*
   Shingles is caused by VZV which is classified as human herpes type III.

7. **Ans. (b) 6 days after onset of rash** *Ref. Park 22/e, p 136*
   "Period of communicability of varicella range from 1 to 2 days before the appearance of rash, and 4 to 5 days there after."
   The patient ceases to be infectious once the lesions have crusted.
   Scabs are not infective
   So, option "a" is wrong.
   Important features of chickenpox
   Causative agent   – Varicella zoster virus (HHV type 3)
   Incubation period   – 14 to 16 days
   Secondary attack rate   – 90%

Rash	
Chickenpox	**Smallpox**
Superficial	Deep seated
Pleomorphic	Only one stage of rash at 1 time
Centripetal	Centrifugal
Unilocular	Multilocular
Dew drop like appearance	Umbilicated
Inflammation (+)nt	No area of inflammation around vesicle
Mostly flexor surface	Mostly extensor surface

8. **Ans. (a), (b) and (e) RSV – Bronchiolitis, HHV5 – Infectious mononucleosis, and VZV – Chickenpox**

Ref. Ananthanarayan 9/e, p 471

> **Remember:** *RSV* is most common cause of bronchiolitis.
> Other causes are:
> – Parainfluenza virus
> – Influenza virus
> – Adenovirus
> – Mycoplasma pneumoniae

9. **Ans. (a) Trigeminal ganglion** *Ref. Ananthanarayan 10/e, p 1355*

> **Site of latency of varicella virus**
> – Dorsal root ganglia (Most frequent) T3-L2
> – Trigeminal ganglia (frequently ophthalmic branch)

10. **Ans. (b) IgG CMV antibodies in blood** *Ref. Nelson 17/e, p 1068; Greenwood 18/e, p 440*

    "IgG antibody test is of little diagnostic value as positive results also reflects maternal antibodies" although its absence exclude the diagnosis of congenital CMV infection."
    .... Nelson

    Diagnosis of congenital CMV infection
    - **Virus isolation**
        - Definitive and best method.
        - Culture: Urine and saliva are best specimen for culture although it can be isolated from buffy coat (blood), bronchoalveolar washing.
        - PCR: Replaced virus isolation for routine detection of CMV infection (Investigation of choice). Blood is the preferred specimen.
    - **Antibody assay**
        - IgG test are not diagnostic as positive results reflects maternal antibodies.
        - IgM test lacks sensitivity and specificity and are unreliable for diagnosis of congenital infection.
    - **Detection in amniotic fluid**
        - Fetal infection can be confirmed by viral isolation from amniotic fluid.
        - Detection of viral genome by PCR in amniotic fluid is equally sensitive (Viral genome > 10^5 genome is a predictor of symptomatic congenital infection).

    > **Remember:** CMV infected cells contain large intranuclear and smaller intracytoplasmic inclusions which are pathognomic for CMV infection.

11. **Ans. (d) Urine** *Ref. Nelson 20/e, p 1592, 3074; Ghai 8/e p272*
    Laboratory Diagnosis of Congenital CMV Infection in Newborns
    - **Definitive diagnosis** of congenital CMV infection is based on isolation of the virus in the first **three weeks** of life because isolation beyond that age may indicate an acquired infection.

    The standard laboratory test for diagnosing congenital CMV infection is polymerase chain reaction (PCR) on saliva or urine (preferred), usually collected and tested for confirmation.
    - It is a very sensitive and specific method of making the diagnosis because there are massive quantities of CMV being excreted in the urine and saliva.
    - The reason for the confirmatory test on **urine** is because most CMV seropositive mothers shed CMV virus in their breast milk.
        - This can cause a false-positive CMV result on saliva collected shortly after the baby has breastfed.

    CMV serology
    - **CMV serology in the newborn is a poor way of identifying congenital CMV infection.**
        - Although the presence of IgM is very specific for fetal and newborn infection, it is not very sensitive. Because the overwhelming infection occurs early on in gestation, the fetus does not mount a significant immune response.

12. **Ans. (b) CMV virus causes B/L temporal lobe infarction** *Ref. Harrison 19/e, p 1192, 20/e, p 1363*
    CNS manifestation of CMV:
    - CMV rarely cause CNS infection.
    - Two forms of CMV encephalitis are seen:
        1. Resemble HIV encephalitis and present as progressive dementia.
        2. Ventriculoencephalitis—Characterized by cranial nerve deficit, nystagmus and ventriculomegally.
    - In immunocompromised patient CMV can also cause subacute progressive polyradiculopathy.

    No where is given that CMV can cause temporal lobe infarction: Hence answer

Other options:
- **Subacute sclerosing panencephalitis**
  - It is a rare chronic progressive demyelinating disease of CNS associated with a chronic permissive infection of brain tissue with measles virus.
- **Progressive multifocal leucoencephalopathy**
  - Progressive disorder characterised pathologically by multifocal areas of demyelination of varying size distributing throughout the CNS caused by JC virus.
- **Spongiform encephalopathy**
  - Caused by prion infection; HIV infection.

13. **Ans. (b) Cytomegalovirus**   *Ref. Harrison 19/e, p 1192, 20/e, p 1363*
    It is a case of diffuse interstitial pneumonitis due to CMV.

    > **Remember:**
    > - **CMV** is the **MC** infection complicating organ transplantation.
    > - **CMV** is **MC** cause of intrauterine infection.
    > - Risk of post-transplant CMV infection is greatest 5-13 weeks after transplant

Infections after Kidney Transplantation			
Period after transplantation			
Infection site	Early (< 1 month)	Middle (1 - 4 months)	Late (> 6 months)
Urinary tract	Bacteria (Escherichia coli, Klebsiella, Enterobacteriaceae, Pseudomonas, Enterococcus) associated with bacteremia and pyelonephritis, Candida	Cytomegalovirus (fever alone is common) BK virus *(nephropathy, graft failure, vasculopathy)*, JC virus.	Bacteria; late infections usually not associated with bacteremia
Lungs	Legionella	**CMV diffuse interstitial** *pneumonitis*, Pneumocystis, Aspergillus, Legionella	Nocardia, Aspergillus, Mucor
Central nervous system		Listeria meningitis, CMV encephalitis, Toxoplasma gondii	CMV retinitis, Listeria meningitis, cryptococcal meningitis, Aspergillus, Nocardia

14. **Ans. (b) Varicella zoster**   *Ref. Ananthanarayan 10/e, p 478*
    "Multinucleated giant cells and type a intranuclear inclusion bodies may be seen in smears prepared by scraping the base of early vesicles (Tzank smears) and stained with toludine blue, Giemsa or Papanicolaou stain"

    > **Note:** Electron microscopy of vesicle fluid can demonstrate the typical virus.

15. **Ans. (d) CMV**   *Ref. Ananthanarayan 10/e, p 479*
    Cytomegalovirus, the largest virus of herpes family are characterized by enlargement of infected cell and prominent intranuclear inclusions.

16. **Ans. (b) CMV**   *Ref. Harrison 20/e, p 1033*
    CMV can get reactivated after transplantation or recipient may become super infected with other strain. The disease however is most severe when the donor is seronegative and recipient is seropositive and there is hematopoietic stem cell transplantation.

17. **Ans. (b) Epidermodysplasia verruciformis**   *Ref. Harrison 19/e, p 1199, 18/e, p 1467*
    Epidermodysplasia verruciformis is a rare inherited disease with numerous flat warts on the hand and feet.
    These individuals have defect in cell mediated immunity and increased susceptibility to human papilloma virus infection.

    > **Remember:** Multiple myeloma is associated with human herpes virus 8, in some cases not with EBV.

18. **Ans. (a) EBV**   *Ref. Ananthanarayan 10/e, p 482*
    Paul Bunnell test is the standard diagnostic procedure of infectious mononucleosis which is caused by EBV.
    Paul Bunnell test detects heterophile antibody.

    Paul Bunnell Test
    Heterophile agglutination test:
    - In this test inactivated serum (56°C for 30 minutes) in doubling dilutions is mixed with equal volumes of a 1% suspension of sheep erythrocytes.

- An agglutination titre of 100 or above is suggestive of infectious mononucleosis.
- For confirmation, differential absorption of agglutinins with guinea pig kidney and ox red cells is necessary
- Infectious mononucleosis antibody is removed by ox red cell but not guinea pig kidney.
- The Paul Bunnell antibody develops early during the course of infectious mononucleosis, and disappears within two months.
- *False-positive:* In patient with lymphoma, hepatitis, malaria, connective tissue disease.

Differential absorption test for Paul-Bunnell antibody		
	Guinea pig kidney	Ox red cells
Normal serum	Absorbed	Not absorbed
Antibody after serum therapy	Absorbed	Not absorbed
Infectious mononucleosis	Not absorbed	Absorbed

Remember:
- MC cause of heterophile antibody (+)ve infectious mononucleosis is **EBV**.
- MC cause of **heterophile antibody (–) ve** infectious mononucleosis is **CMV**.
- Heterophile (–) ve IM is also caused by toxoplasmosis, Listeria, non-infectious stimuli.

19. **Ans. (a) i.e. Heterophile agglutination test** *Ref. Ananthanarayan 10/e, p 482*

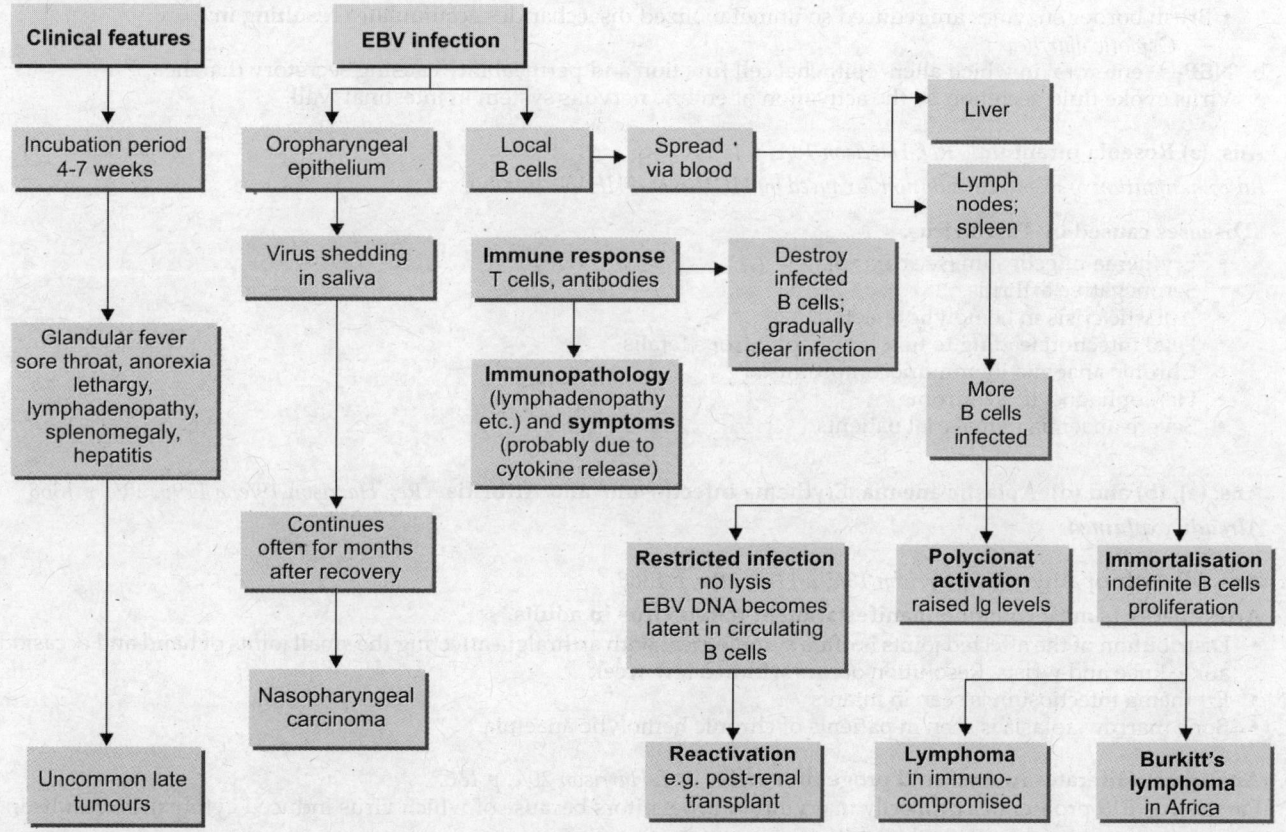

20. **Ans. (d) Polyclonal B-cell activation** *Ref. Harrison 20/e, p 1358; Jawetz 27/e, p 475*
    EBV receptor (CD-21) on the surface of B-cells is also the receptor for the C3d component of complement. So, when B-cells are infected with EBV they become transformed and can proliferate indefinitely.
    This polyclonal activation of B-cells leads to the production of antibodies directed against host cells and viral proteins.
    Thus, this is also not difficult to understand that cellular immunity is more important than humoral immunity in controlling EBV infection.

21. **Ans. (a) Varicella** *Ref. Harrison 20/e, p 1355; Nelson 18/e, p 1365*
    Congenital varicella syndrome is characteristically associated with limb reduction defects (If infection occurs prior to limb bud formation) and scarring of skin.
    Any neonate with limb defect along with skin scarring should be investigated for congenital varicella syndrome.

Limb hypoplasia and congenital varicella
- Limb hypoplasia are seen if infection occurs prior to or during limb bud formation
- *The virus has affinity to tissues that are in a rapid development stage such as the limb buds*
- Fetus infected at 6-12 weeks of gestation appears to have maximal risk of limb hypoplasia
- The remaining of the torso may be entirely normal in appearance

Scarring of Skin (Cicatricial skin lesions)
- Scarring of skin is a common feature of congenital varicella syndrome
- The characteristic cutaneous lesion has been called a **Cicatrix**
- Cicatrix represents zigzag scarring in a dermatomal distribution (and is often associated with atrophy of the affected limb)

> **Note:** Perinatal varicella is associated with mortality rates as high as 30% when maternal disease develop within 5 day before delivery or within 48 h thereafter.

22. **Ans. (b) Rotavirus**   *Ref. Harrison 18/e, p 1591*
    Mechanism of Rotavirus diarrhea:
    a. Rotavirus destroy mature enterocytes of proximal small intestine.
       - Loss of absorptive villi and proliferation of secretory crypt cells
         – *Secretory diarrhea*
       - Brush border enzymes are reduced so unmetabolized disaccharides accumulates resulting in:
         – *Osmotic diarrhea*
    b. NSP_4 = enterotoxin which alters epithelial cell function and permeability causing secretory diarrhea.
    c. Virus evoke fluid secretion by the activation of enteric nervous system in intestinal wall.

23. **Ans. (a) Roseola infantum**   *Ref. Harrison 19/e, p 1195*
    Roseola infantum or exanthem subitum is caused by HHV-6 and HHV-7 (rarely).

    > **Diseases caused by Parvo virus:**
    > - Erythema infectiosum (see color plate)
    > - Seronegative arthritis
    > - Aplastic crisis in hemolytic anaemia
    > - Fetal infection leading to non-immunohydrops fetalis
    > - Chronic anaemia in immunocompromised
    > - Hemophagocytic syndrome
    > - Severe anaemia in malarial patients.

24. **Ans. (a), (b) and (d) Aplastic anemia, Erythema infectiosum and Arthritis**   *Ref. Harrison 19/e, p 1196, 20/e, p 1368*
    Already explained

25. **Ans. (d) Arthropathy**   *Ref. Harrison 19/e, p 1196, 20/e, p 1368*
    Arthropathy is most common manifestation of parvo virus in adults.
    - Distribution of the affected joints is often symmetrical with arthralgia affecting the small joints of hand and occasionally ankle knee and wrists. Resolution occurs within a few week
    - Erythema infectiosum is seen in infants
    - Bone marrow aplasia is seen in patients of chronic hemolytic anaemia.

26. **Ans. (b) Proliferates in erythroid progenitor cells**   *Ref. Harrison 20/e, p 1367*
    Parvovirus B19 proliferates primarily in erythroid progenitors because of which virus induced cytotoxicity results in cessation of red-cell production and leads to transient aplastic crises.
    Parvovirus
    - SS DNA virus
    - **Smallest virus**
    - **Has smallest genome**
    - Only one medically important human parvovirus—Parvovirus B19
    - Transmission is by respiratory route and through blood.
    - Infection is commonly acquired in childhood (5-10 yrs).
    - Most of the infections are asymptomatic.
    - Most common presentation is respiratory infection with an erythematous maculopapular rash and arthralgia → *Erythema infectiosum or fifth disease.*
    - Starts with prominent erythema of cheeks→*slapped cheek disease*

- In human bone marrow Parvovirus-B19 infection is restricted to erythroid progenitor cells.
- *Parvovirus B-19 induces aplastic crisis in children with chronic hemolytic anemias, as in sickle cell disease.*
- Parvovirus B-19 infection during second or third trimester of pregnancy may result in **nonimmune fetal hydrops.** *Transplacental transmission rate is 30% or higher.*
- In **adults**, parvovirus infection commonly causes acute **arthralgia and arthritis.**
- *Parvovirus B-19 is difficult to grow and virus isolation is not used to detect infection.*

27. **Ans. (a, b) and (c) Viral warts usually resolve spontaneously, Plantar warts should not be excised, and Callosity are formed occupationally** *Ref. Harrison 17/e, p 1118; 20/e, p1371; Short case by S. Das 2/e, p 20*

    Warts are patches of hyperkeratotic overgrowth of skin.
    - Three types of warts can be seen:
        a. Common wart
        b. Venereal wart
        c. Senile wart
    - Common wart can be:
        - Verruca vulgaris   = *MC* type
        - Verruca plana   = Flat wart - *MC* type in children
        - Plantar wart   = Verrucaplantaris - painfull

      HPV is the etiological agent of these warts.

    Treatment - Most HPV lesion resolve spontaneously.
    - Cryosurgery is treatment of choice.
    - Surgical excision is not recommended as it leads to scarring and recurrence rate is quite high.

    Other options
    - **Callosity** - Superficial circumscribed yellowish white flat thickened patch of hyperkerotic material. Etiology is mostly occupational.
    - **Corn** - Localised hyperkeratosis of skin.
        - Usually occurs at the pressure site, e.g. on sole, foot and toes.

28. **Ans. (b) Vaccinia** *Ref. Ananthanarayan 10/e, p 467*
    - Vaccinia virus is unique in that it is an artificial virus and does not occur in nature as such.
    - It is used as a vector for development of recombinant vaccines.
    - Its genome can accommodate 25,000 foreign base pairs.
    - Genes encoding antigens of HBV, HIV, rabies and neuropeptides are inserted in it.
    - However it is not useful as vector for human use due to pathogenic effect.

29. **Ans. (d) Both b and c** *Ref. Harrison 20/e, p 1372, 19/e p 1199*
    - *HPV is associated with cervical and oral cancer. In order to reduce the incidence of these potentially lethal malignancy, HPV vaccine has been introduced.*

    HPV vaccines
    - Directed against viruses types that cause anogenital disease and are derived from the expression of the major capsid protein(L) gene in tissue culture.
    - **Currently three vaccines are available**
        1. *Quadrivalent vaccine (Gardasil, Merck):* It contains major capsid protein from low risk types 6 and 11 and high risk types 16 and 18. It is administered to girls and young women 9 - 26 years of age.
        2. *Bivalent (cervarix):* Containing HPV types 16 and 18.
        3. Nine valent vaccine (target 6, 11, 16, 18 plus 31, 33, 45, 52, 58).

    Dose: 3 doses are given in 0; 2nd and 6th month

    Adverse effects: Minimal consists of mild to moderate localized pain, erythema, swelling.

30. **Ans. (d) Transplacental transfer occurs in only 10% of cases.** *Ref. Harrison 19/e, p 1195, 20/e, p 1368*

    Parvovirus B19
    - Member of genus erythrovirus, exclusively infects humans
    - Transmission occurs predominantly via respiratory route, transfusion related transmission also seen.
        - *Pathogenesis* - B19 replicates primarily in erythroid progenitors. This specifically is due to limited tissue distribution of B19 receptor, blood groups antigen (globoside). Resulting in transient aplastic crisis.
            - Other cells bearing B-19 receptor include megakaryocytes, endothelial cells, placenta, myocardium and liver.
    - Transplacental infection is seen in 30% and the risk of fetal loss is 9%. Risk of congenital infection is < 1%.

31. **Ans (a, c) EBV and HPV** *Ref: Harrison 18/e p 656*

Oncogenic Microbes and Parasites	
Organism	**Neoplasm**
Human papilloma virus (Papovaviridae)	Cervical, vulvar, penile cancers, squamous cell carcinoma, oropharyngeal carcinoma
HSV type 2	Cervical carcinoma
Hepatitis B virus (Hepadnaviridae)	Hepatocellular carcinoma
Hepatitis C virus (Flaviviridae)	Hepatocellular carcinoma, Lymphoplasmacytic lymphoma
HTLV – I (Retroviridae)	Adult T-cell leukemia/ lymphoma
HTLV – II (Retroviridae)	T-cell variant of hairy cell leukemia
HTLV – III (Retroviridae)	AIDS related malignancies, NHL, Kaposi sarcoma, SCC (esp of Urogenital tract), Diffuse large B-cell lymphoma Burkitt's lymphoma
Epstein barr virus (Herpesviridae)	Mixed cellularity Hodgkin's, Nasopharyngeal carcinoma (anaplastic), African Burkitt's lymphoma, Post organ transplant lymphoma, Primary CNS diffuse large B-cell lymphoma, Extranodal NK/T cell lymphoma (nasal type)
H. Pylori	Gastric Malt lymphoma, Gastric cancer
Human Herpes virus 8	Primary effusion lymphoma, Multicentric Castleman's disease
Schistosoma hematobium	Bladder cancer (squamous cell)
Clonorchis	Cholongiocarcinoma
Opisthorchis	Cholongiocarcinoma

32. **Ans. (a, b) Herpes simplex virus, Rabies** *Ref. Harrison 18/e, p 3418, 3421*

Viral encephalitis	
Sporadic	**Epidemic**
Herpes virus (HSV-1*, VZV*, EBV*, CMV)	Alpha virus (ECE virus, western equine encephalitis virus)
Rabies	Flaviviruses (West Nile virus*), Japanese encephalitis virus, Pawassan virus, St. Louis encephalitis* virus)
Mumps	Bunyaviruses (California encephalitis virus, La Crosse virus)
Enterovirus	Nipah virus

* Common cause

Nipah virus
- Nipah virus infection is a newly emerging zoonosis that causes severe disease in both animals and humans. The natural host of virus are fruit bats.
- Clinical presentation of nipah virus range from asymptomatic infection to acute respiratory syndrome to fatal encephalitis.
- It can cause in pig and other domestic animals too.
- It was associated with epidemic of encephalitis in Bangladesh in 2004.

33. **Ans. (c) Polyoma BK virus** *Ref. Harrison 20/e, p 1036*

Causes of nephropathy (1 month after renal transplant)
CMV infection (MC) > BK virus infection > JC virus infection

Both BK virus and JC virus belongs to papova viridae.

34. **Ans. (d) Adult T cell lymphoma** *Ref. Harrison 19/e 1476*
Manifestations of HHV-8 Infection
Immunocompetent Individual: Fever and maculopapular rash. Among individuals with intact immunity, chronic asymptomatic infection is the rule, and neoplastic disorders generally develop only after subsequent immunocompromise.
Immunocompromised persons:
a. *Primary infection*: Fever, splenomegaly, lymphoid hyperplasia, pancytopenia, or rapid- onset Kaposi Sarcoma.
b. *Reactivation of latent infection*: Kaposi Sarcoma, Body cavity Lymphoma, Multicentric Castleman's disease.

NEET Pattern Questions

1. **Lymphocytosis with atypical lymphocytes are seen in infection with:** *[Ref. Harrison 20/e, p 1358]*
   a. HSV
   b. HBV
   c. EBV
   d. RSV

   Note: Among atypical lymphocytes CD8+ t-cells are predominant

2. **Paul Bunnell reaction is a type of:**
   a. Agglutination
   b. CF
   c. Precipitation
   d. Flocculation test
   [Ref. Ananthanarayan, 10/e, p482]

3. **Most common Molluscum virus:**
   a. 1
   b. 2
   c. 3
   d. 4

4. **Congenital varicella infection causes all except:**
   a. Macrocephaly
   b. Limb hypoplasia
   c. Cortical atrophy
   d. Cicatrix
   [Ref. Harrison, 20/e, p 1355]

5. **Which pox would not grow in egg, animal cells?**
   a. Cow pox
   b. Vaccinia
   c. Variola
   d. Molluscum
   [Ref. Ananthanarayan, 10/e, p 471]

   Molluscum virus cannot be grown in egg, tissue culture or animals.

6. **Shingles are seen in:** *[Ref. Ananthanarayan, 10/e, p 478]*
   a. IMN
   b. Herpes zoster
   c. Chicken pox
   d. Small pox

7. **HHV-8 causes:**
   a. Burkitt's lymphoma
   b. Nasopharyngeal carcinoma
   c. Kaposi sarcoma
   d. Hepatic carcinoma
   [Ref. Harrison, 20/e, p 1365]

8. **Slapped cheek sign is seen in:**
   a. Parvovirus B19
   b. JC virus
   c. Rota virus
   d. Mumps
   [Ref. Greenwood, 20/e, p 1368]

   B19 cause slapped cheek disease = fifth disease = erythema infectiosum

9. **HHV-6 causes:**
   a. Erythema infectiosum
   b. Kaposi sarcoma
   c. Roseola infantum
   d. Herpangina
   [Ref. Harrison, 20/e, p 1365]

10. **Cause of Herpes Zoster:**
    a. Primary infection with VZV
    b. Recurrent infection with VZV
    c. Reactivation of latent infection of VZV
    d. Multiple infection with VZV
    [Ref. Ananthanarayan, 10/e, p 479]

11. **Most common cause of genital Herpes:**
    a. HSV-1
    b. HSV-2
    c. HSV-3 (VZV)
    d. EBV
    [Ref. Ananthanarayan, 10/e, p 474]

12. **Wrong statement about chicken pox/herpes zoster:**
    a. Caused by VZV
    b. Chicken-pox primary infection
    c. Herpes-zoster recurrent infection
    d. Latent infection in trigeminal ganglion
    [Ref. Ananthanarayan, 10/e, p 477]

13. **CMV belongs to which family of DNA viruses?**
    a. Poxviridae
    b. Herpesviridae
    c. Papovaviridae
    d. Paravoviridae
    [Ref. Ananthanarayan, 10/e, p 480]

14. **True about CMV are all except:**
    a. Most common cause of post-transplantation infection
    b. Most common cause of transplacental infection
    c. A non-enveloped DNA virus
    d. Produces intranuclear inclusions
    [Ref. Ananthanarayan, 10/e, p 472]

    All herpes virus are enveloped virus

15. **Most common pox virus infection in human is:**
    a. Smallpox
    b. Monkeypox
    c. Cowpox
    d. Mulluscum contagiosum *[Ref. Harrison, 20/e, p 1366]*

16. **Most common cause of sporadic encephalitis:**
    a. EBV
    b. HSV
    c. Poliovirus
    d. CMV
    [Ref. Harrison, 20/e, p 1348]

17. **Least common cause of sporadic encephalitis:**
    a. HSV
    b. VZV
    c. Arbovirus
    d. Rhinovirus
    [Ref. Harrison, 20/e, p 1340]

Ans.
1. c. EBV
2. a. Agglutination
3. a. 1
4. a. Macrocephaly
5. d. Molluscum
6. b. Herpes zoster
7. c. Kaposi sarcoma
8. a. Parvovirus B19
9. c. Roseola infantum
10. c. Reactivation...
11. b. HSV-2
12. c. Herpes-zoster...
13. b. Herpesviridae
14. c. A non-enveloped...
15. d. Mulluscum ...
16. b. HSV
17. d. Rhinovirus

Section - B

18. Which of the following belongs to Herpesviridae:
    a. Variola
    b. Adenovirus
    c. HPV
    d. RK virus
    [Ref. Ananthanarayan, 10/e, p 473]

> RK virus is the old name of HHV-7

19. Most sensitive test for diagnosis of infectious mononucleosis:
    a. Monospot test
    b. Paul Bunnell test
    c. Lymphocytosis in peripheral smear
    d. Culture of the virus [Ref. Harrison 20/e, p 1360]

> - Monospot test is more sensitive than classic heterophile test. It is 75% sensitive and 90% specific. False-positive monospot test is seen in connective tissue disease, lymphoma, viral hepatitis and malaria
> - Nucleic acid hybridization is most sensitive means of detecting EBV in patient
> - IgM antibody to VCA is most useful test for diagnosis of infectious mononucleosis

20. HPV-6 most often implicated in causation of:
    a. Cervical cancer
    b. Condyloma acuminata
    c. Flat wart
    d. Common wart [Ref. Greenwood, 18/e, p 455]

21. Herpes simplex virus is:
    a. Single stranded DNA
    b. Double stranded DNA
    c. Single stranded RNA
    d. Double stranded RNA
    [Ref. Ananthanarayan 10/e, p 473]

> Herpes virus produces intranuclear type A inclusion bodies. On chick embryo CAM it produces non-necrotic pocks. Cytopathic changes include well defined foci with heaped up cells and syncytial and giant cell formation.

22. Oropharyngeal carcinoma is caused by:
    a. HBV
    b. CMV
    c. HSV
    d. HPV
    [Ref. Harrison, 20/e, p 1370]

> HPV is associated with invasive cancers of the anus, penis, vulva, vagina, cervix and a subset of oropharyngeal cancers.

23. Which of the herpes virus is included in Biohazard risk group 4?
    a. HSV 1
    b. CMV
    c. EBV
    d. Herpes simiae

> **Biohazard Risk Group IV**
> It includes agents that are likely to cause serious or lethal human disease for which preventive or therapeutic interventions are not usually available.

24. Castleman disease is associated with:
    a. HSV
    b. CMV
    c. EBV
    d. HHV-8
    [Ref. Greenwood, 18/e, p 443]

25. Which of the following is a wrong association?
    a. HPV–CaCx
    b. EBV–Burkitt's lymphoma
    c. HHV 8–Kaposi sarcoma
    d. CMV–Nasopharyngeal carcinoma
    [Ref. Ananthanarayan, 10/e, p 479]

26. EBV enters B-cells through:
    a. CD-1
    b. CD-2
    c. CD-21
    d. CD-19
    [Ref. Ananthanarayan, 10/e, p 481]

27. Human B-cell lymphotropic virus belongs to:
    a. Picorna virus
    b. Pox virus
    c. Reovirus
    d. Herpes virus
    [Ref. Ananthanarayan, 9/e, p 477]

28. Patient present in your clinic. On physical examination, there is bilateral lymphadenopathy, which is tender on palpation. He gave history of sexual contact. He is truck driver by profession. The probable causative agent is: [NEET pattern 2016]
    a. Herpes
    b. LGV
    c. H. ducreyi
    d. Treponema
    [Ref. Park 22/e 308]

Painful vesicles/ulcer single on multiple:	Herpes simplex
Painless ulcer with shotty lymph node:	Syphilis
Painful ulcer with painful bubo:	Chancroid
Painless ulcer with painful inguinal lymphadenopathy:	Lymphogranuloma venereum

29. Most common extra skin manifestation of varicella is involvement of: [NEET pattern 2016]
    a. CNS
    b. Lungs
    c. Kidneys
    d. CVS
    [Ref. Harrison 20/e, p 1355]

> Most common extracutaneous site of involvement in V2V is CNS where the most common manifestation is acute cerebral ataxia and meningeal inflammation.

18. d. RK virus	19. a. Monospot ...	20. b. Condyloma...	21. b. Double ...
22. d. HPV	23. c. EBV	24. d. HHV-8	25. d. CMV-Nasopharyngeal...
26. c. CD-21	27. d. Herpes virus	28. b. LGV	29. a. CNS

DNA Virus

30. All of the following are true about Herpes group of virus *except*: [NEET pattern 2016]
    a. Ether-sensitive
    b. May cause malignancy
    c. HSV II involves below diaphragm
    d. Burkitt's lymphoma involves T-cells
    [Ref. Ananthanarayan, 10/e, p 473; Greenwood 18/e, p 420]

> **Burkitt's lymphoma** = ALL L3.
> • ALL are tumors of relatively mature B cells.

31. All of the following are true about the papovavirus *except*:
    a. They are non-enveloped icosahedral viruses
    b. Produce papilloma
    c. RNA virus
    d. SV-40 is oncogenic [Ref. Ananthanarayan, 10/e p 557]

> Papova virus are nonenveloped; Icosahedral human virus containing Ds DNA as genetic material.
> **Family Papova virus contains 2 genera:**
> 1. Papilloma virus – Contains humans and animal
> 2. Polyoma virus   – Contains SV-40 polyoma viruses

32. Human papillomatosis is caused by:
    a. HSV   b. HPV
    c. HIV   d. HBV
    [Ref. Ananthanarayan, 10/e, p 557]

33. Flat warts is caused by which HP types:
    a. 2, 4   b. 3, 10
    c. 16, 18   d. 5, 8
    [Ref. Harrison 20/e p1371; Greenwood 18/e p456]

> Flat warts (verruca plana) are common among children and occur on the face, neck, chest and flexor surface of the forearm and legs. They are caused by: HPV 3 and HPV 10
> **Note:**
> Common wart: HPV 2, 4 and 7
> Anogenital wart: HPV 6

34. Most common type of HPV associated with cervical cancer: [Ref. Ananthanarayan, 10/e, p 557]
    a. 6, 11   b. 5, 8
    c. 16, 18   d. 6, 8

35. Condyloma accuminatum is caused by:
    a. HSV   b. HPV
    c. HIV   d. VZV
    [Ref. Ananthanarayan, 10/e, p 557]

> Condylomata accuminata or genital wart is a soft pedunculated wart found on the external genitalia is usually due to types 6 and 11, 42-44. It may be transmitted venerally and may occasionally turn malignant.

36. HPV infects which cells first?
    a. Superficial cells epidermis
    b. Basal cells
    c. Subcutaneous cells
    d. Dermal cells [Ref. Harrison, 20/e, p 1370]

> Replication of HPV begins with infection of basal cells later on there is proliferation of all epidermal layers except the basal layer and produces acanthosis, parakeratosis and hyperkeratosis. Koilocytes appear in the granular layer.

37. Bivalent HPV vaccine contains which types?
    a. Type 6, 11
    b. Type 6, 16
    c. Type 16, 18
    d. Type 11, 18
    [Ref. Harrison, 20/e, p 1372]

> **HPV vaccine**
> Component: Virus like particles (VLPs) that consists of the HPV L_1 major capsid protein
> - Bivalent vaccine: Contain HPV-16 and HPV-18
> - Quadrivalent vaccine: HPV-6, 11, 16 and 18
> - Second generation vaccine: HPV 16 and 18, additional oncogenic HPV 31, 33, 45, 52 and 58

38. Which viral gene acts as carcinogen in causing carcinoma cervix?
    a. P24 -gene   b. E-gene
    c. L -gene   d. H -gene
    [Ref. Greenwood, 18/e, p 454]

> **HPV Genome**
> a. Early region:
>   – Two large frames   E1 & E2
>   – Several small frames   E4 – E7
> b. Late region
>   – Two large genes
> • E region encodes pathogenic proteins
> • L region encodes regulator proteins
> • E6 & E7 are the prime oncogenes which integrates with host chromosome (Note: Most HPV associated tumor therefore show integrated rather than episomal virus)

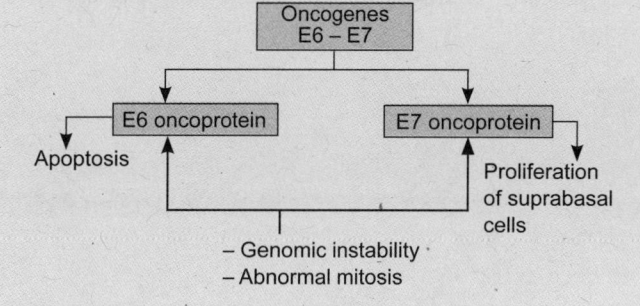

Ans.

30. d. Burkitt's ..	31. c. RNA virus	32. b. HPV	33. b. 3, 10
34. c. 16, 18	35. b. HPV	36. b. Basal cells	37. c. Type 16, 18
38. b. E -gene			

39. **HPV causes which change in cervical epithelial:**
    a. Induction of apoptosis
    b. Induction of necrosis
    c. Immortalization of epithelial cells
    d. None of the above [Ref. Greenwood, 18/e, p 454]

40. **Low risk type of HPV:**
    a. Type-16
    b. Type-6
    c. Type-18
    d. Type-31
    [Ref. Harrison 20/e, p 1370]

41. **E6, E7 genes of which virus are implicated in oncogenesis?**
    a. EBV
    b. CMV
    c. HTLV-1
    d. HPV
    [Ref. Greenwood, 18/e, p 454]

42. **Small pox belongs to which class of poxviruses?**
    a. Parapoxvirus
    b. Capripoxvirus
    c. Leporipox virus
    d. Orthopoxvirus
    [Ref. Harrison, 20/e, p 1366]

43. **Following virus is a pox virus:**
    a. Variola
    b. Coxsackie
    c. ECHO
    d. HSV
    [Ref. Ananthanarayan, 10/e, p 467]

Pox virus Genus
Orthopox virus: Variola, Monkey pox, cowpox, Buffalopox, vaccinia.
Molluscipox virus: Molluscum contagiosum
Parapox virus: Orf pseudocowpox, Deer pox, Seal pox
Yatapox virus: Tanapox

44. **Pharyngoconjunctival fever is caused by:**
    a. Adenovirus 3 and 7
    b. Adenovirus 11, 21
    c. Adenovirus 40, 41
    d. Adenovirus 8, 10 [Ref. Ananthanarayan, 10/e, p 488]

45. **Adenovirus causes all except:**
    a. Hemorrhagic cystitis
    b. Diarrhea
    c. Respiratory tract infection
    d. IMN [Ref. Ananthanarayan, 10/e, p 488]

46. **Brick-shaped virus:** [Ref. Ananthanarayan, 10/e, p468]
    a. Chicken pox
    b. Small pox
    c. CMV
    d. EBV

47. **Suckling mice is used for isolation of:**
    a. Coxsackie virus
    b. Pox
    c. Herpes
    d. Adenovirus [Ref. Ananthanarayan, 10/e, p 434]

Animal cultivation of virus
- Earliest method; Initially virus was inoculated into human volunteers
- White mice is the commonest animal used for this purpose
- Infant mice are very susceptible to cox-sackie and arbovirus
- Mice can be inoculated by several routes: intracerebral, subcutaneous, intraperitoneal or intranasal
- Disadvantage of animal inoculation are that immunity may interfere with viral growth and animal may harbour latent infection

48. **8-year-old girl presents with watery diarrhea. Most likely causative agent:**
    a. Rota virus
    b. V. cholerae
    c. Salmonella
    d. Shigella
    [Ref. Ananthanarayan, 10/e, p 565]

49. **Bollinger bodies are seen in:**
    a. Chickenpox
    b. Cowpox
    c. Fowlpox
    d. Smallpox
    [Ref. Ananthanarayan, 10/e, p 451]

Bollinger bodies are large inclusion bodies seen in fowl pox	
Negribodies	: Rabies
Guarnieri bodies	: Viccinia
Molluscum bodies	: Molluscum contagiosum
Cowdry type A	: Herpes
Cowdry type B	: Polio adenovirus

Ans.
39. c. Immortalization ...
40. b. Type-6
41. d. HPV
42. d. Orthopox virus
43. a. Variola
44. a. Adenovirus 3 and 7
45. d. IMN
46. b. Small pox
47. a. Coxsackie virus
48. a. Rota virus
49. c. Fowlpox

RNA Virus

CHAPTER 25

PICORNAVIRUSES

Icosahedral, nonenveloped positive sense ssRNA viruses, divided into two broad subgroups:

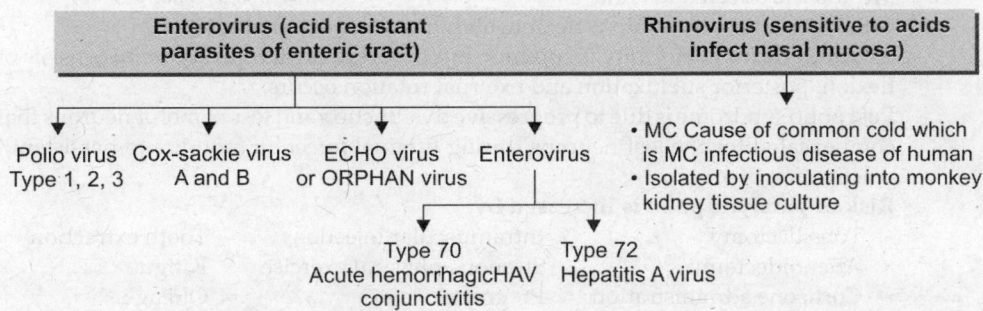

Picornavirus
SS RNA virus family includes:
– Polio   – Coxsackie virus
– Echo virus   – Enterovirus

- Overall coxsackie virus B1 is the most common enterovirus infection followed by echovirus 18, 9 and 6. ... *Harrison 18/e 1593*
  Enterovirus lacks lipid envelope and are stable in acidic environment, including the stomach. They are susceptible to chlorine containing cleansers but resistant to inactivation by standard disinfectants (e.g. alcohol) and can persist for days at room temperature.

POLIO VIRUS

- SS positive sense RNA virus, which does not survive lyophilization.
- *MC* type and most epidemics caused by **Type 1**.
- Epidemic caused by Type 1 and 3 while endemic is caused by Type 2.
- Vaccine induced paralysis is caused by mutated **Type 3**.
- Most **antigenic strain** - Type **2**.
- Two antigen – D or Native (N) antigen and C or heated (H) are identified.
- Anti D antibody is protective and used for measuring potency of injectable vaccine in terms of D antigen units.
- Transmitted by **feco-oral** route.

Pathology:
- Mouth is the portal of entry
- Primary multiplication takes place in oropharynx (tonsil and neck nodes) or intestine (Peyer's patcks)
- Polio virus then spreads along axons of peripheral nerves to the CNS
- **Earliest change** is the degeneration of Nissl bodies (**chromatolysis**) seen mostly in anterior horns of spinal cord (Signs of **lower motor neuron paralysis**).

Earliest neurogenic change of polio: Degeneration of Nissl bodies.

In March 2014 WHO announced the eradication of poliomyelitis from India. The last case of polio in India was reported in 2011

Clinical Features

- I P 7–14 days. Manifest as:
  a. *Inapparent* (**subclinical**) *infection* – *MC* manifestation (95%).
  b. *Abortive polio or minor illness*.
  c. *Nonparalytic polio* - Mimics aseptic meningitis (~1%)
  d. *Paralytic polio* – Least common but severe manifestation (<1%)

Polio Virus
- Most epidemics are due to Type I
- Most antigenic: Type III
- Vaccine induced paralysis: Type II
- MC muscle affected: Quadriceps femoris
- MC muscle undergoes complete paralysis: Tibialis anterior

Paralytic polio
- Can be biphasic (aseptic meningitis → recovery → fever/paralysis)
- Bulbar type paralysis causing dysphagia, difficulty in handling secretions or dysphonia
- Predominant sign - **Descending**; asymmetric; **proximal** more than distal; flaccid paralysis of **legs** (*MC*), arms, abdominal, thoracic or bulbar muscles.
- **Objective sensory** testing usually yields **normal** results.
- MC muscle affected — *Quadriceps*
- MC muscle which undergoes complete paralysis — *Tibialis anterior*
- MC muscle affected in hand — *Opponens pollicis*
- Common deformity at hip is flexion, abduction and external rotation.
- **At knee** - flexion deformity is common but in severe cases *triple deformity* consists of flexion, posterior subluxation and external rotation occurs.
- Post polio syndrome is due to progressive dysfunction and loss of motor neurons that compensated for the lost neurons during original infection (not due to persistent/reactivation of virus).
- **Risk of paralytic polio is increased by:**
    - Tonsillectomy   - Intramuscular injection   - Tooth extraction
    - Adenoidectomy   - Strenous physical exercise - Fatigue
    - Cortisone administration - Pregnancy   - Old age

COXSACKIE VIRUS, ECHO VIRUS AND OTHER ENTEROVIRUSES

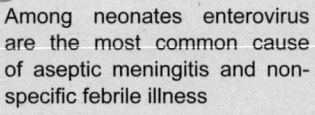

It is necessary to employ suckling mice for the isolation of coxsackie virus

- *MC* clinical **manifestation of enterovirus** infection - Non-specific febrile illness (Summer Grippe) …Harrison 19/e, p 1291
- *MC* cause of **aseptic** meningitis – Enterovirus (ECHO is *MC*)
- *MC* cause of **rubelliform** rash – Echovirus 9
- Transplacental Transmission occurs in coxsackie virus.

Clinical Presentation of Enterovirus			
Manifestation	Coxsackie virus	Enterovirus	Echo
Acute hemorrhagic conjunctivitis (characteristic subconjunctival hemorrhage)	A-24	Ent. 70	–
Aseptic meningitis	Most group A, all B	Ent	E
Encephalitis	A, B	Ent	E
Exanthem	A, B	Ent	E
Generalized disease of newborn	B_{2-5}	–	E
Hand, foot and mouth disease	A, B (commonly by A)	Ent 71	–
Herpangina	A, B (commonly by A)	Ent 71	–
Myocarditis, pericarditis	A, B (commonly B)	–	–
Paralysis	A, B (commonly A)	Ent	–
Pleurodynia (Bornholm disease)	A, B (commonly B)	–	E
Pneumonia	A, B	Ent	E
Juvenile diabetes	B-4	–	–
Orchitis	Coxsackie	–	–
Post viral fatigue syndrome	B	–	–

Among neonates enterovirus are the most common cause of aseptic meningitis and non-specific febrile illness

Echovirus 9 and 16 are frequently associated with fever and exanthem

- Mc clinical manifestation of enterovirus infection: summer grippe
- Mc enterovirus causing aseptic meningitis: Echovirus

Diagnosis of Enterovirus (Including Polio)

- *MC* **procedure** for diagnosis of infection - *Isolation* of enterovirus *in cell culture*.
- Isolation of virus from nasopharyngeal, throat sample, stool is sensitive but not specific (isolation from throat is more specific than from stool).

- Culture of CSF, serum, fluid from body cavities or tissues - less sensitive but specific.
- If CSF culture is negative than stool culture is done within first 2 weeks after onset of symptoms to confirm diagnosis.
- PCR of CSF - Highly sensitive and specific and rapid than culture.
- PCR of serum - Done for disseminated disease.
- Coxsackie virus may require inoculation into special cell-culture lines or into suckling mice.

Treatment

- IV/Intrathecal or intraventricular Ig for chronic enterovirus meningoencephalitis and dermatomyositis in patient with hypo or aggamaglobulinemia.
- *Pleconaril*, a drug once used is not available now.
- Glucocorticoids are contraindicated.

MYXOVIRUS

- Myxovirus is enveloped RNA virus, characterized by ability to adsorb onto mucoprotein receptors on erythrocytes causing hemagglutination.
- It is divided into two families - Orthomyxoviridae and Paramyxoviridae.

Distinguishing features of Orthomyxo and Paramyxovirus		
Features	Orthomyxoviridae	Paramyxoviridae
• *Genome*	Segmented (8 pieces)	Single linear RNA
• *Site of synthesis of Ribonucleo protein*	Nucleus	Cytoplasm
• *Genetic Reassortment*	Present	Absent
• *Antigenic Stability*	Variable	Stable
• *Hemolysis*	Absent	Present
• *Members*	Influenza virus	Measles (Morbillivirus), Mumps, Parainfluenza (Paramyxovirus), Respiratory syncytial virus (pneumovirus)

INFLUENZA

- Typically spherical virus divided into 3 subtypes (A, B, C) which are antigenically distinct.
- Type B and C occur almost exclusively in humans, whereas Influenza A exhibit a broad host range.
- **Antigenic structure**
- It has two types of antigens:
  a. Internal antigen: Type specific, i.e. (A, B, C) and stable.
     - Consists of RNP or soluble (S) antigen and M protein antigen.
     - It also includes envelope lipid antigen which is host specific.
  b. Surface/Viral or V antigen: Strain specific and show antigenic variations (A > B).

Antigenic variation is of 2 types:

(i) *Major antigenic variation or antigenic shift*: It is due to *genetic recombination that is genetic reassortment* between animal and human virus and is **responsible for** *major epidemics or pandemic. Only* shown by type **A. Occurs every 10-15 years**
(ii) *Minor antigenic variation or antigenic drift:* It is due to *point mutation* and **is responsible for** *periodical epidemic.*
  - Shown by type *A* and *B.*
- Type C does not show antigenic variation.
- Major pandemics are associated with antigenic shifts.
- The two viral protein demonstrating antigenic variation are envelope glycoprotein, the hemoglutinin and neurominidase (NA).

Myxovirus
- Enveloped RNA virus family include orthomyxoviridae (influenzae) and paramyxoviridae (measles, mumps, parainfluenzae)
- Influenzae virus exhibit antigenic shift and antigenic drift
- H_1N_1 is the causative agent of most recent pandemic.

- B & C strains mainly seen in human
- A strain mainly infect water based wild birds.

- *V antigen* composed of at least 2 virus coded protein:
  (i) **Hemagglutinin (H):** - Cause hemagglutination. Composed of two polypeptide HA_1 and HA_2.
  - HA protein binds virus particle to susceptible cell and it is the major antigen against which neutralising antibodies are directed.
  (ii) **Neuraminidase (N)** - Is receptor destroying enzyme (RDE) so cause elution.
  - Anti-neuraminidase antibody is not as effective in protection as that of hemagglutinin.
  - It facilitates release of virus particle from infected cell during budding.
  - Viral subtypes are distinguished, according to their surface protein the hemagglutinin and neuraminidase (NA). **16** HA subtype and **9** NA subtype are found

H5 N1 causative agent of avian influenza has GST potential of causing pandemic.

- In world, three types of influenza virus are circulating - A (H_1N_1), A(H_3N_2), and B viruses.
- *New* influenza virus: A (H_5N_1), causative agent of bird flu.
- *Source of Infection* — Usually a case or subclinical.
- *Portal of entry* — Respiratory route
- *Incubation period* — 18-72 hours.
- Virus is readily killed by exposure to heat for 30 min at 56°C.
- Viruses are inactivated by detergents soaps, ethanol, halogens and phenolic compounds.

> **Note:** WHO system of nomenclature of influenza A: Host of origin/geographical origin/strain No/ year of isolation/antigenic description of hemagglutinin and neuraminidase example: swine/ Iowa/3/70 ($H_1 N_1$).

Clinical Features

- There is *no* viremia.
- Respiratory symptoms are prominent but abdominal pain and vomiting may occur in type B infections.
- *MC* complication is *pneumonia*. Mixed viral and bacterial pneumonia being most common.
- **Most serious** complication of influenza *B virus* is Reye's syndrome [also occurs in influenza A and VZ virus].
- Cardiac, neurological complication and gastric flu (with type B) may occur.
- *MC secondary* bacterial pneumonia in influenza - pneumococci. *Staphylococcus haemophilus*.

> **Note:** Influenza deepithelializes the airways and destroy ciliary function allowing bacterial contamination.
> Staphylococci/pseudomonas proteases enhance cleavage of influenza hemagglutinin and thereby facilitate viral replication.

Lab Diagnosis

- Virus isolation — **Best** specimen is *nasopharyngeal* secretion
  - Detected by indirect fluorescent antibody.
  - For primary isolation the most suitable cells are Madin-Darby canine kidney (MDCK) cells.
- RT-PCR is the most sensitive and specific test for detection.
- Rapid influenza diagnostic test: They detect influenza virus antigen. They are specific but are less sensitive.

Prevention

1. **Best** is immunization. Vaccine is recommended only in certain selected population. Vaccine is of following types.
   a. *Killed vaccine*:
   Most commonly used vaccine:
   - Contains H, N antigens
   - Usually one dose given but in patient with no previous immunological response 2 doses given
   - Immunity lasts for only 3-6 months.
   - Vaccine can produce very rarely Guillain-Barre syndrome (ascending paralysis).

b. *Live attenuated vaccines (intra-nasal spray):*
   Administered as nose drops so induce both local and systemic immunity
c. *Newer vaccines:*
   Split virus vaccine (sub-virion vaccine); Neuraminidase specific vaccine (sub-unit vaccine contains only N-antigen); Recombinant vaccine

2. **Antiviral drugs:**
   - For type A virus   :   Amantadine and rimantadine
   - For both A and B   :   Zamamivir, Oseltamivir.

Treatment

- Mainly symptomatic with acetaminophen. Other NSAID should be avoided in patient < 18 years of age due to risk of Reye's syndrome.
- Maintain hydration and provide rest.
- **Specific antiviral:** Neuraminadase inhibitor oseltamivir and zanamivir for both type A & Adamontane agent amantadine and rimantidine for type A if sensitive.

PARAMYXOVIRUS

- Family of enveloped viruses containing single strand of negative sense RNA.
- Resemble orthomyxovirus but are larger and more fragile.
- Enters the body through respiratory system.

Classification and important pathogens of the paramyxoviruses		
Genus	**Human viruses**	**Animal viruses**

Paramyxovirus	Paramyxovirus
	  Parainfluenza viruses types 1, 3
	  Rubulavirus
	  Mumps virus
	  Parainfluenza viruses types 2, 4a, 4b
		Newcastle diseases virus (NDV) (poultry), simian virus 5

Morbillivirus	Measles virus	Canine distemper virus, rinderpest virus, equine morbillivirus, morbilliviruses of seals, dolphins
Pneumovirus	Respiratory syncytial (RS) virus Human metapneumovirus (hMPV)	Turkey rhino-tracheitis virus (avian metapneumovirus)
Henipavirus	Hendra virus* Nipah virus*	Hendra virus Nipah virus
*These viruses cause disease in animals but can cause serious zoonotic human diseases		

MEASLES (RUBEOLA)

- A Morbillivirus
- Nonsegmented, SS RNA paramyxovirus, having *only one* serotype.
- *It cannot* survive outside the human body.
- *Carriers* are *not* known to occur. But subclinical cases occurs.
- Secondary attack rate > 80%.
- Immunity after vaccination and infection is life-long.
- Multinucleated giant cells with inclusion bodies in the nucleus and cytoplasm (*Warthin - Finkeldey Cells*) in respiratory and lymphoid tissue are pathognomic for measles.
- Virion spike carry a haemagglutinin but not a neuraminidase function -F-protein is also a haemolysin.

Measles:
- RNA virus
- Exclusive human pathogen with very high secondary attack rate > 80%
- Warthin–Finkeldey cells are pathognomic
- Koplik spot over buccal mucosa are pathognomonic exanthem

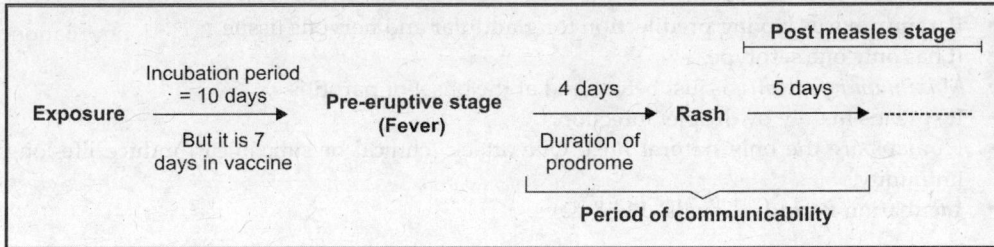

- Measles during pregnancy is not associated with congenital abnormalities.
- However in pregnancy disease is more severe and can lead to abortion, pre-term delivery.

Clinical Features

- *Prodromal/Pre-eruptive stage*: A day or two before the appearance of rash **Koplik's spot** (*bluish white with erythematous halo*) appear on the buccal mucosa opposite the first and second upper molars.
  - It is **pathognomonic enanthem** of measles.
  - It disappears after the onset of rash.
  - Cough, coryza conjunctivitis and increasing fever is there.
- *Eruptive stage:* Rash appears on 4th day from fever. It begins at hairline and behind the ear and spreads downward rapidly. Characteristically it is erythematous, non-pruritic and maculopapular. Fever usually resolves by 4th or 5th day after the onset of rash. Prolong fever suggest complication.
- *Postmeasles stage*

> **Remember:** Modified measles occur in individual with pre-existing partial immunity induced by active or passive immunization.
> In HIV infected individual or cell mediated immunity impaired individual rash may be absent.

Diagnosis

- Best made by demonstration of measles specific IgM in blood or salivary sample.

Complication

- Diarrhea, pneumonia and otitis media are the common complications of measles
- SSPE is the delayed complication of measles, related to prions.

- *MC* complications are - measles associated diarrhea, pneumonia and *otitis media* (**MC** complication **in young children**).
- More *serious* are neurological complication (febrile convulsions, encephalitis and sub-acute sclerosing pan encephalitis i.e. SSPE). Most cases result from immune mediated response to myelin proteins (post infectious encephalomyelitis) and not directly from viral infection.

> **Remember:** Typical measles occur in person who received formalin inactivated measles vaccine in which rash begins peripherally and moves centrally.
> Pneumonia is due to direct invasion of virus.

Prevention

1. Measles Vaccination:
   - *Live attenuated, tissue culture; freeze dried vaccine of HDC - Edmonston - Zagreb strain*; given to child as single subcutaneous dose of 0.5 ml as close to the age of 9 months.
   - Reconstituted in distilled water and should be used within one hour.
   - Measles virus is susceptible to heat and UV radiation, so attenuated measles vaccine must be transported in cold chain.
   - There is no spread of virus from vaccines to contacts.
   - Immunity develops in 11 to 12 days after vaccination.
   - One dose of vaccine give 95% protection.
   - Susceptible contacts may be protected by giving vaccine within 3 days of exposure.
   - Toxic shock syndrome occurs if vaccine is used after 4 hours of opening the vial.
   - Pregnancy is contraindication.
2. Immunoglobulin

> **Remember:** Eradication is achieved when immunization coverage is at least 96%.

MUMPS VIRUS = MYXOVIRUS PAROTIDITIS

Mumps
- Exclusive human pathogen and is the most common cause of parotitis.
- After parotitis, orchitis is the most common manifestation.

- Paramyxovirus having predilection for glandular and nervous tissue.
- It has only one serotype.
- *Maximum infectivity* is just before and at the onset of parotitis.
- It spreads mainly by droplet infection.
- Humans are the only natural host. One attack (clinical or subclinical) induce life-long immunity.
- **Incubation Period** – Usually 14-18 days.

Clinical Features

- *Mumps* is the **most frequent** cause of *parotitis in children* in the age group 5-15 years.
- Usually bilateral parotitis occurs. Submandibular and sublingual gland can also be involved.
- Some patients develop pre-sternal edema.
- Other than parotitis, *orchitis* is the *MC* manifestation among *post-pubertal males*. May lead to testicular atrophy.
- *Aseptic meningitis* is a common manifestation in both children and adults.
- Glucose level in CSF may be abnormally low and this raises suspicion of bacterial meningitis.
- In pregnancy, it does not lead to premature birth or fetal malformation.
- **Diagnosis:** Usually clinical
- *RT PCR* is the most sensitive test for detecting Virus in CSF
- For isolation monkey kidney or HEP2 cells are used.

Prevention

- Single dose of live-attenuated vaccine primarily in susceptible adults especially males who have not had mumps.
- *Combined vaccine* - MMR: At the age of 12-15 month and again at 4-6 years of age.

... Harrison 18/e, p 1610

Parainfluenza virus:
- 2nd MC cause of lower respiratory tract illness
- Most serious manifestation is laryngotrachitis

PARAINFLUENZA VIRUS

- First parainfluenza virus to be discovered - Sendai virus or Hemagglutinating virus of Japan (HVJ) or influenza virus type D.
- It ranks second only to RSV as cause of lower respiratory tract illness.
- It has 4 types - 1, 2, 3, 4.

Clinical Features

- **Most serious** clinical disease is *croup (laryngotracheobronchitis)*.
- Para-influenza **type 1** is *MC* cause of croup in children.
- **Type 3** is important cause of lower respiratory disease (bronchitis, bronchiolitis and pneumonia) in infants.
- In older children and adults, most frequent symptom - common cold or hoarsenss.
- This virus confined to respiratory tract unlike mumps which is a systemic disease.

Diagnosis

- Isolation of virus from throat and nasal swabs by inoculating in primary monkey kidney cell cultures or continuous monkey kidney cell line (LLC-MK2) with trypsin.

- *Respiratory syncytial virus:*
  - SSRNA virus.
  - MC cause of lower RTI
  - MC cause of bronchiotitis

RESPIRATORY SYNCYTIAL VIRUS (RSV)

- An enveloped ssRNA virus.
- Most fragile among all paramyxovirus
- Lack haemagglutinin, hemolysin or neuraminidase.
- Broadly divided into two subgroups, Group A (mild disease) and Group B (severe)
- *MC* cause of *lower respiratory tract disease*.
- *MC* cause of *bronchiolitis seen* among infants between 1 and 6 months of age, peaking between 2 and 3 months of age.
- *MC* manifestation **in infants** rhinorrhea. Most serious manifestation is bronchiolitis.
- RSV is associated with sudden infant death syndrome
- **In adults MC** symptom are *common cold* with *rhinorrhea*, sore throat and cough.
- RSV is transmitted primarily by close contact with contaminated fingers or fomites.
- Incubation period is 4-6 days.
- Immunity is not long lasting.
- Nasal IgA is more protective than serum antibody.
- It produces fine rales; rhonchi, emphysematous change (that is hyperexpansion on chest X-ray) and atelectasis.

Diagnosis

- Specific diagnosis – by isolation of RSV from respiratory secretions (sputum, throat swab, nasopharyngeal wash).

Treatment

- *Oxygen:* Mainstay of therapy.
- *Ribavirin:* For infants who are severely ill or who are at high risk of complications of RSV infection (premature infants and those with bronchopulmonary dysplasia, congenital heart disease and immunosuppression).

HUMAN METAPNEUMOVIRUS

- Discovered in Netherlands in 2001 in bronchiolitis patients
- Closely resemble respiratory syncytial virus in all aspect
- It affects slightly older age group than RSV
- Diagnosis is made by RT-PCR
- Treatment is symptomatic

ROTAVIRUS AND OTHER VIRAL GASTROENTERITIS

- *MC* cause of diarrheal disease in infants and children: *Rotaviurs*
- *MC* agent among older children and adults: Norovirus *(Norwalk like viruses)*

Rotavirus:
- MC cause of diarrhea in infant and children
- Non-enveloped segmental ds RNA virus
- Group A is the most common one
- Produce severe dehydration

ROTAVIRUS

- Non-enveloped, icosahedral virus with **segmented dsRNA (Character of Reovirus family)** so it exhibits *genetic reassortment.*
- VP-6 is major structural protein, which also is the target of commercial immunoassays and determines the group specificity of rotaviruses.
- There are seven major group. **Human illness** is caused *primarily* by **group A** and to a much lesser extent by group B and C.
- Adult diarrhea rota virus (ADRV) belongs to **group B** while **group C** causes pediatric gastroenteritis.
- 10 G serotypes of group A are identified in humans but 5 types *(G1 through G4 and G9)* are common.

Pathogenesis

1. It infects and destroys mature enterocytes in villous epithelium of proximal small intestine causing:
   a. Secretory diarrhea – by ↓ villous epithelium area (by destroying mature enterocytes) + ↑ secretory crypt cells
   b. Osmotic diarrhea – by reducing brush border enzymes thereby accumulation of unmetabolized disaccharides.
2. Secretory diarrhea also results by:
   a. Enterotoxin (=NSP4) which alter epithelial cell function and permeability.
   b. Activation of enteric nervous system in the intestinal wall leads to increased fluid secretion.
   ...*Harrison 20/e, p 1467*

Rotavirus produce secretory diarrhea by ↓ villous epithelium

Clinical Features

- *Incubation period:* 1-3 days.
- It infects all children by 3-5 years. May also infect neonates.
- Peak age - 4 to 23 months.
- Occurs predominantly during the winter months.
- Transmitted predominantly through feco-oral route. Also transmitted by respiratory secretion, person to person, contaminated environmental surface.

- *Severity of dehydration:* Rotavirus > Norovirus > Sapovirus
- *Vomiting* frequently *precedes* the diarrhea.
- Stools are characteristically loose and watery and only infrequently contain red or white cells.
- Rotavirus is associated with respiratory and neurologic features, sudden infant death syndrome, necrotizing enterocolitis, intussusception and diabetes mellitus type I.
- Its infection produces virus specific secretory IgA in intestine and IgA, IgM, IgG in serum which increase with each reinfection, so severe disease is *more common* in first or second infection i.e. in young children

Diagnosis

- As virus is shed in large quantities (10^7–10^{12}/g) in stool, the diagnosis is *confirmed by* detecting viral antigen in feces by Enzyme immunoassays and by detecting viral RNA (by gel electrophoresis, probe hybridization or PCR).
- Human rotavirus does *not grow* readily in cell culture.

Treatment

- Rehydration therapy is given.
- Antibiotics and antimotility agents avoided.
- In immunocompromised children - oral immunoglobulin or colostrum given.

Prevention

- First licensed rotavirus vaccine (Rotashield) was withdrawn due to its association with intussusception.
- Two new live attenuated oral vaccine have been introduced:
  a. Pentavalent bovine human reassortant rotavirus vaccine (RotaTeq) contains G_1, G_2, G_3, G_4 and P(8).
  b. Single attenuated human rotavirus strain (Rotarix) contains $P_1 A(8) G_1$

Norovirus is the MC cause of mild gastroenteritis
Adenovirus, Astrovirus, Torovirus are other enterovirus

OTHER VIRAL GASTROENTERITIS

1. **Norwalk and Related Human Calciviruses:**
   - Small rounded icosahedral ssRNA virus, broadly classified into two genera: *Norovirus* (previously called Norwalk like virus) and *sapovirus* (previously called sapporos like virus).
   - Norovirus is the *MC* infectious agent of mild gastroenteritis in the community and affects all age groups whereas sapoviruses primarily cause gastroenteritis in children.
   - Noroviruses are the major cause of epidemics of gastroenteritis worldwide.

   Pathogenesis:
   - It gets attached on carbohydrates (similar to human histoblood group antigens) of duodenal epithelium of individuals with the secretor phenotype (genetic predisposition to illness).
   - Reversible lesion in upper jejunum, e.g. broadening and blunting of villi, shortening of microvilli, etc.
   - Malabsorption of carbohydrates and fats and decreased brush border enzymes.
   - Adenylate cyclase activity is not altered.
   - Gastric motor function is delayed but histological changes are absent in stomach and colon.

Modes of Transmission:	– Transmission occurs predominantly by fecal-oral route but virus is also present in vomitus. – Also transmitted by aerosolization, contact with contaminated fomites, person to person contact. – Shellfish harvested from fecally contaminated water pose a special risk.

   Clinical Features:
   - *Vomiting* is more common among children where adults usually develop *diarrhea*.
   - Constitutional symptoms like fever, chills and rigor are common.

- *Stools* are characteristically loose and watery without blood, mucus or leukocytes.
- There is paradoxic inverse association between level of antibody and protection from disease that is person with higher level of pre-existing antibody are more susceptible to illness.

Diagnosis:
- PCR for detection of virus in stool and vomitus.
- EIA (Enzyme immunoassays) for detection of virus in stool and serologic response to specific viral antigen.
- It has not yet been propagated in cell cultures.

Treatment:
- Generally not required since it is self-limited.

2. **Adenovirus:** – Enteric adenovirus (40 and 41) are difficult to cultivate in cell lines.
3. **Astrovirus:** – Serotype 1 is *MC*.
4. **Torovirus:** – Cause less vomiting and more bloody diarrhea.
5. **Picobirnaviruses:** – Bi-segmented *double stranded RNA* virus.
   – Cause gastroenteritis *in HIV* infected adults.
6. **Hendra and Nepah viruses:** – Classified under paramyxoviridae family. Cause gastroenteritis in persons in contact with pigs.
7. **SARS-Cov:** (Severe acute respiratory syndrome associated coronavirus).
8. **Enteroviruses, reoviruses, pestiviruses, parvovirus B.**

- Most arboviral disease are transmitted by mosquito:
- Chikungunya is a arboviral disease related to alpha viruses

ARBOVIRUSES = ARTHROPOD BORNE VIRUSES

- The most important arbovirus vectors are mosquitoes followed by ticks.
- Most arbovirus agglutinate red cells (Hemagglutination) but spontaneous elution does not occur.
- Arboviruses have been placed in Toga, Flavi, Bunya, Reo and Rhabdovirus families.
- Arboviruses known to be prevalent in India are:

Group A	Group B		Others
(Alphaviruses)	(Flaviviruses)	Umbre	Chandipura
Sindbis	Dengue	Sathuperi	Chittoor
Chikungunya	Kyasanur Forest disease	African horse sickness	Minnal
	Japanese encephalitis	Venkat puram	Sandfly fever Vellore
	West Nile	Kaisodi	

- *Clinical syndromes of Arbovirues:*
  – **Febrile group:**
    - *MC* group
    - No rash and arthralgia seen
      e.g. Sindbis, Chikungunya, dengue (Types 1-4), Westnile, Sandfly fever, Rift valley fever.
  – **Hemorrhagic fevers (HF):**
    - Dengue, chikungunya, kyasanur forest disease, lassa fever, yellow fever, marburg or ebola HF, hantavirus pulmonary syndrome, HF with renal syndrome, rift valley fever, crimean congo HF, omsk HF.
  – **Encephalitis:**
    - West Nile, Japanese encephalitis.

Rabies:
- Bullet shaped SS RNA virus
- Maldive is the only country where there is no rabies.
- Virus first spread centripetally and then centrifugally.
- Negri bodies are pathognomonic

RHABDOVIRIDAE

- **Bullet shaped**, enveloped viruses with SS RNA genome are known as Rhabdovirus.
- Rhabdoviridae contain two genera:
  (i) Vesiculovirus containing vesicular stomatitis virus, chandipura virus.
  (ii) Lyssavirus containing Rabies virus, Lagos bat, Mokola, Duvenhage.

RABIES VIRUS (LYSSAVIRUS SEROTYPE 1)

- Unsegmented, linear negative, **neurotropic**, RNA virus which causes direct zoonosis of **warm blooded animals** (particularly carnivorous such as dogs, cats, jackals and wolves) including man called as RABIES.
- Serotype 2, 3, 4 are *rabies related virus.*
- Viral genome encodes for five proteins: nucleocapsid, matrix, phosphoprotein, glycoprotein and RNA polymerase.
- It has two major antigens—glycoprotein (G Protein) and nucleocapsid protein.
- Glycoprotein seems to be the only antigen capable of inducing the formation of virus neutralizing (protective) and hemagglutination - inhibiting antibodies.
- Virus excreted in the saliva of rabid animals is called 'street virus' which is pathogenic for all mammals and has long **variable** incubation period.
- *Serial brain to brain passage of Street Virus modifies it into fixed virus which has following characteristics:*
  - Short, fixed and reproducible incubation period.
  - Not form Negri bodies and not multiply in extraneural tissues.
  - Used in the preparation of anti-rabies vaccine.
  - It is pathogenic under certain conditions, e.g. when inadequately inactivated for vaccine production.
- Rabies is only communicable disease of man that is *always fatal.*

> **Remember:** Rabies is dead end infection.

Type of Rabies

(i) **Urban rabies:** Caused by the dog and is responsible for 99% of human cases in India.
(ii) Sylvatic or wild-life rabies.
(iii) Bat rabies.

> **Remember:**
> - In most of the world, dog is the most important vector.
> - Maldives is the only country which does not have human or animal rabies.
> - In India, rabies occur in all parts except Lakshadweep and Andman and Nicobar Islands
> - Most effective natural barrier to rabies - water.

- **Mode of transmission:**
- *Animal bites - MC*
- Licks on abraded skin and abraded or unabraded mucosa.
- Respiratory (aerosol) transmission.
- Person to person - rare
- Also by corneal and organ transplants.

Incubation period: Highly variable depending on the site of bite (i.e. actual distance that the virus has to travel to reach to CNS), severity of bite, etc. It is usually 1-3 months but can be < 2 week or > 1 year.

Clinical Features

- Virus spreads *centripetally* from site of infection (striated muscle) then ascends through nerve associated tissue space, and then spreads *centrifugally* in peripheral autonomic nerves to many tissues.
- Once the virus enters the CNS, it rapidly disseminates to other regions of the CNS via fast axonal transport along neuro-anatomic connections.
- Rabies *prominently infect neurons*, infection of astrocytes is unusual.
- After establishing CNS infection, there is centrifugal spread to other tissues including salivary gland, heart, adrenal gland and skin.
- Salivary gland invasion is *crucial* for transmission of virus.
- Pathological study shows mild inflammatory changes in the CNS with mononuclear cells in leptomeninges, perivascular regions and parenchyma including microglial nodules called *Babes nodules*

...Harrison 19/e, p1301

- Negri bodies are made up of fibrillar matrix and rabies viral particles
- Cell culture vaccine are derived from fixed rabies virus

Rabies virus spread centripetally towards the CNS at a rate of 250 mm/d Via retrograde fast axonal transport to the spinal cord or brainstem.

- Most characteristic pathologic finding in CNS is the formation of cytoplasmic inclusions called **Negri Bodies** (*composed of finely fibrillar matrix and rabies virus particles*) within neurons of Ammon's horn, cerebral cortex, brain stem, hypothalamus, purkinje cells of the cerebellum and dorsal spinal ganglia. However, Negri bodies are not observed in all cases of rabies.
- It has four stages:
  a. *Prodromal period*: Specific symptom is complaint of paresthesia/fasciculation at or around the site of inoculation of virus, fever, headache, lethargy are common constitutional symptoms.
  b. *Encephalitic phase*: Abnormalities of automatic nervous system. Aerophobia (pathognomic) and Hydrophobia (pathognomic and absent in animals) may be seen, hypersalivation, aphasia.
  c. **Manifestation of brain stem dysfunction**: The prominence of early brainstem dysfunction distinguishes it from other viral encephalitis.
  d. *Coma and Death*.
  e. *Paralytic Rabies*: In about 20% of patients cardinal features of encephalitic rabies are lacking. Rather they exhibit early and prominent flaccid paralysis of involved extremity that progress to quadriparesis and death.

> **Remember:** It may be also present as ascending paralysis resembling GBS, most frequently among persons given post-exposure prophylaxis after being bitten by vampire bats

Diagnosis

- Confirmed by antigen detection using immunofluorescence of infected tissue (corneal impression smear, skin biopsy or brain) and by virus isolation from saliva and other secretions.
- The commonly performed direct fluorescent antibody testing of skin biopsy material from posterior neck (where hair follicles are highly innervated) has a sensitivity of 60-80%.

.....*CMDT 2014, p 1320*

Prevention Types of Vaccine

- *Rabies can never be cured but can always be prevented with passive + active immunization. There are various vaccine available:*
(a) Nervous tissue vaccine (NTV)
   – From suckling mouse brain
   – From adult animal tissues (e.g. sheep): Sample type
(b) Duck embryo vaccine (DEV)
   – Not available in India
(c) Cell culture vaccine

Cell culture vaccine	
Human diploid cell (HDC) vaccine: In India it is used for both pre and post exposure prophylaxis (PEP). It is a purified preparation of fixed rabies virus grown on human diploid cell.	**"Second generation" tissue culture (animal cell) vaccines,** i.e. of non human origin, e.g. chick embryo fibroblast, vero cells. The WHO recommended that culture of HDC line should be replaced by culture of animal cell line

Types of Prophylaxis

1. *Post-exposure prophylaxis*: Combined administration of single dose of antirabies serum with a course of vaccine, and local treatment of wound is the *best* specific prophylactic treatment after exposure of man to rabies.
   Indication of Anti-rabies Treatment:
   a. If animal shows sign of rabies within 10 days
   b. Biting animal can't be traced
   c. Unprovoked bites
   d. Laboratory test (fluorescent rabies antibody test or test for negri bodies) of brain of biting animal are positive.
   e. All bites by wild animals.

Class I (slight risk)	Class II (Moderate risk)	Class III (severe risk)
Classification of exposures		
Class I (slight risk)	Class II (Moderate risk)	Class III (severe risk)
• Licks on healthy unbroken skin	• Licks on fresh cuts	• All bites or scratches with oozing of blood on neck, head, face, palm, fingers
• Consumption of unboiled milk of suspected animal	• Scratches with oozing of blood	• Lacerated wounds on any part of body
• Scratches without oozing of blood	• All bites except on head, neck, face, palm, fingers	• Multiple wounds 5 or more in numbers
	• Minor wounds less than 5 in number	• Bites from wild animals

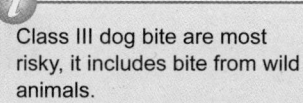

Class III dog bite are most risky, it includes bite from wild animals.

- The optimal form of passive immunisation is human rabies immunoglobulin (20 IU/kg) administered once, the full dose should be infiltrated around the wound. Any remaining amount can be infected intramuscularly at a site distant from wound.
- Along with this active immunization by vaccine (HDCV or purified chick embro cell vaccine) must be administered as per **standard WHO intramuscular regimen**: 0, 3, 7, 14, 28, days and booster on 90 days.

2. *Preexposure prophylaxis*
   - Given to laboratory staff working with rabies virus, veterinarians, etc.
   - Cell culture vaccines on 0, 7, 28 days.
   - If titer of neutralizing antibody in serum taken after 1 month of 3rd dose, is less than 0.5 IU/ml then administer booster until antibodies become demonstrable.

3. *Postexposure treatment of persons who have been vaccinated previously:*
   - If titer of antibody > 0.5 IU/ml and bite is not severe – 2 doses (days 0, 3).
   - If titer of antibody is unknown or bite is severe - 3 doses of HDC on 0, 3, 7 days.

Multiple Choice Questions

Polio and Enterovirus

1. **True about polio:** [AIIMS 08]
   a. Paralytic polio is most common
   b. Only one type exists
   c. Increased muscular activity leads to increased paralysis
   d. Polio drop given only in <3 years

2. **Which of the following is the most common cause of meningoencephalitis in children:** [AI 2011]
   a. Mumps
   b. Arbovirus
   c. HSV
   d. Enterovirus

3. **All are false regarding polio virus except:**
   a. Most cases are symptomatic [AIIMS Nov 07]
   b. Inactivated vaccine given IM
   c. Inactivated polio vaccines are given to child less than 3 years of age
   d. Only one type exists

4. **Acute hemorrhagic conjunctivitis is caused by which enterovirus:** [NEET Pattern 2018]
   a. 69
   b. 72
   c. 70
   d. 71

5. **True Statement about Enteroviruses:** [PGI May 2013]
   a. Composed of segmented RNA genome
   b. Stable at pH 4
   c. Cause pleurodynia
   d. Cause encephalitis
   e. Cause meningitis

Influenza and Parainfluenza

6. **A 70-year-old woman refused to take influenza vaccine, devloped flu. Death happened 1 week after pneumonia. Causes of post influenza pneumonia:** [AIIMS Nov 2014]
   a. Staphylococcus
   b. Measles
   c. Legionella
   d. CMV

7. **H_5N_1 is:** [AI 08]
   a. Bird flu virus
   b. Vaccine for HIV
   c. Causative agent of Japanese enpcehalitis
   d. An eradicated virus

8. **True statement about influenza A virus:** [AIIMS 18]
   a. It has a double stranded segmented RNA
   b. Pandemics are caused by antigenic drifts
   c. Nucleocapsid antibody is not specific
   d. Hemagglutinin and neuraminidase are strain specific

9. **Segmented RNA is found in:** [PGI 13]
   a. Influenza virus
   b. Rabies virus
   c. Herpes virus
   d. Molluscum contagiosum virus

10. **Incubation period less than 10 days seen in:** [PGI 12]
    a. Influenza
    b. Cholera
    c. Plague
    d. Chickenpox
    e. Rabies

Measles, Mumps & Rubella

11. **Most characteristic congenital heart disease in rubella:**
    a. Ventricular septal defect [NEET Pattern 2019]
    b. Coarction of aorta
    c. Pulmonary artery stenosis
    d. Aortic stenosis

12. **Congenital rubella syndrome true association is:** [NEET Pattern 2019]
    a. Cataract, VSD, intracerebral hemorrhage
    b. Retinitis, tetralogy of Fallot, limb hypoplasia
    c. Cicatrism, microcephaly
    d. Hernia, cerebellar atresia, coarction of aorta

13. **True about congenital rubella syndrome:** NEET Pattern 2019
    a. Occur in infection after 20 weeks
    b. More chances of birth defect if infection is acquired late
    c. Leads to chronic infection in the affected child
    d. Caused by a virus that belongs to Toga virus family

14. **With reference to mumps which of the following is true?** [AI 06]
    a. Meningoencephalitis can precede parotitis
    b. Salivary gland involvement is limited to the parotids
    c. The patient is not infectious prior to clinical parotid enlargement
    d. Mumps orchitis frequently leads to infertility

15. **All of the following statements are true about congenital rubella except:** [AI 05]
    a. It is diagnosed when the infant has IgM antibodies at birth
    b. It is diagnosed when IgG antibodies persist for more than 6 months
    c. MC congenital defects are deafness, cardiac malformation and cataract
    d. Infection after 16 weeks of gestation result in major congenital defects

16. **Which of the following is not true about measles?**
    a. High secondary attack [AI 08]
    b. Only one strain causes infection
    c. Not infectious in prodromal period
    d. Infections confer life-long immunity

17. **Which of the following is the 'Least common' complication of measles?** [AIIMS 06]
    a. Diarrhea
    b. Pneumonia
    c. Otitis media
    d. SSPE

18. **Warthin-Finkeldey cells are seen in which infection:** NEET Pattern 2018
    a. Rubella
    b. Chickenpox
    c. Measles
    d. Mumps

Rotavirus & Norovirus

19. A patient comes to your clinic with a complaint of multiple episodes of loose watery stool for 3 days. On probing, you discover that these episodes start after he had ingested shellfish at a local restaurant 3 days back and other people who had food from that restaurant had similar symptoms. What is the most likely cause of viral diarrhea in these adults?: [AIIMS 15]
    a. Adenovirus
    b. Calcivirus
    c. Rotovirus
    d. Norovirus

20. Vaccination causing intussusception: [PGI Dec. 07]
    a. Rotavirus
    b. Parvovirus
    c. Inactivated polio
    d. BCG
    e. Measles

21. Reassortment is typically seen in: [AIIMS Nov 10]
    a. Herpes
    b. Hepadna
    c. Rotavirus
    d. Astrovirus

Rabies

22. Vaccines prepared by embryonated hen's egg are:
    a. Measles
    b. Rabies [PGI 10]
    c. Rubella
    d. Varicella

23. Negro body is seen in: [AI 07]
    a. CMV
    b. Rabies
    c. Inclusion of herpes simplex
    d. EBV

24. For the treatment of case of class III dog bite, all of the following are correct *except*: [AI 05]
    a. Give Ig for passive immunity
    b. Give ARV
    c. Immediately stitch wound under antibiotic coverage
    d. Immediately wash wound with soap and water

25. A 25-year-old girl has admitted to hospital with provisional diagnosis of rabies. The most suitable clinical sample that can confirm the antemortem diagnosis is: [AIIMS 04]
    a. Serum for antivirus IgG antibody
    b. Corneal impression smear for immuno-fluorescence stain
    c. CSF sample for viral culture
    d. Giemsa stain on smear prepared from salivary secretions

26. A boy got unprovoked bite from a neighbour's dog. The animal control authority caught the dog and it was found to be healthy. What will be the next step? [AIIMS May 10, AI 2010]
    a. Test antibody level in the dog
    b. With hold immunization and observe the dog for 10 days for signs of rabies
    c. Start post-exposure prophylaxis
    d. Perform euthanasia for the dog

27. Diagnostic of Rabies: [AIIMS May 10, AI 2010]
    a. Guarneri bodies
    b. Negri bodies
    c. Cowdry Aody
    d. Bollinger bodies

28. A patient presented to the hospital with severe hydrophobia. You suspect rabies obtain corneal scrapings from the patient. What test should be done on this specimen for a diagnosis of Rabies?
    a. RT-PCR for rabies virus [AIIMS 2017]
    b. Negri bodies
    c. Antibodies to rabies virus
    d. Indirect immunofluorescence

29. Bird arthropod man cycle is seen in: NEET Pattern 2019
    a. Malaria
    b. Paragominus
    c. Japanese encephalitis
    d. Plague

Arbovirus

30. Soft tick transmits: [AI 08]
    a. Relapsing fever
    b. KFD
    c. Tick typhus
    d. Tularemia

31. Which of the following viral infections is transmitted by tick? [AI 05]
    a. Japanese encephalitis
    b. Dengue fever
    c. Kyasanur-Forest disease (KFD)
    d. Yellow fever

32. Which is true about arboviral disease? [AI 10]
    a. Yellow fever is endemic in India
    b. Dengue viruses have only one serotype
    c. KFD is transmitted by ticks
    d. Japanese encephalitis is transmitted by Aedes

33. Mark true in following: [AIIMS 08]
    a. Hanta virus pulmonary syndrome is caused by inhalation of rodent urine and feces
    b. Kyasanur forest disease is caused by bite of wild animal
    c. Lyssa virus is transmitted by ticks
    d. Chikungunya is caused by anopheles

34. Most specific for Dengue diagnosis: [AIIMS 08]
    a. IgM ELISA
    b. Tissue culture
    c. CFT
    d. Electron microscopy

35. Which of the following is/are arboviral diseases?
    a. Japanese encephalitis [PGI June 09]
    b. Dengue
    c. Yellow fever
    d. Hand-foot-mouth disease
    e. Rocky mountain spotted fever

36. True about dengue fever: [PGI May 2013]
    a. Caused by 4 serotypes
    b. Effective vaccine is available
    c. Presents with fever and joint pain
    d. Virus belongs to flavivirus genus
    e. Contain segmented RNA

37. In a suspected patient of dengue, all of these are acceptable investigations at day 3 of presentation *except*:
    a. NS1 antigen detection [AIIMS Nov 2016]
    b. Viral culture and isolation in C6/36 cell line
    c. RT-PCR
    d. ELISA for antibody against dengrue virus

Other

38. The most common etiological agent for acute bronchiolitis in infancy is: [AI 06]
    a. Influenza virus
    b. Parainfluenza virus
    c. Rhinovirus
    d. Respiratory syncytial virus

39. The following lesions were seen in a child. The patient is suffering from a disease caused by which of these viruses: [AIIMS 2017]

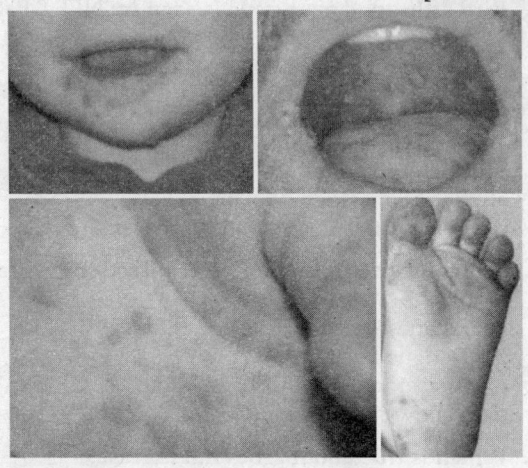

   a. Pox virus
   b. Coxsackie A virus
   c. Herpes simples type 1 virus
   d. Toga virus

40. Laboratory diagnosis of viral respiratory tract infections can be established by all of the following tests except: [AI 09]
    a. Detection of virus specific IgM antibodies in single serum specimen
    b. Demonstration of viral antigens by indirect immunofluorescence assay in nasopharyngeal washings
    c. Isolation of viruses using centrifugation enhanced culture
    d. Detection of viral hemagglutination inhibiting (HAI) antibodies in a single serum specimen

41. Choose the correct matches: [PGI 12]
    a. Mumps-RA 27/3 strain
    b. Rubella-Jeryl-Lynn strain
    c. Measles-Edmonston-Zagreb strain
    d. BCG-Danish 1331 strain

42. Micro-organism used as weapon in biological terrorism:
    a. Smallpox virus   b. Rabies virus   [PGI 09]
    c. Ebola virus   d. Influenza C virus
    e. Human parvovirus

43. All are RNA virus except: [AIIMS 08]
    a. Ebola virus   b. Vesicular stomatitis virus
    c. Simian 40   d. Rabies

44. All are true regarding hantaan virus except:
    a. DNA virus   [PGI 2005]
    b. Carried by rodents
    c. Causes recurrent respiratory infection
    d. Hemorrhagic manifestation may occur

45. New infectious agents are: [PGI 07]
    a. Nipah virus   b. Pneumocystis jeruveci
    c. Corona virus   d. SARS
    e. Prion

46. True about Crimean-Congo haemorrhagic fever:
    a. Zoonosis   [PGI Nov 11]
    b. Develop petechial rashes
    c. Transmitted by mites
    d. Recently disease has been reported in Gujarat
    e. It has high fatality

Explanations and References with Illustrative Answers

1. **Ans. (c) Increased muscular activity leads to increased paralysis** *Ref. Ghai 6/e, p 210; Park 22/e, p 185*

   Predisposing factors for paralytic polio
   - Tonsillectomy
   - Tooth extraction
   - Strenuous physical exercise
   - Cortisone administration
   - Intramuscular injection
   - Adenoidectomy
   - Fatigue

   • Oral polio vaccine is recommended to all children below 5 years.
   • For eradication it is essential to immunize all infants below 6 months.

   Important features of Polio virus
   • Poliovirus, causative agent of polio, is SS positive sense RNA virus having 1, 2 and 3 serotypes.
   • *MC* serotype - *Type 1*
   • *MC* cause of epidemic - Type 1 (epidemics are also caused by Type 3 while endemics are by Type 2)
   • *MC* type associated with paralysis - *Type 1*
   • Most difficult to eradicate Type -1
   • Most antigenic - Type 2
   • *MC* cause of vaccine induced paralysis - *mutated Type - 3*

- **Modes of transmission**
  - *Main route*: Feco-oral route directly or indirectly.
  - *Droplet infection*: May occur in acute phase of disease.
- **Clinical Spectrum**
  - Most vulnerable age is between 6 months and 3 years.
  - M.C clinical presentation – Inapparent / subclinical infection.
  - Most rare clinical presentation – Paralytic polio.
  - Usual cause of death – respiratory insufficiency.
  - Progressive paralysis, coma or convulsions usually indicate cause other than polio.
- **Prevention**
  - Two types of vaccine:
    i. *Inactivated (salk) injectable polio vaccine.*
    ii. *Oral (sabin) live attenuated vaccine:*
       - It provides both local immunity (by producing intestinal IgA) and systemic immunity.
       - Vaccine progeny is excreted in feces and secondary spread occurs to household contacts so non immunized persons are immunized by replacing wild strain by vaccine strain.
       - It results in herd immunity even if only about **66%** of community is immunized.

Mnemonics: = For Live Attenuated Vaccine (TIPS BYE C$_2$MMR)

T	I	P	S
Typhoid oral	Influenza	Plague	Sabin
B	Y	E	
BCG	Yellow Fever	Epidemic typhus	
C2	M	M	R
Chicken pox Cholera	Measles	Mumps	Rubella

Vaccine Derived Poliovirus

- Vaccine associated paralytic poliomyelitis is seen in 4 case/10 lakh birth
- Clinical features are exactly same as that seen with wild poliovirus.
- It is most frequently associated with sabin 3 (60% of cases) followed by sabin 2 and sabin 1.
- In patients with common variable immunodeficiency syndrome, sabin virus replicate for prolong periods, resulting in chronic shedding of vaccine derived poio virus with increased neurovirulence, Such viruses are termed as immunodeficiency associated vaccine derived poliovirus (*iVDPV*).

Note: HIV or AIDS are risk factors for the development of iVDPV.

2. **Ans. (d) Enterovirus** *Ref. Nelson 18/e, p 2521*

"Enterovirus are the most common cause of viral meningitis and meningoencephalitis in children".

Remember:
- Most common cause of sporadic viral encephalitis: HSV-1
- Most common cause of epidemic viral encephalitis: HSV-1

3. **Ans. (b) Inactivated vaccine is given IM** *Ref. Park 22/e, p 188*

Inactivated poliovaccine or IPV (salk type) is given subcutaneously or IM.
Other options
Option a
Most cases of polio are asymptomatic
Option c
- **Dose schedule of IPV:**
  - First dose when infant is 6 weeks old
  - Additional doses are recommended prior to school entry and then every five years until the age of 18.

Option d
- These are three serotypes of polio virus
- Most outbreaks of paralytic polio are due to type 1.

4. **Ans. (c) 70** *Ref. Ananthanarayan 10/e, p 499*
   Acute hemorrhagic conjunctivitis, a pandemic is caused by enterovirus 70
   - EV-70 grows only on human embryonic kidney or HeLa cell lines for primary isolation
   - Coxsackie type A-24 also produce the same diseases

   Causes of acute hemorrhagic conjunctivitis
   - Pneumococci
   - Adenovirus
   - Coxsackie virus 24
   - Enterovirus 70   **mnemonic: PACE**

5. **Ans. (b, c, d, e) Stable at pH 4, Cause pleurodynia, Cause encephalitis, Cause meningitis**
   Ref. Greenwood 18/e, p 489; Ananthanarayan 9/e, p 491

   Let us consider each option
   Option a and b

Property	Enterovirus
Capsid form	Icosohedral
– Polypeptide	VP_1, VP_2, VP_3, VP_4
– RNA type	Single stranded positive sense
– RNA molecular weight	2×10^6
Acid	Stable (pH 3-9)
Optimal temperature	37°C
Density in caesium chloride	1.34

   Option c, d, e

Diseases associated with enterovirus	
Paralysis	Poliovirus, Coxsackie A
Aseptic meningitis	Poliovirus Coxsackie A, Coxsackie B, ECHO
Encephalitis	Poliovirus Coxsackie A, Coxsackie B, ECHO
Fever with rash	Coxsackie A, ECHO
Hand foot and mouth disease	Coxsackie A
Herpangina	Coxsackie A
URI	Coxsackie A
Pneumonia, bronchiolitis	New enterovirus types
Myocarditis, pericarditis	Coxsackie B virus
Acute hemorrhagic conjunctivitis	Cox Sackie A
Bornholm disease	Cox Sackie B virus

6. **Ans. (a) Staphylococcus** *Ref. Harrison 19/e, p 1212; 20/e, p1386*
   Pulmonary complications of influenzae
   a. **Primary influenza viral pneumonia:** Least common but most severe of all pulmonary complications of influenzae Sputum production is generally scanty, but sputum may contain blood. In advanced cases, diffuse rates may be noted X-ray finding shows diffuse interstitial infiltrates. Primary influenzae pneumonia has predilection for individuals with cardiac diseases.
   b. **Secondary bacterial pneumonia:** Characterised by reappearance of fever along with sign and symptoms of bacaterial pneumonia after initial improvement. The commonest bacterial pathogens are S.pneumoniae, staphylococcus aureus, and haemophilus influenzae.
   c. **Mixed bacterial and viral pneumonia:** Most common pneumonic complication after influenza patient may show gradual progression of their acute illness or may show transient improvement followed by clinical exacerbation. Patients with mixed viral and bacterial pneumonia have less wide spread involvement of lung than those with primary viral pneumonia
   d. Worsening and exacerbation of COPD
   e. **Other pulmonary complications:** Worsening of COPD, In children croup, sinusitis as well as otitis media can be there

7. **Ans. (a) Bird flu virus** *Ref. Park 22/e, p 147*
   H_5N_1 **is a type of new influenza virus which is a causative agent of bird flu.**
   - Majority of avian influenza do not infect humans. However, avian H5N1 is a strain with pandemic potential since it ultimately adapt into a strain that is contagious among humans.

8. **Ans. (d) Hemagglutinin and neuraminidase are strain specific** *Ref. Ananthanarayan 10/e, 504' 9/e p 497-498*

Antigenic Structure of Influenza Virus	
Surface/viral or V antigen	**Internal antigen**
• Strain specific	a. Envelop antigen (nucleocapsid) - Host specific
• Shows antigenic variation	b. Membrane (M) antigen - Type specific, i.e. A, B or C

• Two types:
  a Hemagglutination - Antibody against this is protective
  b Neuraminidase - Antibody against this is not protective
	c. Ribonucleoprotein (RNP) or soluble(s) antigen:
	  – Type specific
	  – Stable, i.e. not shows antigenic variation

Antigenic variation	
Antigenic drift or Minor antigenic variation	**Antigenic shift or Major antigenic variation**
Due to point mutation	Due to genetic reassortment
Responsible for epidemic	Responsible for pandemics
Shown by A, B	Only shown by type A

Remember:
- Ds RNA – Reoviridae family (reo, orbi, rota virus), Picobirnaviruses
- Ss DNA – Parvoviridae

9. **Ans. (a) Influenza virus** *Ref. Ananthanarayan 10/e, 503*
   RNA genome of influenza virus is segmented and consist of eight pieces.

Segmented RNA viruses are:		
P – Picobirna viruses	→ ds RNA	
A – Arena viridae	→ ds RNA	
R – Reoviridae	→ ds RNA	**Mnemonic = PARBO**
B – Bunyaviridae	→ ss RNA	
O – Orthomyxoviridae (Influenza)	→ ss RNA	

10. **Ans. (a), (b) and (c) Influenza, Cholera and Plague** *See below:*

Disease	Incubation Period
Pertussis	7 - 14 days
Chicken pox	14 - 16 days
Polio	7 - 14 days
Rubella	2 - 3 weeks (average 18 days)
Mumps	usually 18 days
Influenza	18 - 72 hrs
Diphtheria	2 - 6 days
Menigococcal meningitis	usually 3 - 4 days
Cholera	a few hours up to 5 days (commonly 1 - 2 days)
Rabies	highly variable, commonly 3 - 8 weeks (vary from 4 days to many years)
Plague	
- Bubonic plague	2 - 7 days
- Septicemic plague	2 - 7 days
- Pneumonic plague	1 - 3 days
Tetanus	usually 6 - 10 days
Leprosy	average 3 - 5 years or more

11. **Ans. (a) Ventricular septal defect** *Ref. COGDT 11/e p 275, Harrison 20/e p 1478; Ghai 8/e p 401*
    Congenital rubella syndrome produce following cardiac defects:
    - PDA
    - Peripheral pulmonary stenosis
    - VSD

> **Congenital rubella syndrome**
> - Rubella one of the most teratogenic virus cross the placenta to produce fetal infection
> - Virus produce cytopathic damage to vessels and ischemia in affected fetal organ
> - Congenital damage depends upon the time of exposure to virus. 50-80% of neonates exposed to virus prior to 12 weeks gestation exhibit congenital infection which is rare if infection occurs beyond 18 weeks gestation
> - Congenital anomalies include: Hearing impairment (most common), cataract (including retinopathy), heart-defect (PDA, VSD), microcephaly, pancephalitis, hepatosplenomegaly, thrombocytopenia
> - Diagnosis is made by isolation of virus from throat swabs and RTPCR
> - Infant may excrete virus up to one year.

12. **Ans. (a) Cataract, VSD, intracerebral hemorrhage** *Ref. IGDT 11/e p 275*
    Already explained

13. **Ans. (d) Caused by...** *Ref. Ananthanarayan 10/e, p 558*
    Rubella virus has been classified in the family togaviridae as the only member of genus Rubivirus.

14. **Ans. (a) Meningoencephalitis can precede parotitis** *Ref. Nelson 17/e, p 1035 - 1036*
    Important Points About Mumps
    - *MC* manifestation of mumps - bilateral parotitis.
    - It can also involve submaxillary and sublingual glands but never involved alone.
    - *MC* manifestation (other than parotitis) in post pubertal males is orchitis (sterility is rare). Seen in 20% of cases.
    - Though sterility is rare, subfertility is estimated to occur in 13% of cases of unilateral orchitis and in 30-87 of cases of bilateral orchitis.
    - Oophoritis is far less common than orchitis. It also not lead to sterility.
    - *MC* manifestation (other than parotitis) in children: Aseptic meningitis which may develop before, during or in absence of parotitis.
    - **Period of communicability** – Usually 4-6 days *before onset of symptoms and a week or more* thereafter. Period of maximum infectivity is just before and at onset of parotitis.

    Complications of Mumps
    - *Meningoencephalomyelitis*
       - *MC* complication in childhood.
       - Males are affected *more commonly*.
       - May be either due to primary infection of neuron or post-infectious encephalitis with demyelination.
       - In primary infection it occurs before parotitis while in post-infectious form, it follows parotitis.
       - Parotitis may be absent in some cases.
       - CSF shows lymphocytic pleocytosis.
    - *Orchitis and Epididymitis*
       - These complications are rare in prepubscent age group, while common inadolescent and adults.
       - Infertility is rare even with bilateral orchitis.
    - Pancreatitis, myocarditis, arthritis, thyroiditis, Mastitis, GB syndrome, Transverse myelitis
    - Cerebral ataxia, measles associated deafness, dacryoadenitis are other complications.

15. **Ans. (d) Infection after 16 weeks of gestation results in major congenital defects**
    Ref. Park 21/e, p 140-41; 22/e, p 141-142; Harrison 20/e, p 1477-1479

    Important features of Rubella virus
    - Rubella is RNA virus of *togavirus* family.
    - No known carrier state for postnatally acquired rubella.
    - Infectivity is greatest when rash is erupted.
    - Rubella (*German measles*) is mainly a disease of childhood, particularly 3-10 years.
    - One attack results *life-long immunity*
    - It causes two types of disease:
      a. **Postnatally Acquired Rubella**
         - Virus is shed from pharynx during prodromal phase and continue for about a week after onset.
         - It is invariably self-limited.
         - *Symptoms*
            - Posterior auricular, cervical and suboccipital lymphadenopathy; fever and rash *(begins on face and spreads down the body).*
            - Petechial enanthem on soft plate called *Forschheimer* spots may be seen.
         - **Complications:**
            - Arthritis (*MC* in fingers, wrist or knees) almost exclusively in women.
            - Hemorrhage due to thrombocytopenia and vascular damage.
            - Encephalitis (*in immunosuppressed*)

- **Diagnosis:**
  - Throat swab culture for virus isolation
  - **Serology:** - Most widely used serological test is hemagglutination inhibition test (HAI).
    - 4-fold rise in HI antibody titer in paired sera or presence of IgM in single sera obtained 2-weeks after the rash is **diagnostic** of recent rubella infection.

b. Congenital Rubella Syndrome
- Infectivity as well as severity is more in early pregnancy (*first trimester of <11 weeks*).
- *Classic* triad of *patent ductus arteriosus (cardiac malformation), cataract* and *deafness* is seen.
- Infection in 2nd trimester - may be deafness only.
- >16 wks – no major abnormalities
- **Diagnosis**
  - Isolation of virus in cell cultures of throat samples, urine or other secretions.
  - Detection of IgM in single serum sample shortly after birth.
  - Persistence of Rubella IgG antibodies serum beyond 1 year or rising antibody titer anytime during infancy in an unvaccinated child.
  - Biopsy of tissues/blood/CSF fluid for viral antigen by monoclonal antibodies.
  - Detection of Rubella RNA by in situ hybridization and PCR.
- **Prevention:**
  - **Rubella vaccine:** Live attenuated RA 27/3 vaccine
  - **Strategy:**
    - Immunize all infants at 12-15 mths with MMR and second dose in early childhood
    - Also administer to anyone who is thought to be susceptible to infection and is not pregnant.
    - **Contraindication for Rubella vaccine:** Pregnancy

> **Remember:** Pregnancy should be avoided for at least 3 months after rubella vaccination.

16. **Ans. (c) Not infectious in prodromal period** *Ref. Park 22/e p 138*
    "Measles is highly infectious during the prodromal period and the stage of rash."

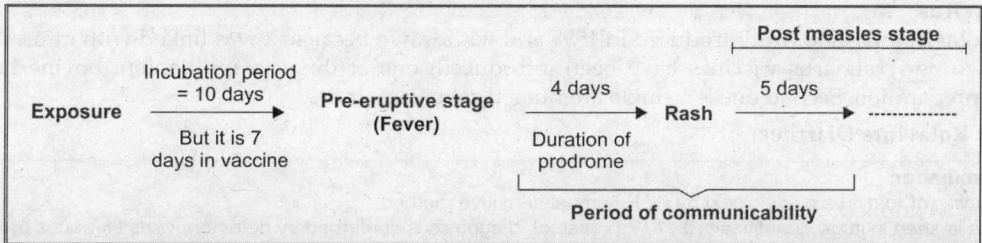

17. **Ans. (d) SSPE** *Ref. Harrison 20/e, p 1476*

Complication of Measles	
• Otitis media (MC) • Pneumonia	Very common in infants with measles May be primary viral pneumonia or bacterial superinfection; frequent reason for hospitalization of adults; measles rash sometimes lacking in immunocompromised patients with measles pneumonia. Primary giant cell *(Hecht's)* pneumonia is seen in immunocompromised
• Croup	Occasionally severe
• Gastroenteritis	Many children with measles develop diarrhea which contributes to malnutrition
• Cervical adenitis	Due to lymphoid hyperplasia as host response to virus; common
• Acute encephalitis	May be mild to severe/fatal; occurs in 1 in 1000 cases of mesles
• Subacute sclerosing panencephalitis (SSPE)	In 1 in 100,000 cases of measles, usually when measles occurred in infancy; seen 5-10 years later. SSPE is a rare progressive disease characterized by seizures and progressive deterioration of cognitive and motor functions and death

18. **Ans. (c) Measles** *Ref. Ananthanarayan 10/e p 518*
    Warthin-Finkeldey cells are multinucleated giant cells found in the lymphoid tissue of patients of measles.

Intracytoplasmic eosinophilic
• Negri bodies in Rabies
• Guarnieri bodies in vaccinia, variola (smallpox)
• Paschen bodies in variola (smallpox)

Contd...

Intracytoplasmic eosinophilic
• Bollinger bodies in fowlpox
• Henderson-Patterson bodies in Molluscum contagiosum
• Eosinophilic inclusion bodies in boid inclusion body disease
Intranuclear eosinophilic (acidophilic)
• Cowdry type A in Herpes simplex virus and Varicella zoster virus
• Torres bodies in Yellow fever
• Cowdry type B in Polio and adenovirus
Intranuclear basophilic-
• Cowdry type B in Adenovirus
• "Owl's eye appearance" in cytomegalovirus
Both intranuclear and intracytoplasmic-
• Warthin–Finkeldey bodies in Measles

19. **Ans. (d) Norovirus** *Ref. Harrison 20/e, p 1463*
"Norovirus may be the most common infectious agent of mild gastroenteritis in the community and affects all age groups."
Norovirus
- Non enveloped, Icosahedral RNA virus
- Infectious dose: 10–100 viral particles
- Route of infection: Feco-oral, aerosolization
- Incubation period: 12–72 h, illness lasts 12–60 h
- *Clinical features*: Loose waters stools without blood, mucous, leucocytes.
- *Diagnosis*: PCR

20. **Ans. (a) Rotavirus** *Ref. Harrison 19/e, p 1289, 20/e, p 1467*
- The first rotavirus vaccine was introduced in 1998 and withdrawn because it was linked with intusssuception.
- In 2006 two new rotavirus vaccines have been introduced, one of this is a multivalent bovine human reassortant rotavirus preparation. Second one is a single attenuated rotavirus strain.

Diagnosis of Rotaviurs Diarrhea

1. **Stool examination**
   - Genotyping of rotavirus nucleic acid by PCR is most sensitive method.
   - As virus is shed in large quantities (10^7-10^{12}g) in stool, diagnosis is confirmed by detecting *virus in faeces* by enzyme immunoassay or viral RNA can be detected by gel electrophoresis, probe hybridization, or PCR.
   - Viral shedding detectable by EIA usually subsides within a week but may persist for >30 days in immunocompromised while PCR detect viral shedding for longer periods.
   - Electron microscopy / immunoelectronmicroscopy is used to see virus in feces. Conc. > 10^6 virus/ml is necessary
   - Serological techniques for demonstration of stool are simple and sensitive. Rotavirus share a common group antigen situated in the inner capsid layer which can be detected by IEM, ELISA or latex agglutination.
   - They do not grow readily on cell culture.
2. **Serology:** IgM or IgG antibodies in the blood are increased.

21. **Ans. (c) Rotavirus** *Ref. Harrison 20/e, p 1465*
Reassortment
Mixing of the genetic material of different strains of a species in to a new combination. Process contributing of re-assortment includes:
- Assortment of chromosomes
- Chromosomal crossover

It is typically seen in influenza virus and rota virus. E.g. If a single host (human or chicken) in infected by two different strains of the influenza virus, then it is possible that new assembled viral particle may have segment from both the strains.

22. **Ans. (b) Rabies** *Ref. Ananthanarayan 10/e p 539*
- **Vaccine that grows in embryonated eggs:**
  - Influenza
  - Yellow fever (17 D strain)
  - Rabies (Flury strain)
  - *Mumps*

- Varicella vaccine grown in chick embryo fibroblast culture.
- Rubella – RA 27/3 vaccine produced in human diploid fibroblast. ... *Park 22/e, p 142*
- No eggs culture vaccine of measles are produced. All are tissue culture vaccine, either chick embryo or human diploid cell line.

23. **Ans. (b) Rabies** *Ref. Ananthanarayan 10/e p 535*
    - Negri bodies are the intracytoplasmic inclusions of rabies virus in the CNS.
    - Negri bodies are distributed throughout the brain particularly in Ammon's horn, the cerebral cortex, the brain stem, the hypothalamus, purkinje cells of cerebellum and the dorsal root spinal ganglia.
    - They are not seen in about 20% cases of rabies and their absence does not rule out the diagnosis.

Inclusion Bodies	
It is of following types:	
a. Intracytoplasmic eosinophilic inclusions:	
Negri bodies	– rabies
Guarnieri bodies	– variola (small pox), vaccinia
Bollinger bodies	– fowlpox
Henderson – Peterson bodies	– molluscum contagiosum
b. Intranuclear acidophilic inclusion bodies:	
Cowdry type A	– herpes, chicken pox, CMV, yellow fever
Torres bodies	– yellow fever
Cowdry type B	– polio virus
c. Both Nuclear and cytoplasmic:	
Warthin Finkeldey	– measles
d. Intranuclear basophilic inclusion bodies:	
Cowdry type B	– adenovirus

24. **Ans. (c) Immediately stitch wound under antibiotic coverage** *Ref. Park 22/e, p 254; 21/e, p 253-254*
    "*Immediate stitching is contraindicated.*"
    - **Combined administration of:** Single dose of anti-rabies serum; Anti-rabies vaccine (ARV) and; Local treatment of wound is the *best* specific prophylactic treatment after exposure of man to rabies (especially in all severe cases, i.e. class III exposures and in all cases of unprovoked bites by wild animals).
    - **Anti-Rabies Serum (*Passive immunity*)** should be given as promptly as possible after sensitivity test, irrespective of interval between exposure and beginning of treatment.
        – It prolongs I.P. if administered soon after exposure to rabies so it is particularly important in class III bites.
        – It is given either as Horse anti-rabies serum (40 IU) or Human rabies immunoglobulin (20 IU) in which part of the dose is given around the wound and rest by IM in gluteal region.
    - **Local Treatment of wound:**
        – It can reduce the chances of developing rabies by up to 80%. It consist of:
            a. Cleansing with plenty of soap and water, preferably under a running tap for at least 5 minutes.
            b. Chemical treatment by virucidal agents either alcohol, tincture 0.01% of aqueous solution of iodine or povidone iodine (not use savlon, cetavlon, carbolic or nitric acid).
            c. *Suturing - Not done immediately* but should be done 24 - 48 hours later.

Classification of Exposures		
Class I (Slight risk)	**Class II (Moderate risk)**	**Class III (Severe risk)**
• Licks on healthy unbroken skin • Consumption of unboiled milk of suspected animal • Scratches without oozing of blood	• Licks on fresh cuts • Scratches with oozing of blood • All bites except on head, neck, face, palm, fingers • Minor wounds less than 5 in number	• All bites or scratches with oozing of blood on neck, head, face, palm, fingers • Lacerated wounds on any part of body • Multiple wounds 5 or more in number • Bites from wild animals

25. **Ans. (b) Corneal impression smear for immunofluorescence stain** *Ref. Ananthanarayan 10/e p 538*
    "*The method most commonly used for diagnosis of rabies is demonstration of rabies virus antigen by immunofluorescence. The specimens tested are corneal smears and skin biopsy (from face or neck) or saliva in live cases, and brain postmortem*".

    Diagnosis of Human Rabies
    - *Specimen*
        (a) *Antemortem* Corneal smears, skin biopsy from face or neck, saliva.
        (b) *Postmortem:* Brain

- Method
  - *Most commonly used* for diagnosis is the demonstration of rabies virus **antigens by immunofluorescence** (direct or using monoclonal antibodies).
  - Demonstration of negri bodies in the brain or spinal cord.
  - *Isolation* of virus by intracerebral inoculation in mice; from the brain, CSF, saliva, urine.
  - Rapid isolation is done by tissue culture cell lines.
  - High titre rabies specific **antibodies in CSF** (Not seen after immunization) by Fluorescent antibody test.
  - Detection of rabies virus RNA in saliva by Reverse transcription PCR.

> **Remember:**
> - Rabies infection terminates in death, not lifelong immunity.
> - Rabies virus has single serotype, i.e. Lyssavirus type 1.
> - Rabies vaccine is killed inactivated vaccine.
>   - Inactivation is commonly done by phenol or Betapropiolactone.

26. **Ans. (b) With hold...** Ref. Harrison 20/e, p1488, 19/e, p 1302-1304

    "*Healthy dogs, cats, or ferrets may be confined and observed for 10 days. Post exposure prophylaxis is not necessary if animal remains healthy. If the animal develop signs of rabies during the observation period, it should be euthanized immediately, and the head should be transported to the laboratory under refrigeration and examined for the presence of rabies virus by DFA testing.*"
    ...Harrison 19/e 1303

    In high risk exposures and in areas where canine rabies is endemic rabies prophylaxis should be initiated without waiting for lab results.

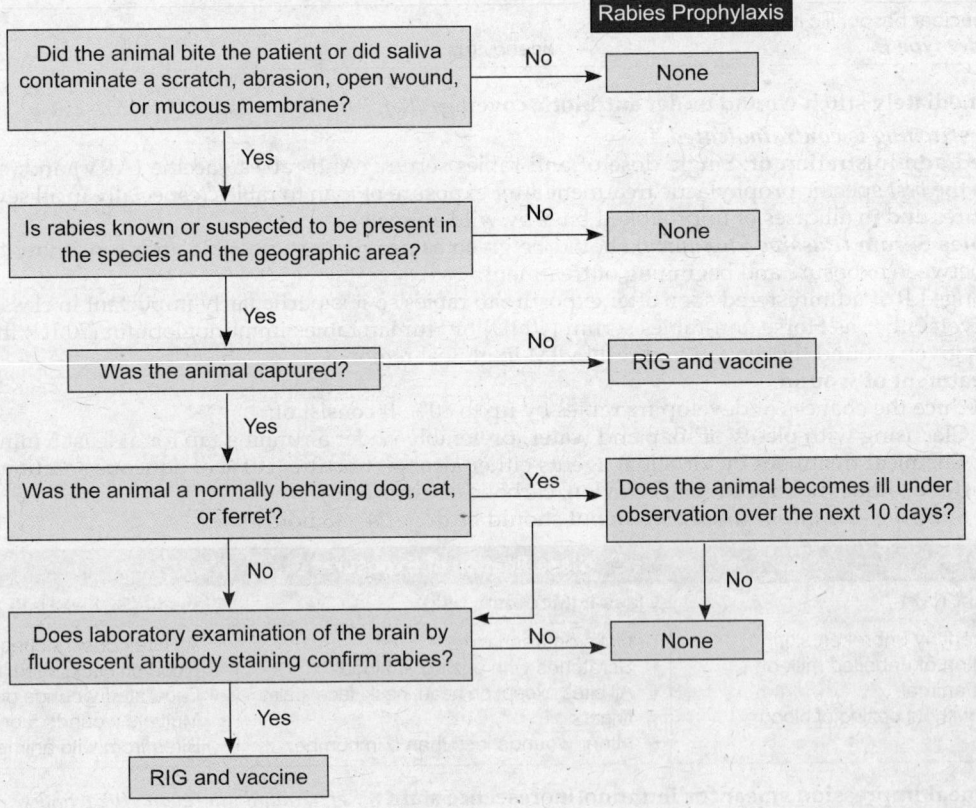

27. **Ans. (b) Negri bodies** Ref. Ananthanarayan 10/e p 535

    Already explained

28. **Ans. (c) Antibodies to rabies virus**

    Corneal Smear test
    - Rabies virus antigen can be detected by simple FAT test on corneal epithelium during the terminal stages.

- The methodology of this test involves the gentle rubbing of that surface of a clean microscope glass slide on each cornea.
- The test is not routinely performed due to its low sensitivity.

Note: Specimen for RT-PCR would be saliva.

29. **Ans. (c) Japanese encephalitis** *Ref. Park 22/e, p 259-260*

   Japanese encephalitis
   - Caused by Group B arbovirus (filovirus)
   - **Vector:** – *Culex tritreniorhynchus* (most important)
     – *C. vishnvi*
     – *C. gelidus.*
   - Cycle is Bird → Arthropod → Man
   - Man is an incidental *'dead end'* host.
   - **Animal host:** – Pigs – major vertebrate host. – not manifest any symptoms so act as amplifiers.
     – Cattles and buffaloes: Act as mosquito attractants.
     – Horses – only domestic animals which show signs of encephalitis.
   - **Birds host** – Pond herons (reservoir host), Cattle egrets, poultry and ducks.
   - *Incubation period in man* – 5-15 days.
   - Average period between onset of illness and death is about 9 days.
   - *Diagnosis* is mainly based on serology using *IgM capture ELISA.*

   Remember: Killed mouse brain vaccine is available by which immunity develops after one month of second dose.

30. **Ans. (a) Relapsing fever** *Ref. Park 22/e, p 712, 725*

Tick borne diseases		
Hard tick	• Tick typhus	• Viral encephalitis
	• Tularemia	• Tick paralysis
	• Human Babesiosis	• Colorado tick fever
	• Viral encephalitis (not Japenese encephalitis which is transmitted by culex)	• Viral hemorrhagic fever (e.g. Kyasanur forest disease)
Soft tick	• Relapsing fever	• Q fever

31. **Ans. (c) Kyasanur Forest disease** *Ref. Park 22/e, p 725*

   Already explained

32. **Ans. (c) KFD is transmitted by ticks** *Ref. Park 22/e, p 262-263*
    - *Yellow fever* is an exotic disease for India, i.e. disease which may be imported in India or India is yellow fever 'receptive' area that is "an area in which yellow fever does not exist but where condition would permit its development if introduced".
    - *Dengue virus* has at least **4 serotypes** (not one).
    - *Japanese encephalitis* is transmitted by *culex* (not Aedes).

   Remember: Other culex transmitted diseases are:
   - Bancroftian filariasis
   - West Nile fever
   - Viral arthritis (epidemic/polyarthritis).

33. **Ans. (a) Hantavirus pulmonary syndrome is caused by inhalation of rodent urine** *Ref. Jawetz 25/e, p 531; Park 22/e, p 262*

   Hantavirus are classified in the hantavirus genus of the Bunyaviridae family. It can cause very serious and often fatal disease.
   (a) Hemorrhagic fever with renal syndrome.
   (b) Hantavirus pulmonary syndrome.
   - Hantavirus are natural pathogen of rodents. Viremia is present in infected rodents and the virus is shed in urine, feces and saliva in high titres. *Transmission from rodent to rodent and rodent to human* is primarily respiratory by inhalation of virus contained in dried excreta.

   Other options:
   - *KFD* is a febrile disease caused by an arbovirus and transmitted to man by bite of infective tick.
   - *Chikungunya fever*-Dengue like disease caused by chikugunya virus and transmitted by Aedes, Culex and Mansonia mosquito.

34. Ans. (a) IgM ELISA   *Ref. Harrison 20/e, p 1508; Park 22/e, p 228-229*

Laboratory diagnosis of Dengue
- Thrombocytopenia (100,000/mm^3 or less)
- *Hemoconcentration:* Hematocrit increased by 20% or more of base line value
- Leukopenia
- Elevation of serum Aminotransferase ($\pm$)
- Antigen detection ELISA or RT PCR or virus isolation in acute phase
- IgM ELISA or paired serology during recovery
- Strip immunochromatographic test of IgM for rapid diagnosis

Remember: IgM appears within 2-5 days of onset of illness and persists for one to three months.

35. Ans. (d) Hand-foot-mouth disease   *Ref. Ananthanarayan 10/e, p 523*

Family	Genus	Important species
Togaviridae	Alphavirus	Chikungunya, Sindbis and Venezuelan equine encephalitis viruses
Flaviviridae	Flavivirus	Japanesse encephalitis, West Nile, Yellow Fever, Dengue types 1, 2, 3, 4, Kyasanur Forest Disease, Omask hemorrhagic fever
Bunyaviridae	Bunyavirus	California encephalitis
	Phlebovirus	Sandfly fever viruses, Rift valley fever virus
	Nairovirus	Crimean Congo hemorrhagic fever viruses, Ganjam virus
	Hantavirus	Hantan, Seoul, Puumala, Prospect Hill, Sin Nombre viruses
Reoviridae	Orbivirus	Colorado tick fever, African horse sickness, Blue tongue viruses
Rhabdoviridae	Vesiculovirus	Vesicular stomatitis virus, Chandipura virus

Remember: Hand, Foot and Mouth Disease (HFMD) is caused by coxsackie A-16, 9; B 1-3; Enterovirus 71: It is an exanthematous fever of young children characterized by papulovesicular lesion on skin and oral mucosa.

36. Ans. (a, c, d) Caused by 4 serotypes, Presents with fever and joint pain, Virus belongs to flavivirus genus
Ref. Ananthanarayan 9/e, p 525; Greenwood 18/e, p 531-532

Dengue Fever
- Caused by four serologically related virus termed dengu 1, 2, 3 4. Out of 4 types, type II is most virulent
- All are enveloped SS RNA virus belongs to flavivirus family
- Diseases is transmitted by *Ae. aegypti mosquito*
- Epidemics of dengue are common in Southeast Asian countries including India, particularly in September-October.
- *IP* : 3-14 days
- Dengue present clinically as fever of sudden onset with headache, retrobullar pain, pain in back and limbs (*break bone fever*), lymphadenopathy and maculopapular rash. The fever is usually biphasic that lasts for 5-7 days
- In some cases (which exhibit hypersensitive or enhance response) dengue may present with hemorrhagic manifestation (dengue hemorrhagic fever) or with shock (dengue shock syndrome)
- Control of dengue is limited to vector control as **no vaccine** is currently available
- *No vertebral hosts other than humans* have been identified.

37. Ans. (d) ELISA for antibody detection against dengue virus

Laboratory diagnosis of Dengue
- *Detection of Virus:* After the onset of illness, the virus can be detected in serum, plasma, circulating blood cells and other tissues for 4–5 days. During the early stages of the disease, virus isolation, nucleic acid or antigen detection can be used to diagnose the infection.
- *Nucleic Acid Amplification Test:* Before day 5 of illness, during the febrile period, dengue infections may be diagnosed by detection of viral RNA by nucleic acid amplification tests (NAAT). Nucleic acid detection assays with excellent performance characteristics may identify dengue viral RNA within 24–48 hours
- *Antigen Detection Test:* Detection of viral antigens by ELISA can be used in first week of disease. NS1 antigen detection kits have now become the commonest method for diagnosis of dengue. After day 5, dengue viruses and antigens disappear from the blood coincident.

- *Serology:* Method of choice at the end of infection. Antibody response to infection differs according to the immune status of the host
    a. *Primary dengue infection* (in persons who have not previously been infected with a flavivirus or immunized with a flavivirus vaccine): IgM antibodies are the first immunoglobulin isotype to appear. They are detectable in 50% of patients by days 3-5 after onset of illness, increasing to 80% by day 5 and 99% by day 10. IgM levels peak about two weeks after the onset of symptoms and then decline generally to undetectable levels over 2–3 months.
    b. *Secondary dengue infection* (a dengue infection in a host that has previously been infected by a dengue virus, or sometimes after non-dengue flavivirus vaccination or infection): Antibody titres rise rapidly the dominant immunoglobulin isotype is IgG and is detectable at high levels.
- To distinguish primary and secondary dengue infections, IgM/IgG antibody ratios are now more commonly used than the haemagglutination-inhibition test (HI)

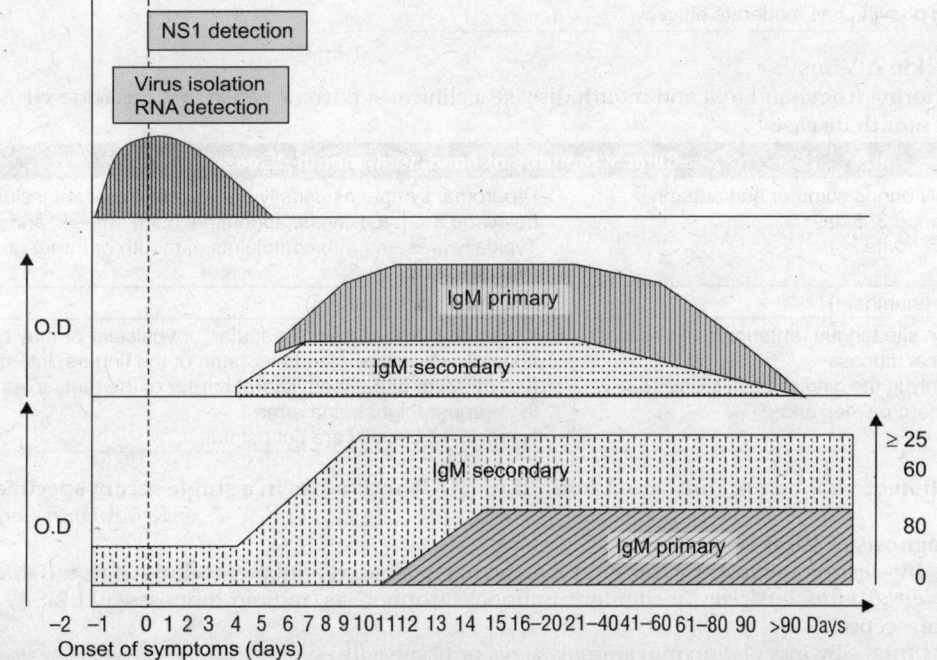

Diagnostic methods	Diagnosis of acute infection	Time to results	Specimen	Time of collection after onset of symptoms
Viral isolation and serotype identification	Confirmed	1-2 weeks	Whole blood, serum, tissues	1-5 days
Nucleic acid detection	Confirmed	1 or 2 days	Tissues, whole blod, serum, plasma	1-5 days
Antigen detection	Not yet determined Confirmed	1 day > 1 day	Serum Tissue for immuno-chemistry	1-6 days NA
IgM ELISA	Probable	1-2 days	Serum, plasma, whole blood	After 5 days
IgM rapid test		30 minutes		
IgG (paired sera) by ELISA, HI or neutralization test	Confirmed	7 days or more	Serum, plasma, whole blood	Acute sena, 1-5 days: convalescent after 15 days

38. **Ans. (d) Respiratory syncytial virus** *Ref. OP Ghai 8/e, p 381; Nelson Pediatrics 17/e, p 1076*
    - RSV is the *most common* cause of bronchiolitis.
    - RSV is the *most common* cause of viral pneumonia in infants.
    RSV
    – RNA virus belonging to family paramyxoviridae.
    – In infants *MC* manfestation is ***bronchiolitis.***
    – In adults *MC* manifestation is ***common cold.***

Cause of Bronchiolitis	
Respiratory syncytial virus (MC)	
Parainfluenza 3, 1, 2	
Adenovirus	
Influenza virus	
Mycoplasma pneumonia (Rarely).	Mnemonic - **My PAIR**
Treatment of Bronchiolitis:	

- In uncomplicated cases, treatment is symptomatic.
- Humidified oxygen is usually indicated for hospitalized infant.
- Epinephrine may be given, however, corticosteroids are not indicated.
- Antiviral drug ribavirin has moderate efficacy.

39. **Ans. (b) Coxsackie A Virus**

The child is suffering from hand foot and mouth disease a clinical syndrome cause by Coxsackie virus

Hand foot and mouth disease

Clinical features of hand, foot, mouth disease	
• Occur typically during summer and autumn • Incubation period 3–5 day • Spread by oral route	• Prodromal symptoms usually are absent if present include fever (generally below 38.3°C), fussiness, abdominal pain, emesis, and diarrhea. • Typically presents with complaints of mouth or throat (in verbal children) or refusal to eat.
Oral lesions (as enanthem)	Skin lesions (as exanthem)
• Most common site tongue (anterior to the faucial pillars) > buccal mucosa • Less commonly in the gingivolabial groove and on the soft and hard palates and	• It may be macular, maculopapular, or vesicular or may be all three • It typically involves: Hands (dorsum of the fingers, interdigital area, palms), feet (dorsum of the toes, lateral border of the feet, soles, heels), buttocks, legs (upper thighs), and arms • Nonpruritic, Usually are not painful,

40. **Ans. (d) Detection of viral hemagglutination inhibiting (HAI) antibodies in a single serum specimen**

Ref. Ananthanarayan 10/e, p 455-457

Laboratory Diagnosis of Viral Disease

- *Microscopy:* By electron microscopy (for viral diarrhea); Fluorescent antibody technique (e.g. Rabies), etc.
- *Demonstration of virus antigen:* By counterimmunoelectrophoresis, radioimmunoassay, ELISA, precipitation in gel immunofluorescence.
- *Isolation of virus:* – By inoculation into animals, eggs or tissue culture.
  – As most viruses are heat labile, refrigeration is essential during transport.
- *Serological diagnosis:*
  – By neutralization, complement fixation, ELISA, Hemagglutination inhibition tests, immunofluorescence.
  – It is essential to examine paired sera (acute and convalescent).
  – Examination of single sample of serum for antibodies is meaningful only when IgM, specific test are done.
  – Serological diagnosis is based on greater than fourfold rise in IgG in convalescent sera when acute and convalescent serum are analyzed at the same time. A simultaneous fall in IgM confirms recent primary viral infection.
  – Paired sera with rising titers of antibody to virus specific antigens and shift from IgM to IgG are generally accepted as diagnostic of acute viral infection.
  – Hemadsorption and hemagglutination assay measure the ability of serum antibodies to inhibit RNA virus induced erythrocyte adsorption or agglutination.

41. **Ans. (c) and (d) Measles - Edmonston zugreb strain and BCG-Danish 1331 strain** *See below:*

Vaccine	Strain
Mumps	Jeryl-Lynn strain
Chicken pox	OKA strain
Measles	HDC-Edmonston-Zagreb strain
Rubella	RA 27/3
BCG	Danish 1331 Strain
Cholera	CVD. 103 - HgR strain
Typhoral	Ty 21-a strain
Yellow fever 17-D	Asibi strain

Non-cultivable viruses:
- Rotavirus (certain strains can grow in tissue culture)
- Norwalk virus
- Molluscum contagiosum
- Hepatitis virus except hepatitis A

42. **Ans. (a) and (c) Smallpox virus and Ebola virus** *Ref. Harrison 18/e, p 1769*

    Bioterrorism agents
    - **Category A:**
      - Anthrax *(Bacillus anthracis)*
      - Botulism *(Clostridium botulinum toxin)*
      - Plague *(Yersinia pestis)*
      - Smallpox *(Variola major)*
      - Tularemia *(Francisella tularensis)*
      - Viral hemorrhagic fevers:

Arenaviruses:	Lassa, New World (Machupo, Junin, Guanarito, and Sabia).
Bunyaviridae:	Crimean Congo, Rift Valley
Filoviridiae:	Ebola, Marburg
Flaviviridae:	Yellow fever, Omsk fever, Kyasanur Forest

    - **Category B:**
      - Brucellosis *(Brucella spp.)*
      - Epsilon toxin of *Clostridium perfringens*
      - Food safety threats (e.g., *Salmonella* spp., *Escherichia coli* 0157: H7, *Shigella*)
      - Glanders *(Burkholderia mallei)*
      - Melioidosis *(B. pseuodmallei)*
      - Psittacosis *(Chalmydia psittaci)*
      - Q fever *(Coxiella burnetii)*
      - Ricin toxin from *Ricinus communis* (castor beans)
      - Staphylococcal enterotoxin B
      - Typhus fever *(Rickettsia prowazekii)*
      - Viral encephalitis [alphaviruses (e.g. Venezuelan, eastern, and western equine encephalitis)]
      - Water safety threats (e.g. *Vibrio cholerae*, *Cryptosporidium parvum*).
    - **Category C:**
      - Emerging infectious diseases threats such as nipah, hantavirus and SARS coronavirus.

43. **Ans. (c) Simian 40** *Ref. Ananthanarayan 9/e, p 552, 562, 10/e, p 569*

    SV 40 = Simian vacuolating virus 40 = Simian virus 40
    - It is a DNA viruses
    - Its family is papoviridae and genera is polyoma virus.
    - It is oncogenic virus, causing cytopathic effects with prominent cytoplasmic vacoulation

    Remember: Simian virises 5, 41 are animal virus antigenically similar to paranfluenza virus type 2

44. **Ans. (a) DNA virus** *Ref. Ananthanarayan 9/e, p 527; 10/e, 532*
    - Hantaan virus is an RNA virus belong to genus Hantavirus and family Bunya viridiae.
    - It causes two syndromes:
      a. *Hemorrhagic fever with renal syndrome (HFRS) or Manchurian epidemic HF or rodent bone nephropathy*
        - It occurs in two forms:
          i. Epidemic nephritis–milder form
          ii. Epidemic hemorrhagic fever–serious form
        - Resembles typhoid, leptospirosis and scrub typhus clinically.
        - Genus hantavirus contain four species–Hantaan, Seoul, puumala and Hill virus.

- They are natural pathogen of rodents so considered as robovirus and not stirctly an arbovirus infection.
- *Major host* for hantaan: Field mice
- Transmission from rodent to rodent and rodent to human is primarily respiratory, by inhalation of virus contained in dried excreta.
- *Diagnosis:* Demonstrating IgM by ELISA or of rising titre of immune adherence hemagglutinating antibodies in paired sera.

b. *Hantavirus pulmonary syndrome*
- Caused by new Hantavirus the *Sin Nombre* (meaning nameless) virus which is associated with deer, mouse and other rodents.
- *No arbovirus* is linked in transmission.
- Transmission occurs by inhalation of virus aerosol in dried rodent feces.

45. **Ans. (a), (c) and (d) Nipah virus, Corona virus and SARS** *Ref. Harrison 18/e, p 1769*

    Already explained, (category C)

46. **Ans. (a, b, d, e) Zoonosis, Develop petechial rashes, Recently disease has been reported in Gujarat, It has high fatality**
    Ref: Ananthanarayan 10/e, p 662, Harrison 20/e, p 1507

    Crimean-Congo Hemorrhagic Fever/CCHF)
    - Tick-borne viral disease, a zoonosis of domestic animals and wild animals, that may affect humans. Usually seen in East and West Africa, is a member of the Bunyaviridae family of RNA viruses.
    - However, in *January 2011*, out break occurred in *Gujarat* that led to few deaths.
    - Human infection is acquired via a tick bite or during the crushing of infected ticks. Domestic animals do not become ill, but do develop viremia.
    - Clinical disease is rare in infected mammals, but commonly *severe in infected humans, with a 30% mortality rate.*
    - Though similar to other HF syndromes, Crimean-Congo HF is associated with extensive live damage.
    - Laboratory values indicate DIC and show elevations in AST. creatine phosphokinase, and bilirubin.
    - Patients with fatal cases generally have more marked changes, even in the early days of illness, and also develop leucocytosis rather than leucopenia.
    - Cattle sheep goat and other domesticated animal acts as natural reservoir.

NEET Pattern Questions

1. **Which is enveloped virus:**
   a. Dengue virus
   b. Norwalk virus
   c. Hep A virus
   d. Adenovirus
   [Ref. Harrison 18/e, p 1433, 1434]

   All RNA virus are enveloped except Picorna, Caliciviridae, Reoviridae, Astrovirus

2. **Non-enveloped ss-RNA virus is:**
   a. Picornavirus
   b. Poxvirus
   c. Retrovirus
   d. Bunyavirus
   [Ref. Ananthanarayan, 10/e, p 490]

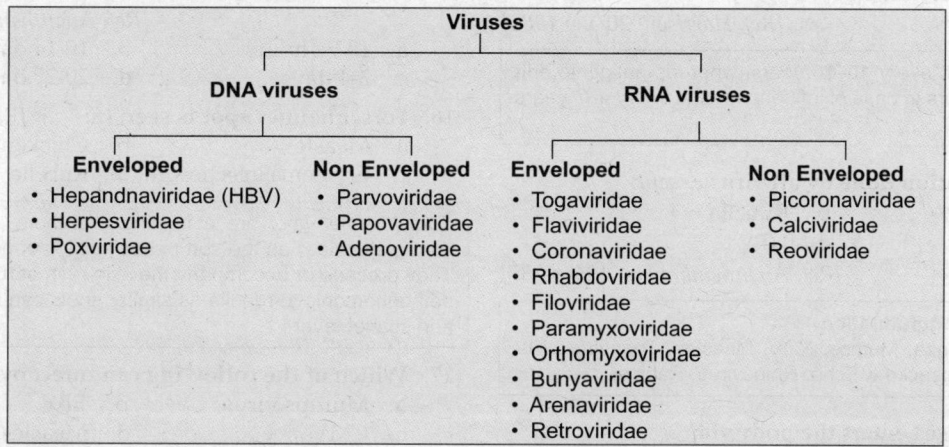

3. **Influenza virus culture is done on:**
   a. Charioallantoic membrane
   b. Allantoic cavity
   c. Yolk sac
   d. All
   Ref. Ananthanarayan, 10/e, p 506]

   Isolation of Influenza Virus
   - Specimen : Throat garglings
   - Tissue : Isolation can be made in eggs or in monkey kidney cell culture. For primary isolation the most suitable cells are Madin-Darby Canine Kidney (MDCK) cells.
   - Procedure : The material is inoculated into the amniotic cavity of 11-13 day old eggs. After inoculation at 35°C for three days the eggs are chilled and the amniotic and allantoic fluids harvested separately. The fluid are then tested for hemagglutination separately.

4. **All oncogenic viruses containing RNA belongs to:**
   a. Picornaviridae
   b. Herpesviridae
   c. Retroviridae
   d. Flaviviridae
   [Ref. Ananthanarayan, 10/e, p 570]

5. **Causative organism of SARS:**
   a. H1 N1
   b. Corona virus
   c. Rotavirus
   d. RSV
   [Ref. Harrison, 20/e, p 883]

   SARS (severe acute respiratory syndrome)
   - Caused by corona virus type IV
   - Identified in 2002
   - Bats and Civets are important animal reservoir
   - Droplet transmission with low mortality

   Middle east respiratory distress syndrome
   - Novel beta corona virus is the causative agents
   - Transmitted from camel through direct or indirect contact
   - Inefficient human to human transmission but carries high mortality.

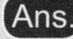 **Ans.**
1. a. Dengue virus
2. a. Picornavirus
3. b. Allantoic cavity
4. c. Retroviridae
5. b. Corona virus

6. **All enveloped helical RNA viruses belong to one large group, which includes all of the following except:**
   a. Influenza
   b. Parainfluenza
   c. Mumps
   d. Herpes
   [Ref. Ananthanarayana 10/e, p 502]

   Influenza, Para-influenza, mumps all belongs to myxovirus

7. **Antigenic shift:**
   a. Occurs every 2-3 years
   b. Gradual change over time
   c. Result from genetic recombination
   d. Occurs in all influenza viruses
   [Ref. Harrison, 20/e, p 1383]

   Antigenic shift occurs every 10–15 years, whereas antigenic drift occurs every 2–3 years in case of influenza A and every 4–7 years in case of influenza B.

8. **Hemagglutination done by all virus except:**
   a. Influenza
   b. Rubella
   c. Measles
   d. HPV
   [Ref. Ananthanarayan, 10/e p 437]

   Virus causing hemogglutination
   Influenza, Parainfluenza, Mumps, NDV, Measles, Togavirus, Rubella, Enterovirus, Cosacke & Echo, Rhinovirus, Rabies.

9. **Paramyxoviruses enters the body via:**
   a. Blood
   b. Respiratory virus
   c. Conjunctiva
   d. Fecal-oral route
   [Ref. Ananthanarayan, 10/e p 503]

10. **Virus which has more than one serotypes:**
    a. Measles
    b. Mumps
    c. Rubella
    d. Influenza
    [Ref. Ananthanarayan, 10/e p 504]

11. **Which influenzae strain, not of human origin and can cause pandemic:** [Ref. Park, 22/e, p 147]
    a. H_1N_1
    b. H_2N_2
    c. H_5N_1
    d. H_9N_1

    H_5N_1 (causative agent of avian influenzae) is a strain with pandemic potential. It has got extremely high mortality.

12. **True about influenza vaccine:** [Ref. Park, 22/e, p 146]
    a. Live vaccine is used most commonly
    b. Live vaccine is given by nasal drops
    c. Killed vaccine is given intramuscular in deltoid
    d. All are correct

13. **Not true about paramyxoviruses:**
    a. Belong to family myxoviridae
    b. Are DNA viruses
    c. Have linear nucleic acid
    d. Antigenically stable [Ref. Ananthanarayan, 10/e, p 512]

14. **Classic triad of congenital rubella includes all except:**
    a. Cataract
    b. Deafness
    c. Retinitis
    d. CHD
    [Ref. Ananthanarayan, 9/e, p 555]

    Classic triad of congenital rubella:
    • Cardiac cardiac defects
    • Cataract
    • Deafness

15. **Incubation period of measles is:**
    [Ref. Ananthanarayan, 10/e, p 518]
    a. 18-72 hours
    b. 10-14 days
    c. 3-4 days
    d. 20-25 days

16. **Forschheimer spot is seen in:** [Ref. Park, 22/e, p 142]
    a. Measles
    b. Chickenpox
    c. Erythema infectiosum
    d. Rubella

    Forschheimer spot are a fleeting exanthem seen as small, red spot (petechiae) on the soft palate in 20% of patients with rubella. They precede or accompany the skin rash of rubella. They are not pathognomonic to rubella as similar spots can be seen in measles and scarlet fever

17. **Which of the following can infect ovary:**
    a. Mumps virus
    b. EBV
    c. CMV
    d. Measles virus
    [Ref. Ananthanarayan, 10/e, p 514]

    Less common complications of mumps:
    Arthritis   Oophiritis   Nephritis
    Pancreatitis   Thyroiditis   Myocarditis

18. **Coxsackie virus is:**
    a. Herpes virus
    b. Pox virus
    c. Enterovirus
    d. Myxovirus
    [Ref. Ananthanarayan, 10/e, p 491]

    • Influenza resistance in society causes:
      – Antigenic drift: By mutation changes its hemagglutirin surface protein
      – Antigenic shift: By segmentation of genome and reassortment of protein
      – Extensive mammalian and avian reservoir.

19. **Herpangina is caused by:**
    a. Enterovirus
    b. Rhinoviruses
    c. Myxovirus
    d. Rabies virus
    [Ref. Ananthanarayan, 10/e, p 497]

    Herpangina is caused by Coxsackie virus group A which is a subtype of enterovirus.

Ans.
6. d. Herpes
7. c. Result from...
8. d. HPV
9. b. Respiratory...
10. d. Influenza
11. c. H_5N_1
12. d. All are correct
13. b. Are DNA viruses
14. c. Retinitis
15. b. 10-14 days
16. d. Rubella
17. a. Mumps virus
18. c. Enterovirus
19. a. Enterovirus

20. Suckling mice is used for isolation of:
    a. Coxsackie virus
    b. Pox
    c. Herpes
    d. Adeno Virus
    [Ref. Ananthanarayan, 10/e, p 498]

21. Hand-foot-mouth disease is caused by:
    a. Coxsackie - A virus
    b. Coxsackie - B virus
    c. EBV
    d. CMV
    [Ref. Ananthanarayan, 10/e p 497]

> Coxsackie virus A16 is the most common cause of HFMD. Enterovirus 71 (EV-71) is the second-most common cause.
> **Hand, foot and mouth disease (HFMD)**
> - Exanthematous fever affecting mainly young children, characterized by clusters of papulovesicular lesions on the skin and oral mucosa.

22. In which of the following virus is shed in stool:
    a. Herpangina
    b. Influenza
    c. Varicella
    d. Smallpox
    [Ref. Ananthanarayan 10/e, p 498]

> Herpangina (vesicular pharyngitis) is a common clinical manifestation of Coxsackie Group A infection in children. It is a severe febrile pharyngitis with headache, vomiting and pain in abdomen. Like all other enterovirus it also spreads through fecoral route.

23. Coxsackie group A commonly causes:
    a. Conjunctivitis
    b. Aseptic meningitis
    c. Hepatitis
    d. Myocarditis
    [Ref. Ananthanarayan 10/e, p 497]

24. False about Polio:
    a. Descending paralysis
    b. Bilateral symmetrical
    c. Non-progressive
    d. LMN type paralysis
    [Ref. Ananthanarayan, 10/e, p 492]

> **Paralysis in polio is asymmetric**
> - Depending on the distribution of paralysis cases are classified as spinal, bulbar or bulbospinal.

25. Diagnosis of polio:
    a. Detection of polio virus in stool
    b. Serology
    c. Limb wasting
    d. AFP
    [Ref. Ananthanarayan, 10/e, p 493]

> Isolation of virus in tissue culture is the best method for diagnosis. Virus can be isolation from blood (1-2 weeks after infection) from throat in early stages of disease, from feces in over 80% of cases in 1st week.

26. Epidemic hemorrhagic conjunctivitis is caused:
    a. HSV
    b. HZV
    c. HIV
    d. Picorna virus
    [Ref. Ananthanarayan, 10/e, p 499]

27. Which of the following is live attenuated vaccine:
    a. Salk polio vaccine
    b. Sabin polio vaccine
    c. Rabies vaccine
    d. KFD vaccine
    [Ref. Ananthanarayan, 10/e, p 496]

28. Most virulent dengue fever strain is:
    [Ref. Park 22/e, p 225]
    a. 1
    b. 2
    c. 3
    d. 4

29. Hemorrhagic fever is caused by:
    a. West-Mile fever
    b. Sandfly fever
    c. Ebola virus
    d. All of the above
    [Ref. Harrison, 20/e, p 1506,-1509]

30. Colorado Tic fever is caused by:
    a. Filoviridae
    b. Reoviridae
    c. Coronaviridae
    d. Calciviridae
    [Ref. Ananthanarayan, 10/e p 564]

> Colorado tick fever is caused by orbivirus which is one of the three genera of reoviridae: Reovirus, orbivirus and rotavirus

31. True about Nipah virus are all *except*:
    a. Is a paramyxovirus
    b. Causes hemorrhagic fever
    c. Emerging infection
    d. Present in India
    [Ref. Jawetz, 27/e p 594]

> **Nipah virus**
> - Zoonotic paramyxovirus that caused outbreaks of severe encephalitis (mortality rate >35%) in Malaysia during 1998.
> - Fruit bats are the natural host.
> **Note**: Hendra virus (an equine virus) is another emerging zoonotic paramyxovirus that caused many horse fatalities and few human fatalities in Australia.

20. a. Coxsachie...	21. a. Coxsackie - A virus	22. a. Herpangina	23. b. Aseptic...
24. b. Bilateral...	25. a. Detection...	26. d. Picorna ...	27. b. Sabin polio vaccine
28. b. 2	29. c. Ebola virus	30. b. Reoviridae	31. d. Present in India

32. **Diagnosis of Dengue fever can be made earlie by:**
    a. Viral culture
    b. NS-1 antigen detection
    c. IgG antibody detection
    d. Nucleic acid test   [Ref. Jawetz, 27/e p 553]

33. **In India, human infections have been reported dengue virus type:**
    a. Types 1 and 2
    b. Types 1 and 3
    c. Types 2 and 4
    d. Type 1 only
    e. All 4 types   [Ref. Park 22/e, p 225]

> In India type I and type II serotypes are common

34. **KFD is transmitted by:**
    a. Fleas   b. Mite
    c. Tick   d. Mosquito
    [Ref. Ananthanarayan, 10/e, p 530]

> KFD infection is transmitted by the bite of ticks, principal being Haemaphysalis spinigera.

35. **Rabies diagnosis is done best by:**
    a. Brain biopsy   b. Blood culture
    c. Electron microscopy   d. None
    [Ref. Harrison 20/e, p 1407]

> - Detection of rabies virus RNA by RT-PCR is highly sensitive and specific so is direct fluorescence antibody.
> - RT-PCR can be performed on fresh saliva, CSF, skin and brain tissues.
> - DFA require biopsy from brain or skin

36. **Ebola virus belongs to:** [Ref. Ananthanarayan, 10/e, p 562]
    a. Picornaviridae   b. Togaviridae
    c. Flaviviridae   d. Filoviridae

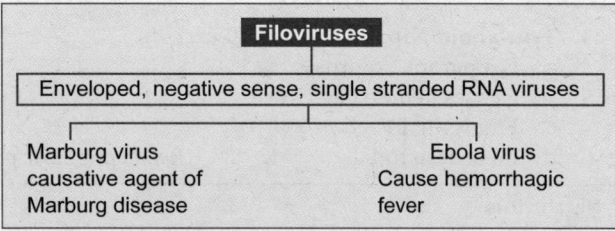

37. **Note true about Japanese encephalitis**
    a. Transmitted by culex mosquito
    b. Caused by group A arbovirus
    c. Pig is amplifier host
    d. Man is incidental host   [Ref. Park, 22/e, p 259]

38. **Appearance of cowdry type A inclusion bodies:**
    a. Granular   b. Circumscribed
    c. In polio   d. None
    [Ref. Ananthanarayan, 10/e, p 451]

> Cowdry classify intranuclear antibodies into two types:
> (a) Cowdry type A: Variable size and granular in appearance
> (b) Cowdry type B: More circumscribed and often multiple e.g. adenovirus and poliovirus

39. **True about rotavirus:**
    a. Is a DNA virus
    b. Has lipid envelop
    c. Older vaccine cause intussusception
    d. All are correct   [Ref. Ananthanarayan, 10/e, p 564]

40. **True about rotavirus vaccine:**
    a. Killed vaccine   [Ref. Greenwood, 18/e, p 565]
    b. Given subcutaneous
    c. Pentavalent vaccine
    d. Should be given before 5 years

41. **Human metapneumovirus is structurally similar to:**
    a. Influenza virus b. Respiratory syncytial virus
    c. Measles virus   d. Rubella virus
    [Ref. Ananthanarayan, 9/e, p 514]

42. **Virus lacking hemagglutinin and nuraminidase but have membrane fusion protein is:**
    a. RSV   b. CMV
    c. HSV   d. Ebestein Barr virs
    [Ref. Anantharayan 10/e, p 516]

> - RSV differs from other paramyxovirus in not possessing hemagglutinin activity and neurominidase activity. So it is non-hemolytic. Its nucleocapsid diameter is also less than that of other paramycovirus.

43. **All are cultivable virus *except*:**
    a. Rotavirus   b. Enterovirus
    c. ECHO virus   d. Coxsackie virus
    [Ref. Ananthanarayana 10/e, p 564]

> **Non-cultivable viruses:**
> - Rotavirus (certain strains can grow in tissue culture)
> - Norwalk virus
> - Mollauscum contagiosum.

44. **Which of the following is a RNA virus:**
    a. Herpes virus   b. Adenovirus
    c. Poxvirus   d. Picornavirus
    [Ref. Ananthanarayana 10/e, p 490]

Ans.
- 32. **d.** Nucleic acid test
- 33. **e.** All 4 types
- 34. **c.** Tick
- 35. **a.** Brain biopsy
- 36. **d.** Filoviridae
- 37. **b.** Caused …
- 38. **a.** Granular
- 39. **c.** Older vaccine…
- 40. **c.** Pentavalent vaccine
- 41. **b.** Respiratory syncytial virus
- 42. **a.** RSV
- 43. **a.** Rotavirus …
- 44. **d.** Picornavirus

CHAPTER 26

Slow Virus Disease

SLOW VIRUS INFECTIONS

They have the Following Characteristics:
- Incubation periods range from months to year.
- Course of illness lasting for months or years with remissions and exacerbations.
- Predilection for central nervous system.
- Absence of immune response or an immune response that does not arrest the disease but may actually contribute to pathogenesis.
- Genetic predisposition.
- Invariable fatal termination.

> **Remember:** MC prion disorder in humans is sporadic form of CJD.

Slow Virus Disease:
- Fatal
- Altered immune response
- Very long incubation period
- MC slow virus disease: CJD

CLASSIFICATION

I. Group A
- Slowly progressive infections of sheep caused by non-oncogenic retroviruses, lentiviruses
  - e.g. visna, maedi

II. Group B = Subacute Spongioform viral encephalopathies
- Comprise prion (infectious protein) diseases of the CNS, scarpie, mink encephalopathy, Kuru and CJD disease collectively known as the subacute spongiform viral emcephalopathies.
- These are chronic progressive degenerative diseases of CNS.
- Pathology consists of progressive vacuolation in the dendritic and axonal process of neurons and extensive astroglial hypertrophy and proliferations which leads to spongiform degeneration in the grey matter. There is no sign of any inflammation or immune response.
- Definitive diagnosis is made by brain biopsy. After biopsy all instruments should be destroyed

Visna: Demyelinating disease of sheep characterized by slow onset paresis that progress to coma

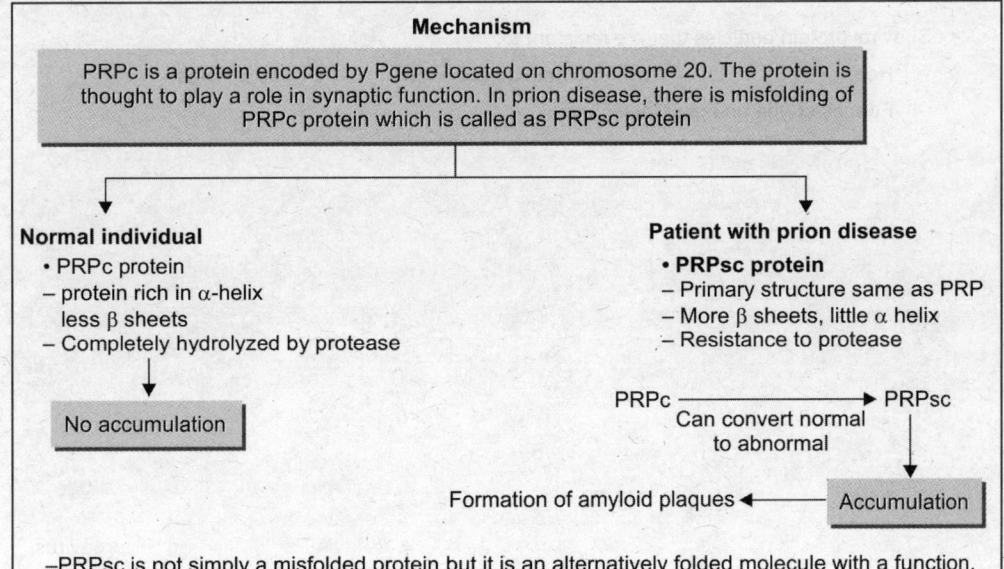

- Subacute sclerosing panencephalitis: Caused by Measles, rubella virus
- Progressive multifocal leukoencephalopathy: Caused by JC virus.

Disease	Etiology
Human	
a. Kuru (meaning tremor)	Infection through ritualistic cannibalism
b. Iatrogenic Creutzfeldt-Jakob disease (CJD)	Infection from prion contaminated human growth hormone, dura mater graft, corneal transplant
c. Variant (CJD)	Infection from bovine prion (Eating BSE infected beef)
d. Familial CJD	Germline mutation in PRNP
e. Sporadic CJD	Somatic mutation or spontaneous conversion of PRPc into PRPsc
f. Fatal familial insomania	Germline mutation in PRNP
g. Gertsmann-Straussler-Scheinker	Germline mutation in PRNP
Animal prion disease, e.g.	
a. Scrapie	
b. Mink encephalopathy	
c. Bovine spongiform encephalopathy (BSE, mad-cow disease).	

III. Group C

Includes two unrelated CNS disease

a. Subacute sclerosing panencephalitis (SSPE)
   - It is delayed sequel to infection with defective measles virus, characterized by slow progressive demyelination in CNS
   - Virus cannot be isolated in routine culture but only by co-cultivation of infected brain cells with susceptible cells of non-neural origin.
   - Antibody is regularly found in CSF and is **pathognomonic.**
   - *SSPE also seen in Rubella infection.*

b. Progressive multifocal leukoencephalopathy (PML)
   - Seen in elderly persons whose immune process is impaired by malignancy or HIV, etc.
   - Caused by JC virus (papovavirus).

   Remember: JC virus also causes Hodgkin's disease of brain.

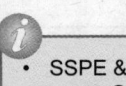

- SSPE & PML belongs to group C prion disease
- Kuru is transmitted due to cannibalism

Prions

- Subviral protein particles that are resistant to:
  - Heat
  - Ionizing and UV radiation
  - DNase & RNase
  - Formaldehyde and glutaraldehyde

Multiple Choice Questions

1. **Prions are:** [AI 08]
   a. Infectious proteins
   b. Made up of bacteria and virus particles
   c. Nuclear material
   d. Can be cultured in cell free media

2. **Prions consist of:** [AIIMS 07]
   a. DNA and RNA
   b. DNA, RNA and proteins
   c. RNA and proteins
   d. Only proteins

3. **True about Prion disease is all except:** [AIIMS 11]
   a. Myoclonus is seen in 10% of the patients
   b. Caused by infectious protein
   c. Brain biopsy is diagnostic
   d. Commonly manifests as dementia

4. **True about prion:** [AIIMS 08]
   a. Are virus coded
   b. Cause misfolding of protein
   c. Cleave protein
   d. Defect in synthesis of protein.

5. **Which of the following is correct about prions?** [AIIMS Nov 2012]
   a. Long incubation period
   b. Destroyed by autoclaving at 121°C
   c. Nucleic acid present
   d. Immunogenic

Explanations and References with Illustrative Answers

1. **Ans. (a) Infectious protein** *Ref. Jawetz 27/e, p 615*

   Prions are infectious protein devoid of nucleic acid.
   - Prions are usually resistant to standard means of inactivation. They are resistant to treatment with formaldehyde, urea, dry heat, boiling. However, they are sensitive to phenol, and autoclaving.
   - Prions infect and propagate by refolding abnormally into a structure which is able to convert normal molecule of protein into the abnormally structure form.
   - Common feature of all prions is conversion of a host encoded sialoglycoprotein into a protease resistant from which then accumulates.

   Various prion disease are as follows:

Kuru	Creutzfeldt-Jakob disease (CJD)
Fatal familial insomnia (FFI)	Gerstmann-Straussler-Scheinker disease (GSS)
Sporadic fatal insomnia (SFI)	Scrapie
Transmissible mink encephalopathy	Bovine spongiform encephalopathy (mad cow disease)
Chronic wasting disease	Feline spongiform encephalopathy
Exotic ungulate encephalopathy	

2. **Ans. (d) Only protein** *Ref. Jawetz 27/e, p 3*

   Already explained, refer Ans. 1

3. **Ans. (a) Myoclonus is seen in 10% of the patients** *Ref. Harrison 20/e, p 3151*
   - Most patients with **CJD** exhibit myoclonus that appears at various times throughout the illness.
   - Prion is proteinaceous infectious particle that lacks nucleic acid and causes slow progressing disease.
   - **MC** human prion disease is sporadic **CJD**.

- **Clinical Features of CJD**
  - Most patient present with deficits in higher cortical function which almost always progress to dementia.
  - 90% patient exhibit myoclonus which persist during sleep in comparison of other involuntary movements.
  - Also present with visual impairment or cerebellar gait, coordination deficit, extrapyramidal dysfunction, pyramidal signs, seizures.
- **Diagnosis**
  - Constellation of dementia, myoclonus and peirodic electrical burst in an afebrile 60 years old patient generally indicates CJD.
  - *Only specific diagnostic test for CJD is measurement of PRPsc*
  - In humans the diagnosis of CJD as established by brain biopsy if PRPsc is detected.
    - There is no abnoramlity on gross examination of brain.
    - Pathologic hallmarks are spongiforms degeneration (in cerebral cortex, putamen, etc.) and Astrocytic gliosis.
    - 10% of CJD patient have amyloid plaques.
  - Sequencing the PRNP gene.
  - CJ finding may be normal or show cortical atrophy.
  - CSF is nearly always normal but may show minimal protein elevation.

4. **Ans (b) Cause misfolding of protein**   *Ref. Greenwood 18/e, p 608, Ananthanarayan 10/e, p 560*
   - Prion is an infectious agent made up of protein. In the presence of prion protein, the normal PRPc protein is converted into an abnormally folded PRPsc protein (protein with more β sheets). ***This PRPc protein is resistant to proteolysis and get accumulated.*** The "alternatively folded" is a better term than misfolded, as the abnormal protein has got alternative function.

5. **Ans. (a) Long incubation period**   *Ref. Greenwood 18/e 607; Harrison 20/e, p 3148*

   Prion are infective proteins, that are resistant to inactivation by:
   - Heat
   - Ionizing radiation
   - DNAase & RNAase
   - Formaldehyde and glutaraldehyde

   Prion disease are characterized by absent immune reaction, long incubation period (*usually around 10 years*).

   Note: Creutzfeldt Jacob disease is the most common prion disease.

NEET Pattern Questions

1. **Which of the following infection agent lacks RNA?**
   a. Virus
   b. Staphylococci
   c. Prions
   d. Cryptococcus
   [Ref. Ananthanarayan, 10/e, p 448]

   > Human prion disease are: CJD, Kuru, Gerstmann- Scheinker (GSS) syndrome, Fatal familial insomnia, Sporadic fatal insomnia

2. **All of the following are prion disease** *except*:
   a. KJD
   b. Subacute spongiform encephalothies
   c. Mink Encephalopathy
   d. Burkitt lymphoma [Ref. Ananthanarayan, 10/e, p 561]

3. **Which prion disease affect human?**
   a. Scrapie
   b. Madcow disease
   c. Kuru
   d. Bovine spongiform encephalopathy
   [Ref. Ananthanarayan, 10/e, p 561]

4. **Which of the following is infectious protein?**
   a. Avidin
   b. Prion
   c. Tau protein
   d. None
   [Ref. Ananthanarayan, 10/e, p 561]

Ans.
1. c. Prions
2. d. Burkitt lymphoma
3. c. Kuru
4. b. Prion

Hepatitis Virus

CHAPTER 27

> **HAV:** Picorna
> **HBV:** Hepadna
> **HCV:** Flavivirus
> **HDV:** Defective
> **HEV:** Calcivirus

Comparative Features of Viral Hepatitis

Feature	HAV	HBV	HCV	HDV	HEV
Family	Picornavirus	Hepadnavirus	Flavivirus	Defective virus	Calcivirus/Alphavirus
Incubation (days)	15-45, mean 40	30-180, mean 60-90	15-160, mean 50	90-180 mean 60-90	14-60,
Onset	Acute	Insidious or acute	Insidious	Insidious or acute	Acute
Transmission					
Fecal-oral	+++	–	–	–	+++
Percutaneous	Unusual	+++	+++	+++	–
Perinatal	–	+++	±	+	–
Sexual	±	++	±	++	–
Clinical					
Severity	Mild	Occasionally severe	Moderate	Occasionally severe	Mild
Fulminant	0.1%	0.1-1%	0.1%	5-20%	1-2%
Progression to chronicity	None	Occasional (1-10%) (90% of neonates)	Common	Common	None
Carrier	None	0.1-30%	1.5-3.2%	Variable	None
Cancer	None	+	+	±	None
Prognosis	Excellent	Worse with age, debility	Moderate	Acute: good Chronic: poor	Good
Prophylaxis	IG Inactivated vaccine	HBIG Recombinant vaccine	None	HBV vaccine None for HBV carriers	Unknown
Therapy	None	Interferon Lamivudine Adefovir	Pegylated interferon plus ribavirin	Interferon ±	None

Other virus causing sporadic hepa,titis

• CMV	• EBV
• HSV	• Rubella virus
• Enterovirus	

Note: Morphologic lesion of all types of viral hepatitis are similar and consist of panlobular infiltration with mononuclear cells, hepatic cell necrosis, kupter cell hyperplasia, cholestatis Liver cell damage consist of hepatic cell degeneration, ballooning of cells, acidophilic degeneration of hepatocytes (forming *councilman or apoptic bodies*).

HEPATITIS A

- *Non-enveloped ssRNA virus* belonging to picorna family.
- Originally called as enterovirus 72.
- Resistant to ether, acid and heat but sensitive to chlorination, boiling for 1 minute, radiation.
- Virion contain four capsid polypeptide designated VP1 to VP4.
- *Only* hepatitis virus that can be cultivated *in vitro*.
- MC cause of acute hepatitis in children.
- *Only* viral hepatitis which can cause spiky fever.
- As the age increases chances of jaundice increases

> **Hepatitis A**
> - Non-enveloped ssRNA virus
> - Over all MC cause of hepatitis
> - Transmitted by feco-oral route
> - Grows only in cells of primate origin

Pathology
- Replication of virus is limited to liver only. But the virus is present in liver, bile, stool and blood during the late incubation period.

Diagnosis
Detection of *IgM anti-HAV* antibody during late incubation period which reaches peak level in *2-3 weeks*.

Treatment
Symptomatic no specific antiviral drug is given.

Prevention
- *Formalin inactivated tissue culture vaccine* is effective.
- Given IM, two doses at 6 month interval
- Vaccine should be given in age > 2 years.
- Provides immunity after 4 weeks of vaccination.
- Immunity last for approx 20 years.

HEPATITIS B (SERUM HEPATITIS)

Most widespread and important type of hepatitis virus.
- *Ds DNA virus belonging to hepadnaviruses family.* Classified as hepa DNA virus type 1.
- *Transmitted parenterally* (sex > perinatal > blood transfusion). Virus is stable and capable of surviving for days on environmental surface. It can be destroyed by sodium hypochlorite or autoclaving.

> DNA polymerase of HBV has both DNA dependent DNA polymerase and RNA dependent reverse transcriptase activities

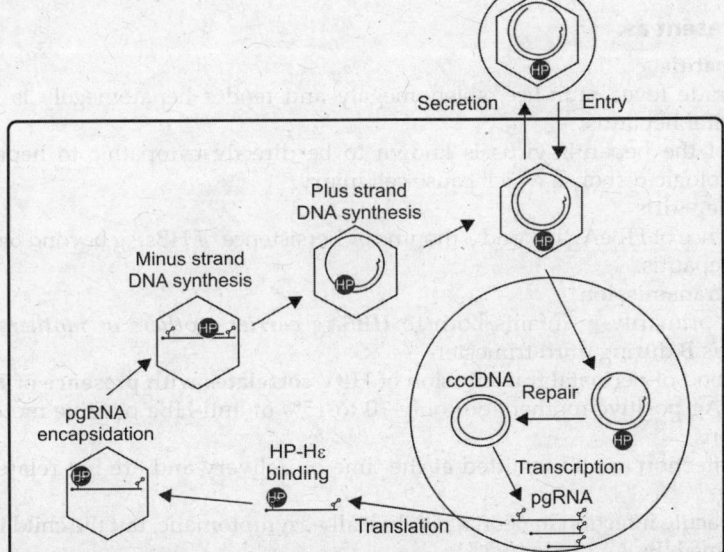

Instead of direct DNA replication, HBV relies on reverse transcription of minus strand DNA from pregenomic RNA intermediate. The plus strand DNA is transcribed from minus strand.

Viral Proteins and Particles

Three particulate form can be seen by electron microscopy:
1. 22 nm spherical or filament form (**MC**). Represent *excess viral envelop protein*.
2. 42 nm double shelled spherical particles. Represent intact HBV virion. (*dane particle*)
3. Smaller spherical or tubular particle. Represent hepatitis B surface antigen (**HBS Ag = Australia Antigen**).

Hepatitis B antigens
- HBeAg: Signal peptide that binds to smooth endoplasmic reticulum
  - Secreted in circulation.

- HBcAg: Lacks signal peptide
  - Not secreted.
- HBsAg: Envelop protein expressed on outer surface of the virion.

HBV Genes and Gene Products

Genes	Regions	Gene products
S	S	Major protein (S)
	S + Pre-S2	Middle protein (M) HBs Ag
	S + Pre-S1 and S2	Large protein (L)
C	C	HbcAg
	C + Pre-C	HbeAg
P (Largest gene)		DNA polymerase
X		**HBx Ag (contributes to carcinogenesis)**

Mutants of HBV

Two types of mutant are found:
- *Hbe Ag Negative phenotype (MC mutant):* Results in severe chronic infection with detectable HBV DNA and anti-HBe Ag but HBe Ag is not detectable.
- *Escape mutant:* Due to change in HBs Ag. Vaccine is not effective against them.

Pathogenesis and Clinical Features

- Cellular immunity plays major role in the pathogenesis.
- HBcAg and HBeAg are the viral target antigen that invites cytotoxic T-cells to destroy HBV infected hepatocytes.

Clinically present as:

1. **Acute hepatitis**
   - Low grade fever, jaundice, splenomegaly and tender hepatomegaly is found in all acute viral hepatitis.
   - None of the hepatitis virus is known to be directly cytopathic to hepatocyte, it is immunologic response which cause cell injury.
2. **Chronic hepatitis**
   - Persistence of HBeAg beyond 3 months or Persistence of HBsAg beyond 6 months after acute hepatitis.
3. **Perinatal transmission**
   - Occurs primarily in infants born to *HBSAg carrier mothers or mothers with acute hepatitis B* during third trimester.
   - Likelihood of perinatal transmission of HBV **correlates with presence of HBeAg;** 90% of HBeAg positive mothers but only 10 to 15% of anti-HBe positive mother transmit infection.
   - Most infection are transmitted at the time of delivery and are not related to breast-feeding.
   - Mostly acute infection in neonate is clinically asymptomatic, but the child is very likely to become HBs Ag carrier (90%).
4. **Extrahepatic manifestation of HBV**
   - Serum sickness like syndrome
   - Glomerulonephritis
   - Polyarteritis nodosa
   - Essential mixed cryoglobulinemia.
5. **Carrier stage**
   - Carriers is more common in patients of:
     - Down's syndrome   – Leukemia
     - Polyarteritis nodosa   – I.V. drug users
     - Lepromatous leprosy   – Hodgkin's disease
     - Chronic renal disease
   - *Carriers of HBs Ag particularly those infected in infancy have high-risk of hepatocellular Ca.*

Hepatitis B
- Ds DNA virus
- Transmitted parenterally, sexually, vertically
- First virological marker detectable: HBsAg
- Diagnostic marker of acute hepatitis B: IgM anti HBC
- Marker of Infectivity: HBe Ag

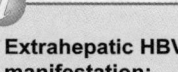

Extrahepatic HBV manifestation:
- Serum sickness
- Glomerulonephritis
- Polyarteritis nodosa
- Cryoglobulinemia

Serology and Diagnosis

A. Serology
- *First virologic marker* detectable is HBsAg.
- **Diagnostic** *marker* of *acute* hepatitis B infection IgM anti-HBc.
- HBcAg is sequestered in HBsAg coat so, it is not routinely detectable.
- Diagnosis in window period is made by AntiHBc.
- **Marker of infectivity - HBe Ag**
- *Titre of HBsAg bears inverse relationship with the degree of cell damage, i.e. titer is very low in acute fulminant hepatitis.*

Carrier stage in HBV
- **Simple carriers**
  – HBs Ag +
  – HBV DNA –
  – Anti HBe –
- **Super carriers**
  – HBs Ag +
  – HBV DNA +
  – HBe Ag +
- **Super carriers are highly infective**

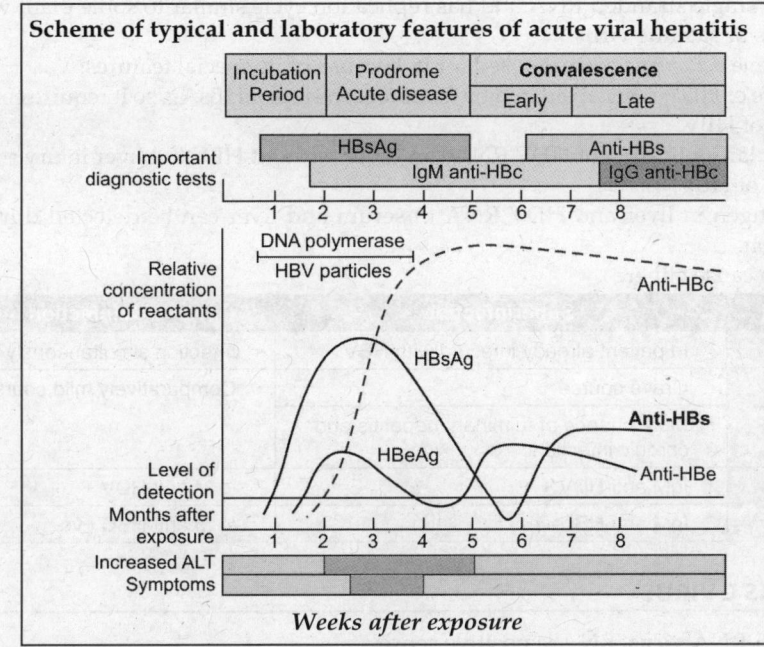

- **Markers of replicative phase:**
  – HBeA   : *Qualitative marker.*
  – HBV DNA   : *Quantitative marker.*
- **Anti-HBSAg**
  – *Protective antibody*
  – Anti-HBSAg without anti-HBc **signifies vaccination.**
  – Anti-HBSAg in presence of IgG anti-HBc signifies recovery of infection.

B. *Liver function test* (done in all case of acute hepatitis).
- ↑ ALT and AST (Level does not correlate with degree of cell damage).
- ↑ Bilirubin
- PT — **Prolonged value** signify hepatocellular necrosis and indicate bad prognosis.

- Quantitative marker of replication: HBV DNA
- HBV vaccine: Non-glycosylated HBs Ag particles with alum as adjuvant

Treatment
- Acute – Antiviral therapy is not used usually.
- In severe acute hepatitis B — Treatment with nucleoside analogue such as lamivudin can be given.

Under ordinary circumstances none of the hepatovirus is known to be directly cytopathic to hepatocytes.

Prevention
- **Genetically engineered vaccine** from yeast consisting of nonglycosylated HBsAg particles.
  Dose: – 3 IM dose (in deltoid not in gluteal)
        – Injections are recommended at 0, 1 and 6 months.
        – *Pregnancy is not contraindication to vaccine.*
- *Postexposure prophylaxis*: Combination of HBIG and hepatitis B vaccine simultaneously at different sites.

- **Perinatal exposure:**
  - Single dose of HBIG 0.5 ml IM at birth followed by complete 3 dose of hepatitis B vaccine.
  - First dose of vaccine should be given within 12 hours of life.

Remember: As hepatitis B can lead to hepatocellular carcinoma, vaccination makes **HCC the only human cancer which is vaccine preventable.**

HEPATITIS D VIRUS = DELTA VIRUS

Hepatitis D
- Defective delta virus
- ssRNA virus
- Can cause both superinfection, coinfection.

Defective virus that require helper function of HBV for its replication.
- Contains single stranded RNA and has replication cycle similar to some plant virus such as viroids or satellite virus.
- A new gene *deltavirus* has proposed for it, because of its special features.
- Delta core of HDV is encapsidated by an outer envelop of HBsAg, so it require cooperative function of HBV.
- Intracellular replication of HDV RNA can occur without HBV but liver injury require the presence of HBV.
- HDV antigen in liver and HDV RNA in serum and liver can be detected during HDV replication.
- HDV can cause either:

Features	Superinfection	Coinfection
Definition	• In patient already infected with HBV	• Infection simultaneously with HBV
Course	• Grave course	• Comparatively mild course
	• More chance of fulminant hepatitis and chronic infection	
Serology	IgM anti-HDV +	Ig M anti-HDV +
	IgM anti-HBc–ve	Ig M anti-HBC +ve

HEPATITIS C VIRUS

- Linear **SS RNA virus.** RNA is positive sense.
- Belongs to gene hepacivirus of family flavivirus.
- **MC virus** associated with transfusion related hepatitis.
- **Cause fatty change in liver.**
- HCV is associated with *Cryoglobulinemia; porphyria cutanea tarda; Idiopathic pulmonary fibrosis; membrane proliferative glomerulonephritis.*

Genome

- Envelope protein coded by hypervariable region varies from isolate-to-isolate and allow the virus to invade host immunity.
- Because of divergence of HCV isolates within a genotype or subtype and within the same host, these intragenotypic differences are referred to *as* quasispecies.
- As HCV replicate via RNA dependent RNA polymerase which does not require DNA intermediate, so HCV never integrate with host genome.
- HCV entry into hepatocyte occur via CD-81 receptor.

Presence of anti HCV in serum without HCV RNA signifies recovery from HCV infection.
...CMDT 2014, p 650

Serology and Diagnosis

- Assays of **HCV RNA** are the most sensitive test for HCV infection and represent the *gold standard for diagnosis* of hepatitis C (*HCV RNA detection has supplanted RIBA in most clinical settings*).
- Two types of Amplification techniques can be used to detect HCV RNA.
  - *Branched chain complementary DNA (b DNA) assay.*
  - *Reverse transcriptase PCR or TMA:* It is more sensitive than b DNA assay.
- Anti-HCV antibody are not be detectable in acute phase and are not sensitive.
- **Anti-HCV are** not protective so chance of chronicity is very high.

Treatment

- In typical case of hepatitis C recovery is rare; *progression to chronic hepatitis is the rule.*
- Antiviral therapy with interferon alpha reduce the rate of chronicity.
- *Duration of infection* is the single most important variable which determine interferon responsiveness.

CHRONIC HEPATITIS C

Clinical features:
- *Fatigue* is *MC* symptom jaundice is rare.
- Extrahepatic manifestations may be seen.

Lab features:
- Aminotransferase fluctuate between high-to-high normal value.
- Both ALT and AST increase with ALT > AST.
- But when cirrhosis develop AST becomes greater than ALT
- **LKM1 - Antibody may be seen in cases of HCV.**

Treatment:
- Combination therapy of pegylated interferon plus Ribavirin is now standard therapy.
- **Liver transplantation -** When cirrhosis develops.

> **Remember:**
> - Progression of liver disease is more likely in patients older age, longer duration of infection, advanced histologic stage and grade, HIV infection and obesity, increased hepatic iron.
> - Chronic hepatitis C is MC indication of liver transplantation.
> - Best prognostic indicator in chronic hepatitis C is liver histology.
>
> .... Harrison, 19/e, p 2041

> **Hepatitis C**
> - ssRNA virus belong to flavi virus family
> - MC cause of transfusion hepatitis
> - HCV RNA assay are the most sensitive test for diagnosis (RT PCR and b DNA assay)

HEPATITIS E VIRUS

- Epidemic *hepatitis or enterically transmitted non-A, non-B hepatitis.*
- Non-enveloped *SS RNA* virus belonging to Hepeviridae family.   ..... *Jawetz, 27/e, p 498*
- Hepatitis of hepatitis *E. virus* is characteristically *associated with cholestasis.*
- *Most important* **cause of fulminant hepatitis in pregnancy.**
- In India it is the most common form of acute hepatitis of **adults (Overall most common is Hepatitis A).**

> Hepatitis E: ssRNA virus causing fulminant hepatitis in pregnant female

HEPATITIS G VIRUS

- Blood-borne RNA virus.

| Important points about chronic hepatitis ||||
Type of hepatitis	Diagnostic test (s)	Autoantibodies	Treatment
Chronic hepatitis B	HBsAg, IgG anti-HBc, HBeAg, HBV DNA	Uncommon	IFN-α, lamivudine
Chronic hepatitis C	Anti-HCV, HCV RNA	Anti-LKMI	PEG-IFN-α Plus ribavirin
Chronic hepatitis D	Anti-HDV, HDV RNA, HBsAg, IgG anti-HBc	Anti-LKM3	IFN-α

- **Other viral infections associated with hepatitis**
    - CMV
    - HSV
    - VZV
    - Measles
    - EBV
    - Lassa fever
    - Yellow fever
    - Marburg
    - Coxsackie virus
    - Enterovirus

> Hepatitis G: Blood borne RNA virus

Multiple Choice Questions

Hepatitis A

1. Which of the following hepatitis virus is cultivable:
   a. Hepatitis A   b. Hepatitis B   [AIIMS 07]
   c. Hepatitis D   d. Hepatitis E

Hepatitis B and D

2. Australia antigen in hepatitis B virus refers to:
   [NEET Pattern 2018]
   a. HBsAg   b. HBcAg
   c. HBeAg   d. HBnAg

3. Serology of a young man shows HBsAg, however HBeAg is negative with normal levels of AST and ALT. He is asymptomatic. What is the next line of management?
   a. Wait and watch   [AI 08]
   b. Antivirus
   c. Immunoglobulins
   d. Liver transplant

4. Which of the following hepatitis virus have significant perinatal transmission?   [AI 12]
   a. HEV   b. HCV
   c. HBV   d. HAV

5. The replication cycle of a virus is depicted below. Identify the virus?   [AIIMS 2017]

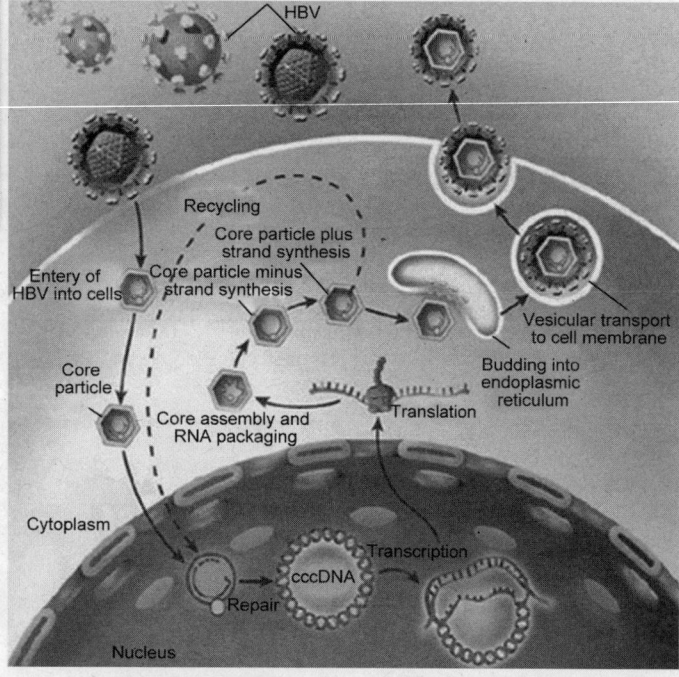

   a. Herpes simplex virus   b. Hepatitis B virus
   c. HIV   d. Influenza virus

6. Marker for acute hepatitis B is: [AIIMS 07]
   a. HBV DNA polymerase
   b. IgG anti HBc
   c. Core antigen (HbcAg)
   d. Anti-HbsAg

7. In a patient of active chronic hepatitis B all are seen except: [AIIMS 07]
   a. HbsAg
   b. IgM anti-HBcAg
   c. HbeAg
   d. Anti-HbsAg

8. A 30-years-old patient presented with history of jaundice for 10 days. His liver function tests showed bilirubin of 10 mg/dl, SGOT/SGPT - 1100/1450, serum alkaline phosphatase–240 IU. He was positive for HbsAg. What should be the confirmatory test to establish acute hepatitis B infection?
   a. IgM Anti-HBc antibody   [AIIMS 06]
   b. HbeAg
   c. HBV DNA by PCR
   d. Anti-HBc antibody

9. A 30-years-old lady delivered a healthy baby at 37 weeks of gestation. She was a known case of chronic hepatitis B infection. She was positive for HBsAg but negative for HBeAg. Which of the following is the most appropriate treatment for the baby?   [AIIMS 05]
   a. Both active and passive immunization soon after birth
   b. Passive immunization soon after birth and active immunization at 1 year of age
   c. Only passive immunization soon after birth
   d. Only active immunization soon after birth

10. A 30-years man presented with nausea, fever and jaundice of 5 days duration. The biochemical tests revealed a bilirubin of 6.7 mg/dl (conjugated 5.0 mg/dl) with SGOT/SGPT (AST/ALT) of 1230/900 IU/ml. The serological tests showed presence of HBs Ag IgM anti-HBc and HBeAg. The most likely diagnosis: [AIIMS-05]
    a. Chronic hepatitis B infection with high infectivity
    b. Acute hepatitis B infection with high infectivity
    c. Chronic hepatitis B infection with low infectivity
    d. Acute hepatitis B infection with low infectivity

11. Which of the following hepatitis virus is a DNA virus?
    [PGI 09]
    a. Hepatitis C virus   b. Hepatitis B virus
    c. Delta agent   d. Hepatitis E virus

12. Acute hepatitis B can be earliest diagnosed by:
    [AIIMS 18]
    a. IgM anti-HBcab   b. HBsAg
    c. IgG anti-HBcAb   d. Anti-HBsAb

13. If a patient was immunized with hepatitis B vaccine, which of the following is seen in serum? [PGI 06]
    a. HBeAg
    b. HBsAg
    c. Anti-HBs antibody
    d. Anti-HBe antibody
    e. Anti-HBc antibody

14. Which of these is not a marker of active replicative phase of chronic hepatitis B? [AIIMS 08]
    a. HBV DNA
    b. HBV DNA polymerase
    c. Anti-HBC
    d. AST and ALT

15. About hepatitis B, false statement is: [AIIMS 10, 12]
    a. Vertical transmission is more important than horizontal
    b. Communicable period lasts for months
    c. Virus can be found in blood 1 month before jaundice
    d. Age of onset determines the prognosis

16. Reverse transcriptase is a RNA dependent DNA polymerase. Which of the following use it? [AIIMS 16]
    a. Hepatitis A virus
    b. Hepatitis B virus
    c. Hepatitis E virus
    d. Hepatitis C virus

17. Cryoglobulinemia is seen in infection with which hepatitis virus: [NEET Pattern 2018]
    a. HAV   b. HBV
    c. HCV   d. HDV

Hepatitis C

18. Chronic liver disease is caused by: [AIIMS 08]
    a. Hepatitis B
    b. Hepatitis A
    c. Hepatitis C
    d. Hepatitis E

19. Hepatitis C virus true finding is: [AIIMS 10]
    a. Spreads along feco-oral route
    b. Antibody to HCV may not be seen in acute stage
    c. Does not cause chronic hepatitis
    d. It cannot be cultured

20. HCV is: [PGI 05]
    a. Enveloped RNA virus
    b. Unenveloped RNA virus
    c. Unenveloped positive strand RNA
    d. Unenveloped negative strand RNA
    e. DNA virus

Hepatitis E

21. A young pregnant woman presents with fulminant hepatic failure. The most likely etiological agent is:
    a. Hepatitis B virus
    b. Hepatitis C virus [AI 04]
    c. Hepatitis E virus
    d. Hepatitis A virus

22. With which of the following of viral hepatitis infection in pregnancy, the maternal mortality the highest: [AIIMS 06]
    a. Hepatitis A
    b. Hepatitis B
    c. Hepatitis C
    d. Hepatitis E

23. Which of the following is calcivirus? [PGI 09]
    a. HEV
    b. HBV
    c. HCV
    d. HAV

24. Hepatitis virus without envelope: [AIIMS 2018]
    a. HAV   b. HBV
    c. HCV   d. HDV

Explanations and References with Illustrative Answers

1. **Ans. (a) Hepatitis A** *Ref. Ananthanarayan 10/e, p 545*

   HAV can be grown in some human and simian cell cultures and is the only human hepatitis virus which can be cultured easily in vitro. It has also been cloned.

   > **Remember:**
   > - HAV is the hepatitis virus
   >   – That causes spiky fever
   >   – Show no perinatal transmission
   > The risk of transmitting HAV is greatest from 2 weeks before to 1 week after the onset of Jaundice.

2. **Ans. (a) HBsAg** *Ref. Ananthanarayan 10/e, p 547*

   Structure of hepatitis B virus

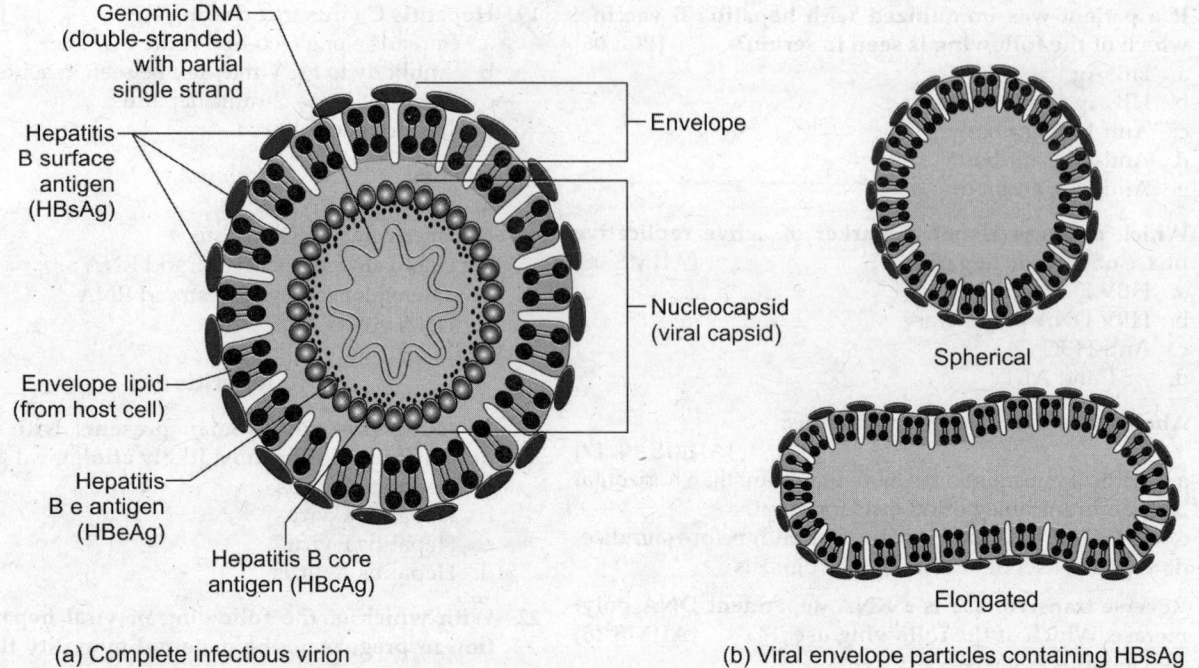

(a) Complete infectious virion   (b) Viral envelope particles containing HBsAg

Note: HBsAg is called Australia antigen because it was first identified in the serum of an a individual named Aboriginal Australian.

3. **Ans. (a) Wait and watch**   *Ref. Harrison 20/e, p 2363*
   - In hepatitis B, among previously healthy adult who present with clinically apparent acute hepatitis recovery occurs in 99% therefore, antiviral therapy is not likely to improve the rate of recovery and is not required.
   - In this case also patient is virtually asymptomatic, so no treatment is required.

   Note: In rare instance of severe acute hepatitis treatment is done with nucleoside analogue (entecavir, tenofovir) at oral dose.

4. **Ans. (c) HBV**   *Ref. Harrison 20/e, p 2355*

Perinatal transmission of various hepatitis virus					
HAV	HBV	HCV	HDV	HEV	Hepatitis G
–	+++	+/–	+	–	++

Transmission	
Parenterally	**Feco-oral**
Hepatitis B	Hepatitis A
Hepatitis C	Hepatitis E
Hepatitis D	
Hepatitis G	

- **HBV is *MC* hepatitis virus that is transmitted perinatally.**
- *Most important* **factor** that determine perinatal transmission is HBeAg (risk 90%).
- *MC* **time** of perinatal transmission is at the **time of delivery**.
- *MC* **presentation** in neonate is asymptomatic **HBsAg carrier.**
- *Most effective* **treatment** of neonatal infection is HBIg immediately after delivery followed by complete 3 dose immunization by HBsAg vaccine. First dose within first 12 hours of life.

5. **Ans. (b) Hepatitis B virus**   *Ref: Harrison 20/e, p 2346*
   Life cycle of Hepatitis B virus

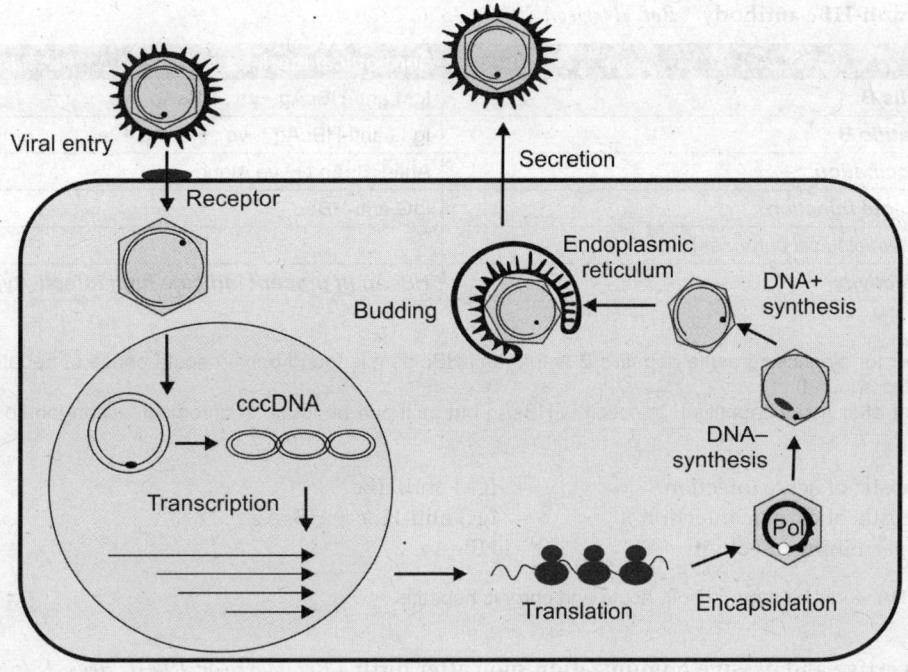

6. **Ans. (a) HBV DNA polymerase** *Ref. Jawetz 27/e p 503*
   - DNA polymerase activity, HBV DNA and HBeAg which are representative of viremic stage of hepatitis B, appears early in the incubation period, concurrently or shortly after the first appearance of HBsAg.
   - Thus, from these lines it is clear that DNA polymerase is a marker of HBV infection. However, it is elevated in both acute and chronic active hepatitis. As there is no other correct option, this can be taken as correct.

   DNA polymerase of HBV has two activities:
   - DNA dependent DNA polymerase.
   - RNA dependent Reverse transcriptase.

   Note: Hepatitis core antigen never appears in serum as it remain inside hepatocyte (intrahepatic)

7. **Ans. (b) IgM anti-HBcAg** *Ref. Harrison 19/e, p 2032, 20/e, p 2350*

   IgM anti-HBcAg is seen in acute hepatitis not in chronic active.

   Marker of chronic active hepatitis: HBsAg+, IgG anti-HBcAg, HBV DNA+, HBeAg+
   There is confusion in *option d* (Anti-HbsAg) also:

   Harrison 17/e, p 1943 writes: – 10-20% of person with chronic HBV infection may harbor low level Anti-HBs. This antibody is not directed against common variant a, but against heterotopic subtype determinant.

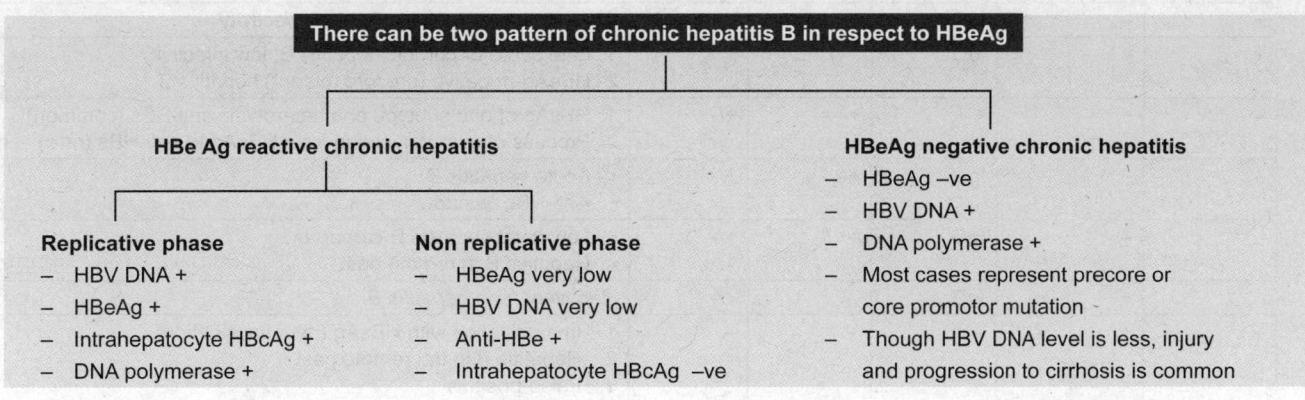

8. **Ans. (a) IgM anti-HBc antibody** *Ref. Harrison 20/e, p 2350, 2360*

Types	Serological markers of HBV
Acute hepatitis B	IgM anti-HBcAg +ve ; HBsAg +ve
Chronic hepatitis B	Ig G anti-HBcAg +ve ; HBsAg +ve
Marker of vaccination	Anti-HBsAg (+) ve Alone
Marker of remote infection	IgG anti-HBc
(Used for epidemiological purposes)	
Marker of infectivity	HBeAg **(If present indicate high infectivity)**

Remember:
- Best marker for diagnosing acute hepatitis B is IgM anti-HBc as it is found only in acute phase of hepatitis B (In chronic hepatitis IgG anti-HBc is found).
- First marker after acute hepatitis B infection is HBsAg but as it can be found in chronic infection too so, it is not reliable of acute infection.

- Test diagnostic of acute infection   – IgM anti-HBc
- Test diagnostic of chronic infection   – IgG anti-HBc + HBsAg
- Test for determining infectivity   – HBeAg.

Note: HBV DNA would be there in both acute and chronic hepatitis

9. **Ans. (a) Both active and passive immunization soon after birth** *Ref. Harrison 19/e, p 2013, 18/e, p 2547*

   Perinatal Transmission of Hepatitis B
   - Likelyhood of perinatal transmission of HBV *correlates* with **presence of HBeAg.** 90% of HBeAg +ve and only 10-15% of anti-HBe +ve mother transmit infection.
   - Most infection are transmitted at the time of delivery.
   - Acute infection in neonate is clinically asymptomatic but the child is likely to become HBsAg carrier and have *high risk of developing hepatocellular carcinoma.*

   Treatment of perinatal exposure:
   – *For all infant born to HBsAg positive mother:*
   – *A single dose of HBIG* should be given intramuscularly in thigh *soon after birth.*
   – Followed by complete course of three injections of recombinant *hepatitis B vaccine* with first dose *to be given with in the first 12 hour of life.*
   – Subsequent dose of active immunization should be given after 1 month and 6 months.

10. **Ans. (b) Acute hepatitis B infection with high infectivity** *Ref. Harrison 20/e, p 2360*

    See the following table, **Do not try to learn it, just try to understand.**

Commonly Encountered Serologic Patterns of Hepatitis B Infection					
HBsAg	**Anti-HBs**	**Anti-HBc**	**HBeAg**	**Anti-HBe**	**Interpretation**
+	–	IgM	+	–	Acute hepatitis B, high infectivity
+	–	IgG	+	–	Chronic active Hepatitis B, high infectivity
+	–	IgG	–	+	1. Late acute or chronic hepatitis B, low infectivity 2. HBeAg-negative (precore mutant) hepatitis B
+	+	+	+/–	+/–	1. HBsAg of one subtype and heterotypic anti-HBs (common) 2. Process of seroconversion from HBsAg to anti-HBs (rare)
–	–	IgM	+/–	+/–	• Acute hepatitis B • Anti-HBc "window"
–	–	IgG	–	+/–	• Low-level hepatitis B carrier or • Hepatitis B in remote past
–	+	IgG	–	+/–	*Recovery from hepatitis B*
–	+	–	–	–	1. Immunization with HBsAg (after vaccination) 2. Hepatitis B in the remote past 3. False-positive

11. Ans. (b) Hepatitis B virus *Ref. Harrison 20/e, p 2347*

Virus	Morphology and genome	Family
HAV	Non-enveloped RNA SS+	**P**icorna virus
HBV	DNA	**H**epadna virus
HCV	Enveloped RNA SS+	**F**lavivirus
HDV	Enveloped RNA SS−	**D**efective virus
HEV	Nonenveloped RNA SS+	**H**epeviridae

+ = Positive strand   − = Negative strand

Mnemonic: **pH Fall Dangerous Hai**

12. Ans. (b) HBsAg *Ref. Harrison 20/e, p 2360, 2350*

Here question is about the earliest diagnostic marker, **which is no doubt HBsAg.**
- HBsAg in absence of IgM anti-HBc or IgG anti-HBc indicates early acute infection.

So, go with **HBsAg.**

> **Remember:**
> - Dignostic marker of Acute hepatitis B   – IgM anti-HBC
> - Earliest marker of Acute hepatitis B   – HBsAg.
> - Diagnosis of HBV infection is usually made by HBsAg (Australia antigen).
>   In cases where HBsAg is too low diagnosis can be established by the presence of IgM anti-HBc ...*Harrison 17/e, p 1942*

13. Ans. (c) Anti-HBs antibody *Ref. Harrison 20/e, p 2360*

Already explained see answer 10

14. Ans. (c) Anti-HBC *Ref. Jawetz 24/e, p 475, Harrison 20/e, p 2350*

Anti-HBC has no relation with viral replication
- HBV DNA, HBV DNA polymerase represent active viral replication
- Level of HBV DNA correlates well with the degree of liver injury as suggested by raised AST, ALT
- It is not compulsory in chronic active hepatitis that HBeAg is positive. Infact HBeAg negative chronic hepatitis B is more dangerous.

15. Ans. (a) Vertical transmission is more important than horizontal *Ref. CMDT 2014/e, p 646; Park 22/e, p 193*

Epidemiology of HBV
- Endemic throughout the world
- Based on the carrier stage, countries can be divided into three categories:
  a. *High Endemicity:*   (> 8%) Vertical transmission is more common
  b. *Intermediate Endemicity:* (2-8%) India belongs to this category. Vertical = Horizontal transmission
  c. *Low Endemicity:*   (<2%) European countries. Horizontal transmission is more common
- **Mode of transmission:** Inoculation of infected blood or blood products, sexual contacts, vertical (Mother to fetus). Overall greatest number of cases results from heterosexual transmission. In India blood transfusion related infections are equally common.
- **Period of communicability:** Virus is present in body secretions and blood during the incubation period (for a month before jaundice) and acute phase of disease.
- Period of communicability is usually several months (occasionally years in chronic carriers) or until disappearance of HBsAg.
- *Outome* of HBV infection is age dependent with chances of acute hepatitis is *directly proportional to age* and occurs in 1% of perinatal, 10% of early childhood and 30% of late (> 5 years age) HBV infection.
- Development of *chronic* HBV infection is *inversely related to age* and occurs in 95% of infants infected perinatally, 5-10% infected after 5 years of age.

> **Remember:** Period of infectivity for HAV: 2 weeks before and 1 week after the onset of jaundice.

16. Ans. (b) Hepatitis B virus

See below: DNA polymerase of HBV has both DNA-dependent DNA polymerase and RNA-dependent reverse transcriptase activities.

> **Note:** Instead of DNA replication directly from a DNA template, hepadnaviruses rely on reverse transcription (effected by the DNA polymerase) of minus-strand DNA from a "pregenomic" RNA intermediate. Then plus-strand DNA is transcribed from the minus strand DNA template by the DNA-dependent DNA polymerase and converted in the hepatocyte nucleus to a covalently closed circular DNA, which serves as a template for messenger RNA and pregenomic RNA.

17. Ans. (c) HCV   *Ref. Harrison 19/e, p 2354*

See, the following line.

"HCV is a pathogenic factor in cryoglobulinemia and membranoproliferative GN and may be related to lichen planus, Autoimmune thyroiditis; Lymphocytic sialadenitis; Idiopathic pulmonary fibrosis; Porphyria cutanea tarda; Monoclonal gammopathies and lymphoma, increase risk of Type II diabetes mellitus."....CMDT

Now *see Harrison 17/e, p 1963*

> **Remember:**
> - LKM 1 antibody – Hepatitis C
> - LKM 2 antibody – Drug induced hepatitis
> - LKM 3 antibody – Hepatitis D

Extrahepatic Manifestations of Viral hepatitis			
Hepatitis A	**Hepatitis B**	**Hepatitis C**	**Hepatitis E**
—	• Glomerulonephritis • Nephrotic syndrome • Polyarteritis nodosa	• Essential mixed cryoglobulinemia • Glomerulonephritis • Lichen planus • Thyroiditis • Sialedenitis • Porphyria cutanea tarda • Lymphoma	• Rare neurological manifestations

Essential mixed cryoglobulinemia is a immunological disorder characterized by arthritis, cutaneous vasculitis and occasionally glomerulonephritis. Disease is mediated by circulating immune complexes of more than one immunological class.

18. Ans. (c) Hepatitis C   *Ref. Harrison 20/e, p 2362*

Decreasing order of progression to chronicity

	HCV	> HDV	> HBV	> HAV = HEV
Frequency of Chronicity	70-80%	5-20%	1-10% 90% of neonates	None (0.1%)

> **Remember:**
> - HCV is MC cause of chronic hepatitis.
> - Chronic hepatitis C is MC indication of liver transplantation.

19. Ans. (b) Antibody to HCV may not be seen in acute stage   *Ref. Harrison, 20/e, p 2361; CMDT 2014 p 654*

Anti HCV can be detected is acute hepatitis during the initial phase of elevated aminotransferase activity. The antibody however may never become detectable in 5-10% of patients with acute hepatitis C; Level of anti HCV become undetectable after recovery (which is very rare).

- Assays for **HCV RNA** are most sensitive test for HCV infection and represent **gold standard** in diagnosis.

> **Note:** In chronic hepatitis C, anti HCV is detectable in > 95% of cases.

Other options
- Only hepatitis virus that can be cultured *in vitro* is HAV. But other hepatitis virus can be cloned in *E. coli*.
- In *option "d"* it is not clear whether they are asking culturability *in vitro* or *in vivo* (clonability) so, this option may be partially correct.
- HCV is transmitted parenterally.

20. **Ans. (a) Enveloped RNA virus** *Ref. Harrison 20e, p 2352*

    Hepatitis C virus
    - Enveloped virus belonging to hepacivirus family. Contains SSRNA genome which is positive sense
    - HCV genome contains a single, large open reading frame (CRF) gene that codes for a virus polyprotein of ~ 3000 aminoacids which is cleaved after translation to yield 10 viral proteins.

21. **Ans. (c) Hepatitis E virus** *Ref. Harrison 20/e, p 2353; COGDT 9/e, p 439, 18/e, p 2540*

    Hepatitis E Virus
    - Hepavirus of family hepeviridae
    - Infected patient secret virus in stool, bile
    - Transmitted fecoorally IP 5-7 weeks
    - Most case occur in young and middle aged adults
    - Unique feature is the clinical severity and high care fatality rate (20–60%) in pregnant female particularly in last trimester.
    - Carrier state is prevalent in pigs
    - HEV can be demonstrated by immune electron microscopy (IEM) in the bile and feces of patients.

    Learn the following characteristics:

HAV	Cause spiky fever
HBV	Only hepatitis virus which is DNA virus, may cause cytopathic effect
HCV	Cause fatty change
HDV	Defective virus
HEV	Cause fulminant hepatitis in pregnant woman; associated with cholestasis.

    Remember: HEV – ss RNA virus belonging to alpha virus family. Transmitted feco-orally.
    – Secondary person-to-person transmission is rare (C/F to other enteric born infection).

22. **Ans. (d) Hepatitis E** *Ref. Harrison 20/e, p 2353*

    MC cause of *fulminant hepatitis* in pregnancy - Hepatitis E.
    MC cause of *hepatic encephalopathy* in pregnancy is - Hepatitis E.

23. **Ans. (a) HEV** *Ref. Ananthanarayan, 9/e, p 550*

    According to *Ananthanarayan 9/e, p 550*
    "HEV has been classified in genus herpes virus under family caliciviridae."
    But according to *Harrison 18/e 2543*
    "HEV although resembling calicivirus is sufficiently distinct from any known agent to merit a new classification of its own as a unique genus; Hepevirus with in the family Hepeviridae."

24. **Ans. (a) HAV** *Ref. Harrison 19/e, p 2006, 18/e, p 2539*

    HAV is a nonenveloped ss RNA virus of picorna family

NEET Pattern Questions

1. **True about HCV include all *except*:**
   a. Highest rate of chronicity among all hepatitis viruses
   b. Can be cultured
   c. Diagnosed by detection of HCV RNA
   d. Transmitted through transfusion of infected food
   [Ref. Ananthanarayan, 10/e, p 553]

   > HCV virus can not be grown in culture, but has been cloned in E. coli.

2. **All of the following hepatitis virus can be transmitted through blood *except*:**
   a. Hepatitis B
   b. Hepatitis C
   c. Hepatitis D
   d. Hepatitis E   [Ref. Ananthanarayan, 10/e, p 555]

3. **Commonest causes of acute hepatitis in India:**
   a. Hepatitis B
   b. Hepatitis B + D
   c. Hepatitis C
   d. Hepatitis A   [Ref. Park 22/e, p 191]

4. **HBV and HDV false is:**
   a. Both can infect simultaneously
   b. HDV can cause more serious infection due to super infection
   c. HDV can not infect in absence of HBV
   d. Both are DNA virus   [Ananthanarayan, 10/e, p 553]

5. **Serological testing of a patient shows HBsAg, IgM HBc and HBeAg positive. The patient has:**
   a. Chronic hepatitis B with low infectivity
   b. Acute hepatitis B with high infectivity
   c. Chronic hepatitis B with high infectivity
   d. Acute on chronic hepatitis
   [Harrison, 20/e, p 2360]

6. **Hepatitis C virus is:**
   a. Togavirus   b. Flavivirus
   c. Filovirus   d. Retrovirus
   [Ananthanarayan, 9/e, p 549]

7. **Which is ssRNA unenveloped virus:**
   a. HBV   b. HEV
   c. HCV   d. None
   [Ananthanarayan, 10/e, p 554]

8. **HDV is:**
   a. SS RNA virus
   b. SS DNA virus
   c. DS RNA virus
   d. DS DNA virus   [Ananthanarayan, 10/e, p 553]

   > HDV is a defective SSRNA virus

9. **First antibody to appear in hepatitis:**
   a. IgM anti HBe
   b. IgM anti HBc
   c. IgG anti HBe
   d. IgM anti HBs   [Ananthanarayan, 10/e, p 2350]

10. **All cause viral hepatitis *except*:**
    a. Measles   b. EBV
    c. Rhinovirus   d. Reovirus
    [Ananthanarayan, 9/e, p 541, 560]

    > Reovirus have not been proved to cause any human disease.

11. **Best test to diagnose prodrome of Hepatitis A:**
    a. HAV in blood
    b. IgG anti-HAV
    c. IgM anti-HAV
    d. HAV in stool   [Harrison, 20/e, p 2347]

12. **Hepatitis E usually affects:**
    a. Children
    b. Adults
    c. Old age
    d. Toddlers   [Harrison, 20/e, p 2353, 2358]

    > In Asia most infections occur in young adults and are usually linked to genotype 1 and 2. In non-endemic areas genotype 3 and 4 are predominant and seen mainly in older males (>60 years).

13. **Which flavivirus causes hepatitis in human?**
    a. Hepatitis A
    b. Hepatitis B
    c. Hepatitis C
    d. Hepatitis D   [Jawetz, 27/e, p 496]

14. **E antigen (HBeAg) of hepatitis B virus is a product of which gene?**   [Ananthanarayan, 10/e, p 548]
    a. S   b. C
    c. P   d. X

1. b. Can be cultured	2. d. Hepatitis E	3. d. Hepatitis A	4. d. Both are DNA virus	5. b. Acute hepatitis B
6. b. Flavivirus	7. b. HEV	8. a. SS RNA virus	9. b. IgM anti HBc	10. d. Reovirus
11. c. IgM anti-HAV	12. b. Adults	13. c. Hepatitis C	14. b. C	

15. DNA polymerase of HBV is encoded by which of the following?
    a. S gene b. C gene
    c. P gene d. X gene
    [Ananthanarayan, 10/e, p 548]

16. Super carrier of HBV shows following serum markers:
    a. HBsAg
    b. HbsAg + HBV DNA
    c. HbsAG + HBeAg + HBV DNA
    d. Anti-BHsAg + HBV DNA

17. Defective hepatitis virus is:
    a. HAV b. HBV
    c. HCV d. HDV
    [Ananthanarayan, 10/e, p 553]

18. Which is not parenterally transmitted?
    a. HAV b. HBV
    c. HCV d. HDV
    [Ananthanarayan, 10/e, p 555]

19. Infectivity of HBV is indicated by:
    a. HBeAg b. HBsAg
    c. HBcAg d. Anti-HBc
    [Ananthanarayan, 10/e, p 551]

20. Hepatitis A virus is:
    a. Flavivirus
    b. Calcivirus
    c. Enterovirus
    d. Defective virus [Ananthanarayan, 10/e, p 544]

21. Marker for acute viral hepatitis caused by HBV:
    a. IgM anti-HBc Ag
    b. IgG anti-HBc Ag
    c. IgM anti-HBs Ag
    d. IgG anti-HBs Ag [Harrison, 20/e, p 2350]

22. Which of the following does not indicate Hepatitis B replication?
    a. HBcAg b. HBeAg
    c. HBV DNA d. Viral copies
    [Harrison, 20/e, p 2350]

23. Councilman body is seen in:
    a. Molluscum contagiosum
    b. Rabies
    c. Granuloma inguinale
    d. Viral hepatitis [Harrison, 20/e, p 235]

24. HAV is not destroyed by:
    a. 0.5 ppm chlorine
    b. 1:4000 formalin
    c. UV radiation
    d. Boiling at 100°C for 5 minutes
    [Ref. Ananthanarayan 10/e, p 545, 9/e, p 541]

> HAV is inactivated by boiling for one minute; 1:4000 of maldehyde at 37°C for 72 hours and chlorine 1 ppm for 30 min. It is not affected by anionic detergents, ether

25. Choose the false statement regarding hepatitis G virus:
    a. Also called GB virus
    b. Blood-borne RNA virus
    c. Mostly infected with C virus
    d. Responds to Lamivudine
    [Ref. Ananthanarayan 10/e, p 554]

> **Hepatitis G virus:**
> - RNA virus belonging to flavivirus family
> - Mode of transmission is same as that of HCV, i.e. blood borne
> - Also called as GB virus
> - Prevalence is higher in patient infected with HIV and HCV

26. HBV present in India is:
    a. Adw b. Ayw
    c. Adr d. Ayr
    [Ref. Ananthanarayan 10/e, p 547]

> - HBsAg exhibit antigenic diversity. It contains two different antigenic components:
>   a. Common group reactive antigen 'a'
>   b. Two pair of type specific antigen d-y, w-r
> - Thus, there can be four antigenic subtypes.
>   1. ayw- Common in West Asia, Northen India, Western India.
>   2. Adw- Common in Europe and Australia
>   3. Adr: Found in South and East India
>   4. Ayr: Rarest

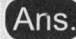

15. c. P gene	16. c. HbsAG + HBeAg + HBV DNA	17. d. HDV	18. a. HAV
19. a. HBcAg	20. c. Enterovirus	21. a. IgM anti-HBc Ag	22. a. HBcAg
23. d. Viral hepatitis	24. a. 0.5 ppm ...	25. d. Responds ...	26. b and c...

CHAPTER 28

HIV and Other Retrovirus

- Discovered in 1983 by Luc Montagenier who called it as lymphadenopathy associated virus. The term HIV was given on 1986.
- Causative agent of **AIDS** = Slim disease.
- Belongs to *family **retroviridae**; subfamily **lentiviridae**.*
- Two types are found HIV 1 and HIV 2. **HIV 1 is most common cause** of **AIDS in world.**
- HIV 1 is more virulent than HIV 2.
- *Pan troglodyte troglodytes species of chimpanzees are natural reservoir of HIV 1.*

.... Harrison, 19/e, 1216

HIV:
- SS RNA virus belongs to retroviridae, subfamily lentiviridae.
- Two types HIV1 (more common) and HIV 2
- Main genes are:
  - gag (determine core and shell)
  - env (determine envelope)
  - pol (determine polymerase)
- HIV1: Three groups group M (most common) N and O
- There are 9 subtypes of M group, subtype C being most common.
- **Mnemonic:** Learn as 1 MC

Retroviridae	
Oncoviridae (oncogenic viruses)	– RNA tumor virus group (HTLV 1, HTLV 2 Rous sarcoma virus).
Lentiviridae	– HIV 1, HIV 2 – Visna virus – Feline immunodeficiency virus
Spumavirinae foamy virus	– Simian foamy virus – Human foamy virus

MORPHOLOGY AND REPLICATION CYCLE

- Spherical *enveloped* virus. Nucleocapsid has *icosahedral* structure.
- Virus contain *external spikes formed by the* **two major envelope protein** *— the external gp 120* and *transmembrane gp - 41.* gp 120 is the major envelope antigen.
- Genome is composed of two identical single stranded positive sense RNA copies.
- *Main genes are:*

  gag – Determines *the core and shell of virus.* Codes for precursor protein p55 which is cleaved into three proteins p15, p18 and p24.

  env – Determines *the synthesis of envelope glycoprotein.* gp 160 which is then cleaved into gp 120 and gp 41.

  pol – Codes for *polymerase reverse transcriptase* and other viral enzymes.

Note: Reverse transcriptase is RNA dependent DNA polymerase.
Inviral envelope lipid is derived from host cell membrane and glycoprotein are virus coded.

Major Antigens of HIV
Envelope antigen
Gp 120 : Spike antigen
Gp 41 : Transmembrane pedicle protein
Shell antigen
P18 : Nucleocapsid protein
Core antigen
P24 : Principal core antigen
P15, P55 : Other core antigen
Polymerase antigen:
P31, P51, P66

Other genes are: tat, rev, jej, vif, vpu, vpx, vpr, LTR.
- The major difference between genomes of **HIV 1** and **HIV 2** is HIV 2 lacks vpu gene and has vpx gene which is not present in HIV 1.

Antigenic variation and molecular heterogeneity
- *HIV is highly mutable virus.*
- The variability of HIV is believed to be due to error prone nature of reverse transcription.

- There are three groups of HIV -1.
  - **Group M *(Most of infection)*, Group O and Group N.** There are *nine subtypes* of M group:

..... Harrison 20/e, p 1396
  - Subtype C is *most prevalent* worldwide.
  - *In India and China* also subtype **C** *is most prevalent.*
  - In Europe, Australia and America subtype B is predominant.
- It is not uncommon to find recombinants form (CRF). CRF (circulating recombinant form) are generated by infection of a individual with two subtype which then recombine and create a virus with selective advantage. AE form is most prevalent CRF.

Note: The AIDS pandemic virus is primarily caused by HIV-1 M. group virus.

MODES OF TRANSMISSION

A. Sexual transmission

- The *most common* **mode** of transmission worldwide is **heterosexual transmission**.
- Chance of infection from *male to female* is **twice** as from *female to male*.
- The overall risk of transmission ranges from 0.04-0.38% per coital act for female to male and 0.08 to 0.6 per act for male to female per act. Risk of HIV transmission via unprotected anal intercourse was estimated to be 1.4% for both men and women.

B. Transmission by blood and blood products

- 2nd most common mode
- Transmission of whole blood. Packed red cells, platelets, leucocytes and plasma are all capable of transmitting HIV infection.
- Hyperimmunoglobulin, hepatitis B immunoglobulin, plasma derived hepatitis B vaccine and Rh immunoglobulin *have not been* associated with transmission of HIV infection.
- Risk of getting HIV infection from **transfusion of a unit of infected blood is > 95%.**

C. Maternal fetal transmission: Risk is 30%

- Third most common mode
- Occurs *most commonly* in perinatal period.
- Cesarean section decrease risk of transmission.
- The probabilities of transmission of HIV from mother to child were 23–30% before birth, 50–65% during birth and 12–20% via breastfeeding
- Risk of infection is high if the mother is newly infected or if she has already developed AIDS.
- *Vitamin A deficiency* increase risk of transmission.
- Exclusive breastfeeding carries lower risk of transmission than mixed feeding.

..... Harrison 20/e, p 1402

- Presence of mastitis, low maternal CD4+ T cells counts and maternal vitamin A deficiency increase risk of transmission.

D. Transmission by other body fluids:

- HIV can be isolated in low titres from saliva, but *saliva can not transmit* HIV infection *due to presence* of endogenous antiviral factors of which most important *is secretory leukocyte protease inhibitor (SLPI).*

> **Mode of Transmission:**
> - Sexual: MC, but risk of transmission is least.
> - Blood and blood product: Carries (>95%) highest risk of transmission
> - Vertical (risk is 30%).
> - Sexual → Blood/blood products → Perinatal

LIFE CYCLE

- *Replication begins* with the high affinity **binding of gp120 with CD-4** (Present on CD4 + T cells and monocyte macrophage lineage cells). After binding with CD-4, gp120 undergoes conformational change that facilitates binding of coreceptor. The major coreceptor for HIV-1 are CCR-5 (receptor for chemokine RANTES, MIP1a and MIP1β) and CXCR-4 (the receptor for chemokine SDF-1)
- Strains of HIV that utilize **CCR-5 as coreceptor**, usually infect *macrophages* and are referred as R-5 virus.
- Strains of HIV that utilize **CXC R4** usually infects *lymphocytes* and are referred as X-4 virus.
- Many viral strains are dual tropic (utilize both CCR-5 and CXCR-4) which are referred as R5X4 virus.
- After fusion, HIV genome RNA is uncoated and internalized into target cell. The reverse transcriptase catalyze the reverse transcription of RNA to DNA. DNA so formed integrates with host cell chromosome through the action of virus encoded enzyme integrase.

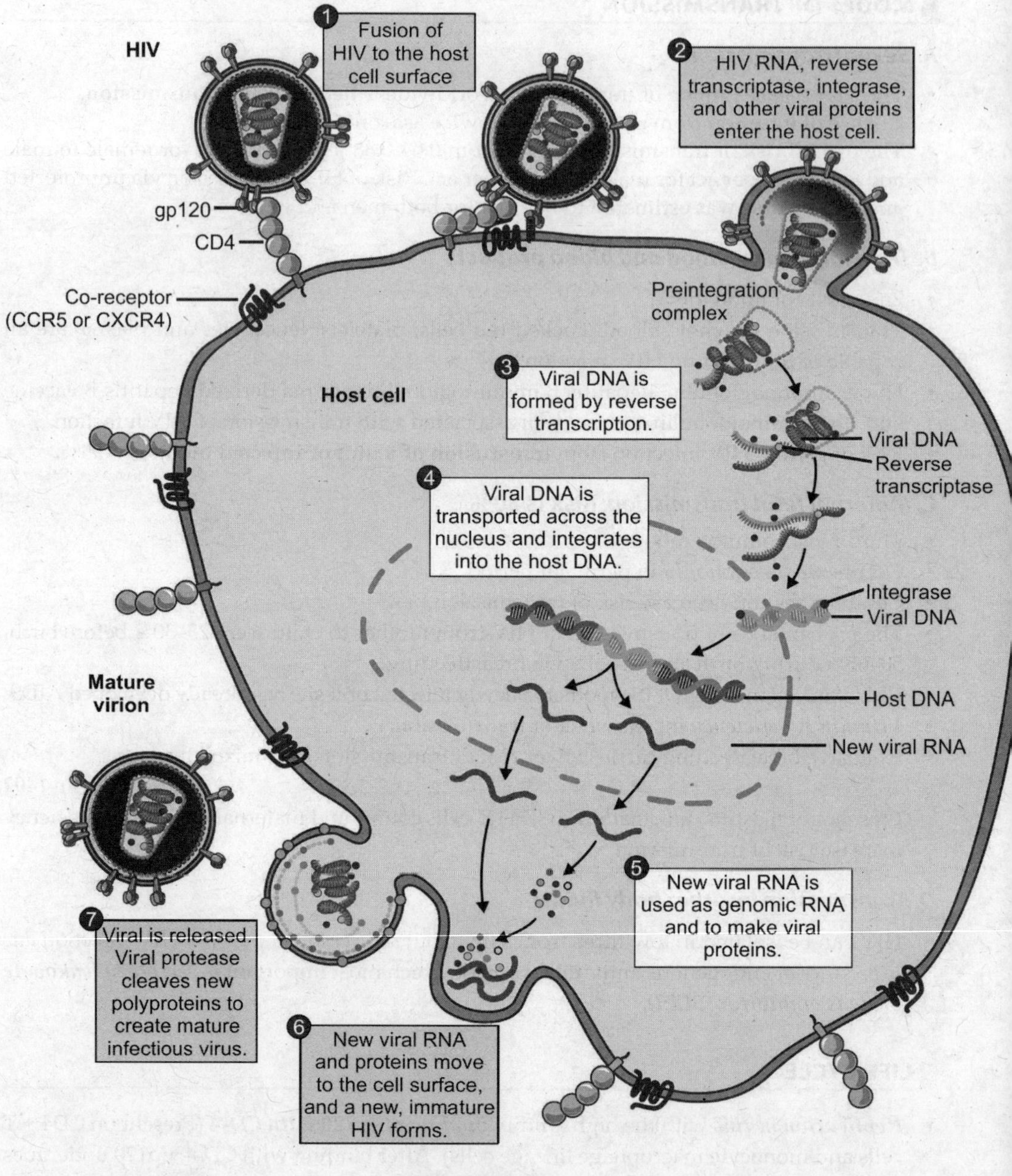

Life cycle of HIV

PATHOGENESIS

- The hallmark of HIV disease is a profound immunodeficiency due to quantitative and qualitative deficiency of helper or inducer T cells (CD4 - T cells).
- *Primary HIV infection and Initial Viremia:*
  - Dendritic cells play an important role in the initiation of HIV infection due to presence of lectin called DC-SIGN which binds with high affinity to HIV envelope.
- *Chronic and Persistent Infection:*
  - Establishment of chronic infection is due to the ability of virus to mutate.
  - Evolution of mutants that escape control by CD8 + cytolytic T lymphocytes is critical for progression of HIV infection.
  - Another mechanism is the down regulation of HLA class 1 molecules resulting in lack of ability of CD8 + CTL to kill the infected target cell.

Pathogenesis:
- Quantitative and qualitative deficiency of helper or inducer T cell
- Co-receptor for HIV CCR-5 and CXCR4

- *Cellular target of HIV:*
  - **CD 4 + Helper = Inducer T cell** *(Primary target)*
  - Monocyte - Macrophages (10-15%)
  - Dendritic, Langerhans cells
  - Few B cells (5-10%).

CLINICAL FEATURES

Cellular targets of HIV:
- T cells CD4, Monocyte-Macrophage, dendritic Langerhans cells, Few B cells

- **Acute HIV infection** with in 3-6 weeks of infection.
  - Infectious mononucleosis like symptoms.
  - In most patient it is followed by prolonged period of clinical latency.
- **Asymptomatic stage** = Latent infection:
  - Median time of asymptomatic stage is ~ *10 years*.
  - Rate of *disease progression* can be directly correlated with *HIV RNA levels*.
  - During this stage rate of CD4 + T cell decline is ≈ 50 µl/yr.
  - Any HIV infected individual with CD4 + T cell count < 200/µl has AIDS by definition.
- **Persistent generalized lymphadenopathy:** Presence of enlarged lymph nodes at least 1 cm in diameter in two or more non-contiguous extra-inguinal sites, that persist for atleast three months without any other attributable cause.
- **AIDS related complex: (ARC):** ARC includes patients with considerable immunodeficiency suffering from various constitutional symptoms or minor opportunistic infection.
- **Symptomatic Disease: AIDS**

- Asymptomatic stage of HIV last for about 10 years
- Any HIV + individual with CD4 + T cell count < 200/µl has AIDS by definition

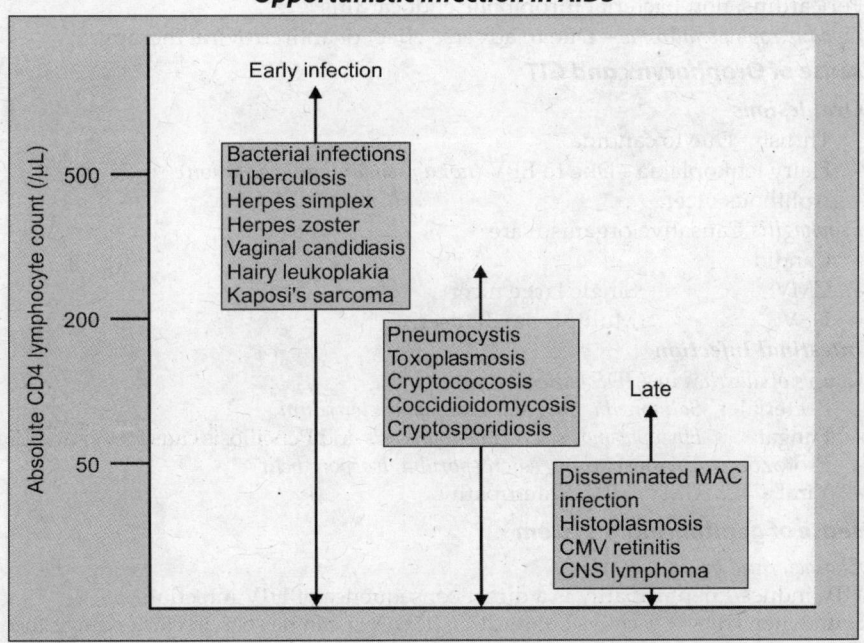

AIDS

AIDS can lead to infection/disturbance in almost every organ system.

A. Disease of Respiratory System
- **Sinusitis**
  - *Most commonly* maxillary sinus is involved. *MC* causative organism are **H. influenzae** and **Streptococcus**.
- **Pulmonary manifestation**
  - *MC* pulmonary manifestation is pneumonia. The *most common* cause of pneumonia is *P. carinii*.
  - Pneumocystis pneumonia present with fever, cough and shortness of breath but hypoxemia may be severe.

Clinical Manifestation:
- **Respiratory:** MC is pneumonia. MC cause P. carini.
- **Meningitis:** MC cause cryptococcus
- **Esophagitis:** MC cause Candida
- **Blindness:** MC cause CMV retinitis

- Chest X-ray shows diffuse or perihilar infiltrate (characteristic of *P. carnii*) but only in 2/3rd of patient. Chest X-ray might be normal in 10-15% of cases.
- Large pleural effusion are uncommon and its presence suggest some other cause
- Definitive diagnosis is made by direct fluoroscence antibody (DFA) test of induced sputum.
  - MC bacterial cause of pneumonia in HIV patient are H. influenzae, streptococci.
  - Tuberculosis-HIV increase risk of developing active TB by factor of 100. Can be seen even in high CD-4 count. Affect upper lobe (when CD-4 count is high), diffuse or lower lobe when CD-4 count is low. ...Harrison 19/e 1254
- *In India, mycobacterium tuberculosis is **MC** opportunistic infection in **AIDS** patient.*
  - Atypical mycobacterial infection – **MC** are *M. avium* or *M. intracellulare* species (MAC) occur *when CD-4 < 50/μl.*
  - Mostly present as disseminated infection.
- **Fungal infection-** Coccidiodes immunitis; *Aspergillosis; Histoplasmosis.*
- *Idiopathic interstitial pneumonia*
- Lymphoid interstitial pneumonia (LIP) and nonspecific intestinal pneumonitis.

B. Disease of CVS

It includes:
- *HIV associated cardiomyopathy*—Dilated cardiomyopathy associated with CHF due to direct consequence of HIV infection.
- Pericardial effusion, cardiac tamponade
- Pericarditis, non-bacterial thrombolic endocarditis
- *Lipodystrophy syndrome* – Due to adverse effect of antiretroviral therapy.

C. Disease of Oropharynx and GIT

- *Oral lesions*
  - Thrush - Due to candida
  - Hairy leukoplakia - Due to EBV *(not a premalignant condition)*
  - Aphthous ulcer.
- *Esophagitis* Causative organism are:
  - Candida
  - CMV: Single large ulcer
  - HSV: Multiple small ulcer.
- *Intestinal Infection*
  Causes of diarrhea in AIDS patient.
  - Bacterial : Salmonella, Shigella, Campylobacter jejuni.
  - Fungal : Histoplasmosis, Coccidiodomycosis and Pencillosis cause fever and diarrhea.
  - Protozoa : Cryptosporidia, Microsporidia, Isospora belli
  - Viral : CMV, HIV, Enteropathy

D. Disease of genitourinary system

- *Characterized by proteinuria*
- HIV induced nephropathy is a direct consequence of HIV infection
- Seen when CD-4 + T cell is below 20%, however can be seen in earlier stage too
- Diagnosis is made by biopsy which shows focal segmental glomerulosclerosis (80%) and mesangial proliferation.

E. Disease of Hematopoietic system

- *Anemia*—**MC** hematologic abnormality.
- *Thrombocytopenia*—Due to platelet specific antibody or as a direct result of HIV on megakaryocytes.
- *Lymphadenopathy and Leukopenia.*

F. Dermatologic disease

- Dermatologic problems occur in >90% of patients with HIV infection.
- Folliculitis is the most prevalent dermatologic disorder in patients with HIV infection. Seen when CD4 + T cell counts < 200 cells/μl.
- Seborrheic dermatitis occurs in up to 50% of patient with HIV infection.

Contd...

CDC Stage 3 (AIDS)-defining opportunistic illnesses in HIV infection
Lymphoma, primary, of brain
Mycobacterium avium complex or *Mycobacterium kansasil*, disseminated or extrapulmonary
Mycobacterium tuberculosis of any site, pulmonary,[b] disseminated, or extrapulmonary
Mycobacterium, other species or unidentified species, disseminated or extrapulmonary
Pneumocystis jirovecii (previously known as *Pneumocystis carinii*) pneumonia
Pneumonia, recurrent[b]
Progressive multifocal leukoencephalopathy
Salmonella septicaemia, recurrent
Toxoplasmosis of brain, onset at age >1 month
Wasting syndrome attributed to HIV

[a]Only among children age <6 years.
[b]Only among adults, adolescents, and children age ≥6 years.

CDC HIV infection stages 1-3 based on age-specific CD4+T Lymphocyte count or CD4+T lymphocyte percentage of total lymphocytes[a]						
Age on Date of CD4 T+ Lymphocyte Test						
	<1 year		1-5 Years		6 Years through adult	
Stage[a]	Cells/μL	%	Cells/μL	%	Cells/μL	%
1	≥1500	≥34	≥1000	≥30	≥500	≥26
2	750–1499	26–33	500–999	22–99	200–499	14–25
3	<750	<26	<500	<22	<200	<14

[a]The stage is based primarily on the CD4+T lymphocyte count; the CD4+T lymphocyte count takes precedence over the CD4+T lymphocyte percentage, and the percentage is considered only if the count is missing.

LABORATORY DIAGNOSIS

Laboratory diagnosis	
Demonstration of Antibody	**Demonstration of HIV or its components**
• ELISA **(sensitive and best screening test)**	• **Antigen detection** p-24 is earliest virus marker to appear in blood
• Western blot (specific) (demonstrate antibody to products of all major HIV gene)	• **Virus isolation**—By cultivation of patient lymphocyte with uninfected lymphocyte in present of IL-2

• Modern 4th generation EIA kit combines antibody detection with p24 antigen assay	• PCR—Gold standard for diagnosis in all stages of HIV
	  – DNA PCR; RNA PCR, RT PCR
	  – *RT PCR is most sensitive and best.*

- RT PCR is used as a diagnostic and prognostic tool and has become a technique of choice for studies of sequence diversity and microbial resistance to antiretroviral agents.
- **Nucleic acid amplification detection:** Reverse transcriptase PCR, branched DNA (b DNA) and nucleic acid sequence based amplification. (NSABA)
- **Among all RTPCR is most sensitive which can detect upto 40 copies/mL.**

Characteristics of Tests for Direct Detection of HIV

Test	Technique	Sensitivity
Immune complex-dissociated p24 antigen capture assay	Measurement of levels of HIV-1 core protein in an EIA-based format following dissociation of antigen-antibody complexes by weak acid treatment	Positive in 50% of patients; detects down to 15 pg/mL of p 24 protein
HIV RNA by PCR	PCR amplification of cDNA generated from viral RNA (target amplification)	Reliable to 40 copies/mL of HIV RNA
HIV RNA by bDNA	Measurement of levels of particle-associated HIV RNA in nucleic acid capture assay employing signal amplification	Reliable to 50 copies/mL of HIV RNA
HIV RNA by NASBA	Isothermic nucleic acid amplification with internal controls	Reliable to 80 copies/mL of HIV RNA

Note: In patients in whom HIV infection is suspected, the appropriate initial test is the EIA. In case of strong suspicion and to make early diagnosis p24 antigen detection is recommended.

Serological tests in the diagnosis of HIV-1 or HIV-2 infection

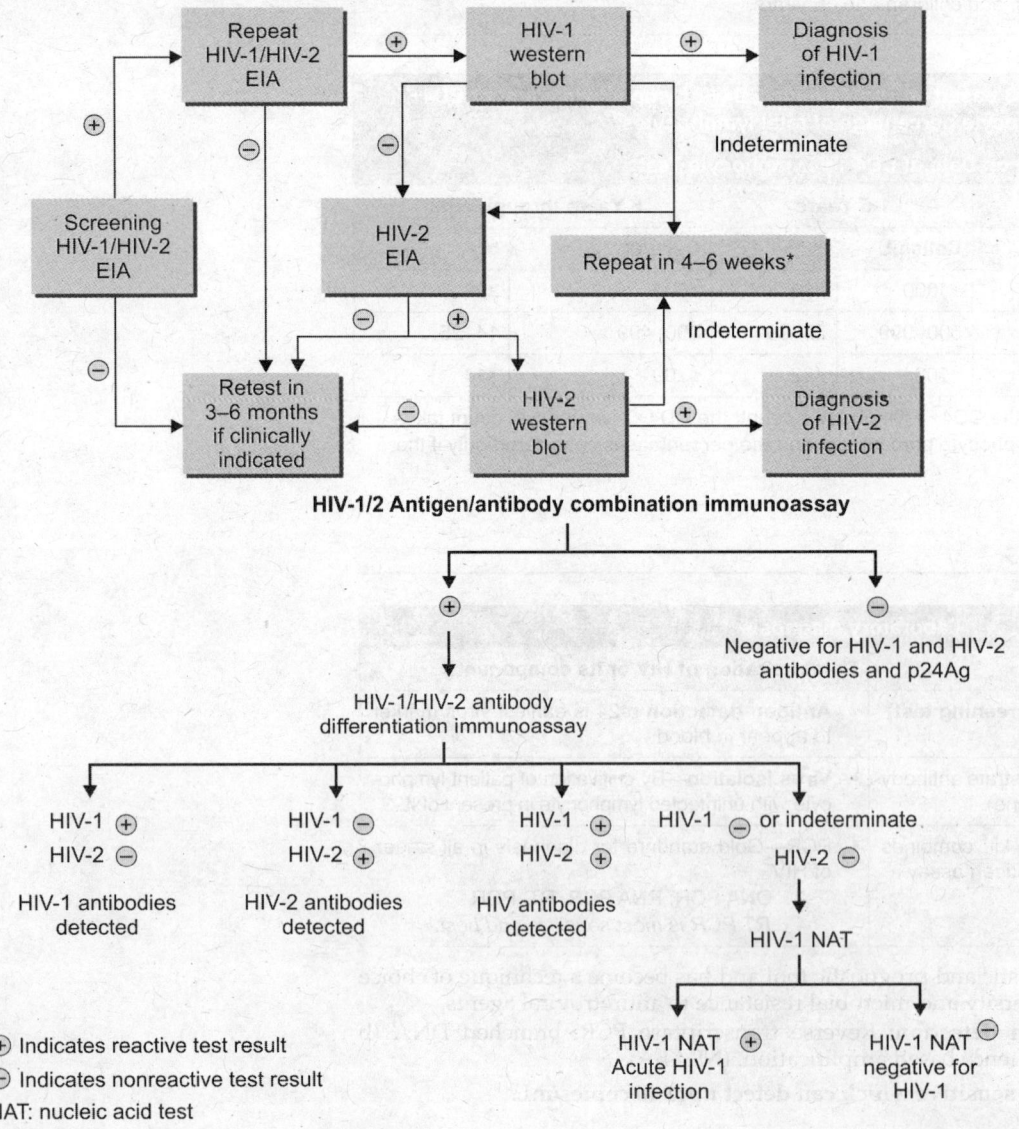

⊕ Indicates reactive test result
⊖ Indicates nonreactive test result
NAT: nucleic acid test

Diagnosis of HIV Infection in Newborn

- The presence of anti-HIV antibody (ELISA) is not diagnostic of infection until after 18 month of age.
- Diagnosis during first few month of life is made by detection of HIV DNA with PCR (Best).
- Other methods are p-24 antigen detection and HIV culture.

Lab Monitoring of Patient with HIV Infection

- *CD4 + T cell count* – Best indication of immediate state of immunologic competence of patient with HIV infection.
- *HIV RNA determination* – By RT PCR and bDNA assay.
- Determine disease progression. Should be monitored every 3-4 months.
- *HIV resistance testing.*

TREATMENT

As per WHO recommendations 2010	
When to start	All adolescents and adults including pregnant women with HIV infection and CD4 counts of ≤350 cells/mm^3, should start ART, regardless of the presence or absence of clinical symptoms. Those with severe or advanced clinical disease (WHO clinical stage 3 or 4) should start ART irrespective of their CD4 cell count.
What to be given	*(see table below)*
Laboratory monitoring	All patients should have access to CD4 cell-count testing to optimize pre-ART care and ART management. HIVRNA (viral-load) testing is recommended to confirm suspected treatment failure. Drug toxicity monitoring should be symptom-directed.

Target Population	Preferred options
Adults and adolescents	AZT or TDF+ 3TC or FTC + EFV or NVP
Pregnant women	AZT + 3TC + EFV or NVP
HIV/TB coinfection	AZT or TDF + 3TC or FTC + EFV
HIV/HBV coinfection	TDF + 3TC or FTC + EFV or NVP

Nucleoside reverse transcriptase inhibitor (NRTI)	Protease inhibitors	Non-nucleoside reverse transcriptase inhibitors (NNRT I)
AZT = Zidovudine	Ritonavir	Delaviridine
ddI = Didanosine	Indinavir (IDV)	Nevirapine (NVP)
ddC = Zalcitabine	Nelfinavir	Efavirenz (EFV)
d4T = Stavudine	Saquinavir (SQV)	
3TC = Lamivudine	**Mnemonic: RIN shakti**	
TDF = Tenofovir		
ABC = Abocavir		

WHO recommendations for initiating antiretroviral treatment in infants and children				
Criteria to start ART in infants and children				
Age	Infants	1-3 years	3-5 years	> 5 years
% CD4	All	< 20	< 20	< 20
Absolute CD4*	-	< 750 mm^3	< 350 mm^3	As in adults

* Absolute CD4 count is naturally less constant and more age-dependent than % CD4; it is not therefore appropriate to define a single threshold

- Irrespective of CD4, ART should be given to all infants
- For post exposure prophylaxis Zidovudine, lamuvidine and nelfinavir should be administered for four weeks

Treatment of opportunistic Infection		
Infection	1st line treatment	Alternative treatment
• Pneumocystic jeroveci	Trimethoprime + Sulphamethoxazole	Pentamidine
• Toxoplasmosis	Pyrimethamine + Sulphadiazine	Pyrimethamine + lindamycin
• Cryptococcus	Amphotericin + Flucytosine	Amphotericin
• Candida – Mucosal – Systemic	Clotrimazole/Flucytosine Amphotericin	Ketoconazole
• CMV	Gancyclovir	Foscarnet
• H simplex – Oral – Encephalitis	Acyclovir Acyclovir	Vidarabine
• Herpes zoster – Local – Disseminated	Acyclovir Acyclovir	– Vidarabine

POSTEXPOSURE PROPHYLACTIC TREATMENT

- Antiretroviral drugs started with hours following accidental exposure reduce the chances aquiring infection by 75%. Following regimen is recommended.
  - A combination of two nucleoside analogues reverse transcriptase inhibitor *(mostly zidovudine + lamivudine)* for 4 weeks for routine exposure.
  - For high-risk exposure or if the source individual has advanced AIDS protease inhibitor nelfinavir should be added.
- Clinically all cases are considered high-risk and high-risk regime is given to all cases.
- If the source individual has failed on zidovudine + lamivudine combination than stavudine + didinosine should be used instead of AZT + lamivudine.

OTHER RETROVIRUS

Human T cell lymphotropic virus 1 (HTLV - 1):
- Also called as adult T cell lymphoma virus type I (ATLV 1)
- Causative agent of
  - Adult T cell lymphoma
  - Tropical spastic paraparesis.

Human T cells lymphotropic virus II (HTLV - 2):
- Thought to be as a virus searching for disease.
- Associated with some cases of T cell variant of hairy cell leukemia.

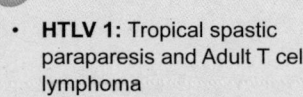
- **HTLV 1:** Tropical spastic paraparesis and Adult T cell lymphoma
- **HTLV 2:** Virus searching for disease

Multiple Choice Questions

1. **Not a AIDS defining illness:** [NEET pattern 2019]
   a. Pulmonary tuberculosis
   b. Primary lymphoma of brain
   c. Disseminated salmonellosis
   d. Tertiary syphilis

2. **True about HIV in pregnancy:** [NEET Pattern 2019]
   a. Pregnancy perse has maximum effect on disease progression
   b. Post natal transmission is rare
   c. Oxytocin and amniotomy is indicated
   d. Transmission risk is to fetus is directly proportional to maternal viral load

3. **HIV can be detected and confirmed by:** [AI 05]
   a. Polymerase chain reaction (PCR)
   b. Reverse transcriptase - PCR
   c. Real time PCR
   d. Mimic PCR

4. **Which one of following is true regarding HIV infection?** [AI 12]
   a. Following needle stick injury infectivity is reduced by administration of nucleoside analogues
   b. CD4 counts are the best predictors of disease progression
   c. Infected T cells survive for a month in infected patients
   d. In latent phase HIV has minimal replication

5. **HIV virus has:** [NEET pattern 2018]
   a. Single stranded positive DNA
   b. Single stranded negative RNA
   c. Double stranded DNA
   d. Double stranded RNA

6. **Regarding HIV infection, not true is:** [AIIMS 07]
   a. p24 is used for early diagnosis
   b. Lysis of infected CD4 cells is seen
   c. Dendritic cells do not support replication
   d. Macrophage is a reservoir for the virus

7. **A patient with HIV has diarrhea with AFB +ve organism in stool. The most likely organism is:** [AI 09]
   a. *Mycobacterium avium intracellulare*
   b. *Mycobacterium TB*
   c. *Mycobacterium leprae*
   d. *Mycoplasmas*

8. **A patient comes to hospital with a history of sore throat, diarrhea and sexual contact 2 weeks before the best investigation to rule out HIV is:** [AI 10]
   a. p24 antigen assay
   b. ELISA
   c. Western blot
   d. Lymph node biopsy

9. **Which is NOT AIDS defining illness?** [PGI June 09]
   a. *Oropharynx candidiasis*
   b. *CMV retinitis*
   c. *Primary CNS lymphoma*
   d. *Kaposi's sarcoma*
   e. *Cryptococcosis*

10. **Most common genital lesion in HIV patient is:** [AI 2010]
    a. *Chlamydia*
    b. *Herpes*
    c. *Syphilis*
    d. *Candida*

11. **HIV virus was discovered in:** [AIIMS May 2014]
    a. 1976
    b. 1983
    c. 1996
    d. 1988

12. **A person with AIDS related complex is most likely suffering from:** [AI 12]
    a. Opportunistic infection
    b. Cancer related to AIDS
    c. Generalized lymphadenopathy
    d. Herpes zoster

13. **In HIV window period indicates:** [AIIMS 07]
    a. Time period between infection and onset of symptoms
    b. Time period between infection and detection of antibodies against HIV
    c. Time between infection and treatment
    d. Time between treatment and death

14. **A known HIV positive patient is admitted in an isolation ward after an abdominal surgery following an accident. The resident doctor who changed his dressing the next day found it to be soaked in blood. Which of the following would be the right method of choice of discarding the dressing?** [AIIMS 05]
    a. Pour 1% hypochlorite on the dressing material and send it for incineration in a appropriate bag
    b. Pour 5% hypochlorite on the dressing material and send it for incineration in a appropriate bag
    c. Put the dressing material directly in an appropriate bag and send for incineration
    d. Pour 2% lysol on the dressing material and send it for incineration in a appropriate bag

15. **Tissue of origin of Kaposi's sarcoma is:** [AIIMS 05]
    a. Lymphoid
    b. Vascular
    c. Neural
    d. Muscular

16. Which of the following lesion is associated with HIV infection: [AIIMS 14]
    a. Hairy leukoplakia   b. Erythroplakia
    c. Oral lichen planus d. Bullous pemphigoid

17. All of the following methods are used for the diagnosis of HIV infection in a 2 month old child *except*: [AIIMS 08]
    a. DNA PCR   b. Viral culture
    c. HIV ELISA   d. p24 antigen assay

18. Which of the following gene is present in HIV genome? [PGI 06]
    a. Gag   b. Tat
    c. p500   d. Kinase
    e. P24

19. Which of the following is an AIDS defining criteria according to WHO? [PGI 11]
    a. Generalized lymphadenopathy
    b. Fever, weight loss and fatigue
    c. *Pneumocystis carinii* pneumonia
    d. *Mycobacterium avium* infection
    e. Persistent diarrhea

20. Persistent diarrhea in AIDS is caused by A/E: [PGI 12]
    a. *Microsporidia*   b. *Cryptosporidium parvum*
    c. *Cryptococcus*   d. *Isospora belli*
    e. *Giardia lambia*

21. Receptor for HIV? [AI 09]
    a. CD4   b. CD3
    c. CD5   d. CD56

22. CNS lesion in HIV is commonly caused by: [PGI June 09]
    a. *Cryptococcus*   b. *Toxoplasma*
    c. *Neurocysticercosis* d. *Mucormycosis*
    e. Lyme disease

Explanations and References with Illustrative Answers

1. **Ans. (d) Tertiary syphilis**   *Ref. Harrison 20/e, p 1394*
   Syphilis is not a AIDS defining illness
   Please refer theory portion for the list of AIDS defining illness

2. **Ans. (d) Transmission risk is to fetus is directly proportional to maternal viral load**   *Ref. COGDT 11/e p 720*
   Higher rates of transmission have been reported to be associated with many factors the best documented is presence of high maternal levels of plasma viremia, with the risk increasing linearly with the level of maternal plasma viremia.

   Factors affecting mother to child transmission

Viral	Viral genotype and phenotype (more with subtype E)
	Viral resistance
	Viral load (directly proportional)
Maternal	Maternal immunological status (inversely proportional to maternal CD4 count)
	Maternal nutritional status (more with vitamin A deficiency)
	Behavioural factors (cigarette smoking increase risk)
	Antiretroviral treatment
Obstetrical	Prolonged rupture of membranes (> 4 hours)
	Mode of delivery
	Intrapartum haemorrhage
	Obstetrical procedures
	Invasive fetal monitoring
Fetal	Prematurity
	Genetic
	Multiple pregnancy
Infant	Breastfeeding
	Gastrointestinal tract factors
	Immature immune system

Obstetrical factors

Most consistent one is prolong rupture of membrane. Duration of labour is not as important one.

Duration of ruptured membranes of over four hours nearly doubled the risk of infection, regardless of the eventual mode of delivery

Possible strategies for the prevention of mother-to-child transmission of HIV

- Termination of pregnancy
- Behavioural interventions
  - Reduction in the frequency of unprotected sexual intercourse during pregnancy
  - Reduction in the number of sexual partners during pregnancy
  - Lifestyle changes, including avoidance of drug use and smoking in pregnancy
- Therapeutic interventions
  - Antiretroviral therapy: zidovudine alone or combination,
  - Long- or short-course Vitamin A and other micronutrients
  - Immunotherapy
  - Treatment of STD
- Obstetric interventions
  - Avoidance of invasive tests
  - Birth canal cleansing
  - Caesarean section delivery

3. **Ans. (b) Reverse transcriptase PCR**   *Ref. Harrison 20/e, p 1424*

Laboratory diagnosis of AIDS

a. **Virus Isolation**
   - HIV can be cultured from lymphocytes of peripheral blood. The number of circulating infected cells vary with the stage of disease. High titres are found in advanced stage. The most sensitive virus isolation technique is to co-cultivate the test sample with uninfected nitrogen stimulated blood mononuclear cells. Viral growth is confirmed by testing culture supernatant fluid (after 7-14 days) for viral reverse transcriptase activity or for virus specific antigens.
   - Due to the time it requires, virus isolation is seldom used for diagnosis of AIDS. It is mainly indicated for lab characterization of virus and to determine clinical stage; as plasma viremia is a better correlate of clinical stage than the presence of any antibody.
   - For determining clinical stage too, *viral nucleic acid* load estimation is rapid and has replaced virus culture.

b. **Serology**
   - *Enzyme linked immunoassay* has a sensitivity and specificity above 98%. It is cheap and yield rapid result; these properties makes ELISA screening test of choice.
   - When EIA tests are used for screening population with low prevalence of HIV infection, a positive test must be confirmed by a repeat test. If the repeat test is reactive, a confirmation test is performed to rule due false positive EIA result.
   - Most commercial EIA Kit contains antigen from both HIV-1 and HIV-2
   - Conditions associated with false positive EIA include antibodies to class II antigens (may be seen during pregnancy, post-transplantation), auto antibodies, hepatic disease, recent influenza vaccination, and acute viral infection.
   - *Most widely used confirmation assay* is **western blot** in which antibody to specific viral proteins can be detected. Antibodies to viral core protein p24 or envelope glycoproteins gp41, gp120 or gp160 are most commonly detected.
   - The mean time for seroconversion after HIV infection is 3-4 weeks, virtually all HIV infected individuals have detectable antibodies within 6 months. Means both ELISA and westernblot yield false negative result during the **window period** (*an interval required for seroconversion after HIV infections*) which usually range from 3 weeks - 6 months. Antiretroviral therapy during window period also delays seroconversion. X-linked agammaglobinemia is another condition in which antibody test may yield false negative result.

c. **Detection of viral nucleic acid or Antigens**
   - RT PCR, DNAPCR and bDNA assays are commonly used to estimate viral RNA in clinical specimen.
   - RT-PCR uses an enzymatic method to amplify HIV RNA
   - bDNA assays amplifies viral RNA by sequential oligonucleotide hybridization steps

   These molecular test are very sensitive and can be used for both diagnosis and plasma viral load estimation i.e. prognosis.
   - Low level of circulating HIV-1 p24 antigen can be detected in plasma soon after infection. The antigen often become undetectable after formation of antibodies (because p-24 antigen is complexed with p24 antibody), but may reappear late in the course of infection. *This reappearance indicates a poor prognosis.*

4. **Ans. (a) Following needle stick injury infectivity is reduced by administration of nucleoside analogues**
   Ref. Harrison 20/e, p 1460-1461; Park 22/e, p 327

   "Four week treatment with AZT monotherapy after needle stick exposure to HIV among health care worker decreases the chance of their becoming infected by 79%."

   Guidelines for postexposure prophylaxis
   I. A combination of two nucleoside analogue reverse transcriptase inhibitors for 4 weeks for less severe exposures.
   II. A combination of two nucleoside analogue RT inhibitor plus a protease inhibitor given for 4 weeks for more severe exposure.

   Most clinical administer 2nd reginen in all cases

   > **Factor associated with increased risk of occupational transmission**
   > - Deep injury.
   > - Presence of visible blood on the instrument causing the exposure.
   > - Injury with the device that has been placed in vein or artery of source patient.
   > - Terminal illness of source patient.
   > - Lack of postexposure antiretroviral therapy in exposed health care worker.
   > - TB is another infection common to HIV infected population that can be transmitted to health care workers following needle stick. For this reason all healthcare workers should check there PPD status and receive 6 months of isoniazid treatment if their skin test is positive.

   Other Options

   Option 'b'
   - *Best predictor to disease progression is HIV RNA estimation (not CD 4 + count.)*   Harrison 20/e, p 1421, 1458
   - CD 4 + count are the *best* indicator of immediate state of immunologic competence.
   - Following initiation of therapy one should expect at least 1 log(10 fold) reduction in plasma HIV RNA level with HIV RNA level reaching < 50/mL with in 6 months.

   Option 'd'
   - **Clinical latency versus microbial latency**
     – Clinical latency should not be confused with microbial latency since virus replication is present in most patient.

   So, *option 'd'* is wrong.

   > **Remember: Test for monitoring of patient with HIV infection:**
   > - CD 4 + T cell count
   > - HIV RNA determination—Best by RT-PCR
   > - HIV resistance testing.

5. **Ans. (a) Single stranded positive RNA**   *Ref. Ananthanarayan 10/e, p 575*

Classification of HIV (= HTLV III)		
Family	–	Retroviridae
Subfamily	–	Lenti virus
Genome	–	ss RNA positive sense.

   - Virion contain **lipoprotein envelope** and nucleocapsid is icosahedral in shape.
   - ***Characteristic feature of retrovirus*** is presence of reverse transcriptase enzyme.
     – Viral RNA is transcribed by this enzyme first in to ss DNA then to dsDNA which gets integrated with host cell.
     – Thus in contrast to central dogma flow of information is RNA → DNA → RNA

6. **Ans. (c) Dendritic cells do not support replication**   *Ref. Ananthanarayan 10/e, p 577; Harrison 20/e, p 1405*
   - **Cellular target of HIV**
     – CD 4+ lymphocyte and CD 4 + cells of monocyte and macrophage lineage are principal target of HIV.
     – Circulating dendritic cells—play important role in initiation of HIV infection.
     – Epidermal langerhans' cells.
     – 5 - 10% of B lymphocyte.   ..... *Ananthanarayan, 10/e, p 574*
     – Alveolar macrophages in the lung
     – Langerhans cells in the dermis
     – Glial cells and microglia in the CNS
     – Follicular dendritic cells from tonsils can be infected by HIV without the involvement of CD 4.

   ...*Ananthanarayan 10/e, p 577*

- Degree of cytopathicity of HIV for cells of the monocyte lineage *is low,* and HIV can replicate extensively in cells of monocyte lineage. Hence play a role in dissemination of HIV in the body and can serve as reservoir of HIV infection.

..... Harrison, 19/e, p 1238

Immunological abnormalities in HIV infection
I. Features that characterize AIDS   • Lymphopenia   • Selective T cell deficiency — Reduction in number of T4 (CD4) cells, Inversion of T4: T8 ratio.   • Decreased delayed hypersensitivity on skin testing   • Hypergammaglobulinemia — predominantly IgG and IgA; and IgM also in children.   • Polyclonal activation of B cells and increased spontaneous secretion of Ig.
II. Other consistently observed features   • Decreased in vitro lymphocyte proliferative response to mitogens and antigens.   • Decreased cytotoxic response by T cells and NK cells   • Decreased antibody response to new antigens.   • Altered monocyte/macrophage function.   • Elevated levels of immune complexes in serum.

7. **Ans. (a)** *Mycobacterium avium intracellulare*   *Ref. Harrison 19/e, p 1254, 20/e, p 1434*

   MAC infection in AIDS patients
   - MAC infection is the late complication of HIV infection occur when CD 4< 50/µl.
   - *MC* presentation is disseminated disease with fever weight loss and night sweats. Other clinical features are:
     – Abdominal pain
     – Diarrhea
     – Lymphadenopathy.
   - Diagnosis is made by demonstration of long, slender AFB in sputum, stool, blood or bone marrow.
   - **Treatment:** *Clarithromycin + Ethambutol is treatment of choice.*

8. **Ans. (a)** p24 antigen assay   *Ref. Ananthanarayan 10/e, p 582*

   The major core antigen p24 is the earliest virus marker to appear in blood and is the one tested for.
   - p24 antigen assay is the most useful screening test for acute HIV syndrome as p24 antigen assay can detect those in windows period also.
   - After appearance of IgM, p24 antigen disappears and remain undetectable, P24 antigen reappears when severe disease set in.

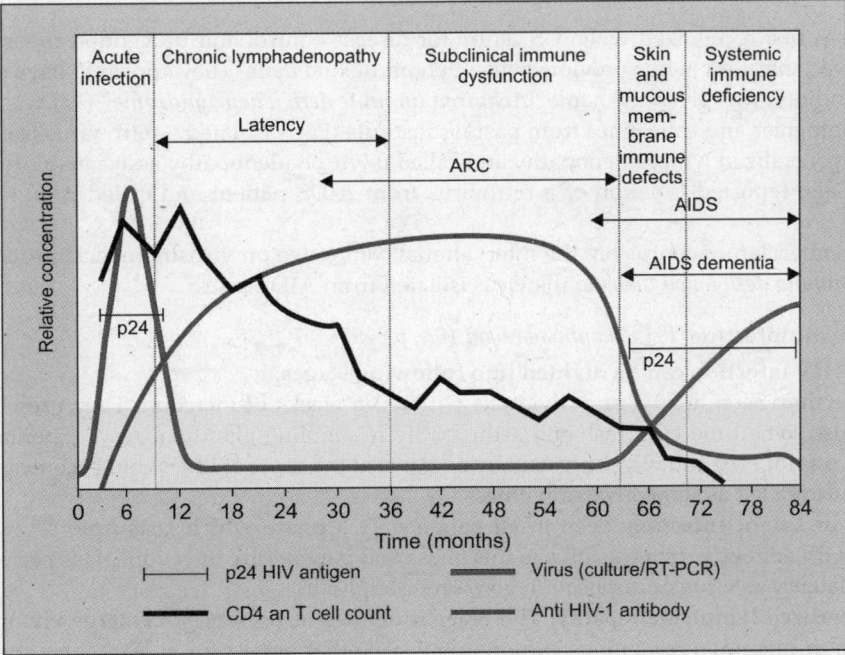

- Sequence of appearance of p24 antigen and antibodies after a massive HIV infection with time course of immune response, viremia, and disease resulting from HIV 1 infection.

9. **Ans. (a) Oropharynx candidiasis** *Ref. Harrison 20/e, p 1394, Park 22/e, p 322*
   Candidiasis of bronchi, trachea, lung, oesophagus comes under AIDS defining criteria.
   Infections listed in the AIDS surveillance case definition
   - Candidiasis of bronchi, trachea, lungs, oesophagus
   - Coccidioidomycosis, disseminated or extrapulmonary
   - Cryptococcosis, extrapulmonary
   - Cryptosporidiosis, chronic, intestinal (> 1 month's duration)
   - Cytomegalovirus disease (other than liver, spleen, or nodes)
   - Cytomegalovirus retinitis (with loss of vision)
   - Encephalopathy, HIV-related
   - Herpes simplex: chronic ulcer(s) (> 1 month's duration); orbronchitis, pneumonia, or esophagitis
   - Disseminated or extrapulmonary histoplasmosis
   - Isosporiasis, chronic intestinal (>1 month's duration)
   - Mycobacterium avium complex or M.kansosil, disseminated or extrapulmonary
   - Mycobacterium tuberculosis, any site (pulmonary or extrapulmonary)
   - Mycobacterium, other species or unidentified species, disseminated or extrapulmonary.
   - Pneumonocystis jiroveci pneumonia
   - Salmonella septicemia, recurrent
   - Toxoplasmosis of brain
   - Wasting syndrome due to HIV

10. **Ans. (b) Herpes** *Ref. Harrison 20/e, p 1442*
    See below
    - Herpes simplex (in developed world) and chancroid (in Africa) are the most common cause of genital ulceration in HIV infected patients.

    > **Note:** Clinical manifestations of genital herpes are more severe and persistent in HIV infected individual.
    > Most common presentation of syphilis in the HIV infected patient is that of condylomata lata, a form of secondary syphilis.

11. **Ans. (b) 1983** *Ref. Ananthanarayan 8/e, p 570*
    History of HIV
    - In 1981 AIDS was first recognized when US centre for disease control and prevention reported the unexplain occurrences of P. jiroveci infection in five previously health homosexual male. They appear to have lost their immunocompetence. So the condition was given the name *"Acquired immune deficiency syndrome"* (AIDS).
    - In 1983 Lue montognier and colleagues from pasteur institute, Paris isolated a retro virus from a West African patient with persistent generalized lymphadenopathy and called it lymphadenopathy associated virus (LAV).
    - In 1984 Ader Gallo reported isolation of a retrovirus from AIDS patient and called it human T-cell lymphotrophic virus III.
    - To reduce the nomenclature confusion, the intervational committee on virus nomenclature in 1886 decided a generic name *human immuno deficiency virus* to the virus isolated from AIDS cases.

12. **Ans. (a) Opportunistic infection** *Ref. Ananthanarayan 10/e, p 579*
    Natural course of HIV infection can be divided into following stages:
    a. **Acute HIV infection:** Seen in 30% of individuals within 3-6 weeks of infection. They present with low grade fever, headache, malaise some time with rash and arthropathy resembling glandular fever. Spontaneous resolution occurs within weeks. Tests for HIV antibodies are usually negative at the onset of illness but become positive during its course. So this stage is also called as seroconversion illness.
    b. **Asymptomatic or Latent Infection:** Seen in all patients. This phase which lasts upto several years, patient remain asymptomatic. HIV antibody test is positive in this phase and patients are infectious. This period of clinical latency does not mean viral latency as virus multiplication goes on throughout.
    c. **Persistent generalized lymphadenopathy:** This stage is defined as presence of enlarged lymph nodes at least 1 cm in diameter in two or more non-contagious extrainguinal sites, that persist for at least three months, in absence of any current illness or medication that may cause lymphadenopathy.

d. **AIDS related complex:** This group include patients with considerable immunodeficiency suffering from various constitutional symptoms or minor opportunistic infections like oral candidiasis herpes zoster, hairy cell leukoplakia.
e. **AIDS:** This is the endstage representing the irreversible breakdown of immunodefence mechanisms leading to progressive opportunistic infection and malignancies.

> **Remember:**
> - During the period of clinical latency 10 billion HIV particles are produced and destroyed every day.
> - Half life of virus in plasma is about 6 hours.
> - Virus life cycle *(from the time of infection of a cell to the production of new progeny that infect the next cell)* averages 2.6 days

13. **Ans. (b) Time period between infection and detection of antibodies** *Ref. Ananthanarayan 10/e, p 582*

    Window period is the period between infection and detection (diagnosis).
    - This range from 3 weeks - 2 months for antibody detection
    - Detection by p24 antigen has decreased this to 16 days and subsequently to 12 days with nucleic acid testing.

14. **Ans. (c) Put the dressing material directly in an appropriate bag and send for incineration** *Ref. Park 22/e, p 738*

    This type of waste belongs to category 6 of biomedical waste disposal method for this category is direct incineration without chemical treatment.

Categories of Biomedical Waste in India		
Option	**Waste category**	**Treatment and disposal**
Category No. 1	Human Anatomical Waste (Human tissues, organs body parts)	Incineration/deep burial[2]
Category No. 2	Animal Waste (Animal tissue, organs, body parts blood and experimental animals used in research, waste generated by veterinary hospitals colleges.	Incineration/deep burial[2]
Category No. 3	Microbiology and Biotechnology Waste (Waste from laboratory cultures, stock or specimens of micro-organisms, live or attenuated vaccines, human and animal cell culture used in research and infectious agents from research and industrial laboratories, waste from production of biologicals, toxins, dishes and devices and for transfer of cultures)	Local autoclaving/microwaving/incineration
Category No. 4	Waste sharps (needle, syringes, scar pels, blades, glass, etc. that may cause puncture and cuts. This includes both used and unused sharps)	Disinfection (chemical treatment ≅ autoclaving/microwaving and mutation/shredding)
Category No. 5	Discarded medicines and cytotoxic drugs (wastes comprising of outdated, contaminated and discarded medicines)	Incineration ≅ destruction and drugs disposal in secured landfills
Category No. 6	Solid waste (items contaminated with blood, and fluids including cotton, dressings, soiled plaster casts, linen, beddings, other material contaminated with blood)	Incineration ≅ autoclaving/microwaving
Category No. 7	Solid waste (wastes generated from disposable items other than the waste sharps such as tubings, catheters, intravenous sets, etc.)	Disinfection by chemical treatment ≅≅ autoclaving /microwaving and mutilation/shredding ##
Category No. 8	Liquid waste (waste generated from laboratory and washing, cleaning, housekeeping and disinfecting activities)	Disinfection by chemical treatment ≅≅ and discharge into drains
Category No. 9	Incineration ash (ash from incineration of any biomedical waste)	Disposal in municipal landfill
Category No. 10	Chemicals used in production of biologicals, chemicals used in disinfection, as insecticides, etc.	Chemical treatment ≅≅ and discharge into drains for liquids and secured landfill for solids.

≅≅ Chemical treatment using at least 1% hypochlorine solution or any other equipment chemical reagent. It must be ensured that chemical treatment ensures disinfection.
Multilation/shredding must be such so as to prevent unauthorized reuse.
≅ There will be no chemical pretreatment before incineration. Chlorinated plastics shall not be incinerated.
2 Deep burial shall be an option available only in towns with population less than lakhs and in rural areas.

Color coding and type of container for disposal of biomedical wastes		
Color coding	Type of container	Waste category
Yellow	Plastic bag	Cat. 1, Cat. 2, and Cat. 3, Cat. 6
Red	Disinfected container/plastic bag	Cat. 3, Cat. 6, Cat. 7
Blue/White translucent	Plastic bag/puncture proof container	Cat. 4, Cat. 7
Black	Plastic bag	Cat. 5, Cat. 9 and Cat. 10 (solid)

15. **Ans. (b) Vascular** *Ref. Harrison 20/e, p 1421*

Kaposi's sarcoma is a multicentric neoplasm of vascular origin consisting of multiple vascular nodules appearing in skin, mucous membrane and viscera.

Feature of Kaposi's sarcoma:
- Can develop at any stage of HIV infection, even in presence of normal CD-4 count.
- It is a manifestation *of* excess proliferation of spindle cells that are believed to be vascular origin.

..... *Harrison 18/e, p 1564*

- Development of KS is associated with Human herpes virus 8 or HHV - 8 is etiologic agent of KS.
- Clinically KS often appear in sun exposed areas, particularly tip of nose. The initial lesion is a small raised reddish purple nodule on skin (*MC* appear as raised nodules).
- LN involvement does not signify poor prognosis.

Treatment
- *Observation and optimization of antiretroviral therapy.*
- *Single or limited number of lesions*   – Radiation
  – Intralesional vinblastine and Cryotherapy.
- *Extensive disease* Initial therapy: – Interferon - α (if CD 4 + T cells > 150/μl)
  – Liposomal daunorubicin.
  – Subsequent therapy: – Liposomal doxorubicin
  – Paclitaxel and Radiation treatment.
  – Combination chemotherapy
  – Radiation treatment

16. **Ans. (a) Hairy leukoplakia** *Ref. Harrison 20/e, p 1435*

	Oral lesions in AIDS Patient	
1.	Hairy leukoplakia	– Caused by EBV – White frond like lesion along lateral border of tongue – **Not a premalignant condition** – Treatment : Topical podophylin or systemic acyclovir.
2.	Thrush	– Caused by Candida – White chesy exudate on erythematous mucosa in post oropharynx – **Most commonly** seen on soft palate – Diagnosed by direct examination of scraping for pseudohyphal elements.
3.	Aphthous ulcer	– Painful ulcer of unknown etiology over posterior oropharynx – Thalidomide is an effective treatment.

17. **Ans. (c) HIV ELISA** *Ref. CPDT 16/e, p 55*

HIV ELISA is not useful for diagnosing HIV infection in newborn because IgG antibody of mother which has been transferred to neonate gives false positive result.

Diagnosis of HIV in newborn:	1.	Detection of HIV DNA or RNA by PCR (Most effective)
	2.	HIV culture
	3.	HIV p24 antigen assay.

18. **Ans. (a) and (b) Gag and Tat** *Ref. Ananthanarayan 10/e, p 575*

Genes of HIV
Genes coding for structural protein
gag gene — determine the core and shell of virus pol gene — codes for reverse transcriptase and other enzymes endonuclease env gene — encodes the envelope glycoprotein
Regulatory gene
tat gene – enhance expression of all viral gene nef gene – down regulating viral replication rev gene – enhancing expression of structural protein vif gene – influence infectivity of viral particle vpu gene – (present only in HIV - 1) ⎤   ⎬ Enhance maturation and release of progeny vpx gene – (present only in HIV - 2) ⎦ vpr gene – stimulate promoter region of virus LTR sequence – Giving promoter, enhancer, integration signal Note: Detection of type specific sequences vpu and vpx is useful in distinguishing between HIV-1 and HIV-2.

Fungal infection in AIDS patient are:
- ***Pneumocystis carinii*** (*MC opportunistic infection in HIV patient*)
- ***Cryptococcus neoformans*** (*MC cause of meningitis in HIV patient*)
- *Histoplasma*
- *Penicillium marneffei*
- *Coccidiodes immitis*
- *Aspergillosis* (pseudomembraneous bracheobronchitis in AIDS patient).
- *Sporothrix.*

Note: Cryptosporidium is a parasite not a fungus.

19. **Ans. (a, b, c, d) and (e) All are correct options** *Ref. Park 22/e, p 322-323*
    Guys, please see AIDS defining criteria from theory portion.

20. **Ans. (c) and (e) *Cryptococcus*; and *Giardia lambia*** *Ref. Harrison 19/e, p 1257, 20/e, p 1435*

Cause of diarrhea in HIV patient		
Bacterial	**Fungal**	**Parasitic**
– Shigella	– Histoplasmosis	– Cryptosporidia
– Salmonella	– Penicillosis	– Microsporidia
– Campylobacter	– Coccidioidomycosis	– Isospora belli

21. **Ans. (a) CD4** *Ref. Ananthanarayan 10/e, p 577*
    The specific receptor of HIV virus is CD-4 antigen

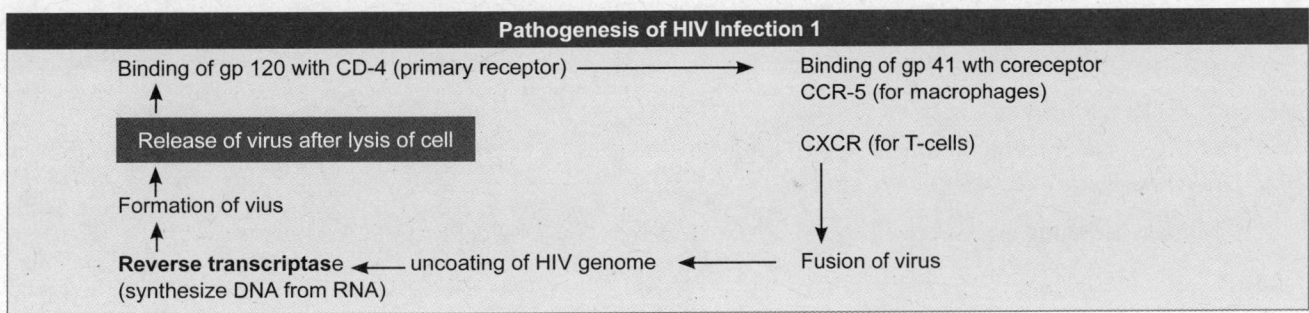

22. Ans. (a,b) *Cryptococcus, Toxoplasma* *Ref. Harrison 19/e, p 1263, 20/e, p 1443*

Neurologic disease in patients with HIV infection	
Opportunistic infections • Toxoplasmosis • Cryptococcosis • Progressive multifocal leukoencephalopathy • Cytomegalovirus • Syphilis • Mycobacterium tuberculosis • HTLV 1 infection **Neoplasms** • Primary CNS lymphoma • Kaposi's sarcoma **Result of HIV-1 infection** • Aseptic meningitis • HIV-associated neurocognitive impairment, including HIV encephalopathy/AIDS dementia complex	**Myelopathy** • Vacuolar myelopathy • Pure sensory ataxia • Paresthesia/dysesthesia **Peripheral neuropathy** • Acute inflammatory demyelinating polyneuropathy (Guillain-Barré syndrome) • Chronic inflammatory demyelinating polyneuropathy (CIDP) Monoeuritis multiplex • Distal symmetric polyneuropathy **Myopathy**

Remember:
- MC cause of meningitis in AIDS patient: Cryptococcus
  - Seizures in AIDS patient can be due to HIV encephalopathy (MC), cerebral toxoplasmosis, cryptococcal meningitis (8%) CNS lymphoma (15-30%), progressive multifocal leukoencephalopathy.

NEET Pattern Questions

1. Which of the following is most sensitive for diagnosis of HIV? **[NEET Pattern 2018]**
   a. RT PCR
   b. bDNA assay
   c. NASBA
   d. P24 detection
   [Ref. Harrison 20/e, p 1426]

   > RT PCR can detect as less as 40 copies/ml of HIV RNA, where bDNA assay and NASBA detects when conc. is more than 50 copies/ml and 80 copies/ml respectively.

2. HIV can infect all *except*:
   a. Circulating dendritic cells
   b. CD4 T lymphocytes
   c. Macrophages
   d. Cytotoxic T cells   *[Ref. Ananthanarayan, 10/e, p 577]*

3. Co-receptor for R5 variant of HIV virus:
   a. Integrin
   b. CCR 5
   c. CXCR 4
   d. P 53
   [Ref. Harrison 20/e, p 1413]

4. An HIV patient developed goitre. On examination there was non-tender diffuse enlargement of thyroid. All of the following can be cause of it, *except*:
   a. Toxoplasma
   b. Cryptococcus
   c. Aspergillus
   d. Pneumocystic   *[Ref. Harrison 20/e, 1440]*

   > In an HIV patient thyroid functions may be altered in 10-15% patients. Both hypo and hyperthyroidism may be seen though the former is more common.
   > In advance HIV disease infection of thyroid may occur with opportunistic pathogens including P. jiroveci, CMV, mycobacteria, Toxoplasma gondii and cryptococcus neoformans.

5. Binding of gp 120 causes:
   a. Infection of target cell
   b. Facilitation of co-receptor
   c. Fusing of virus and target cell
   d. None   *[Ref. Ananthanarayan, 10/e, p 577]*

   > The replication cycle of HIV begins with the high affinity bindings of the gp 120 protein to CD4 molecule on host cell. After binding gp 120 protein undergoes confirmational changes that facilitate binding of one of two major co-receptor (CCR-5, CXCR4).

6. What is p24:
   a. Envelope antigen in HIV
   b. Core antigen in HIV
   c. Genome of HIV
   d. Shell antigen   *[Ref. Ananthanarayan, 10/e, p 575]*

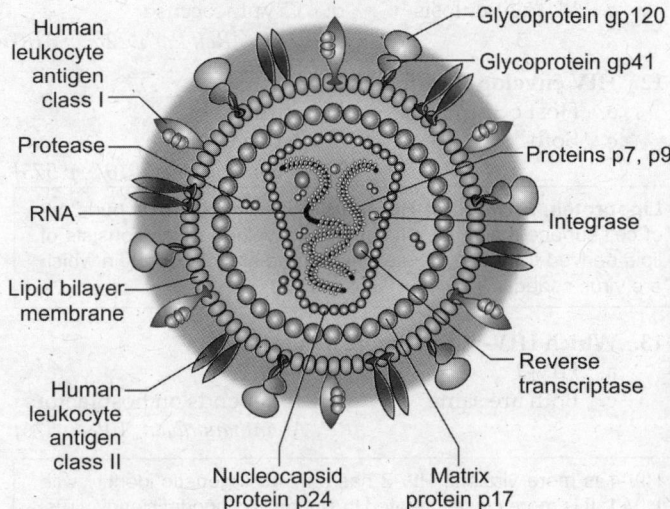

Human immunodeficiency virus
Baltimore group VI (ssRNA-RT)

7. Nef gene in HIV is for use:
   a. Enhancing the expression of genes
   b. Enhancing viral replication
   c. Decreasing viral replication
   d. Maturation   *[Ref. Ananthanarayan, 10/e, p 575]*

8. Most sensitive test for HIV infection:
   a. Western blot
   b. ELISA
   c. Agglutination test
   d. CFT
   [Ref. Harrison, 20/e, p 1424]

9. HTLV extra gene is:
   a. Gag
   b. Pol
   c. Env
   d. Tex

   > Some retrovirus such as HTLV and HIV carry a fourth gene tex or tat after env gene. This is a transactivating gene that regulates the function of viral gene.

Ans.
1. **a.** RT PCR
2. **d.** Cytotoxic T cells
3. **b.** CCR5
4. **c.** Aspergillus
5. **b.** Facilitation of...
6. **b.** Core anthigen...
7. **c.** Decreasing viral...
8. **a.** Western blot
9. **d.** Tex

Self-Assessment and Review of Microbiology and Immunology

10. **The chance that a health worker gets HIV from an accidental needle prick is:**
    a. 1%
    b. 10%
    c. 95%
    d. 100%
    [Ref. Harrison, 20/e, p 1401]

> HIV transmission following skin puncture from a needle or a sharp object that was contaminated with blood from a person with documented HIV infection is 0.3% and after a mucous membrane exposure is 0.09%

11. **Most common opportunistic infection in HIV, globally:**
    a. P. jiroveci
    b. Candida
    c. M. tuberculosis
    d. Cryptococcus
    [Ref. Park, 22/e, p 318]

12. **HIV envelop is formed by:**
    a. Host cell
    b. Virus
    c. Both
    d. None
    [Ref. Ananthanarayan, 10/e, p 575]

> **Lipoprotein Envelop of HIV virus:** When naked virus buds out of cell surface it acquire a lipoprotein envelope which consists of lipid derived from the host cell membrane and glycoprotein which are virus coded.

13. **Which HIV-virus is more dangerous:**
    a. HIV-1
    b. HIV-2
    c. Both are same
    d. It depends on host factors
    [Ref. Ananthanarayan, 10/e, p 576]

> HIV-1 is more virulent. HIV-2 has only 40% genetic identity with HIV-1. It is more closely related to simian immunodeficiency virus.

14. **Which of the following is not seen in HIV patient with CD4 countless than 100/ml, who has non productive cough?**
    a. Mycobacterium tuberculosis
    b. Pneumocystis carinii
    c. Mycoplasma pneumoniae
    d. Cryptococcal infection
    [Ref. Ananthanarayan 8/e p 576, Harrison 19/e p 1250]

> **Opportunistic infection in HIV patient when CD4 < 100/µl**
> - Coccidiodomycosis
> - Disseminated MAC
> - CMV retinitis
> - Cryptosporidiosis
> - Histoplasmosis
> - CVS Lymphoma

15. **A person has unprotected sex 3 weeks back. To rule out HIV infection the best test is:**
    a. P24 antigen assay [Ref. Ananthanarayan, 10/e, p 580]
    b. ELISA
    c. Western blot
    d. Lymph node biopsy

> **P24 capture assay**
> - ELISA which uses anti-p24 antibody as solid phase.
> - Test in useful in patient with recent exposure
> - Positive in about 30% of HIV infected person

16. **HTLV-1 is also known as:**
    a. HIV
    b. ATLV
    c. RSV
    d. ALV
    [Ref. Harrison 20/e p 1390]

17. **A HIV mother delivers a baby. All are true except:**
    a. Risk of HIV in the baby is up to 90%
    b. HIV infection cannot be diagnosed in the baby with available methods
    c. AIDS can be transmitted from mother to child during delivery
    d. Breastfeeding can transmit AIDS
    [Ref. Harrison 20/e p 1402]

> In the absence of prophylactic antiretroviral treatment the probability of transmission of HIV from mother to fetus ranges from 15 to 25% in developed country and 25 to 35% in developing countries. ..... Harrison, p 1223
> **Relative proportion of mother to child transmission are:**
> 23 to 30% – In utero
> 50 to 65% – During birth
> 12 to 20% – Breastfeeding.

Ans.
10. a. 1%
11. c. M. tuberculosis
12. c. Both
13. a. HIV-1
14. c. Mycoplasma pneumoniae
15. a. P24 antigen assay
16. b. ATLV
17. a. Risk of HIV in the baby is up to 90%

SECTION B

UNIT III

Mycology

- Superficial and Subcutaneous Mycosis
- Yeast and Yeast-like Fungus
- Aspergillus and Mucormycosis
- Dimorphic Fungi

Superficial and Subcutaneous Mycosis

CHAPTER 29

DERMATOPHYTES

- Filamentous fungi (Mould) that infect only superficial keratinized tissues – skin, hair and nail.
- Causative agent of *Ringworm or Tinea or Dermatophytoses*.
- Not involve living tissues.
- *It classified in to 3 genera* on the base of morphology of macroconidia – (*Trichophyton, Microsporum, Epidermophyton*).
- *In lesion,* it form *hyphae* and *arthrospores*.
- *In culture* it form *septate hyphae* and *asexual* spores (micro and macroconidia) with powdery and pigmented colonies.
- They are *differentiated* mainly by *nature of macroconidia*.
- In some species of dermatophytes sexual reproductive state has been discovered and all dermatophyte with a sexual form belong to telemorphic genus *Arthroderma*.
- *Culture media: Sabauraud's agar.*

Dermatophytes:
Infect keratinised tissue only.
Includes:
- Trichophyton: Infect hair, skin and nail
- Microsporum: Infect hair and skin
- Epidermophyton: Infect skin and nail only.

Clinical Features

- Local inflammation is due to irritation by fungal products and hypersensitivity reaction.
- Transmission occurs from *infected to uninfected person often by brushes, combs and towels*.

Features	Trichophyton	Microsporum	Epidermophyton
Site	Infect hair, skin and nail	Hair and skin only	Skin and nail only
Mnemonic	Trishna	Mi skin hairs	Epi ski nai
Colony	Powdery, pigmented	Cotton like pigmented	Powdery greenish yellow
Spores			
• Microconidia	Abundant	Relatively scanty	Absent
• Macroconidia	Pencil or Cylindrical shaped, relatively scanty	Multicellular Spindle or fusiform shaped and is predominant spore	Club-shaped or pear-shaped multicellular

- Clinically ringworm is classified depending on the site involved, e.g. *Tinea capitis* infect scalp and hair.
- *MC species* infecting human being – *T. rubrum*.

> **Note:** *Dermatomycosis:* Sometime used as synonym of dermatophytoses, truely it includes the cutaneous manifestation of other systemic mycosis also (e.g. Candida)

Dermatophytids: Hypersenstivity to fungal antigens result in sterile vesicular lesions sometimes seen in sites distant from the ringworm. These lesions may follow antifungal therapy and can be confused with drug allergy.

Lab Diagnosis

- *KOH mounts:* Scrapings from edges of ringworm lesions + 10% KOH. Microscopy reveals branched septate hypae.
- *UV light (Wood's lamp):* To facilitate selection of infected hair for examination (*infected hair appears fluorescent*). Two types of hair infection may be seen:
  - *Ectothrix* - Arthrospores form sheath around the hair.
  - *Endothrix* - Spores are inside the hair shaft.
- *Culture:* Sabouraud's medium (with antibiotics and cycloheximide)

Treatment

- Topical antifungal agents, Oral griseofulvin is **DOC**.

SUBCUTANEOUS MYCOSIS

- Principally seen in tropical and subtropical areas
- Most frequent predisposing factor is trauma
- Includes:
  - Mycotic mycetoma
  - Chromomycosis (chromoblastomycosis and phaeohyphomycosis)
  - Sporotrichosis
  - Rhinosporidiosis
  - Subcutaneous phycomycosis

MYCETOMA

- Chronic slowly progressive post traumatic infections of the subcutaneous tissue

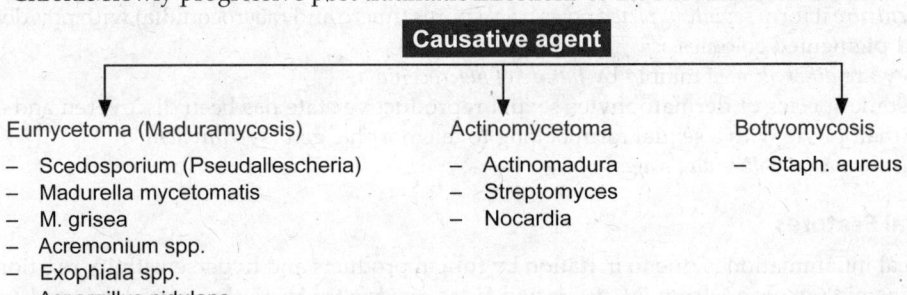

Eumycetoma (Maduramycosis)	Actinomycetoma	Botryomycosis
- Scedosporium (Pseudallescheria)	- Actinomadura	- Staph. aureus
- Madurella mycetomatis	- Streptomyces	
- M. grisea	- Nocardia	
- Acremonium spp.		
- Exophiala spp.		
- Aspergillus nidulans		
- Fusarium spp.		

- **Clinical Presentation**
  - Small subcutaneous swelling after minor trauma. Swelling gradually enlarges, burrowing deeper tissue and tracking to the surface as multiple sinuses, discharging viscid, seropurulent fluid containing granules. The lesions are characteristically painless.
- **Diagnosis:** Based on examination of granules
  - Granules are actually microcolonies of the agents
  - Growth of organism on culture on SDA at 37°C or room temperature helps in establishing diagnosis of eumycetoma
- Treatment: Surgery is the mainstay in eumycetoma

Chromomycosis

Group of clinical manifestations caused by various dematiaceous (pigmented) fungi: Includes:
a. Chromoblastomycosis (verrucous dermatitis): **MC** form of chromomycosis
   - Characterized by warty, cutaneous nodules which resemble the florets of cauliflower.
   - Disease is confined to subcutaneous tissue of the feet and lower leg
   - Causative agent are genera of Fonsecaea, Exophiala dermatidis, Phialophora and Clodophialophora
   - Diagnosis is made by presence of fungus as round on irregular dark brown yeast like bodies with septae called sclerotic bodies (See color plate, pg xxxiv for related image)
b. **Phaeophycomycosis**
   - Localized on systemic infections caused by Phialophora, Clodosporium
   - Site of lesion may be cutaneous, subcutaneous, deeper tissue, on organs like brain or lung.
   - Sclerotic bodies are absent.

Subcutaneous zygomycosis (entomophthoromycoses)
   - Originally reported from Indonesia
   - Caused by conidobolus coronatus and Basidiobolus ranarum. Both are saphrophytic
   - Disease is characterized by painless subcutaneous nodule which enlarge to involve whole limb on large areas of body
   - Diagnosis is made by histopathological examination which shows sharp broad segmented hyphae with beak like projections

Multiple Choice Questions

1. *T. capitis* (endothrix) is caused by: [PGI 00]
   a. *Epidermophyton*
   b. *T. tonsurans*
   c. *T. violaceum*
   d. *Microsporum*

2. Kerion is caused by: [PGI 98]
   a. *Candida*
   b. *Streptococcus*
   c. Dermatophytes
   d. Herpes

3. *Tinea cruris* is caused by: [PGI 97]
   a. *Epidermophyton*   b. *Trichophyton*
   c. *Microsporum*   d. *Candida*

4. A female had a thorn prick 5 years ago. She presented with a slowly growing 2 × 2 cm verrucous lesion which on KOH mount showed the following image: [AIMS 17]

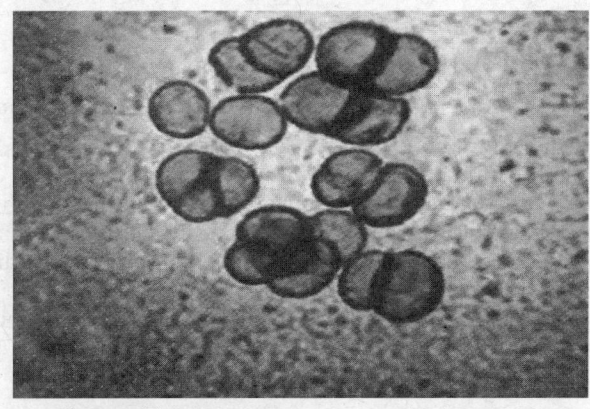

   a. Chromoblastomycosis
   b. Blastomycosis
   c. Sporotrichosis
   d. Phaeophycomycosis

Explanations and References with Illustrative Answers

1. **Ans. (b) and (c)** *T. tonsurans* and *T. violaceum*   Ref. Ananthnarayan, 9/e, p 597; 10/e, p 601

Dermatophytoses	Common causative agents
Tinea capitis	Microsporum, Trichophyton most species
Favus	T. schoenleinii T. violaceum, M. gypseum
Tinea barbae	T. rubrum, T. mentagrophytes, T. verrucosum
Tinea imbricata	T. concentricum
Tinea corporis	T. rubrum and any other dermatophyte
T. cruris (Tock itch)	E. floccosum, T. rubrum
T. pedis (Athlete foot)	T. rubrum, E. floccosum
Ectothrix hair infection	Microsporum species, T. rubrum
Endothrix hair infection	T. schoenleinii, T. tonsurans, T. violaceum

2. **Ans. (c)** Dermatophytes   *Ref. Dashore Manual of Skin, p 26*

   Kerion
   - The fungal infection of scalp caused by *microsporum or trichophyton* species.
   - Inflammatory boggy swelling covering small or large areas of scalp in which hair are loose and fallout or can be easily epilated.
   - Commonly caused by zoophilic dermatophytes like *T. mentagrophytes* and *T. verrucosum*.
   - Follicular scarring and partial alopecia is common after severe kerion.

Favus
- Chronic type of ringworm in which dense crusts (scutula) develop in hair follicles leading to alopecia and scarring

   Remember: Both kerion and favus are type of *Tinea captis*.

3. **Ans. (a) and (b) Epidermophyton and Trichophyton** *Ref. Ananthnarayan 10/e, p 601*
   Already explained, refer Ans. 1

4. **Ans. (a) Chromoblastomycosis** *Ref. Ananthanarayan 10/e p 605*
   Verrucous lesion (cauliflower like) with sclerotic bodies point towards chromblastomycosis
   Important point about chromblastomycosis
   - Commonest form of chromomycosis
   - Usually affects barefoot agriculture workers and wood cutter
   - Lesion consists of warty cutaneous nodules which resemble florets of a cauliflower.
   - Caused by Fonsecaes genera, Exophiala dermatidis, Phialophora and Cladophialophora.
   - Infections caused by F. Pedrosoi and P. verrucosa disseminate to other areas like brain.
   - Sclerotic bodies are diagnostic which can be seen in KOH mount or in tissue sections or by culture on Sabouraud Agar.

NEET Pattern Questions

1. **Dermatophytids are:**
   a. Fungal hyphae in skin
   b. Vegitative fungal cells in keratinised tissue
   c. Cutaneous lesions secondary to hypersensitivity to fungal antigens
   d. Dead fungal tissue   [Ref. Ananthanarayan 10/e, p 601]

> Dermatophytids are the cutaneous lesions secondary to hypersensitivity to fungal antigens. The reaction may follow oral antifungal therapy

2. **Regarding fungal cell wall all are true *except*:**
   a. Contains chitin
   b. Prevent osmotic damage
   c. Azoles act on them
   d. Does not contain peptidoglycan
   [Ref. Book of General Microbiology 2/e, p 58]

> Fungi possess rigid cell wall which is composed polysaccharide homopolymers such as glucans and chitin, rather than peptidoglycan (a component of bacterial all wall)
> - Functions of fungal cell wall
>   - Gives shape and farm
>   - Protects against mechanical injury
>   - Protects against osmotic lysin
> - Drugs acting on fungal cell wall: Amphotericin and Nystatin, Hamycin, Natamycin, Caspofungin.
> - Azoles inhibit ergosterol synthesis and interfere membrane function

3. **Tinea pedis is caused by which of the following?**
   a. E. floccosum
   b. M. furfur
   c. M. canis
   d. E. werneckii   [Ref. Ananthanarayan 10/e, p 601]

> Tinea pedis is most prevalent of all dermatophytoses and usually occur as chronic infection of toe webs. It is caused by *T. rubrun* and *E. floccosum*.

4. **Sclerotic bodies are associated with:**
   a. Mycetoma
   b. Chromoblastomycosis
   c. Sporotrichosis
   d. Rhinosporidiosis   [Ref. Ananthanarayan 10/e, p 605]

> **Chromoblastomycosis**
> - Most common form of chromomycosis
> - Lesion consist of warty, cutaneous nodules which resemble the florets of a cauliflower
> - Most common fungi responsible are species of the genera Fonsecaea and Cladophialophora
> - Histologically the lesion show the presence of the fungus as round or irregular dark brown yeast like bodies with septae called sclerotic bodies.

5. **Pityriasis versicolor is caused by:**
   a. E. floccosum
   b. M. gypseum
   c. M. furfur
   d. T. tansurans
   [Ref. Ananthanarayan 10/e, p 600, 9/e, p 595]

> **Pityriasis versicolor**
> - Chronic asymptomatic involvement of the stratum corneum characterised by discrete or confluent macular areas of discoloration or depigmentation
> - Causative agent is a lipolytic, yeast-like fungus pityrosporum orbicular (Malassezia furfur)

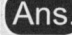 **Ans.**
1. c. Cutaneous lesions...
2. c. Azoles act on them
3. a. E. floccosum
4. b. Chromoblastomycosis
5. c. M. furfur

Yeast and Yeast-like Fungus

CHAPTER 30

CRYPTOCOCCUS NEOFORMANS

Cryptococcus:
- Only pathogenic yeast and is characterized by thick polysaccharide capsule.
- Pathogenic cryptococcus grows at 37°C whereas others do not
- Most common predisposing factor: AIDS
- Meningoencephalitis is the most important manifestation

- Only yeast which is pathogenic (Infact most life threatening fungal pathogen). Only deep mycosis which is common in India. Also called as European blastomycosis.
- Characterized by a thick polysaccharide capsule which can be stained by India Ink.
  ...... *Ananthanarayan 10/e, p 617*
- There are two species, *C. neoformans* and *C. gattii* which can cause cryptococcosis in humans. *C. gattii* to rare and may infect normal individual.
- *C. neoformans* is found in feces of pigeon and other birds whereas *C. gatti* inhabits eucalyptus tree.
- *C. neoformans* occurs in two varieties *grubii* and *neoformans* which correlates with *serotype A* and *D* respectively.

Morphology

- **Cell wall** is Gram-positive.
- All species of cryptococcus are encapsulated and possess urease.
- *C. neoformans* differs from nonpathogenic species of *Cryptococcus* by its ability to grow at 37°C and the production of laccase, a phenol oxidase which catalyses formation of melanin, and its ability to produce urease.
  ...... *Jawetz 27/e, p 688*
- Virulence factors:
  – Polysaccharide capsule
  – Ability to make melanin
  – Elaboration of enzymes (phospholipase and urease).

- Commonest site of clinical manifestation: CNS
- Primary site of infection: Lungs

Pathogenesis and Pathology

- *MC predisposing factor* for cryptococcosis: **AIDS** (risk increase when CD4 <200/ul).
- Most infections in immunocompromised patient are caused by serotype A.
- Infection is acquired by inhalation of the fungus into lung, which is frequently asymptomatic. However, in immunocompromised state there is hematogenous spread from lung to brain which leads to meningoencephalitis.
- Cryptococci are best seen in tissue by staining with *methenamine silver or periodic acid* Schiff.
- Infection can occur by pigeon dropping (Containing serotypes A & D) or eucalyptus tree (Containing serotype B).

- In addition to their capsular serotypes, the two species differ in their genotypes, ecology.

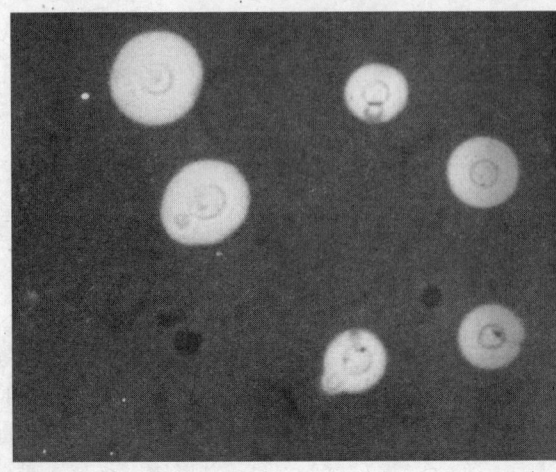

Clinical Manifestation

- Most patient present with meningoencephalitis, though primary site of infection is lung.
- *C. neoformis* is *MC* cause of *meningitis in* **AIDS** patient.
- *C. meningitis* may not show meningismus, which is seen in bacterial meningitis and it may be associated with sudden vision loss.
- In cryptococcal meningitis CSF examination reveals evidence of chronic meningitis with mononuclear pleocytosis and increased protein level and reduced glucose level.
- Focal lesions called cryptococcomas are *more common* in previously normal patient.
- These lesions are located *MC* at **basal ganglia** or the head of caudate nucleus.
- Cryptococcomas are *best* seen with *MRI*.
- *Cryptococcus* in **AIDS** patient has less sign and symptoms.
- Headache is *MC* symptom.
- Uncommon manifestation of cryptococcus include, skin lesions resembling mollascum contagiosum, lymphadenopathy, palatal and glossal ulcers, arthritis, prostatitis, myocarditis.

Diagnosis

- Lumbar puncture is single most useful *diagnostic test*. Visualization of capsules of fungal cells in CSF is a useful rapid diagnostic technique.
- *Indian Ink preparation* is the *method of choice for detecting cryptococci in CSF as the cryptococcal capsule excludes ink particle.*
- Culture of CSF and blood for C. neoformans
- *Latex agglutination* – Approx 90% of patient with cryptococcal meningitis including all AIDS patient, have capsular antigen detectable in CSF. However this is less useful in diagnosis of pulmonary disease.

Treatment

	Type of disease	Preferred treatment	Alternative
i.	Disease in AIDS Patient	Amphotericin B	Itraconazole
ii.	Disease in non AIDS Patient		
	– Meningitis	Amphotericin B	Switch over to fluconazole when patient condition has improved
	– Pulmonary disease		
	Immunocompromised Patient	Amphotericin B	Switch over to fluconazole when patient condition has improved
	Normal	Fluconazole	Itraconazole

CANDIDA

Candidiasis is *MC* systemic mycosis.
- *MC* agent responsible is *Candida albicans*. Now incidence of *C. glabrata* is also increasing.
- All pathogenic *Candida* are commensals of humans particularly in mouth, stool and vagina.

Morphology

- Gram-positive fungi
- They grow as budding yeast cells but they can also form pseudohyphae (except *C. glabrata* which does not) both in culture and in tissues.
- *Candida albicans* is dimorphic as it also forms true hyphae *[other species of Candida are not dimorphic].* ... *Jawetz 27/e, p 684*
- *C. albicans* is identified on basis of their ability to form of large thick walled spores *(diagnostic)* called *chlamydospores* on nutritionally deficient media or corn meal agar at 20°C.
- *C. albicans* form germ tubes *[Reynolds Braude Phenomenon].*
- *Accurate identification* of *Candida* species other than *C. albicans* require biochemical tests.

Candida
- Most common systemic mycosis
- Candida albicans is the most common pathogenic candida
- Candida albicans form chlamydospores at 20°C on corn meal agar
- Diabetes is the most common risk factor.

Pathogenesis

- Invasive candidiasis is usually preceded by ↑ colonization in mouth, vagina due to broad spectrum antibiotics.
- Innate immunity is the most important defence mechanism against hematogeneously disseminated candidiasis and neutrophil is the most important component of this defense.
- Majority of non-albicans vagina species enter the blood through intravascular catheterization.
- In its most serious form Candida form microabscess and small microabscess in major organs.

Clinical Manifestation

I. Cutaneous and mucosal candidiasis:
- **Risk factors** association with superficial candidiasis are:
  - AIDS
  - Pregnancy
  - **Diabetes** (MC)
  - Infants and elders
  - Oral contraceptives
  - Trauma
  - Steroids

It includes the following

A. Oral thrush
- Painless discrete and confluent adherent white plaques on the oral and pharyngeal mucosa, common in AIDS at CD4 <50/µl, bottle fed infants, debilitated patient.
- Cutaneous candidiasis may be **intertriginous** (erythematous scaling or moist lesion) or **paronychial** (seen in occupation which require frequent immersion of hands in water).

B. Esophageal candidiasis:
- Most lesion are in distal 3rd of esophagus. Diagnosed by biopsy.

C. Vulvovaginal candidiasis:
- Mostly in 3rd trimester of pregnancy.

D. Chronic mucocutaneous candidiasis:
- Mostly onset is in early childhood and association with cellular immunodeficiencies and endocrinopathy. Present as hyperkeratotic skin lesion, partial alopecia, and both oral and vaginal thrush.

II. Deeply Invasive (systemic) candidiasis:

Risk factor for invasive candidiasis
- Prolonged neutropenia
- Recent surgery
- Broad spectrum antibiotic therapy
- Presence of intravascular catheters
- Intravenous drug use

- Hematogenous seeding (candidemia) is common to retina, kidney, spleen, liver.
- *In immunocompetent patient*- U/L or B/L white retinal exudates appear within 2 weeks of onset of candidemia. Most cases of ocular involvement occur in non neutropenic patient.
- *Hepatosplenic candidiasis* (Chronic disseminated candidiasis) usually occur in patient with acute leukemia. originates from intestinal seeding of portal and venous circulation. Mostly occur in neutropenic patient.
- *Candida* can cause arthritis of knee in patient who have received *chronic glucocorticoid* injections in joint.
- Endocarditis in previously damaged or prosthetic valve.
- Brain, chorioretina, heart and kidneys are commonly infected.

Diagnosis

i. *Superficial candidiasis*: Demonstration of pseudohyphae or hyphae on wet smear with confirmation by culture or staining (Gram's, PAS, Methenamine silver).
ii. *Invasive candidiasis*: Diagnosed by histologic section of biopsies or by culture of CSF, blood, joint fluid. C. albicans is identified by production of germ tubes or chlamydospores.
   - A rapid method for identifying Candida albicans is based on its ability to form germ tubes within two hours when incubated in human serum at 37°C (Reynolds–Braude Phenomenon)

- Diabetes is the most common risk factor for mucocutaneous candidiasis
- Neutropenia is the most prominent risk factors for invasive candidiasis

- (1-3)-β-D-glucan (BDG) testing: Cell wall polysaccharide, (1-3)-β-D-glucan is found in most fungi with the notable exception of cryptococci, the zygomycetes and Blastomyces dermatidis. BDG can be detected in patient serum in case of invasive fungal infection caused by any fungi containing BDG in its cell wall.

Treatment

	Type	Preferred	Alternative
i.	**Mucocutaneous**		
	• Cutaneous	Topical azoles	Topical nystatin
	• Vulvovaginal	Azole cream or oral fluconazole	Nystatin suppository
	• Oropharyngeal	Clotrimazole or fluconazole	Nystatin
	• Esophageal	Fluconazole or itraconazole	
ii.	**Deeply invasive**		
	• Non-neutropenic	Fluconazole or amphotericin B	
	• Neutropenic	Amphotericin B	
iii.	***Candida* endophthalmitis**	IV polyene + flucytosine	

PNEUMOCYSTIS INFECTION

- Opportunistic fungal pulmonary pathogen, lacks ergosterol so not susceptible to antifungal which inhibit ergosterol synthesis.
- Human isolate – *P. jiroveci*; *P. carinii* is found in rats.   ... *Harrison 18/e, p 1671, 20/e p1547*
- **Most prominent antigen**: Major surface glycoprotein which shows antigenic variation and facilitates its adherence.
- Other important antigen is 35-55kDa - which acts as marker of infection.
- In tissues P. Jiroveci occur in two distinct forms:
  - Thin walled trophozoites.
  - Thick walled spherical or elliptical cysts which contain four to eight nuclei. Cyst can be stained with silver stain. toulidine blue, calcoflour white.
- Molecular studies have clearly placed *P. carnii* among the fungi with a close relationship to ascomycetis.
- The classification is based on analysis of gene sequences for ribosomal RNA, mitochondrial proteins, and major enzymes.
- The cell wall of *P. carnii* contain B glucon similar to other fungi.
- In contrast to most fungus *P. carnii* lacks ergosterol and is not susceptible to ergosterol inhibiting antifungal drugs.

> **Remember:** *P. carnii* (now called *P. jeroveci*) is **MC oppurtunistic infection** in AIDS patient.

Pneumocystis
P. jiroveci is the human isolate
- Major surface glycoprotein in the most important antigen
- AIDS is the most common predisposing factor
- PCR is the most sensitive technique for diagnosis.

Pneumocystic pneumonia
– Transmission: Air borne, person to person
– CXR: Bilateral diffuse perihilar infiltrates

Pathogenesis and Pathology

- Defects in CMI and humoral immunity predispose for its reactivation or reinfection, e.g. In HIV infection occur when **CD4 + T cell count <200/μl**.
- Principal host effector cells – Alveolar macrophage.
- *Transmission* – Airborne; person-to-person.
- **In alveoli:** – It attaches to **type I cells** (extracellular) and damages it.
  - Hypertrophy of type II cells occur, causing surfactant abnormalities.
  - Increase IL-8 and neutrophil in BAL fluid.
  - Alveoli gets filled with typical foamy vacuolated exudate.
- **Malnourished infants exhibit an intense** plasma cell interstitial infiltrate seen (so earlier called as *Interstitial plasma cell pneumoniae*).

P-carinii produce interstitial pneumonia

> **Risk Factors for *Pneumocystis pneumonia***
> - HIV
> - Immunosuppressive therapy particularly glucocorticoids for cancer
> - Organ transplantation
> - Children with primary immunodeficiency disease and premature malnourished infants.

Clinical Feature

- **Symptom** – Dyspnea, fever, non-productive cough.
- **Sign** – Tachypnea tachycardia and cyanosis but lung auscultation reveals few abnormalities.
- Risk for extrapulmonary spread increase with: Administration of aerosolized pentamidine.
- *MC* extrapulmonary site: **Lymph node**, spleen, liver, bone marrow.
- Most widely used prognostic factor is degree of hypoxemia.

Pathology

- Alveoli becomes filled with proteinoceous material resulting in increased alveolar capillary injury and surfactant abnormalities.

Diagnosis

1. **Definitive diagnosis by histopathologic detection by:**
   a. Staining – Methenamine silver, toludine blue stain cell wall while *Wright-Giemsa stain the nuceli*.
      – Immunofluorescence with monoclonal antibodies; more sensitive.
   b. DNA amplification by PCR – *most sensitive*.
2. **Specimen collection**
   a. *Fiberoptic bronchoscopy with BAL* (which is more sensitive than sputum induction) is the mainstay of diagnosis.
   b. *Transbronchial biopsy and open lung biopsy* – *only when* diagnosis cannot be made by BAL.
3. **Chest X-ray**
   - Classic findings include:
     – B/L diffuse infiltrate in perihilar region.
     – Nodular densities, cavitary lesion, Pneumothorax can also occur.
     – ↑*Frequency of upper lobe infiltrate in patient who take aerosolized pentamidine*.
4. **CT:** *Diagnostic modality* shows diffuse ground glass opacity

Treatment

- *DOC cotrimoxazole* for all forms of pneumocystosis including extrapulmonary disease.
- Alternative for mild to moderate case – Trimethoprim + dapsone and clindamycin + primaquine.
- Alternative for moderate to severe – Pentamidine slow IV.
- Adjunctive therapy – Glucocorticoid in HIV patient with moderate to severe pneumocystosis whose pulmonary function deteriorates on taking anti-pneumocystis drugs.

Prophylaxis

- *DOC* for HIV primary and secondary (both HIV and Non HIV) prophylaxis is cotrimoxazole.
- Alternative Dapsone
- In HIV prophylaxis is indicated when:
  – $CD_4 + <200/\mu l$
  – History of oropharyngeal candidiasis.

Multiple Choice Questions

Cryptococcus

1. The capsule of *Cryptococcus neoformans* in a CSF sample is best seen by: [NEET Pattern 2019]
   a. Gram's stain
   b. Indian ink preparation
   c. Giemsa stain
   d. Methanamine-silver stain

2. The most common organism amongst the following that cause acute meningitis in an AIDS patient is: [AI 05]
   a. *Streptococcus pneumoniae*
   b. *Streptococcus agalactiae*
   c. *Cryptococcus neoformans*
   d. *Listeria monocytogenes*

3. Neurotrophic fungus is/are: [PGI 12]
   a. *Cryptococcus neoformans*
   b. Histoplasmosis
   c. *Trichophyton*
   d. *Candida*
   e. Aspergillosis

4. A patient presented with headache and projectile vomiting along with alteration in sensorium. The following parasite demonstrated on India ink staining. What is the likely diagnosis: [PGI 05]

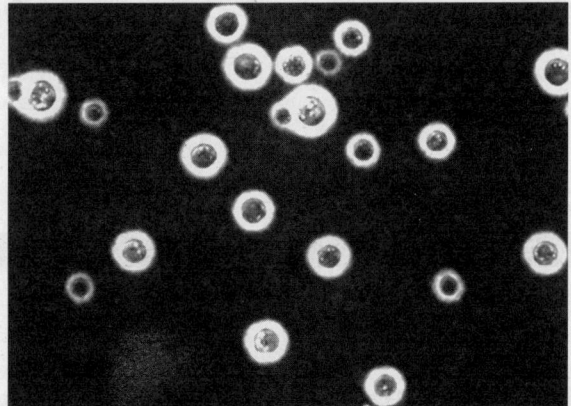

   a. Cryptococcus
   b. Blastomyces
   c. Histoplasma
   d. Coccidioides

5. 1-3 beta-D-glucan assay for fungi is not used for?
   a. Aspergillus species [AIIMS 2017]
   b. Candida species
   c. Cryptococcus species
   d. Pneumocystis jirovecii

Candida

6. An HIV positive female has an indurated ulcer over the tongue. Laboratory findings show growth in cornmeal agar at 20 degrees, microscopy showing hyphae and growth in human serum at 37 degrees show budding yeasts. The probable cause is: [AIIMS 06]
   a. *Candida albicans*
   b. Histoplasmosis
   c. Blastomycosis
   d. Coccidioidomycosis
   e. Mucormycosis

7. Most common fungal infection in febrile neutropenia is: [AI 11]
   a. Aspergillus niger
   b. Candida
   c. Mucormycosis
   d. Aspergillus fumigatus

8. Which among the following is the most common fungal infection seen in immunocompromised patients: [AIIMS 10, AI 2011]
   a. Aspergillus
   b. Cryptococcus
   c. Candida
   d. Penicillium marneffei

9. The infection that is spreading to the newborn by caregivers? [AIIMS May 2014]
   a. Candida albicans
   b. Candia galbrata
   c. Candida parapsilosis
   d. Candida tropicans

Pneumocystis

10. *Pneumocystis Jiroveci*: [AI 08]
    a. Associated with CMV
    b. Diagnosis is by sputum microscopy
    c. Seen only in immunocompromised patients
    d. Always associated with pneumatocele

Others

11. Which dye is most suitable for fungus demonstration in biopsy: [AIIMS 06]
    a. Alizarin red
    b. Verhoff dye
    c. Masson's trichrome
    d. PAS

12. All are yeast like fungus *except*: [AIIMS 97, PGI 06]
    a. *Cryptococcus*
    b. *Candida*
    c. *Trichophyton*
    d. None of the above

13. Endemic fungal infection is caused is by all of the following *except*: [PGI 05]
    a. *Coccidioides immitis*
    b. *Cryptococcus*
    c. *Penicillium*
    d. *Aspergillus*
    e. *Blastomyces*

14. Which of the following are difficult to isolate from culture: [PGI 09]
    a. *Candida*
    b. *Dermatophytes*
    c. *Cryptococcus*
    d. *Malassezia furfur*
    e. *Coccidioidomycosis*

15. Maltese cross in polarizing microscopy is seen in:
    a. Cryptococcus neoformans [AIIMS 10]
    b. Penicillium marneffi
    c. Blastomyces
    d. Candida albicans

16. Rhinosporidium seeberi belongs to: [AIIMS 2017]
    a. Fungus
    b. Bacteria
    c. Aquatic protistan protozoa
    d. Virus

Explanations and References with Illustrative Answers

1. **Ans. (b) Indian Ink preparation** Ref. Ananthanarayan 10/e, p 617; Harrison 20/e, 1328
   - *Cryptococcus neoformans* is the only pathogenic yeast.
   - Within the host and on certain culture media, it is surrounded by a large polysaccharide capsule.
   - Capsule stands out in **India Ink preparation.** ... Ananthanarayan 8/e, p 610
   - ***Indian Ink smears remains the method of choice for detecting Cryptococcus in "CSF".*** ... Harrison 20/e, p 1327
   - Cryptococci are best seen in tissue by staining with methenamine silver or periodic acid Schiff (They stain the fungus itself not capsule).
   - Mucicarmine staining of tissue is diagnostic but demonstrable only in few cases.
   - Cryptococcal antigen (CRAg) detection is sensitive and specific test for meningitis. This test is based on serologic detection of cryptococcal polysaccharide. However test is often negative in pulmonary cryptococcosis.

Diagnosis of cryptococcal disease		
Meningoencephalitis	**Pulmonary Cryptococcus**	**Cutaneous Cryptococcus**
– Lumbar puncture is **most useful** test	– Mimics malignancy	– Biopsy
– India ink smear of CSF reveals encapsulated yeast in more than half of cases	– Biopsy is required for diagnosis	
– 90% of patient have capsular antigen detectable in CSF by latex agglutination		
– CSF culture is definitive diagnostic test		

Note: MRI is more sensitive than CT in finding central nervous system cryptococcomas. ... *CMDT 2014 p1485*

2. **Ans. (c) *Cryptococcus neoformans*** Ref. Harrison 19/e, p 1346, 20/e, p 1526 - 1527
   - *C. neoformans* is MC cause of meningitis in AIDS patient.
   - Generally occurs when CD4+ T cell count **<100/μl.**
   - Diagnosis is made by identification of *C. neoformans* by India Ink or by detection of cryptococcal antigen by latex agglutination test.
   - Strongly +ve result on muciramine staining of tissue is *diagnostic.*

Predisposing factors of *Cryptococcus*	
• AIDS	• Hodgkin' Hematological malignancy
• Solid organ transplant recipient	• Cortiocosteroid therapy
• Sarcoidosis.	

Note: Among HIV(+)ve individuals, those with a decreased percentage of B-cells expressing IgM may be at a greater risk for cryptococcosis. *Treatment:* Patient with AIDS and high risk patient: I.V Amphotericin B followed by fluconazole for maintenance.

3. **Ans. (a), (b), (d) and (e) *Cryptococcus neoformans*; Histoplasmosis; Candida; and Aspergillosis** Ref. Harrison 20/e, p 2492

Fungus causing CNS infection:	– Cryptococcus	– Coccidioidomycosis	– Aspergillus
	– Histoplasmosis	– Blastomycosis	– Candidiasis
	– Sporothrix schenckii		

4. **Ans. (a) Cryptococcus** Ref. Jawetz 27/e, p 687
   This is a characteristic image of cryptococcus capsule when stained under India ink.

5. **Ans. (c) *Cryptococcus species*** Ref. Journal of Clinical Microbiology 2013 Nov. 3478-3484
   - **β-D-glucan** is the component of fungal cell-wall of all fungus (*except* cryptococcus, zygomycetes and blastomyces dermatidis) which is detectable in case of invasive infection.
   - Currently **Fungitell assay** is a FDA approved **β-DG** assay which is positive in invasive candidiasis, Aspergillism and pneumocystis jirovecii.
   - False positive reaction may be seen with certain hemodialysis filters, beta lactam antimicrobials and immunoglobulins.

Beta-(1.2)-D-glucan (BG)	
Present in	**Absent in**
• Candida spp • Aspergilllus spp • Fusarium spp • Acremonium spp • Pneumocystis jirovecii • Sporothrix schenkii • Coccidioides immitis • Histoplasma capsulatum • Blastomyces dermatitidis • Trichosporon spp • Saccharomyces cerevisiae	• Cryptococcus (capsule captures Beta (1,3) D glucan before it is released into the bloodstream) • Zygomycetes (Adsidia, Mucor, Rhizopus) • Blastomyces dermatitidis

6. **Ans. (a) *Candida albicans*** *Ref. Harrison 19/e, p 1342, 20/e, p 1530*

   "*This is a case of oral thrush secondary to candidiasis*"
   - *C. albicans* is a dimorphic fungi which occur both as yeast and moulds (with hyphae).
   - In HIV oral thrush occurs when CD4 <50/µl.

   Characteristic feature of *Candida*
   - Candidiasis is **MC** systemic mycosis.
   - *Gram-positive* fungi characterized by their ability to form *pseudohyphae*.
   - Grows rapidly at 25 to 37°C.
   - Candida *albicans* (not other species) can also form true hyphae so is dimorphic.
   - *Candida albicans* is identified on the basis of their ability to form germ tubes in serum or by formation of thick walled spores called *chlamydospores* on nutritionally deficient media.

7. **Ans. (b) *Candida*** *Ref. CMDT 2014, p 1233, 492*

   Neutropenia ↑ chance of following infection.

Bacterial	Fungal	Viral
Gram – ve enteric pathogens **(MC)** Pseudomonas Gram +ve cocci (particularly *Staph. aureus*; *Staph epidermidis*, and viridans streptococci)	Candida **(MC)** Aspergillus Pneumocystis carnii	Herpes zoster CMV Respiratory syncytial virus Influenza virus

   Organism cause infection in granulocytopenic patients *Ref. Harrison 17/e, p 535*

   - ***Gram-positive cocci***
     - Staphylococcus epidermidis
     - Staphylococcus aureus
     - Viridans Streptococcus
     - Enterococcus faecalis
     - Streptococcus pneumoniae
   - ***Gram-positive bacilli***
     - Diphtheroids
     - JK bacillus
   - ***Gram-negative bacilli***
     - Escherichia coli
     - Klebsiella spp.
     - Non-aeruginosa Pseudomonas spp.
     - Enterobacter spp.
     - Serratia spp.
     - Acinetobacter spp.
     - Citrobacter spp.
   - ***Fungi***
     - Candida spp.

8. **Ans. (c) *Candida*** *Ref. DR Arora 2/e, p 671; Clinical Mycology by Elias J Anaessie 2/e, p 2, 11, 631; Harrison, 20/e, p 1529*

   Candidiasis is the commonest mycosis involving skin, its appendeges, mucosa and internal organs.
   Oral thrush and vulvovaginal candidiasis are commonest manifestation of candida in immunocompetent.

   Other important points:
   - Aspergillus is the most common fungal sinus infection in immunocompetent patients ...*Clinical Mycology by Elias J Anaessie 2/e, p 631*
   - Candida is the most common cause of nosocomial fungal infection ...*Clinical Mycology by Elias J Anaessie 2/e, P No. 2*
   - Cryptococcus neoformans is the most common cause of community associated opportunistic fungal infection
     ....*Clinical Mycology by Elias J Anaessie 2/e, P No. 11*
   - Cryptococcus neoformans is the most life threatening fungal pathogen.

9. **Ans. (c) Candida Paraspilosis** *Ref. Clin Microbiol Rev. Oct 2008; 21(4): 606–625.*
   Candida parapsilosis is an emerging major human pathogen that has dramatically increased in significance and prevalence over the past 2 decades, such that C. parapsilosis is now the second leading causes of invasive candidal disease.
   - Individuals at the highest risk for severe infection include neonates and patients in intensive care units. *C. parapsilosis* infections are especially associated with hyperalimentation solutions, prosthetic devices, and indwelling catheters, as well as the nosocomial spread of disease **through the hands of health care workers**.
   - Factors involved in disease pathogenesis include the secretion of hydrolytic enzymes, adhesion to prosthetics, and biofilm formation.

   Important Points about Candida parapsilosis
   - Candida species are presently the fourth leading cause of nosocomial bloodstream infection.
   - Candida albicans is the most frequent isolate from blood cultures followed by Candida parapsilosis
   - C. parapsilosis does not form true hyphae and exists in either a yeast phase or a pseudohyphal form.
   - C. parapsilosis is notorious for its capacity to grow in total parenteral nutrition and to form biofilms on catheters and other implanted devices, for nosocomial spread by hand carriage.
   - C. parapsilosis is of special concern in critically ill neonates, causing more than one-quarter of all invasive fungal infections in low-birth-weight infants. Additionally, it is the predominant fungal organism isolated in many neonatal intensive care units (NICUs), where it is often associated with neonatal mortality
   - C. parapsilosis is also a normal human commensal, and it is one of the fungi most frequently isolated from the subungual space of human hands
   - C. parapsilosis fungemia can lead to seeding of tissues, resulting in deep-seated infections, and has a mortality rate ranging from 4% to 45%
   - Compared to C. albicans, C. parapsilosis more frequently caused fungemia among neonates, in patients with intravenous lines or vascular catheters, who had received prior antifungal agents, were on parenteral nutrition, or had undergone transplantation.

10. **Ans. (b) Diagnosis...** *Ref. Harrison 20/e, p 1547*

    Pneumocystis Jiroveci
    - Human isolate of Pneumocystis which is associated with severe pneumonia in immunocompromised state particularly AIDS (PcP).
    - *P. jiroveci* is an extracellular pathogen. Growth in the lung is limited to surfactant layer above alveolar epithelium.
    - Serologic evidence suggest that most individuals are infected in early childhood (thus option "c" is wrong) but the pneumonia is seen only in immunocompromised state.
    - Diagnosis is made by detection of organism in proper specimen.
    - **Specimen for *P. carnii* pneumonia (PcP)**
      - *Sputum:* Quick and non invasive.
      - *Broncho-alveolar lavage (BAL) fluid:* Mainstay of pneumocystis diagnosis.
      - *Transbronchial biopsy:* If diagnosis cannot be made by BAL.
    - The overt infection is an *acute interstitial plasma cell pneumonia* that occurs with high frequency among two groups:
      - As epidemic of primary infection among premature or debilitated or marasmic infant of hospital wards in underdeveloped countries.
      - As sporadic cases among older children and adults who have an abnormal cellular immune status.

11. **Ans. (d) PAS** *Ref. Ananthanarayan 10/e, p 596*

    "The periodic acid Schiff (PAS) and methenamine silver are valuable methods for the demonstration of fungal elements in tissue or biopsy section."

    > **Remember:**
    > - Sabaraud's glucose agar (pH - 5.4), czapek - Dox medium and corn meal agar are most commonly used media in mycology.
    > - GMS (Gomorris methenamine silver) stain is best fungal stain for biopsy section.

12. **Ans. (c) Trichophyton** *Ref. Chakraborty 2/e, p 611, 622*

    Trichophyton is dermatophyton which comes under mould.

Morphological Classification of Fungi	
Yeast	**Yeast-like fungi** (Grow partly as yeast and partly as chain of elongated budding cells forming pseudohyphae)
– Cryptococcus neoformans	– Candida

Morphological Classification of Fungi			
Moulds (Filamentous fungi)- Forms true hyphae		**Dimorphic fungi (Grows either as yeast or as filament)**	
– Dermatophyte – Zygomycetes – *Malassezia furfur* – Pseudoallescheria species	– Aspergillus – Penicillium – Madurella species – Philaphora species	– *Sporothrix schenckii* – *Histoplasma capsulatum* – *Paracoccidioides brasiliensis* – *Candida albicans* (no other spices of *Candida*) **Mnemonic –SBH Ca Powerful Personal Computer**	– **B**lastomyces dermatitides – **C**occidioides immitis – **P**enicilium marneffi

13. **Ans. (b), (c) and (d)** *Cryptococcus; Penicillium; and Aspergillus*   *Ref. Jawetz 27/e, p 674*

    Endemic mycosis includes fungal infection which are restricted to specific geographical area.
    It includes:
    - Histoplasmosis (USA)
    - Coccidioidomycosis (USA)
    - Blastomycosis *(North American blastomycosis)*
    - Paracoccidioidomycosis *(South American Blastomycosis).*

Fungal Disease in Human		
Superficial Mycoses	**Subcutaneous Mycoses**	**Systemic Mycoses**
– Dermatophytes (includes trichophyton, microsporum, epidermophyton – *Candida* – Ptyriasis/Tinea versicolor – Tinea nigra	– Mycotic mycetoma – Chromoblastomycosis – Sporotrichosis – Subcutaneous phycomycosis	– Blastomycosis – Coccidiomycosis – Paracoccidioidomycosis – Histoplasmosis – Opportunistic infections (cryptococcus, aspergillus etc.)

14. **Ans. (d)** *Malassezia furfur*   *Ref. Harrison, 20/e, p 1545; Ananthanarayan, 10/e, p 600*
    - *Malassezia furfur* (causative agent of *Tinea versicolor*) were not usually cultured in the clinical laboratory.
    - *Cryptococcus, candida, dermatophytes* and *Coccidioides* are culturable.

    Note: Now most species can be cultured by adding exogenous lipid in the Sabouraud Agar.

    Other important feature of Malassezia:
    - Part of normal flora of human skin.
    - **Dimorphic:** Colonizes skin as yeast, transform to mold phase when cause disease in tissue.
    - Lipophilic yeast and require lipid in the medium for growth.
    - Causative agent of Tinea versicolor and catheter associated sepsis (particularly in infants receiving IV lipid).
    - Diagnosis is confirmed by direct microscopic examination of scrappings of infected cells treated with 10-12% KOH with calcoflour white: short unbranced hyphae and spherical cells are observed.
    - On inspection with woodlight lesion either do not fluoroscence or appear yellow green.

15. **Ans. (a)** *Cryptococcus neoformans*   *See below*
    Medical conditions showing maltese cross

    Infections:
    - Babseia
    - Paracoccidioides
    - Cryptococcus
    - Malassezia sp.

    Lab medicine:
    - Urinalysis: 'Maltese crosses' shaped cast are seen in patients of nephrotic syndrome, eclampsia, renal toxicity, fat embolism, after crush injury and in Fabry's disease—due to aggregates of glycosphingolipids

    Orthopaedics:
    - Arthroscopic fluid following local trauma

16. **Ans. (a)** Fungus   *Ref. Ananthanarayan 10/e, p 607*
    Rhinosporiduim seeberi
    - Lower aquatic fungi forming spores
    - Natural habitat is reservoir water and perhaps soil contaminated with that water.
    - Once infected organism produce a polypoidal mass lesion in the affected area, commonest site being nose, nasopharynx, tonsil, eye.

    Diagnosis:
    Can not be cultivated in artificial media. Histologically the lesion is composed of large number of fungal spores embeded in stroma of connective tissue and capillaries.
    Treatment: Excision of the polyp is the treatment of choice.

NEET Pattern Questions

1. Virulence factor of cryptococcus includes all, except:
   a. Polysaccharide capsule
   b. Production of protease
   c. Ability to make melanin
   d. Urease production [Ref. Harrison, 20/e, p 1527]

2. Pneumocystic carnii infects:
   a. Human
   b. Monkey
   c. Rat
   d. Cats [Ref. Harrison, 18/e, p 1671]

P. carnii infects rats; P. jiroveci infects human

3. Renauld Braud phenomenon is seen is:
   a. Candida albicans
   b. Candida pscitasi
   c. Histoplasma
   d. Cryptococcus [Ref. AA, 10/e, p 616]

Candida albicans forms germ tube when incubated at 37° C in human serum (Reynolds- Braude phenomenon). This property is used for rapid diagnosis of C. albicans.

4. Which of the following is only yeast:
   a. Candida
   b. Mucor
   c. Rhizopus
   d. Cryptococcus [Ref. AA, 10/e, p 617]

Candida is a yeast-like fungus.

5. True about cryptococcus are all except:
   a. Primarily infects lung
   b. Urease negative
   c. India-ink is used
   d. All are true [Ref. Harrison, 20/e, p 1527]

Cryptococcus is urease positive fungus.

6. Most common organism causing fungal infection of oral cavity:
   a. Candida
   b. Blastomycosis
   c. Aspergillosis
   d. Cryptococcus [Ref. Harrison, 20/e, p 1529]

7. All are true about candida except:
   a. Pseudohyphae seen
   b. Produce chlamydospore
   c. It is a mould
   d. It is a dimorphic fungus [Ref. Ananthanarayan, 10/e, p 615]

Candida produce pseudomycelia, both in tissue and in culture. Chlamydospore is the thickwalled big resting spore produced by ascomycota (candida); Basidomycota (Panus); It is the life stage which survives in unfavourable conditions.

8. Type of pneumonia in P. jiroveci:
   a. Lobar pneumonia
   b. Interstitial pneumonia
   c. Bronchopneumonia
   d. Any of the above [Ref. Harrison, 20/e, p 1547]

9. Germ tube test is diagnostic for:
   a. Candida albicans
   b. Cryptococcus neoformans
   c. Histoplasma capsulum
   d. Coccidioidomycosis [Ref. Ananthanarayana 10/e, p 616]

10. Which of the following feature is used for identification of *Cryptococcus neoformans*?
    a. Oxidase +ve
    b. Dextran fermentation
    c. Hydrolyse urea
    d. Ability to grow at 42°C [Ref. Ananthanarayan 10/e, p 616]

The ability to grow at 37°C and hydrolyse urea differentiates C. neoformans from non- pathogenic cryptococci.

11. The most common type of deep mycosis in India is:
    a. Blastomycosis
    b. Histoplasmosis
    c. Coccidioidomycosis
    d. Cryptococcus [Ref. Ananthanarayan 8/e, p 610]

12. Which fungal infection is commonest in neutropenia:
    a. Candida
    b. Histoplasma
    c. Aspergillus niger
    d. Aspergillus fumigatus [CMDT 14 p 1233]

Ans.
1. b. Production of pro...
2. c. Rat
3. a. Candida...
4. d. Cryptococcus
5. b. Urease...
6. a. Candida
7. c. It is a mould
8. b. Interstitial pneu...
9. a. Candida albicans
10. c. Hydrolyse...
11. d. *Cryptococcus*
12. a. *Candida*

Aspergillus and Mucormycosis

CHAPTER 31

ASPERGILLUS

- Mold with septate hyphae with characteristic dichotomous branching and irregular outline.
- MC cause of aspergillosis: *A fumigatus*.
- Aspergillus hyphae are hyaline, narrow and septate with branching at 45°; no yeast forms are present in infected tissue. Hyphae can be seen in cytology or microscopy preparation.
- Out of many species of Aspergillus, only those species that grow at 37°C can cause invasive infection. Although some species without this capability can cause allergic syndromes.

... *Harrison 20/e, p 1532*

Aspergillosis: Collective term to describe all disorders (both allergic and invasive) caused by any of the species of Aspergillus.
A. fumigatus is responsible for most cases of invasive disease. *A. favus* is prevalent in sinus and skin infection. *A. terreus* cause invasive infection with poor prognosis.

Types of Aspergillosis

A. Respiratory disease
1. *In healthy person*: Self limited pneumonitis by massive inhalation of spores.
2. *With underlying lung disease*:
   - Allergic bronchopulmonary aspergillosis in patient with asthma, cystic fibrosis: present with wheeze, central bronchiectasis etc.
   - Endobronchial saprophytic pulmonary aspergillosis (Aspergilloma = fungus ball) in cyst or cavity of TB, sarcoidosis, bronchiectasis, histoplasmosis.
   - Often present with hemoptysis. There is no invasion.

B. Superficial infection
- Sinusitis, otomycosis (usually by *A.niger, A. fumigatus*), keratitis etc.
- Otomycosis is *MC* human disease caused by Aspergillus.
- MC radiologic finding is bilateral diffuse or focal pulmonary infiltrates with tendency to cavitate.

Note: Fungi causing corneal ulcer
- Aspergillus (MC)
- Fusarium
- Candida

C. Disseminated (invasive) Aspergillosis
- *Lung invasion confined almost entirely to immunosuppressed patients:* granulocyte count < 500/ml *[MC risk factor: acute leukemia and recipients of tissue transplants]*.
  - Invasion in neutropenic is characterized by hyphal invasion of blood vessels, thrombosis, necrosis and hemorrhagic infarction.
  - **Earliest CT finding**: One or more small pulmonary nodules; *Halo sign* (Hazy rim around infarcted tissue), *Crescent* sign (seen when Bone marrow function recovers) can be seen.
- In HIV patient, *MC* site of aspergillosis: **lung**
- Occur in HIV when **$CD_4+ < 50/\mu l$**, characterized by B/L diffuse or focal infiltrate with a tendency to cavitate.

- Mold with septate hyphae: Aspergillus
- Mold with aseptate hyphae: Rhizopus
- MC cause of aspergillosis: A. fumigatus
- MC human disease caused by aspergillus: Otomycosis

Primary risk factors for invasive aspergillosis are profound neutropenia and glucocorticoid use

Diagnosis

1. *Microscopy*:
   - Even a single isolate of Aspergillus in KOH mount of sputum of neutropenic patient or hematopoietic stem-cell transplant recipient with pneumonia particularly child or non-smoker suggest diagnosis of invasive disease.
   - PAS stain biopsy of lung, nose, paranasal sinus or sites of dissemination can also be used.
2. *Culture:*
   - Velvety to powdery surface of colony. Ability of *A.fumigatus* to grow at 45°C helps to distinguish it from other species.
   - Culture may be negative or few colonies in aspergilloma or invasive disease.

Treatment

Type of disease	Preferred treatment
Fungus ball	Lobectomy
Allergic bronchopulmonary aspergillosis	Short course of glucocorticoids
Invasive aspergillosis	Voriconazole, Amphotericin B

Multiple Choice Questions

1. In a patient, corneal scraping reveals narrow angled septate hyphae. Which of the following is the likely etiologic agent? [Neet Pattern 2018]
   a. Mucor
   b. Aspergillus
   c. Histoplasma
   d. Candida

2. Which of the following is the most common etiological agent in paranasal sinus mycoses? [AIIMS 06]
   a. Aspergillus spp.
   b. Histoplasma
   c. Conidiobolus coronatus
   d. Candida albicans

3. An early diabetic has left sided orbital cellulitis CT scan of paranasal sinus shows evidence of left maxillary sinusitis. Gram stained smear of the orbital exudate shows irregularly branching septate hyphae. The following is most likely etiological agent: [AIIMS 08]
   a. Aspergillus
   b. Rhizopus
   c. Mucor
   d. Candida

4. In HIV infected individual Gram stain of lung aspirate shows yeast like morphology. All of the following are the most likely diagnosis *except*: [AIIMS 05]
   a. Candida tropicalis
   b. Cryptococcus neoformans
   c. Penicillium marneffi
   d. Aspergillus fumigatus

5. Mucor mycosis all *except*: [AI 09]
   a. Angio-invasion
   b. Lymph invasion
   c. Septate hyphae
   d. Long term deferoxamine therapy is predisposing factor

6. A young woman complains of recurrent rhinitis, nasal discharge and bilateral nasal blockage since one year. She also had history of allergy and asthma. On examination, multiple polyps with mucosal thickening and impacted secretions are seen in nasal cavities. Biopsy was taken and the material on culture showed many hyphae with dichotomous branching typically at 45 degree. Which of the following is most likely organism responsible? [AI 2010]
   a. Rhizopus
   b. Aspergillus
   c. Mucor
   d. Candida

7. A diabetic patient present with bloody nasal discharge, orbital swelling and pain. Culture of periorbital pus showed branching septate hyphae. Which of the following is the most probable organism involved? [AI 2010]
   a. Mucor
   b. Candida
   c. Aspergillus
   d. Rhizopus

8. Aflatoxin is produced by: [AI 2011]
   a. Aspergillus flavus
   b. Candida
   c. Aspergillus niger
   d. Penicillum

9. Indentify the fungal organism in this slide stained with Gomori methenamine silver stain: [AIIMS 2017]

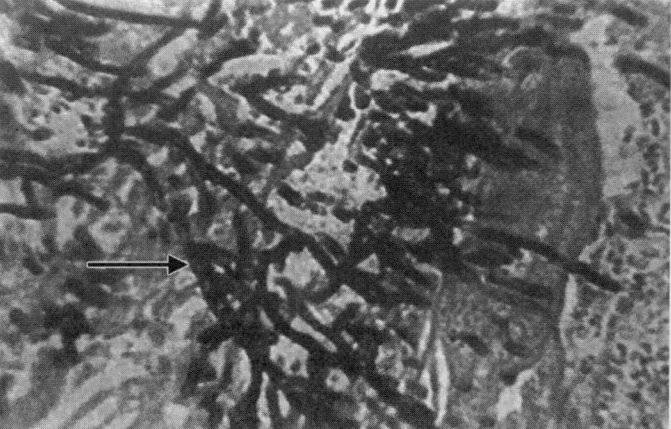

   a. Acute angle branching, Rhizopus
   b. Right angle branching, Aspergillus
   c. Acute angle branching aspergillus
   d. Right angle branching mucor

Explanations and References with Illustrative Answers

1. **Ans. (b) *Aspergillus*** Ref. Ananthanarayan 10/e, p 613; Harrison 20/e, p 1533
   - *Aspergillus* is mold with septate hyphae with branching at 45°.
   - Asexual conidia are arranged in chain, carried on elongated cells called sterigmata borne on expanded ends of conidiophores.
   - *Aspergillus fumigatus* is MC cause of **aspergillosis**.
   - Commonest human disease caused by **aspergillosis** is otomycosis.
   - *Aspergillus* infection is characterized by hyphae invasion of blood vessel, thrombosis, necrosis, and hemorrhagic infarction.

Other options:	• Mucor	– Broad nonseptate hyphae in tissue
	• Histoplasma	– Dimorphic fungi
	• Candida	– Characterised by presence of pseudohyphae.

Remember: Aspergillus is MC cause of fungal corneal ulcer.

2. **Ans. (a)** *Aspergillus spp.* Ref. Dhingra 3/e, p 241
   Many different fungal species are found to involve the paranasal sinuses, the common being *Aspergillus*; Alternaria; Mucor or Rhizopus.

Varieties of fungal infection of sinuses	
• Fungus ball	Implantation of fungus in a healthy sinus Maxillary sinus is most commonly involved Treatment is surgical removal with no antifungal therapy.
• Allergic fungal sinusitis	There is no invasion of sinus mucosa by fungus CT shows mucosal thickening with hyperdense area Treatment is endoscopic surgical drainage with pre- and postoperative systemic steroids
• Chronic invasive	Fungus invades into sinus mucosa CT shows thickened mucosa with opacification of sinus and bone erosion Treatment is endoscopic surgical removal followed by antifungal therapy.
• Fulminant fungal sinusitis	Acute presentation mostly seen in immunocompromised or diabetic individuals *Most common* fungus associated are mucor and aspergillosis.

3. **Ans. (a)** *Aspergillus* Ref. Ananthanarayan 10/e, p 613, 9/e, p 609; Harrison 20/e, p 1535
   "Presence of branched septate hyphae in a patient of orbital cellulitis (occur as complication of sinusitis) suggest Aspergillus."
   Aspergillus Sinusitis occur in three forms:
   1. Ball of hyphae may form in chronically obstructed paranasal sinus, without tissue invasion.
   2. A chronic fibrosing granulomatous inflammation begin in sinus and spread slowly to the orbit and brain.
   3. Allergic fungal sinusitis
   Mucor and Rhizopus belong to family Zygomycetes and have non-septate hyphae.

4. **Ans. (d)** *Aspergillus fumigatus* Ref. Harrison 20/e, p 1532, Ananthanarayan 10/e, p 614
   Aspergillus is a mould with septate hyphae (not have yeast-like morphology).
   Another confusing option is *option "c"*.
   Penicillum marneffi:
   • It is a dimorphic fungi, appearing as small yeast cells in tissue and as a mould in culture.
   • It is a leading cause of opportunistic infection in patients of late stage HIV.
   Candida is a group of yeast-like fungus except C. albicans which is dimorphic.

Respiratory infection in AIDS patients		
Bacterial	**Fungal**	**Viral**
S. pneumoniae (MC) H. influenzae M. tuberculosis Mycobacteria avium complex	P. carnii (MC) Penicillium marneffi Aspergillus Histoplasmosis Candida and Cryptococcus	CMV

5. **Ans. (c)** Septate hyphae Ref. Harrison 20/e, p 1537
   Causative agent of Mucormycosis: • Rhizopus • Rhizomucor • Cunninghamella.
   They are molds and have non-septate hyphae.

Predisposing factors	
• Recipient of organ transplant	• Hematologic malignancy
• Who are receiving long term desferoxamine therapy	• Diabetics
• Treatment with steroid or cytotoxic drugs	• Chronic renal failure.

Important features of Mucormycosis:
- Vascular invasion by hyphae is a prominent feature.
- Ischemic or hemorrhagic necrosis is foremost histologic findings.

Clinical Manifestations
- *Nose and paranasal sinus infection:*
  - Present with bloody nasal discharge with low grade fever and sinus pain followed in few days by double vision.
  - On examination nasal turbinate of involved side may be dusky red or necrotic.
  - Fungal invasion of ophthalmic artery or orbit may lead to blindness.
  - Coma may occur by direct invasion.
  - Cavernous sinus thrombosis.
- *Pulmonary mucormycosis:*
  - Manifest as progressive severe pneumonia.
  - Hematogenous spread to other areas
- *Cutaneous Mucormycosis:*
  - More common than disease at other site and develop after traumatic injury in which wound are contaminated with dirt.
- *GI invasion:*
  - Present as one or more ulcer which tends to perforate.

Diagnosis
- Microscopic examination and culture of biopsy are essential and swabs are insufficient.
- Organism appears as broad ribbon-like, usually non-septate hyphae with branch at right angles.

Treatment: Wide surgical debridement and intravenous amphotericin B is indicated.

6. **Ans. (b)** *Aspergillus*   *Ref. Harrison 20/e, p 1535; AA 10/e, p 612*

A fungi with septate hyphae in asthmatic patient can be none other than aspergillus, and this is a case of ***allergic bronchopulmonary aspergillosis***

Allergic bronchopulmonary Aspergillosis
- Seen in atopic individual with elevated IgE levels following sensitization to inhaled aspergillus spores
- In bronchopulmonary aspergillosis, fungus grows within the lumen of bronchioles, which may be occluded. The condition get worsened after development of hypersensitivity to the fungus
- **Diagnosis** is made by an elevated IgE, a positive skin prick test to *A. fumigatus* or detection of *Aspergillus* specific IgE and IgG. Central bronchiectasis is characteristic
- Aspergillus hyphae are hyaline, narrow and septate with branching at 45°; no yeast forms are present in infected tissue. Hyphae can be seen in cytology or microscopy preparation.

> **Remember: *Aspergillus* can cause:**
> - Allergic bronchopulmonary aspergillosis
> - Invasive aspergillosis
> - Endocarditis
> - Paranasal granuloma
> - Intracavitary aspergilloma (fungus ball)
> - Cutaneous aspergillosis
> - Cerebral aspergillosis
> - Superficial aspergilloma

7. **Ans. (c)** *Aspergillus*   *Ref. Harrison 20/e, p 1533*
- Presence of branching septate hyphae in culture suggests the diagnosis of aspergillosis (Mucor and Rhizopus have nonseptate hyphae).
- **Mucor and Aspergillus species** are the most common opportunistic agents causing orbital fungal infections. They usually involve the orbit by direct extension from nasal cavity and paranasal sinuses through bone destruction.

Histomorphical characteristics		
Characteristic	**Aspergillus**	**Zygomycetes (Mucor/Rhizopus)**
• *Diameter*	Narrow (3-6 μm)	Wide (5-20 μm)
• *Caliber*	Uniform	Varying
• *Branching*	Regular, 45° acute angle (dichotomous)	Random, right angle
• *Branching orientation*	Parallel or radial	Random
• *Hyphae*	Usually septate	Usually non-septate

8. **Ans. (a) *Aspergillus flavus***   *Ref. Ananthanarayan 10/e, p 618*

Aflatoxins are produced primarily by filamentous fungi, Aspergillus flavus and Aspergillus parasiticus.

Mycotic Poisoning	
Mycetism	**Myotoxicosis**

• Eaten Fungus itself produce toxic effects
• Cause GI disease, dermatitis
• Hallucinogenic agents (d-lysergic acid, Psilocybin) produced by psilocybe species have been used for medicinal purpose
	• Fungal toxins contaminate some articles of food examples include:
	  – Aflatoxin produced by Aspergillus flavus
	  – Ergotoxicosis produced by claviceps purpura

Aflatoxin: MC Mycotoxicosis
- It is frequently found in moldy foods, like ground nut, corn, peas
- It is highly toxic to animals, birds and human beings
- It has got carcinogenic effect in liver.

9. **Ans. (c) Acute angle branching aspergillus**   *Ref. Ananthanarayan 10/e p 594*

As mentioned earlier Aspergillus hyphae are septate and they branch at acute angle.

Differential diagnosis of fungal hyphae				
	Aspergillus species	**Zygomycetes species**	**Fusarian species**	**Pseudallescheria Boydii**
Width	3–6 µm	5–25 µm	3–8 µm	2–5 µm
Outline	Parallel	Irregular	Parallel	Parallel
Branching pattern	Dichotomous Acute angle, 45°	At 90° angle	Right angle, occasionally 45°	Haphazard
Septation	Frequent	Inconspicuous	Frequent	Frequent
Reproductive structures in tissue	Present where infected areas communicates with air	Absent	Sometimes present	—
Angioinvasive structure in tissue	Yes	Yes	Yes	—

NEET Pattern Questions

1. **Which of the following is an aseptate fungus?**
   a. Aspergillus
   b. Candida
   c. Nocardia
   d. Rhizopus
   [Ref. Greenwood 18/e 639]

2. **Bronchopulmonary aspergillosis is mediated by:**
   a. Type I hypersensitivity
   b. Type III hypersensitivity
   c. Type II hypersensitivity
   d. Both a and b   [Ref. Ananthanarayan 10/e 612]

   ABPA is mediated either by type I hypersensitivity or type III hypersensitivity (extrinsic alveolitis) or combined type I and type III hypersensitivity

3. **Aseptate hyphae is not seen in:**
   a. Rhizopus
   b. Mucor
   c. Aspergillus
   d. None   [Ref. Ananthanarayan 10/e 613]

   Aspergillus hyphae are hyaline, narrow and septate with branching at 45°; no yeast forms are present in infected tissue.

4. **Aseptate hyphae are seen in:**
   a. Phycomycetes
   b. Ascomycetes
   c. Basidiomycetes
   d. Deuteromycetes   [Ref. Ananthanarayan 10/e 594]

   Phycomycetes are lower fungi that have non septate hyphae and form endogenous asexual spores called sporangiospores.

Ans. 1. d. Rhizopus   2. d. Both a and b   3. c. Aspergillus   4. a. Phycomycetes

CHAPTER 32

Dimorphic Fungi

- **Dimorphic fungus occur in 2 forms:**
  1. **Yeast form = parasitic phase**
     In host tissues and on cultures at 37°C (enriched agar).
  2. **Spores and filamentous (mould) form = saprophytic phase**
     In soil and culture at 22-25°C or Sabouraud's agar at room temperature.
- Disease by all of them are restricted to specific areas of endemicity.
- **Dimorphic fungus are:** *Candida albicans*, *Histoplasma*, *Sporothrix schenckii*, Blastomycosis, Coccidioidomycosis, Paracoccidioidomycosis, Penicillium marneffei.

Mnemonic	= Senior Boys Hostel Ca Powerful Personal Computer.
	= His Pen Can Blast Spores of Coccido and Paracoccido

HISTOPLASMA CAPSULATUM

Histoplasma
- Non-capsulated, intracellular fungus with septate hyphae
- Source of infection: inhalation of spores
- Clinically histoplasmosis mimics TB

- *Non-capsulated* intracellular (in macrophages) fungus with septate hyphae. Cause primarily a disease of reticuloendothelial system.

Source of Infection

- Inhalation of spores present in moist surface of alkaline soil enriched by dropping of birds and bats.

Pathology

It forms 2 types of asexual spores, large tuberculate macroconidia and smaller elliptical microconidia. Microconidia reach the alveoli and initiate granulomatous reaction.

Histoplasma is also called Darling disease or cave's disease

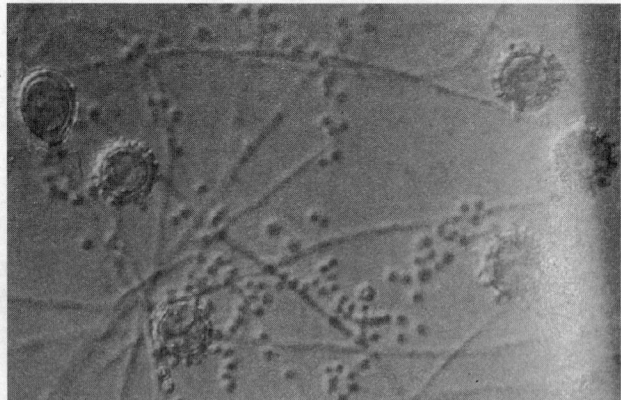

Clinical Features

Tuberculate spores are characteristic of Histoplasma

1. Majority of infections are asymptomatic or mild *(acute primary pulmonary histoplasmosis)*.
   - Cough, fever, malaise, and chest X-ray finding of hilar adenopathy due to caseation necrosis or calcification (which mimics TB) with or without 1 or more areas of pneumonitis are typical features.
2. Small proportion of patient *(who lack history of acute primary pulmonary disease)* develop progressive disease in either form:
   - Chronic pulmonary histoplasmosis or chronic fibrocavitary pneumonia.
   - Disseminated disease: Among immunosuppressed and user of TNF α antagonist infliximab. It mimics disseminated TB.

Diagnosis

Culture (Preferred method):
- *Tuberculate spore is diagnostic*
- Sputum culture – For chronic pulmonary histoplasmosis.
- Culture of bone marrow, mucosal lesion, liver and BAL fluid are diagnostically useful in disseminated histoplasmosis.
- Blood culture is best performed by lysis centrifugation method.

Treatment

Disease	Preferred treatment	Alternative
Acute pulmonary	None	
Chronic pulmonary	Itraconazole	Amphotericin B
Disseminated severe illness • CNS involvement • Immunocompromised	Itraconazole Amphotericin B	Amphotericin B

BLASTOMYCOSIS (=NORTH AMERICAN BLASTOMYCOSIS)

B. dermatitidis is Dimorphic fungi with septate hyphae forming *conidiophores bearing single globose to piriform conidia.* Most cases are found in North America.

Source of infection: Inhalation of conidia from warm moist soil of wooden areas.

Clinical Features

It has marked predilection for lungs, skin and bone.
- Majority of patient, have chronically progressive course and minority have self limited pneumonia.
- Cutaneous disease is usually on the face or other exposed parts of the body in the form of elevated ulcerative lesions.

Diagnosis

Demonstration of fungus in culture of sputum, pus or urine.

Treatment

- Rapid progression or severe illness → Amphotericin B
- CNS disease → Amphotericin B
- Mild to moderate and no CNS disease → Itraconazole

Blastomycosis
- Dimorphic fungi with septate hyphae shows predilection for lungs, skin and bones

Coccidioidomycosis
- Dimorphic fungi with septate hyphae
- Clinically present with influenzae like illness

COCCIDIOIDOMYCOSIS

- *C. immitis is Dimorphic fungi with septate hyphae* forming barrel shaped (arthrospores) or arthroconidia and non-budding spherules with endospores (tissue form).
- It is present in soil and rodents.
- Infection is acquired by inhalation of dust containing arthospore.
- Majority of person develop asymptomatic respiratory infection.
- Some develop self limited influenza like fever known as *valley fever* or *desert rheumatism*.
- Very few develops coccidiodal granuloma often with caseation necrosis.

Diagnosis

a. Sputum, urine and pus should be examined by wet smear and culture (arthrospores are formed in chain from alternate cells of septate hyphae).
b. On *biopsy* appearance of *mature spherule is diagnostic.*
c. Serological test are very helpful.

PARACOCCIDIODES BRASILLIENSIS

- Dimorphic fungi with septate hyphae + rare globose conidia and chlamydospores.
- Tissue form: Yeast with characteristic multiple budding.
- Causative agent of *'South American Blastomycosis'* in which *pulmonary infection spreads hematogenously to* mucosa of mouth; nose; lymph node; skin and other internal organs (e.g. adrenal, GIT).
- Ulcerative granuloma of buccal and nasal mucosa are prominent feature of disease.

Diagnosis

Culture of sputum, pus and mucosal lesion are often diagnostic.

Treatment

- Mild disease - Itraconazole
- Advanced disease - Amphotericin B

SPOROTHRIX

Sporothrix schenckii is thermally **dimorphic fungi** causing subcutaneous mycoses (**Note:** Other dimorphic fungi cause systemic mycosis).

Colonies are blackish (variation in pigmentation) and shiny but becomes wrinkled and fuzzy with age.

Sporothrix
Dimorphic fungi causing subcutaneous mycosis in the form of multiple ulcers

Source of Infection

Acquired from inoculation via thorn pricks of rose, sphagnum moss etc. into subcutaneous tissue through minor trauma.

Clinical Features

- Most cases occur in upper limb.
- Usual site of infection: extremity (facial lesion in case of children).
- Sporotrichosis is characterized by development of nodules on skin, subcutaneous tissue and in lymph nodes, which soften and break to form indolent ulcers.
- It is of following types:

  a. *Plaque sporotrichosis*: Non-tender lesion confined to site of inoculation.
  b. *Lymphangiitis sporotrichosis*: It is **MC** manifestation in which secondary lesion are seen along the lymphatic channels. These small painless nodules may ulcerate and exudate pus.
  c. **Extracutaneous sporotrichosis**: Portal is probably lung. Pulmonary sporotrichosis is usually present as single chronic cavitary upper lobe lesion.

Diagnosis

- *Culture* (most reliable) of pus, joint fluid, sputum or skin biopsy in which septate hyphae carrying flower like cluster of small conidia is seen.
- In tissue – Fungus is seen as 'cigar shaped yeast' yeast cell without mycelia.
- Sometimes '*Asteroid Bodies*' can be seen which is formed due to antigen-antibody reaction.

Treatment

- Cutaneous sporotrichosis – **DOC** Itraconazole
- Alternative potassium iodide
- Extracutaneous sporotrichosis – IV Amphotericin B is drug of choice
- Alternative Itraconazole.

Multiple Choice Questions

1. A series of ulcers in lower extremities in sub-Himalayan area is often caused by: **[AI 2012]**
   a. *Trichophyton rubrum* b. *Pseudallescheria boydii*
   c. *Cladosporium species* d. *Sporothrix schenckii*

2. What is true about Histoplasmosis? **[AIIMS 08]**
   a. In early stages it is indistinguishable from TB
   b. Blood culture is not diagnostic
   c. Hyphal forms are infectious form
   d. Person to person spread occurs by droplet infection

3. Which of the following is not a dimorphic fungus **[AIIMS 2017]**
   a. Penicillium marneffei
   b. Pneumocystis jirovecii
   c. Blastomyces dermatitidis
   d. Histoplasma capsulatum

4. HIV patient presented with fever and diarrhea for 3 weeks. Patient was started on sulphamethoxazole-trimethoprim. His diarrhea responded but he continued to have fever. Bone marrow aspirate showed the following picture. What is not correct for the fungal organism?

   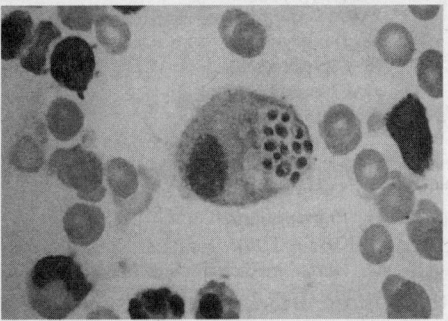

   a. It is an intracellular yeast **[AIIMS 2017]**
   b. It does not grow on SDA medium
   c. In can cause disseminated infection
   d. Infective agent is spores

5. All are dimorphic, except: **[AIIMS May 09]**
   a. Blastomyces
   b. Histoplasma
   c. Penicillium marneffei
   d. Phialophora

6. A gardener has multiple vesicles on hand and multiple eruptions along the lymphatic. Most common fungus responsible is: **[AIIMS 08, 12]**
   a. *Sporothrix schenckii*
   b. *Clasdosporium*
   c. *Histoplasma*
   d. *Candida*

7. Which of the following is/are dimorphic fungi? **[PGI 2017]**
   a. Cryptococcus neoformans
   b. Histoplasma capsulatum
   c. Aspergillus species
   d. Penicillium marneffei
   e. Rhizopus species

Explanations and References with Illustrative Answers

1. **Ans. (d) Sporothrix schenckii** *Ref. Harrison 20/e, 1542*

   Important Features of Sporothrix
   - Thermally dimorphic fungus lives as saprophyte on plants.
   - Infection results from inoculation into subcutaneous tissue after minor trauma.
   - Nursery worker, florist, gardeners acquire the illness from roses, and other plants.
   - Usual manifestation is nearly painless red papule at the site of inoculation, over the next several weeks similar nodules forms along proximal lymphatic channels. The nodules may ulcerate. Thus series of ulcer may form.

   Diagnosis:
   - In skin lesion the organism is hard to find.
   - Culture of pus or a skin biopsy is preferred method of diagnosis.

   Treatment:
   - Potassium iodide
   - Itraconazole.

2. **Ans. (a) In early stages it is indistinguishable from TB** *Ref. Harrison 20/e, p 1519*

   Clinical manifestation of Histoplasma
   1. Majority of infections are asymptomatic or mild (acute primary pulmonary histoplasmosis).
      - Cough, fever, malaise. Chest X-ray shows hilar adenopathy due to caseation necrosis or calcification (which mimics TB) with or without 1 or more areas of pneumonitis.
   2. Small proportion of patient (who lack history of acute primary pulmonary disease) develop progressive disease in either form:
      - Chronic pulmonary histoplasmosis or chronic fibrocavitary pneumonia.
      - Disseminated disease: Among immunosuppressed and user of TNF α antagonist infliximab. It mimics disseminated TB.

   > **Other Options:**
   > - Fungal culture is the gold standard diagnostic test for histoplasmosis.
   > - Mycelia are the naturally infectious forms.
   > - Infection occurs through aerosolization of bird or at dropping.

3. **Ans. (b)** *Pneumocystis Jirovecii*   ...*Ref. Harrison 20/e, p 1515*

   Dimorphic fungus
   - Fungus which occur in two forms:
     - *Yeast form* - In host tissue and on culture at 37°C.
     - *Filamentous (mold) form* - In soil and culture at 22 - 25°C or Sabouraud's agar at room temperature.

   Dimorphic fungus are:

   > - *Sporothrix schenckii*
   > - *Blastomyces*
   > - Coccidioidomycosis
   > - *Candida albicans* (not other species of candida)
   > - *Penicillium marneffei*
   > - *Histoplasma*
   > - Paracoccidioidomycosis
   >
   > **Mnemonic: SBH Ca P**owerful **P**ersonal **C**omputer

   > **Remember:** Candida as a whole is not dimorphic only *Candida albicans* is dimorphic.

4. **Ans. (b) It does not grow**   ...*Ref. Ananthanarayan 10/e p 610; Harrison 20/e p 1515*

   This is a case of progressive disseminated histoplasmosis (PDH) revealing intracellular yeast.
   - PDH is typically seen in immunocompromised individuals who account for ~ 70% of cases. Risk factors include AIDS (CD9+ < 200/μl), extremes of age, immunosuppressive medication
   - Clinical spectrum range from acute rapid fatal course (respiratory failure, shock) to more common subacute course (fever, weight loss, splenomegaly and thrombocytopenia)
   - **Diagnosis:** Fungal culture. On sabouraud or other agar plates at room temperature, white cottony, mycelial growth appears with large (8-20 μ) thick walled, spherical spores with tubercle. These tuberculate spores are diagnostic
   Serology: Rapid and most commonly adopted method. The two routine methodologies are complement fixation and immunodiffusion.

   > **Note:** In healed histoplasmosis, calcified mediastinal nodes or lung parenchymal nodules may erode through wall of airways and cause hemoptysis and expectoration of calcified material. This condition is called broncholithiosis.

5. **Ans. (d)** *Phialophora*   *Ref. Harrison 20/e, p 1515*
   Already explained

   > **Remember:** Phialophora is a dermatiaceous (pigmented fungi) soil fungi which can cause subcutaneous or intramuscular lesion with abscess or cysts containing masses of brown hyphae.

6. **Ans. (a)** *Sporothrix schenckii*   *Ref. Harrison 20/e, p 1542*
   Already explained

7. **Ans. is (b) and (d) Histoplasma capsulatum and Penicillium marneffei**   *Ref. Harrison 20/e, p 1515*
   Already explained

NEET Pattern Questions

1. **Dimorphic fungi behaves like yeast at:**
   a. < 10°C
   b. Body temperature
   c. > 40°C
   d. In vitro
   [Ref. Ananthanarayan, 10/e 594]

   > Dimorphic fungi grows as yeast in culture at 37°C and in tissues

2. **Darling disease is caused by:**
   a. Histoplasma
   b. Candida
   c. Cryptococcus
   d. Rhizopus
   [Ref. Ananthanarayan, 10/e 608]

   > Histoplasmosis is also known as Darling disease or Caves disease or Caver's disease. (As it was originally described by darling).

3. **Dimorphic fungus:**
   a. Candida
   b. Histoplasma
   c. Rhizopus
   d. Mucor
   [Ref. Harrison, 10/e 1515]

4. **All of the following are dimorphic fungi, except:**
   a. Sporotricum
   b. Blastomycetes
   c. Histoplasma
   d. Cryptococcus
   [Ref. Ananthanarayan 9/e p 590]

5. **Not true about Histoplasma capsulatum:**
   a. Dimorphic fungus
   b. May mimic TB
   c. Capsulated
   d. Mostly asymptomatic
   [Ref. Harrison, 20/e 1518]

6. **Asteroid bodies are seen in:**
   a. Cryptococcosis
   b. Histoplasmosis
   c. Sporotrichosis
   d. Aspergillosis
   [Ref. Ananthanarayan, 10/e 606]

   > Asteroid bodies are the characteristic feature of sporotrichosis. They are seen on histological examination of tissue sections stained by methenamine silver stain. They are rounded or oval, basophilic, yeast-like body 3-5 mm in diameter.

7. **"Tuberculate spores" are characteristic features of:**
   a. Candida
   b. Histoplasma
   c. Coccidioidomyces
   d. Cryptococcus
   [Ref. Ananthanarayan, 10/e 610]

Ans.
1. b. Body temperature
2. a. Histoplasma
3. b. Histoplasma
4. d. Cryptococcus
5. c. Capsulated
6. c. Sporotrichosis
7. b. Histoplasma

SECTION B

UNIT IV

Parasitology

- Basics of Parasitology
- Protozoa
- Helminths

Basics of Parasitology

CHAPTER 33

PARASITE

Ectoparasites: Parasite inhabiting the body surface only, e.g. lice, ticks, mites. The term infestation is used in context of ectoparasites.
Endoparasites: Parasite, living inside the body.

HOST

a. **Definitive host:** Host in which adult stage lives or the **sexual** mode of reproduction takes place.
b. **Intermediate host:** Species in which the larval stage of parasite lives or **asexual** reproduction takes place.
c. **Paratenic host:** A host in which parasite remains viable without development or multiplication. Such host is also called as transport host.

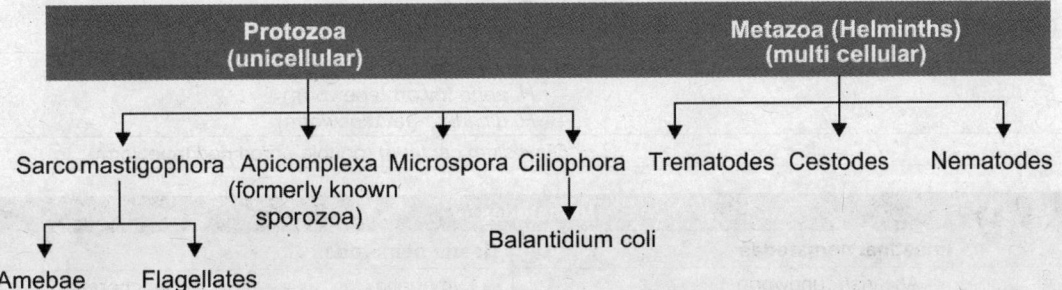

Amebae	
Amebae of alimentary canal	**Pathogenic free living amebae (Brain parasite)**
• Entameba histolytica	• Naegleria fowleri
• Entameba coli	• Acanthameba
	• Balamuthia

Flagellates	
Intestinal flagellates	**Hemoflagellates (Kinetoplastidia)**
• Giardia lamblia	• Trypanosoma
• Trichomonas	• Leishmania

Sporozoa (Apicomplexa)		
Apicomplexa: Members possess a structure called as apical complex, at some stage of their life cycle. Apical complex serve as organ of attachment. They are tissue parasites.		
• Plasmodium	• Toxoplasma gondii	• Sarcocystis
• Isospora belli	• Cryptosporidium parvum	• Babesia
• Cyclospora		

Trematodes (Flukes)	
Dioecious blood flukes (Schistosomes) **[infection by cercarial penetration]**	**Hermaphrodites flukes** **[infection by ingestion of cercaria]**
• S. hematobium/bilharziasis hematobium [live in vesical and pelvic venous plexus]	Biliary tract (liver flukes) - Clonorchis sinensis - Fasciola hepatica - Opisthorchis species
• S. mansoni/ Intestinal bilharziasis [live in inferior mesenteric vein]	Intestinal flukes - Small intestine → *Fasciolopsis, buski,* etc - Large intestine → Gastrodiscoides hominis
• S. japonicum/oriental schistosomiasis/ Katyama disease [live in superior mesenteric vein]	• Lung flukes (*Paragominus westermani*)

Cestodes (Tapeworms)	
Operculated eggs, ciliated larvae	**Non-operculated eggs** **Non-ciliated larvae (bladder worms)**
• Fish tapeworm (*Diphyllobothrium latum*)	• Taenia T. saginata (Beef tapeworm) T. solium (Pork tapeworm)
• Sparganum	• Echinococcus - E. granulosus (Dog tapeworm) - E. multilocularis
	• Hymenolepsis - H. nana (dwarf tapeworm) - H. diminuta (rat tapeworm)
	• Dipylidium caninum (double pored dog tapeworm)

Nematodes			
Intestinal nematodes		**Tissue nematodes**	
• Small intestine	- Ascaris/roundworm - Hookworm/Ancyclostoma - Necator - Strongyloides - Trichinella	• Lymphatic	- Wuchereria - Brugia
		• Subcutaneous	- Loa-loa - Onchocerca - Dracunculus (Guinea worm/ serpent worm)
• Large intestine	- Enterobius (Pinworm/ threadworm/ seatworm) - Trichuris (Whipworm)	• Mesentery • Conjunctiva	- Mansonelia - Loa-loa

Nematodes can also be Classified as

- **On the basis of mode of infection**
  1. *By ingestion*
     a. Eggs - *Enterobius, Ascaris, Trichuris*   `Mnemonic:` **EAT**
     b. Larvae within intermediate host — *Dracunculus*
     c. Encysted larvae in muscle — *Trichinella.*
  2. *By penetration of skin* - *Ancylostoma, Necator, Strongyloides*   `Mnemonic:` **ANS**
  3. *By blood sucking insects* — Filariae
  4. *By inhalation of Dust Containing eggs* - *Ascaris, Enterobius.*
- **Based on whether they lay eggs or larvae:**
  1. *Oviparous* = Laying eggs
     a Unsegmented eggs : *Ascaris, Trichuris*
     b. Segmented eggs : *Ancylostoma, Necator*   `Mnemonic:` **ANS**
     c. Eggs containing larvae : *Enterobius*

2. *Viviparous = Producing larvae*
   - Trichinella
   - Brugia
   - Wuchereria
   - Dracunculus.
3. *Ovoviviparous* (laying eggs containing fully formed larvae which hatch out immediately)
   - Strongyloides

Two Intermediate hosts are seen in:

- *Paragonimus westermani* (Lung fluke)
- *Diphyllobothrium latum* (Fish tape worm)
- *Clonorchis sinesis* (Chinese tapeworm)
- *Metagonimus yokogawai.*

Man is intermediate (Secondary) host in:

- *Plasmodium*
- *Toxoplasma gondii*
- *Sarcocystis lindemanni*
- *T. solium* (man also act as definitive host).
- *Echinococcus granulosus* [*dog tapeworm/ hydatid worm/Taenia echinococcus*]

> **Note:** In other parasitic infection, man act as definitive (primary) host.

Auto-Infection occurs in:

- **C**ryptosporidium parvum
- **H**. nana
- **E**. vermicularis   Mnemonic: **CHEST**
- **T**. solium
- **S**trongyloides stercoralis.

Eggs float (eggs can be demonstrated) in concentrated saturated solution:

- *E. granulosus*
- *H. nana*
- All nematodes (but not unfertilized egg of *Ascaris*).

Charcot Leyden crystal seen in:

- *E. histolytica* (amoebic dysentery)
- Whipworm dysentery
- *Ascaris* pneumonia
- Bronchial asthma.

Worms that crawl out:

- *Enterobius vermicularis*
- *T. saginata.*

Worms which do not multiply in host:

- *Ancylostoma duodenale*
- *Enterobius vermicularis*
- *W. bancrofti.*

Parasites associated with malignancy:

- Clonorchis ⎤
- Opisthorchis ⎦ Bile duct carcinoma
- *Schistosoma hematobium* - bladder carcinoma.

Premunition (immunity to reinfection) seen in:
- Syphilis
- Cutaneous leishmaniasis.
- Hyper/Holoendemic malarial area

Cystic stage is absent in:
- Dientamoeba fragilis
- Entamoeba gingivalis
- Trichomonas vaginalis
- Trichomonas intestinalis.

Undulating membrane seen in:
- Trichomonas species
- Hemoflagellates

IMPORTANT FACTS

Only *'Protozoan'* parasite found in lumen of human small intestine — *Giardia lamblia*
Only *'Ciliate protozoan'* Parasite of man — *Balantidium coli*
Parthenogenic worm (female is able to produce fertile eggs or larvae without meeting with males): *Strongyloides stercoralis*
Largest protozoa: Balantidum coli
Smallest intestinal amoeba: Dientamoeba fragilis
Smallest and most common tapeworm found in human intestine: *H. nana*
Largest helminth: T. saginata (beef tapeworm)
Largest liver fluke: F. hepatica
Largest trematode: infecting man: *Fasciolopsis buski*
Largest nematode: Ascaris (roundworm)
Smallest nematode: Trichinella
MC protozoan parasite: Toxoplasma gondii

Dogs are responsible for transmission of:
- Hydatid disease
- Toxocara canis
- L. donovani infantum

Eggs needs development in soil:
- Ancylostoma duodenale
- Ascaris
- Trichuris (whipworm)
- S. stercoralis.

Sputum examination done for:
- Rhabditiform larva of *Ascaris*
- Golden brown - eggs of paragonimus
- Filariform larva of *Strongyloides, Ancylostoma*
- *Entamoeba histolytica* (due to hepatobronchial fistula).
- *Paragoninus westermani*

Cutaneous larva Migrans caused by:
- Necator americanus
- Sparganosis

Basics of Parasitology

- *Gnathostomiasis*
- Hypoderma and gastrophilus.
- Loa-loa and *Dicrofilaria*
- *Ancylostoma braziliense, A. caninum, A. duodenale*
- *Fasciola* and *Paragonimus*
- *Strongyloides stercoralis* (larva currens/racing larvae).

Visceral Larva Migrans caused by:
- Dog ascarid *Toxocara canis* (**MC**)
- Cat ascarid *T. cati*
- Anisakis (Large ascarid)
- *Gnathostoma.*

Worms Pass through lung during its life cycle:
- Schisto. hematobium (Lung act as 2nd filter)
- Paragonimus
- Echinococcus
- Strong. sterocoralis
- A. duodenale
- Ascaris.

Intracellular Parasites:
- *Leishmania* (amastigote form)
- *Babesia*
- *Plasmodium*
- *Toxoplasma gondii*
- *Sarcocystis.*
- *Trypanosoma cruzi* (amastigote form)

NEUROPARASITES

Protozoa	Helminthes		Ecotopic ova
	Larvae of cestodes	Nematodes	
• E. histolytica	• T. solium	• Visceral larva migrans	• Schistosoma sp (hematobium)
• Naegleria	• E. granulosus	• Ascaris lumbricoides	• F. hepatica
• Acanthamoeba	• Multiceps sp.	• Strongyloides stercoralis	• Heterophyes hyterophyes
• Trypanosoma		• Gnathostoma spinigerum	
• P. falciparum			
• T. gondii			

Protozian parasites causing diarrhea	
• Giardia lamblia	• Entamoeba histolytica
• Cyclospora cayetanensis	• Cryptosporidium parvum
• Isospora belli	

Protozoa parasites detected in peripheral blood film
- Trypanosoma cruzi
- Tryanosoma brucei rhodesiense
- Trypanosoma brucei gambiense
- Leishmania spp.
- Plasmodium spp.
- Babesia spp.

Protozoa transmitted by sexual contact
- Trichomonas vaginalis
- Giardia Iamblia
- Entamoeba histolytica

Parasites which can be transmitted from mother to fetus
- Toxoplasma gondii
- Plasmodium spp.
- Trypanosoms cruzi

Acid fast parasitic organisms
- Microsporidia (spore)
- Cyclospora cayetanensis (oocyst)
- Isospora belli (oocyst)
- Cryptosporidium parvum (oocyst)

Parasites causing opportunistic infections in immunocompromised patients (HIV-positive cases)
- Microporidia
- Cyclospora cayetanensis
- Isospora belli
- Cryptosporidium parvum
- Toxoplasma gondii
- Strongyloides stercoralis
- Entamoeba histolytica

Parasites which can be cultured in laboratory	
• Balantidium coli	• Entamoeba histolytica
• Acanthamoeba spp.	• Giardia lamblia
• Trichomonas vaginalis	• Trypanosoma spp.
• Leishmania spp.	

- Longest cestode infecting man: Diphyllobothrium latum
- Smallest cestode infecting man: Hymenolepis nana
- Largest trematode infecting humans: *Fasciolopsis buski*
- Smallest trematode infecting humans: *Heterophyes*

Parasites with aquatic vegetations as the source of infection	
• Fasciola hepatica	• Fasciolopsis buski
• Gastrodiscoides hominis	• Watsonius watsoni

Parasites with bile stained eggs	
• Ascaris lumbricoides	• Clonorchis sinensis
• Trichuris trichiura	• Fasciola hepatica
• Taenia solium	• Fasciolopsis buski
• Taenia saginata	

Parasites found in urine
- Wuchereria bancrofti
- Schistosoma hematobium
- Trichomonas vaginalis

Parasites found in cerebrospinal fluid	
Protozoa	**Helminths**
• Trypanosoma brucei spp.	• Angiostrongylus cantonensis
• Naegleria	
• Acanthamoeba spp.	

Parasites found in peripheral blood film	
Protozoa	**Nematodes**
• Plasmodium spp.	• Wuchereria bancrofti
• Babesis spp.	• Brugia spp.
• Leishmania spp.	• Loa loa
• Tryponosoma spp.	• Mansonella ozzardi

Parasites with mosquito as Intermediate host
• Wuchereria bancrofti
• Brugia spp.
• Mansonella spp.
• Dirofilaria spp.

Helminths requiring no intermediate host
• Ancylostoma duodenale
• Necator americanus
• Ascaris lumbricoides
• Trichuris trichiura
• Enterobius vermicularis
• Hymenolepis nana

Small Intestinal Parasites		
Protozoa	Nematodes	Cestodes
• Giardia lamblia	• Strongyloides stercoralis	• Diphyllobothrium latum
• Isospora belli	• Ascaris lumbricoides	• Taenia solium
• Cyclospora caytenensis	• Ancylostoma duodenale	• Taenia saginata saginata
• Sarcocystis hominis and suihominis	• Necator americanus	• Taenia saginata asiatica
	• Trichinella spiralis	• Hymenolepis nana
	• Trichostrongylus spp.	
	• Capillaria philippinensis	

IMPORTANT POINTS ABOUT MALARIA

- Infective forms for human is sporozoites in saliva of mosquito.
- Infective forms for mosquito is gametocytes in human blood. At least 12 gametocytes per cubic mm of blood must be present to infect mosquito.
  - Gametocytes are maximum in number during the early stages of infections (may exceed 1000 per cubic mm of blood).
  - Nonmotile zygote converted into motile ookinete in about 18-24 hours.
- Human reservoir is one who harbors the sexual forms (gametocytes) of the parasite.
- Only animal reservoir is chimpanzees.

CHAPTER 34

Protozoa

- Single-celled eukaryotic microorganisms belonging to kingdom protista.
- Represent earliest form of animal life.

> Phylum microspora contains intracellular protozoan parasites which affect immunocompromised individuals only.

> Largest protozoan Parasite: Balantidium coli

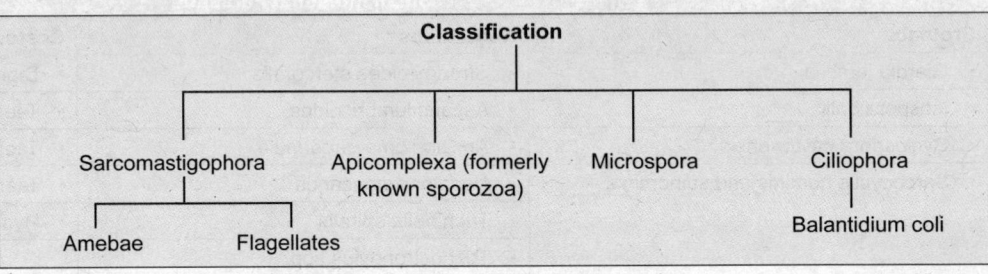

AMEBAE

ENTAMOEBA HISTOLYTICA

> E. histolytica
> - Infective stage: cyst
> - Tissue stage: trophozoite

- Found in human colon, as commensal, but sometimes invades the intestinal tissue and becomes pathogen.
  - It has 3 stages:
    a. **Trophozoite or Vegetative** or Amoeboid form
       - It is the only form present in tissue. Actively motile growing, feeding stage.
       - It can't initiate infection.
    b. **Pre-cystic stage**
       - Encystment occur in intestinal lumen only (not in feces or nor in tissues).
       - Contain no RBC and other ingested food particles.
    c. **Cystic stage**
       - Mature Quadrinucleate cyst: *Infective stage*
       - It is present *only in lumen* of colon and in mushy or formed feces.
       - When stained with iodine, nuclear chromatin and karyosome appears bright yellow while chromidial bars are unstained.

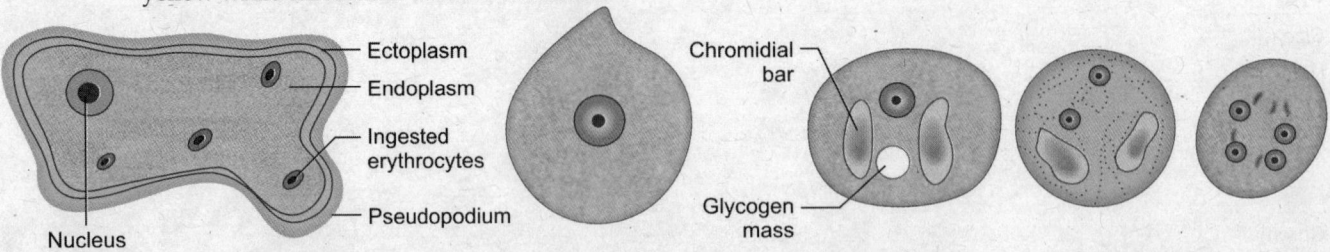

> Fecooral is the commonest mode of transmission. Beside drinking less common modes include oral, Oral sex, blood products.

Life Cycle

- Infective form is mature cyst passed in the feces of convalescent and carriers.
- Cyst ingested through contaminated food, resist gastric acidity due to presence of cyst wall. In small intestine, trypsine lyse the cyst wall and quadrinucleate amoeba comes out. This stage is called as metacyst. Nuclei of metacyst immediately undergo division to form eight nuclei which gets mature to form 8 small amoebae.

- From small intestine trophozoite are carried to caecum where they lodge in the glandular crypts and undergo reproduction by binary fission. Some develop into precystic form and cysts which are then passed in feces to repeat the cycle.

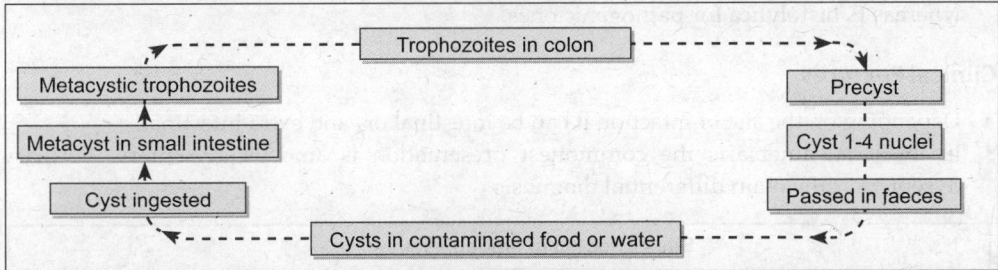

Life cycle of E. histolytica

Note:
- Optimum habitat for metacystic trophozoites is the caecal mucosa.
- Cyst stage is found only in colon, not in extraintestinal sites.

Differential features of intestinal entamoeba			
Features	**E. histolytica**	**E. hartmanni**	**E. coli**
Trophozoite			
Size (μm)	12–60	4–12	20–50
Motility	Active	Active	Sluggish
Pseudopodia	Finger shaped, rapidly extruded	Finger shaped, rapidly extruded	Short, blunt, slowly extruded
Cytoplasm	*Clearly defined into* endoplasm and ectoplasm	Clearly defined into ectoplasm and endoplasm	Not defined
Inclusions	*Red blood cells present*, no bacteria	Bacteria and other particles, no red blood cells	Bacteria and other particles, no red blood cell
Nucleus	Not clearly visible in unstained films; It is *eccentric*	Not clearly visible in unstained films	Visible in unstained films
Karyosome	Small, *central*	Small, eccentric	Large, *eccentric*
Nuclear membrane	Delicate, with *fine chromatin dots*	Coarse chromatin granules	Thick, with coarse chromatin
Cyst			
Size (μm)	10–15	5–10	10–30
Nuclei in mature cyst	4, central karyosome	4	8, eccentric karyosome
Glycogen mass	Seen in uninucleate, but not in quadrinucleate stage	Seen in uninucleate, but not in quadrinucleate stage	Seen up to quadrinucleate stage
Chromatidial bars	1-4, with rounded ends	Often numerous, shape irregular	Splinter like with angular ends

Pathogenicity

- In only 10% of total cases infected, intestinal invasion occurs, in rest of the cases entamoeba resides as commensal.
- Similarly not all strains of E. histolytical are pathogenic. Amoebic cysteine proteinase is a virulent factor which is present in pathogenic strains.

Virulence factors.
- Cystine Proteinase
- Amoebic Lectin
- Ionophore Proteins

- Based on isoenzymes E. histolytica can be classified into 22 zymodemes of these only 9 are invasive and rest are non-invasive commensals.
- It has been proposed to use the new species as E.dispar for nonpathogenic entamoebae whereas E. histolytica for pathogenic ones.

Clinical Features

- Depending on the site of infection it can be intestinal or/and extra intestinal.
- In intestinal amebiasis the commonest presentation is amoebic dysentery. Bacillary dysentery is the main differential diagnosis

> - Most infections are asymptomatic

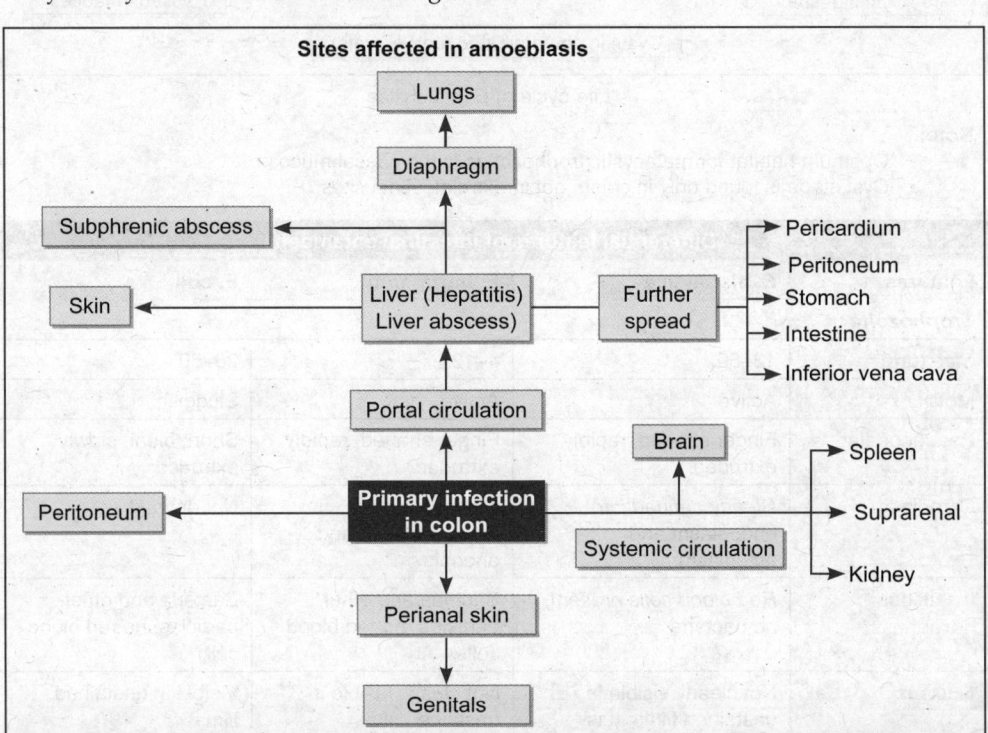

Sites affected in amoebiasis

Feature	Amoebic dysentery	Bacillary dysentery
Organism	E. histolytica	Shigella, Salmonella enterica
Macroscopic		
Number	6-8 motions a day	Over 10 motions a day
Amount (volume)	Relatively copious	Small amount
Appearance and amount	Blood mucus, semi formed	Blood mucus, mainly watery
Odour	Offensive (fishy odour)	Odourless
Colour	Dark red (altered blood)	Bright red (fresh blood)
Reaction	Acidic	Alkaline
Consistency	Not adherent to the container	Adherent to the container
RBCs	In clumps	Usually discrete
Pus cells	Few	Numerous
Macrophages	Few	Numerous, many of them contain RBCs (may be mistaken for E. histolytica)
Charcot-Leyden (C-L) crystals	Present	Absent
Pyknotic bodies	Present	Absent

Contd...

Contd…

Feature	Amoebic dysentery	Bacillary dysentery
Ghost cells	Absent	Present
Parasites seen	Trophozoites of *E. histolytica*	Absent
Bacteria seen	Many motile bacteria	Scanty, nonmotile (*Shigella* is non motile bacteria)
Signs & symptoms		
Abdominal tenderness	Mild and localized	More and generalized
Fever	Afebrile to mild	Mild to moderate

Diagnosis

- Definitive diagnosis of amoebiasis requires demonstration of actively motile trophozoite of entamoeba in freshly passed stool.
- Serology is helpful in diagnosis of extraintestinal amoebiasis, but not in intestinal amoebiasis.
  - Indirect hemogglutination (IHA) and latex agglutination (LA) are the sensitive serological test, whereas gel precipitation test are specific one.
- *DNA PCR* is the most sensitive and specific method for identifying E. histolytica.

Treatment

a. **Luminal amoebicides:** Diloxamide furoate, iodoquinol, paromomycin. Effective in amoebic colitis.
b. **Tissue Amoebicides:** Emetine, chloroquine, effective in extraintestinal amoebiasis. Metronidazole is effective in both conditions.

ENTAMOEBA GINGIVALIS

A commensal amoeba found in mouth, of unhygienic human. Entamoeba gingivalis characteristically lacks cystic stage. Transmitted by direct oral contacts.

PATHOGENIC FREE LIVING AMOEBA

a. **Acanthamoeba:**
   - Causative agent of granulomatous amoebic meningoencephalitis and chronic amoebic keratitis.
   - **A. culbertsoni** is the species most often responsible.
   - Infection is acquired by inhalation, ingestion or through traumatised skin.
   - Both trophozoites and cysts are infective.
   - Differs from naegleria in not having flagillar stage and in forming cyst in tissues.

b. **Naegleria fowleri:**
   - Heat loving (thermophilic amoebae) that lives in low oxygen tension. Only species of genus naegleria which infects man.
   - Causative agent of *primary amoebic meningoencephalitis*
   - Human infection is acquired by water containing cyst comes in, contact with nasal mucosa usually while swimming or diving.
   - Amoeba invades nasal mucosa and enters brain via olfactory nerve.
   - Disease is usually fatal.
   - **Treatment:** Metronidazole and tinidazole.

c. **Balamuthia Mandrillaris**
   Leptomikid free living amoeba that cause granulomatous encephalitis in both immunocompromised and healthy individuals.

Amoebic Ulcer:
- Flask shaped ulcer with pin head centre and raised edges.
- Multiple
- Most numerous in caecum followed by sigmoido-rectal region

- Granulomatous meningoencephalitis. Caused by Acanthamoeba (commonly) and Balamuthia. Usually seen in immunodeficient patient.
- Primary Amoebic Meningoencephalitis (PAM): Cause by free living amoeba naegleria.
- Chronic Amoebic Keratitis (CAK): Caused by Acanthamoeba.
- PAM and CAK usually affect healthy individual.

FLAGELLATES

GIARDIA

- An intestinal flagellates, and perhaps the **most common intestinal** protozoan pathogen.
  ...*Paniker 7/e 30*
- Infective form: Mature cyst (10-100 cysts)
- Produce diarrhea by causing abnormalities in villous architectures, and hence fat malabsorption.
- Lives in crypts of duodenum and jejunum. It does not invade mucosa.
- Infection is acquired by ingestion of cyst in contaminated food and water.

> - **Overall** most common protozoan parasite: Toxoplasma gondii
> - Protozoan parasite found in the lumen of **small intestine**: Giardia lamblia

LEISHMANIA

- Obligate intracellular hemo flagellate protozoan, causing kala-azar.
- Disease is vector borne with *sandfly* as *vector*.
- **L. donovani** is the causative agent of *visceral leishmaniasis,* whereas **L. tropica** is the major causative agent of cutaneous and/or *mucocutaneous leishmaniasis.*
- L. donovani occurs in two forms: The amastigate form (LD body) in humans
  Promastigate form in sandfly and in artificial culture.
- Human acquires the infection by the bite of sandfly (P. argentipes). Most infections are sub-clinical, and only 3% develop kala-azar syndrome.
- **I.P. is 2-6 months:** Cutaneous lesion at the site of bite is usually absent in Indians
- **Pathology:** – Kala-azar results from reticuloendotheliosis, spleen is the organ most affected. Hepatomegaly may also be there
  – The resulting blockade of reticuloendothelial system results in marked depression of cell mediated immunity. As a response there is over production of immunoglobulins.

> - Leishmania: Obligate intracellular protozoan

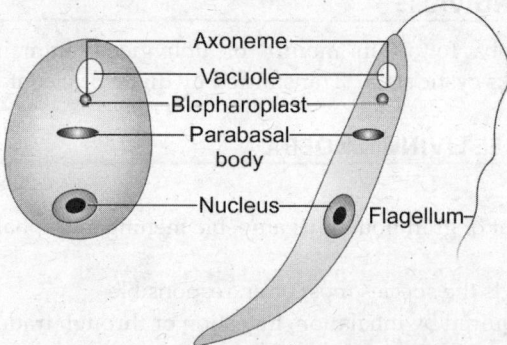

- **Diagnosis:** Demonstration of amastigotes in smears of tissue aspirates is the gold standard for visceral leishmaniasis
- **Culture:** For culturing tissue material or blood NNN medium is adopted

Treatment

- Sodium stibogluconate is the treatment of choice.

TRYPANSOMA CRUZI

- A hemoflagellate protozoan parasite, cause Chaga's disease
- Produce muscle fibrosis and destruct neural tissue that control tone of hollow organs thus produces myopathy, megaoesophagus, mega colon
- Intermediate host: Reduvid bug (vector)
- Definite host : Man
- In humans T. cruzi exists in both amastigote and trypomastigote form

- Infective stage: Metecyclic trypomastigotes
- Diagnosis: Demonstration of T. cruzi in blood on tissues on by serology

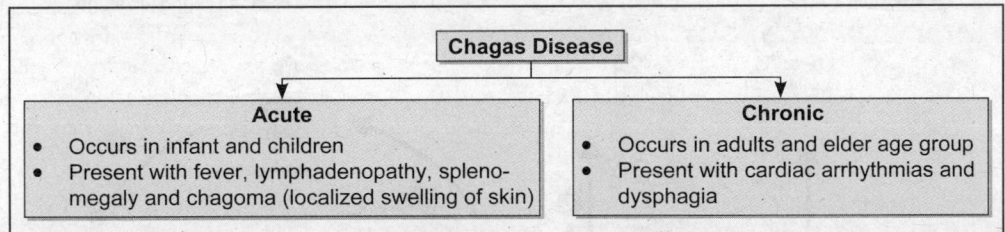

Differences between various morphological stages of hemoflagellates				
	Amastigote	**Promastigote**	**Epimastigote**	**Trypomastigote**
Morphological characteristics	Rounded or ovoid, without any external flagellum. The nucleus, kinetoplast, and axial filaments can be seen.	Lanceolate in shape. Kinetoplast is anterior to the nucleus (antenuclear kinetoplast). There is no undulating membrane	Elongated, with the kinetoplast placed more posteriorly, close to and in front of the nucleus (juxtanuclear kinetoplast). Undulating membrane present	This stage is elongated, spindle shaped with a central nucleus. The kinetoplast is posterior to the nucleus (postnuclear kinetoplast) and situated at the posterior end of the body. Undulating membrane present
Seen in	*Trypanosoma cruzi* and Leishmania as intracellular form	It is the infective stage of *Leishmania*	It is the form in which *Trypanosoma brucei* occur in salivary gland of the vector setse fly and *Trypanosoma cruzi* in the midgut of the vector reduviid bug. Note: This stage is lacking in *Leishmania*	This is the infective stage of trypanosomes. Note: This stage is lacking in *Leishmania*

N: Nucleus; P: Parabasal body; B: Blepharoplast; A: Axoneme; U: Undulating membrane; F: Flagellum.

COCCIDIA

- Unicellular protozoa belonging to phylum *Apicomplexa*
- **Toxoplasma gondii is the prototype**
- *Toxoplasma* is an *obligate intracellular coccidian parasite* which completes its life cycle in two hosts:
  a. **Definitive host:** Cats and other feline in which both sexual and asexual cycle takes place
  b. **Intermediate hosts:** Man and other mammals in which only the asexual cycle takes place
- Life cycle can also be divided in to enteric and exoenteric cycle. Enteric cycle occurs in cat and other felines in small intestine.
- *Exoenteric cycle* occurs in humans and other mammals who acquired infection after eating uncooked or undercooked infected meat (lamb, pork), ingestion of mature oocytes through food water or finger contaminated with cat feces; as congenital infection, through infected blood. Human infection is a dead end for parasite.
- Ingested sporozoites and bradyzoites multiply asexually to form tachyzoites which continue to multiply and spread locally by lymphatic system and blood.
- Some tachyzoites also spread to distance extraintestinal organs like brain, eye liner, spleen and skeleted muscles.

Congenital parasitic infection
- Toxoplasma gondii
- Plasmodium spp.
- Trypanosoma cruzi

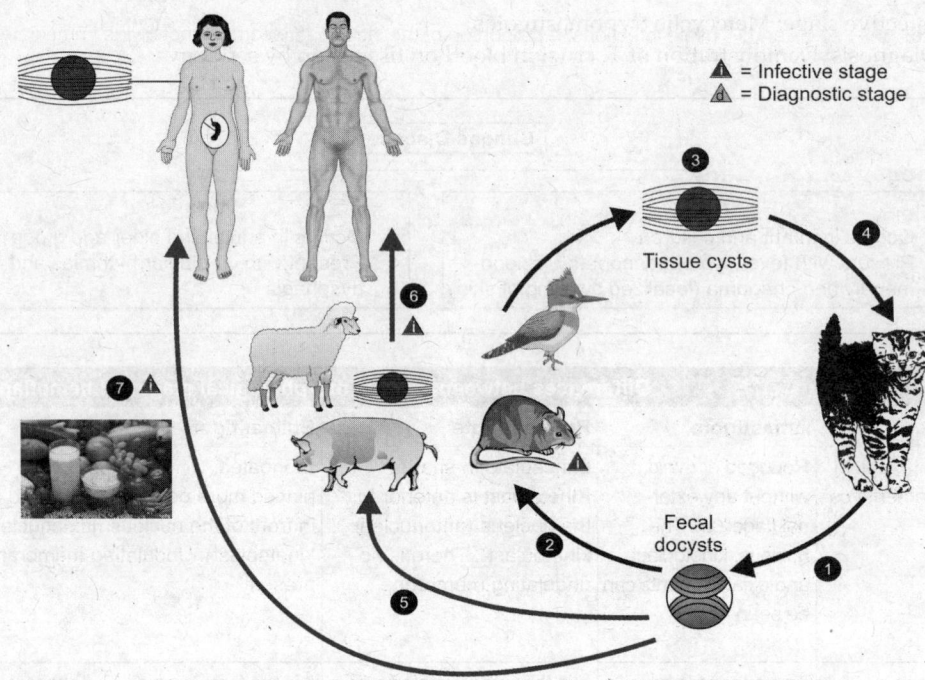

1. Infected cat shed oocyst for 1-2 weeks. Oocysts take 1-5 days to sporulate in the environment and become infective.
2. Intermediate hosts (including birds and rodents) become infected after ingesting soil, water or plant material contaminated with oocysts
3. Oocysts transform into tachyzoites shortly after ingestion and get localize in neural and muscle tissue and develop into tissue cyst bradyzoites.
4. Cats become infected after consuming intermediate hosts harboring tissue cysts or directly by ingestion of sporulated oocysts.
5-7. Humans can become infected by any of several routes:
    – Eating undercooked meat of animals harboring tissue cysts (6)
    – Consuming food or water contaminated with cat feces or by contaminated environmental samples (such as fecal-contaminated soil or changing the litter box of a pet cat) (7).
- In the human host, the parasites form tissue cysts, most commonly in skeletal muscle, myocardium, brain, and eyes; these cysts may remain throughout the life of the host.
- Diagnosis is usually achieved by serology, although tissue cysts may be observed in stained biopsy specimens.
- Diagnosis of congenital infections can be achieved by detecting *T. gondii* DNA in amniotic fluid using molecular methods, such as PCR.

Clinical Features

- **Immunocompetent:** Mostly asymptomatic commonest manifestation is lymphadenopathy (cervical area is most commonly affected)
    – In eyes (occular toxoplasmosis) is present as uveitis, choroiditis, or chorioretinitis
- **Immunocompromised:** Involvement of brain is most common (clinically present as encephalitis, altered mental status).
- Congenital toxoplasmosis

PLASMODIUM

- Causative agent of malaria.
- Four species of plasmodia cause malaria in man viz: P. vivax, P. falciparum, P. malaria, and P. ovale. P vivax and P. falciparum being the most common.
- Discovered by Alphonse Lavaran, a French Army surgeon. Ronald Ross established the mode of transmission of disease in Secunderabad India. Both of them were awarded Nobel Prize.
- **Vector:** In human malaria is transmitted by the female anopheles mosquito.

- A sexual stage: Human
- Sexual stage: Mosquito
- P. vivax and P. falciparum are the commonest cause of malaria in India.

Note: In P. vivax and P. ovale infections, a proportion of the intrahepatic form do not divide immediately but remain dormant for a period ranging from 3 weeks to a year or longer. These dormant forms, or "hypnozoites" are the cause of the relapses that characterize infection with these two species. Person with gametocyte in blood is a carrier of reservoir of malaria.

Pathogenesis and Clinical Features

- Merozoites released after rupture of hepatocytes, enters the RBC.
- Glycophorin acts as receptor for merozoites in RBC.
- Parasite feeds on the hemoglobin of the erythrocyte; however it does not metabolise hemoglobin completely and leaves behind a haematin-globin pigment called as malaria pigment (*also called as haemozoin pigment*). Rupture of mature schizont release huge variety of pyrogens which are responsible for febrile response of malaria. Clinically presenting as:
  - Fever (MC), myalgia, headache
  - Seizures can be seen with any malaria, but generalized seizure are specifically associated with falciparum malaria.
  - Coma is characteristic and ominous feature of falciparum malaria.

> **Protozoa detected in blood:**
> - Trypanosoma
> - Plasmodium
> - Babesia
> - Leishmania

Note: Duration of erythrocytic schizogony varies according to plasmodium species (48 hour is falciparum, ovale and vivax, 72 hrs. in malariae), pre-erythrocytic schizogony doesn't produce clinical illness.

Life Cycle of Plasmodium

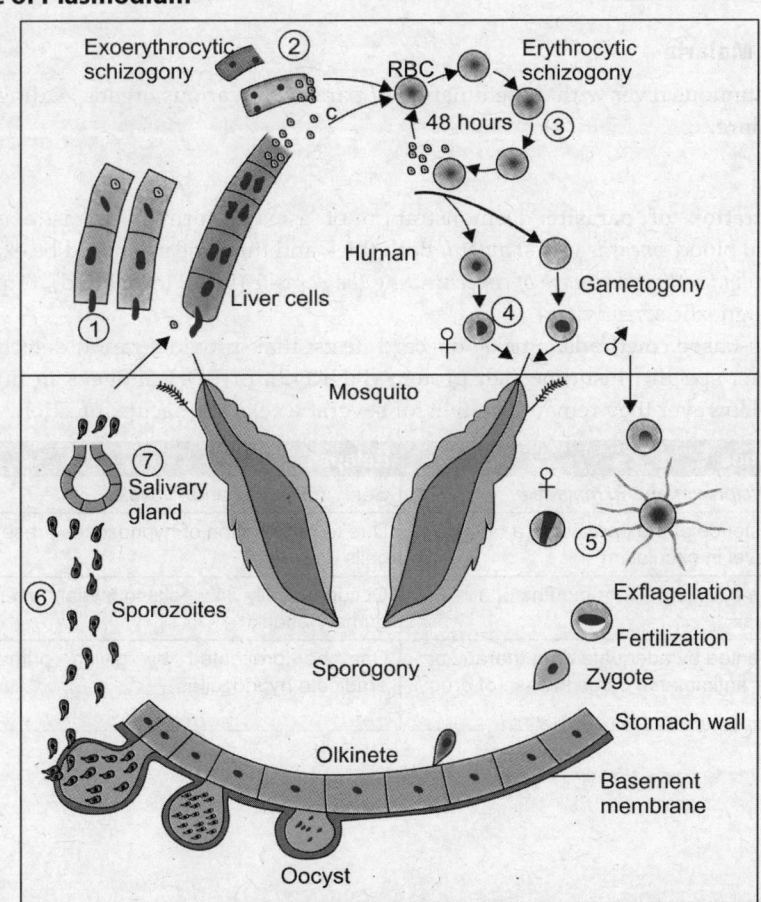

> P. falciparum: Malignant tertian = Pernicious malariae
> P. Ovale: Ovale tertian
> P. vivax: Benign tertian
> P. malariae: Quartan malaria

Life cycle of Plasmodium vivax

1. Sporozoites from the salivary gland of female mosquito are injected into skin capillaries when the mosquito bites humans.

2. They enter liver cells to initiate exoerythrocytic schizogony to form merozoites which infect red blood cells, to initiate the cycle of erythrocytic schizogony which is repeated every 48 hours.
3. Some merozoites initiate gametogony, forming male and female gametocytes.
4. Mosquito ingests gametocytes in its blood meal. Male gametocyte undergoes exflagellation.
5. One male, gamete fertilises female gamete to form zygote. It develops into the motile ookinete, which penetrates the stomach wall and becomes the oocyst inside which sporozoites develop.
6. Sporozoites released by rupture of mature oocyst enter the haemocoele and reach the salivary glands of the mosquito.

Black Waters Fever

- Sometimes seen in falciparum malaria, particularly in patients who experienced repeated infections and inadequate quinine treatment.
- Clinical features include bilious vomiting and prostration with passage of dark red and blackish urine.
- Pathogenesis include massive intravascular hemolysis secondary to anti-erythrocyte antibodies.
- Complications include renal failure, acute hepatic failure and circulatory collapse.

Algid Malaria

- Malaria characterized by peripheral circulatory failure, rapid thready pulse with low BP and cold clammy skin.

Septicemic Malaria

- High continuous fever with dissemination of parasite to various organs leading to multi-organ failure.

Diagnosis

a. **Demonstration of parasite:** Demonstration of asexual form of parasite in stained peripheral blood *smear is gold standard*. Both thick and thin smears should be examined.
   - *Thick film has the advantage of concentrating the parasite* (by 40 to 100 fold), thus enhance the diagnostic sensitivity.
b. **Antibody-based methods:** Sticks or card tests that provide rapid detection of P. falciparum, specific, histidine rich protein (PjHRP-2), or LDH antigens in finger prick method. However they remain positive for several weeks after acute infection.

Recrudescence	Relapse
Seen in P. *falciparum* and P. *malariae*	Seen in P. *vivax* and P. *ovale*
Due to persistence of the parasite at a subclinical level in circulation	Due to reactivation of hypnozoites present in liver cells
Occurs within a few weeks or months of a previous attack	Occurs usually 24 weeks to 5 years after the primary attack
Can be prevented by adequate drug therapy or use of newer antimalarial drugs in case of drug resistance	Can be prevented by giving primaquine to eradicate hypnozoites

Multiple Choice Questions

Amebae

1. All are true about entamoeba histolytica except:
   [AIIMS Nov 2014]
   a. Stool trophozoites are essential for diagnosis
   b. Mostly asymptomatic
   c. Cause disease in brain, liver
   d. Infection does not provide immunity

2. Which of the following cause flasked shaped ulcer?
   [NEET Pattern 2019]
   a. Entamoeba
   b. Giardis
   c. Enterobius
   d. Salmonella

3. Acute primary amoebic meningoencephalitis true is:
   [AIIMS 08]
   a. Meningitis caused by *Acanthamoeba* species is acute in nature
   b. Diagnosed by trophozoite in CSF
   c. Caused by feco-oral transmission
   d. More common in tropical climate

4. A patient presents with lower gastrointestinal bleed. Sigmoidoscopy shows ulcers in the sigmoid. Biopsy from this area shows flask-shaped ulcers. Which of the following is the most appropriate treatment?
   a. Intravenous ceftriaxone [AIIMS 05]
   b. Intravenous metronidazole
   c. Intravenous steroids and sulphasalazine
   d. Hydrocortisone enemas

5. Invasive amoebiasis can be best diagnosed by:
   [AIIMS 01]
   a. ELISA
   b. Counter current immunoelectrophoresis
   c. Indirect hemagglutination test
   d. Complement fixation test

6. The following life cycle depicts which parasites:
   [AIIMS 17]

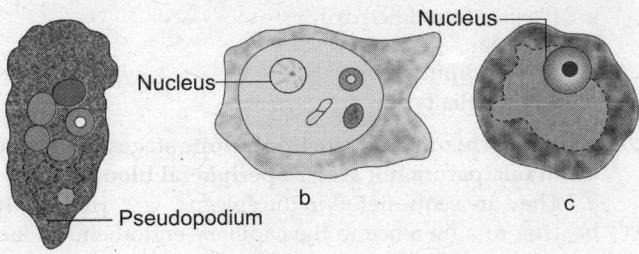
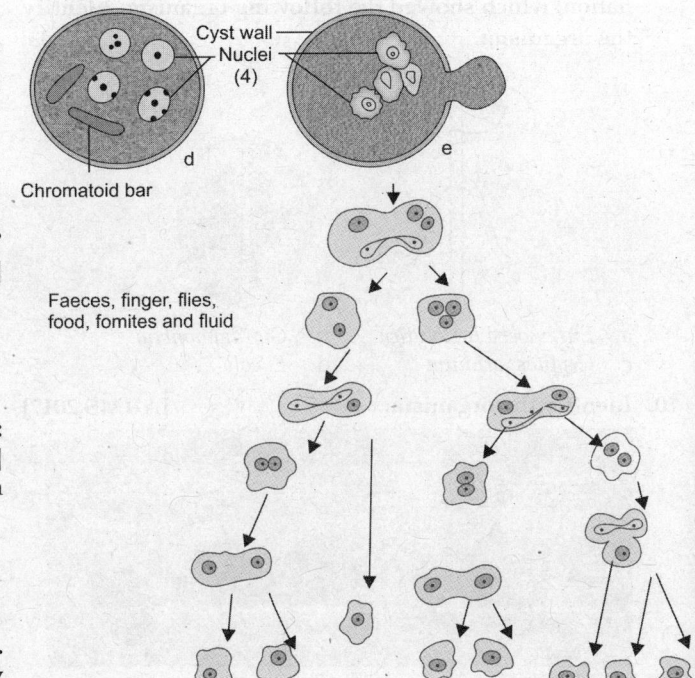

   a. B. coli
   b. E. histolytica
   c. A. duodenale
   d. E. vermicularis

7. A 30-year-old patient treated with features of acute meningoencephalitis in casualty. His CSF on wet mount microscopy revealed motile unicellular microorganisms. The most likely organism is: [AIIMS 05]
   a. *Naegleria fowleri*
   b. *Acanthamoeba castellani*
   c. *Entamoeba histolytica*
   d. *Trypanosoma cruzi*

8. Transmission of amoebiasis occurs by all except:
   [AIIMS Nov 10]
   a. Cockroach
   b. Feco oral
   c. Oro rectal
   d. Vertical transmission

Flagellates

9. An anxious mother brought her 4-year-old daughter to the pediatrician. The girl was passing loose bulky stools for the past 20 days. This was often associated with pain in abdomen. The pediatrician suggested the stool examination, which showed the following organism. Identify the organism: [AI 03]

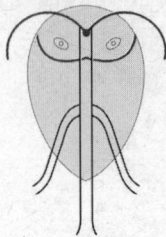 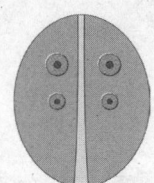

   a. Entamoeba histolytica   b. Giardia lamblia
   c. Cryptosporidium   d. E. coli

10. Identify the organism: [AIIMS 2017]

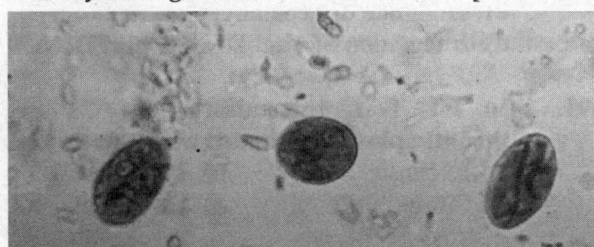

   a. Giardia intestinalis
   b. Entamoeba dispar
   c. Cryptosporidium hominis
   d. Balantidium coli

11. Vector of Kala-azar is: [AIIMS 07]
   a. Flea   b. Tsetse fly
   c. Sand fly   d. Mite

12. Parasite causing encephalitis are all except: [NEET Pattern 2018]
   a. Entamoeba histolytica b. T. gondii
   c. Angiostrongylus cantonensis
   d. T. cruzi

13. Reduvid bug is a vector for the transmission of: [AIIMS 05]
   a. Relapsing fever   b. Lyme's disease
   c. Scrub typhus   d. Chagas disease

14. Which of the following infestations leads to malabsorption? [AI 06; AIIMS 04]
   a. Giardia lamblia   b. Ascaris lumbricoides
   c. Necator americana   d. Ancylostoma duodenale

15. Which of the following is true about *Giardia lamblia*?
   a. Malabsorption commonly seen [PGI 05]
   b. Trophozoite form is binucleate pear shaped
   c. Diarrhea is seen
   d. Jejunal wash fluid is diagnostic
   e. Is a free living nematode

16. True about visceral leishmaniasis: [PGI May 2013]
   a. Neutropenia
   b. Eosinophilia
   c. Hyper gamma globulinemia
   d. Skin hyperpigmentation
   e. Lymphadenopathy

17. Classic presentation of congenital toxoplasmosis: [NEET Pattern 2019]
   a. Hydrocephalus, cerebral calcification, chorioretinitis
   b. Saddle nose, cardiac defects
   c. Chorioretinitis, cicatrissim, limb hypoplasia
   d. VACTERL anomalies, hypospadias sternal defect

Sporozoa

18. All of the following statements about toxoplasmosis are true except: [AI 01]
   a. Oocyst in freshly passed cat's faeces is not infective
   b. May spread by organ transplantation
   c. Maternal infection after 6 months has high risk of transmission
   d. Arthralgia, sore throat and abdominal pain are the most common manifestation

19. A 15-year-old boy presented with fever and chills for 3 days. On examination he was found to have delayed skin pinch time and dry oral mucosa. A peripheral blood smear revealed the following picture. Identify the pathogen involved: [AIIMS 16]

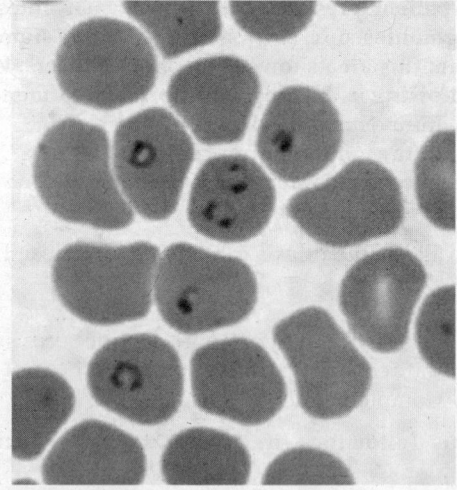

   a. Plasmodium falciparum
   b. Babesia
   c. Plasmodium vivax
   d. Salmonella typhi

20. Why are schizont and late trophozoite stages of Plasmodium falciparum not seen in peripheral blood smear?
   a. They are sequestered in the spleen [AIIMS 16]
   b. Due to adherence to the capillary endothelium, they are not seen in peripheral blood
   c. Due to antigen-antibody reaction and removal
   d. They are seen in mosquito blood

21. Which one of the following is detected by the antigen detection test used for the diagnosis of *P. falciparum* malaria?
    a. Circum sporozoite protein [AIIMS 14]
    b. Merozoite surface antigen
    c. Histidine rich protein I (HRP I)
    d. Histidine rich protein II (HRP II)

22. The plasmodium species known for relapse in malaria is:
    a. *P. falciparum* and *P. vivax* [AIIMS 2017]
    b. *P. vivax* and *P. ovale*
    c. *P. vivax* and *P. malariae*
    d. *P. malariae* and *P. ovale*

23. Toxoplasmosis in the foetus can be best confirmed by: [AIIMS 13]
    a. IgM antibodies against *Toxoplasma* in the mother
    b. IgM antibodies against *Toxoplasma* in the foetus
    c. IgG antibodies against *Toxoplasma* in the mother
    d. IgG antibodies against *Toxoplasma* in the foetus

24. A 35-year-old male suffering from sudden onset of high grade fever. On malarial slide examination all stages of parasites are seen with schizonts of 20 microns size with 14-20 merozoites per cell and yellow brown pigment. The diagnosis is: [PGI 12]
    a. *Plasmodium falciparum*   b. *Plasmodium vivax*
    c. *Plasmodium malariae*   d. *Plasmodium ovale*

25. True about Toxoplasma gondii: [PGI 11]
    a. Direct spread by blood/urine is main mode of transmission
    b. Cerebellum is MC site of brain involvement
    c. Isolation of parasite from blood is very easy
    d. Laboratory test are useful for making diagnosis
    e. Infection is severe and progressive in immunocompromised host

26. Stages seen in peripheral smear of *falciparum* malaria:
    a. Schizonts   b. Gametocytes   [PGI 05]
    c. Accole trophozoite d. Ring form

27. *P. falciparum* causes: [PGI 05]
    a. Thrombocytopenia   b. DIC
    c. Hemolysis   d. Hematemesis

28. Babesiosis true statement is [AIIMS 2018]
    a. Caused by babesia microti
    b. Resides in WBC
    c. Chloroquine is drug of choice
    d. It is a filarial parasite

29. True about *Cryptosporidium parvum*: [NEET Pattern 2019]
    a. Affect only in immunocompromised patient
    b. It is one of the common opportunistic infection in AIDS
    c. Cyst size 12-15 mm
    d. Treatment is metronidazole

30. *Acid fast* organism with oocyte of size 5 μm on stool examination, causing diarrhoea in HIV positive patient:
    a. *Cryptosporidium*   b. *Isospora belli* [AIIMS May 09]
    c. *Microsoporidia*   d. *Blastocystis hominii*

31. Which is the infective stage for mosquito in case of plasmodium vivax: [AIIMS Nov 09]
    a. Gametocyte   b. Sporozoite
    c. Zygote   d. Merozoite

32. Which is not true about fluorescent antibody detection test for diagnosis of *falciparum*? [AIIMS 08]
    a. It is a immunochromatographic test
    b. Detects aldolase antigens
    c. Detects LDH antigens
    d. Detects histidine rich proteins 1

33. Congenital toxoplasmosis not true: [AIIMS May 09]
    a. IgA is more sensitive than IgM
    b. An increase in IgM beyond 1st week of life is diagnostic
    c. IgG is diagnostic
    d. Dye test is used

34. In HIV patient with malabsorption, fever, chronic diarrhea, with acid fast positive organism, What is causative agent? [AIIMS May 10]
    a. Giardia   b. Microsporidia
    c. Isospora   d. E. histolytica

Miscellaneous

35. Parasitic encephalitis is caused by: [PGI 05]
    a. *Ascaris*   b. *Naegleria*
    c. *Acanthamoeba* d. *Balamuthia*
    e. *Entamoeba*

36. About microsporidia all of the following are false except:
    a. It is a fungus   b. It is a protozoa [PGI 05]
    c. It is a bacteria d. It is trematoda
    e. It is associated with diarrhoea in HIV patients

37. A patient complains of diarrhea, stool examination shows ova of size <100 μm, which of the following can not be the cause: [AIIMS May 2013]
    a. Cryptosporidium   b. Opisthorchis viverni
    c. Isospora   d. E. histolytica

38. Rk39 dip stick kit was found to be positive, the treatment of choice is: [AIIMS 2018]
    a. Amphotericin B   b. Albendazole
    c. Doxycycline   d. Praziquantel

Explanations and References with Illustrative Answers

1. **Ans. (a) Stool trophozoites are essential for diagnosis** *Ref. Paniker 7/e, p 21*

   Diagnosis of intestinal amoebiasis is suggested by presence of cyst or dead trophozoite in stool.

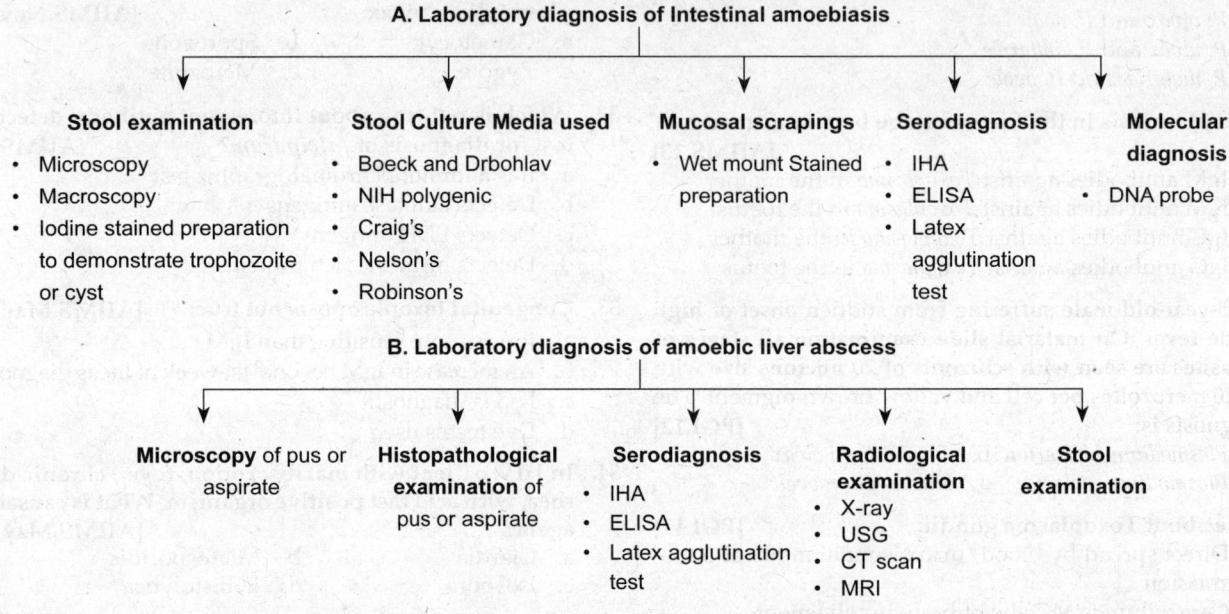

   Note: Stool culture is a sensitive method for diagnosing chronic and asymptomatic amoebiasis

2. **Ans. (a) Entamoeba** *Ref. Paniker 7/e, p 18*

   Typical amoebic ulcer is flask shaped in cross section with mouth and neck being narrow and base large and rounded. 8 small trophozoites (=amoebulae or metacystic trophozoites) are released per infective cyst causing:

Primary amoebiasis	Secondary intestinal lesion	Chronic infection	Invasive amoebiasis
• **MC** site caecum	• **MC** in cecum, appendix or nearby ascending colon	• Occurs when organism travel to ileocaecal valve and terminal ileum	• Extraintestinal infection is metastatic through portal circulation
• Lesion with Pinhead sized center and raised edges	• It occurs due to extension from primary lesion	• Sigmoid colon and rectum are favoured site • Amoeboma may form	• MC form is amebic hepatitis or liver abscess
• Flask shaped ulcers with narrow neck and broad base				
• Mucosa surface between ulcer is normal				
• Ulcer is not premalignant				

- Intestinal amoebiasis present usually as amoebic dysentery.
- Contents of amoebic abscess is called as *anchovy paste*.
- **MC** complication of amoeba liver abscess is *Pleuropulmonary involvement*.

	Typhoid fever	Bacillary dysentery	Intestinal amebiasis
Location	Lower ileum and cecum	Sigmoid, rectum	Cecum
Inflammation	Typhoid granuloma	Fibrinous-pseudomembrane	Necrosis
Ulcer	Longitudinal ulcer	Map-like ulcer	Flask-like ulcer
Clinical	Continued fever, diarrhea, disorientation, Bradycardia	Bloody mucoid diarrhea, tenesmus	Reddish-brown hue (likened to anchovy paste) diarrhea

Protozoa

3. **Ans. (b) Diagnosis by trophozoite in CSF** *Ref. Paniker 7/e, p 25 - 26; Harrison 19/e, p 1367*
Acute primary amoebic meningoencephalitis (PAM) is caused by Naegleria fowleri
Naegleria

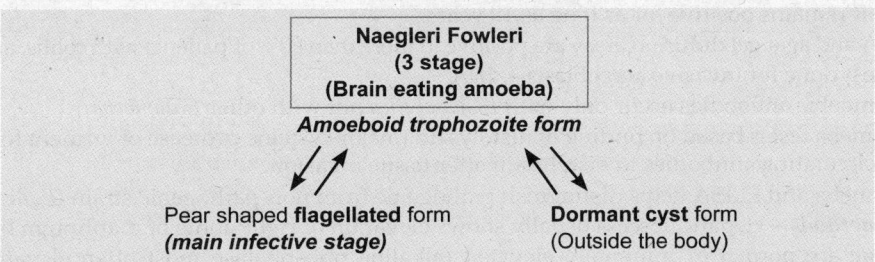

Route of transmission
- It is seen in fresh water lake.
- Aspiration of water contaminated with trophozoites or cysts or inhalation of cyst leading to invasion of olfactory neuroepithelium, then into meninges and brain.

Clinical features
- *Commonly seen* in *otherwise* healthy children or young adults who often report recent swimming in lakes or heated swimming pools.
- Parosmia/anosmia, headache, high fever, nausea, vomiting, meningismus.
- Photophobia and palsies of 3rd, 4rh and 6th cranial nerves are common.
- Seizures, coma and most patient die within a week.

Diagnosis
- Detection of motile trophozoites in wet mounts of fresh spinal fluid.
- Bacterial meningitis *without any bacteria on* Gram's staining/antigen detection assay and culture.

Treatment
- Amphotericin
- Rifampicin may be added.

> **Remember: Other Pathogenic free living amoebae**
> i. Acanthamoeba spp. – Causing chronic granulomatous amoebic encephalitis (GAE), chronic amoebic keratitis (associated with use of contact lens).
> ii. Balamuthia – Cause meningoencephalitis in both immunocompromised and immunocompetent host particularly children and adult.

4. **Ans. (b) Intravenous metronidazole** *Ref. Harrison 17/e, p 1278, 18/e, p 1686, 19/e p 1366*
It is case of intestinal amoebiasis in the form of amoebic dysentry.

Drug Therapy for Amebiasis		
Asymptomatic carrier (Luminal agents)	**Acute colitis**	**Amebic liver abscess**
• Iodoquinol • Paromomycin	• Metronidazole plus Luminal agent	• Metronidazole or Tinidazole or tinidazole or ornidazole plus Luminal agent

5. **Ans. (a) ELISA** *Ref. Harrison 19/e, p 1366 - 1367, 18/e, p 1685; Paniker 7/e, p 21*
Diagnosis of Amoebiasis
Specimen
- Faecal fluid for examination of trophozoite.
- Formed feces for cysts.
- Scrapings and biopsies – *most commonly* by colonoscopy.
- Liver abscess aspirate for trophozoites *(as cyst are absent in tissues)* from edge of abscess, not the necrotic center.
- Blood for serologic test and cell counts.

i. *Fecal findings suggestive of amoebic colitis* - positive test for heme, paucity of neutrophils, *amoebic cyst or hematophagous trophozoite (definitive)*. Examine at least 3 fresh stool specimen.
ii. *Culture* - Diphasic Locke-egg, Monophasic TYGSM and Robinson's media are used.
iii. *Trophozoites in biopsy* specimen from colonic mass confirm the diagnosis of amoeboma.
PCR assay for entamoeba DNA is most sensitive and specific method for identifying E. histolytica
Stool diagnostic test based on the detection of the Gal/GalNAC lectin of E.histolytica compare favorably with the PCR
Harrison 19/e, p 1366

UNIT-IV: Parasitology

iv. *Serology: (Becomes positive only in invasive amoebiasis)*
   - Is primarily for extra-intestinal amoebiasis when stools are often negative.
   - *Most commonly* done by indirect hemagglutination assay (IHA) but it can't distinguish recent from past infection since it remains positive for as long as 10 years.
   - ELISA and agar gel diffusion assay are positive in more than 90% of patients with colitis, amoebomas or liver abscess.
   - *MC* test done for invasive amoebiasis – *IHA*
   - Antamoebic antibodies occur only with *E. histolytica* not with other *Entamoeba*.
   - Enzymeba test is based on finding of histolysain (major cysteine protease of virulent form) in the intestine (stool) plus circulating antibodies to histolysain after tissue invasion.
   - Enzymeba and ELISA helps distinguish pathogenic from non-pathogenic strain (*E. dispar*) in a stool specimen.
v. **Radiation methods** – Hepatic abscess usually shows elevation of right dome of diaphragm by US, CT, MRI, etc.
vi. **Liver enzyme** are normal or minimally elevated (alkaline phosphatase most often elevated) even with large liver abscess.

6. **Ans. (b) E. histolytica** *Ref. Paniker 7/e, p 16*
   Quadrinucleate cyst suggest E. histolytica.

7. **Ans. (a) *Naegleria fowleri*** *Ref. Paniker 7/e, p 26 - 27; Harrison 19/e, p 1367, 18/e, p 1686*
   It is a typical presentation of meningitis caused by Naegleria fowleri.
   Let's consider other options:
   Acanthamoeba
   - No flagellated stage
   - Trophozoite Cyst (Formed in tissue) **(Infective stage)**
   - Encephalitis occurs typically in chronically ill or debilitated patient (lymphoproliferative disorder, chemotherapy, etc) and features of CNS lesion often mimics space occupying lesion.
   - Infection reaches the CNS hematogenously from primary focus in the sinuses, skin nodules/ulcers and lungs.
   Diagnosis:
   - Demonstration of trophozoites and cyst on wet mount of CSF.
   - Culture on non-nutrient agar plates seeded with *E.coli*.

   Entamoeba histolytica
   Brain may occasionally involve (<0.1%), result from hematogenous spread from amoebic lesions of colon.
   ... *Harrison 19/e, p 1365*
   Trypanosoma cruzi
   Neurologic sign are not common but meningoencephalitis have been reported especially in children < 2 years old.
   ... *Harrison 18/e, p 1717*
   So, from above description it is clear that patient of 30 year (young adult with no chronic disease and no GI symptoms) with meningoencephalitis and motile unicellular (all protozoan are unicellular) microorganism on wet mount; is a typical case of PAM of Naegleri fowleri.

8. **Ans. (d) Vertical transmission** *Ref. Paniker 6/e, p 14, 16*
   Epidemiological features of amoebiasis
   Adults > children
   Males > females
   Infective stage–Quadrinucleate cyst
   Source of infection – carrier or asymptomatic cyst passer
   Route of transmission   – Fecooral
   Mode of transmission   – Contaminated food and water
   Mechanical vectors   – Flies and cockroaches
   Sexual transmission   – Occur in homosexuals (*gay bowel disease*)

   > **Remember:** Parasites transmitted transplacentally (vertical transmission) are:
   > Toxoplasmosis
   > Plasmodium
   > T. Cruzi

9. **Ans. (b) Giardia lamblia** *Ref. Paniker 7/e, p 30*
   It is typical figure of ***trophozoite and cyst of Giardia lamblia*** which is the *MC* intestinal protozoan parasite.

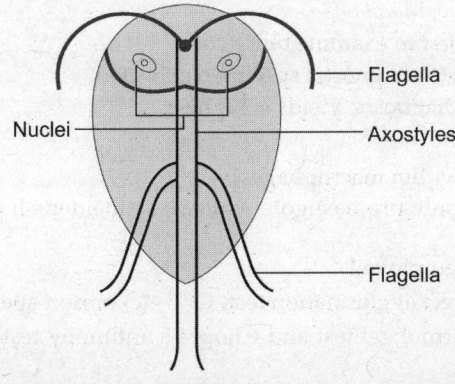 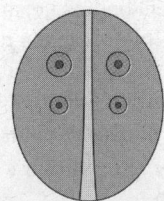

Trophozoite	Cyst
• Pyriform/Heart/Tennis or badminton racket shaped	• Encystation occur in colon
• Bilateral symmetrical and has large concave sucking disc; 2 axostyles; 2 parabasal or median bodies; 4 pairs of flagella; **2 nuclei** with prominent central karyosomes	– Ovoid with hyaline cyst wall
	– Mature cyst has **4 nuclei (= infective stage)**
	– Passed in stool and *is infectious*
• Divides by longitudinal binary fission	– Infective dose is as few as 10 cyst
• Passed in stool but **not infectious**	
• Motility resemble "*falling leaf*"	

Giardia lamblia
- Intestinal flagellate, the only protozoan parasite found in the lumen of human small intestine (Duodenum and upper jejunum).
- Infection is acquired by ingestion of cysts in contaminated food and water.
- It does not invade tissue (so no RBC and pus cells in faeces) but remains attached to epithelial surface by sucking disc which may cause abnormalities of villous architecture and loss of brush border enzymic activities leading to self limited mucus diarrhoea; malabsorption like syndrome; weight loss; abdominal cramps. Occasionally cause biliary colic and jaundice. ... *Paniker 6/e, p 38*
- **Diagnosis:** Detection of cysts (encystation occur in colon) as well as trophozoite (die outside so not infectious) in stool sample or in duodenal aspiration by enterotest if biliary symptoms predominate.
- Detection of antigen by ELISA or immunochromatographic strip test.
- Giardiasis is a cause of traveller's diarrhoea.
- **Treatment:** DOC – Metronidazole/tinidazole
  Alternative – quinacrine hydrochloride and furazolidone.

10. **Ans. (a) Giardia intestinalis** *Ref. Paniker 7/e, p 30; Jawetz 27/e p 710*

    Already explained (See color plate, pg xxxvifb for related image) for details

11. **Ans. (c) Sand fly** *Ref. Harrison 19/e, p 1389; Paniker 7/e, p 51 - 54*

    Visceral Leishmaniasis/Kala-azar

    "Beside the bite of Sand fly (P. argentipes), it is also transmitted by blood transfusion, sexual contact, inoculation and congenitally."

    Important points about visceral Leishmaniasis/Kalaazar
    - Caused by *L. donovani*:
    - *MC* organ affected: **spleen.**
    - Progressive emaciation, irregular fever sometimes hectic, hepatosplenomegaly, bone marrow infiltration epistaxis, bleeding, cancrum oris, pneumonia may occur.
    - Some develops post-kalaazar dermal leishmaniasis (PKDL) characterized by skin lesion mostly on face.
    - Usually develop about an year on two, after recovery from systemic illness
    - PKDL occur in 10-20% cases and it is seen mainly in India.
    - Relapse of visceral lesion can also occur.

Diagnosis

- *Specimen:*
  Peripheral blood — *Best* to examine buffy coat.
  Bone marrow aspirate — *MC* diagnostic specimen collected.
  Spleen aspirates — Diagnostic yields is highest.

1. *Demonstration of parasites by:*
   - Microscopy [LD bodies i.e. amastigote seen within macrophages].
   - Culture in NNN or Tobie's medium shows only promastigote while in Schneider's liquid tissue culture amastigote form also seen.
   - Animal inoculation – Hamster is the animal employed.
2. *Demonstration of antibodies by* using specific (direct agglutination test, CFT etc) or non-specific (WKK) antigen.
3. *Nonspecific serum test* (Napier's aldehyde or Formol gel test and Chopra's antimony test) **based on increased globulin content** of serum.
4. *Absence of hypersensitivity to* leishmanial antigen, i.e. Montenegro (leishmanin) skin test is negative in kala-azar.
5. *Others lab findings* – Anemia, leucopenia, neutropenia, thrombocytopenia with hypergammaglobulinaemia and reversal of albumin: globulin ratio.

Treatment:	– First line therapy	- Pentavalent antimony
		- Amphotericin B lipid formulation
	– Alternative	- Amphotericin B (deoxy cholate), paromomycin sulfate, pentamidine isethionate, miltefosine.

12. **Ans. (a) Entamoeba** *Ref. Harrison 20/e, p 994*
    Parasites causing encephalitis are:
    - *Toxoplasma gondii* (rarely)
    - *Trypanosoma cruzi* (occasionally)
    - *Angiostrongylus cantonensis* (eosinophilic meningoencephalitis)
    - *Acanthamoeba* (Granulomatous amoebic encephalitis)
    - *Naegleria fowleri* (Primary amebic meningoencephalitis)
    - *Balamuthia*.

13. **Ans. (d) Chagas disease** *Ref. Paniker 7/e, p 46; Park 22/e p724*

Hemoflagellate	Vector	Disease	Infective stage for man
Trypanosomes			
i. *T. brucei gambiense and T. brucei rhodesiense*	Tse-Tse fly	African trypanosomiasis (sleeping sickness)	Metacyclic trypomastigote by inoculative route of fly
ii. *T. cruzi* (Intracellular)	Reduvid bug or triatomine bug	Chaga's disease (South American trypanosomiasis)	Metacyclic trypomastigote by rubbing faces into wound made by bite of bug (Stercorarian transmission)
Leishmania – In man, amastigote form present in macrophage forming LD (Leishmania donovani) body			
i. L. donovani	Female Sandfly (P. argentipes)	Visceral leishmaniasis (= kala azar)	Promastigote form by bite of fly
ii. L. Tropica	P. sargenti and P. papatasi	Cutaneous leishmaniasis (=oriental sore)	Promastigote form by bite of fly
iii. L. braziliensis	Sandfly	Mucocutaneous leishmaniasis	Promastigote form by bite of fly

14. **Ans. (a) Giardia lamblia** *Ref. Ghai 6/e, p 252; Harrison 19/e, p 1405, 18/e, p 1730*

    Remember:
    - *Ascaris lumbricoides* in small intestine usually cause no symptoms. In children it may cause pain and intestinal obstruction sometimes complicated by perforation, intussusception or volvulus.
    - Migration to aberrant site can cause biliary colic, cholecystitis, cholangitis, pancreatitis or rarely intrahepatic abscess.
    - Intestinal phase of *A. duodenale* cause epigastric pain, inflammatory diarrhea and iron deficiency anemia.

Protozoa

15. **Ans. (a, b, c) and (d) Malabsorption commonly seen, Trophozoite form is binucleate pear shaped, Diarrhea is seen and Jejunal wash fluid is diagnostic** *Ref. Paniker 7/e, p 30 - 33; Jawetz 27/e, p 709 - 710*
    Already explained

    > **Remember:**
    > - Giardia lamblia lives in the duodenum and upper jejunum and is the only protozoan parasite found in the lumen of human small intestine.

16. **Ans. (a, d, e) Neutropenia, Skin hyperpigmentation, Lymphadenopathy** *Ref. Harrison 20/e, p 1594*
    Manifestations of visceral leishmaniasis
    - Moderate to high grade fever with chills & rigor
    - *Lymphadenopathy:* Lymphadenopathy is common in most endemic regions of the world except the Indian subcontinent
    - *Organomegaly:* Splenomegaly occurs by 2nd week of illness followed by hepatomegally (moderate)
    - *Hyperpigmentation:* Patient loose weights feel weak and the skin gradually develops dark discoloration due to hyper-pigmentation
    - *Hematological:* Anemia, hypoalbunemia, thrombocytopenia, leukopenia.

17. **Ans. (a) i.e., Hydrocephalus** ...*Ref. Harrison 20/e, p 1612*
    Toxoplasma gondii
    - It is *obligate intracellular* sporozoan.
    - It has three forms:
      1. *Trophozoites*:
         - It can invade any nucleated cell (i.e. not **RBC**) and replicate by endodyogeny or internal budding. This rapidly multiplying trophozoite is known as tachyzoites. It can be seen extracellularly also.
         - Crescentic parasites distend the cells which are called as pseudocyst or pseudocolony. It is differentiating from true tissue cyst by its staining property.
         - Stained by Giemsa.
         - It is *non-infective*.
         - It is formed during acute phase.
      2. *Tissue cyst*:
         - It is formed during chronic phase in various organs but persist principally in central nervous system and muscles.
         - Cyst contain slowly multiplying rounded parasite called Bradyzoites.
         - It is stained by silver stains.
      3. *Oocyst*:
         - It develops *only* in intestine of definitive host.
         - It contains two sporocysts with sporozoites inside.

    - **Mode of transmission:**
      - Usually by ingestion of either sporulated oocyst from contaminated soil, food, water or bradyzoites from undercooked meat (ingestion of even single cyst can produce infection).
        Also transmitted by blood transfusion and organ transplantation and transplacentally.

    - **Clinical features:**
      - Human toxoplasmosis is zoonosis (Anthropo-Zoonoses). It is of following types:
        a. *Toxoplasmosis in immunocompetent person*: Mostly asymptomatic.
           - **MC** manifestation: *Cervical lymphadenopathy* which is generalized in 20-30%.
           - Headache, fever, myalgia, splenomegaly often present.
           - Meningoencephalitis, myocarditis, pneumonitis, chorioretinitis are rare.
        b. *Toxoplasmosis in immunocompromised person*:
           - **MC** site is **CNS** (usually brainstem).
           - **MC** symptom: Altered mental status.
        c. *Congenital toxoplasmosis*
           - Occurs only when mother gets primary toxoplasmosis infection whether clinical or asymptomatic during pregnancy or <6 months before conception (i.e. no risk if acquired > 6 months before conception).

- As gestational age is increased, risk of transmission to fetus increased, i.e. max. in 3rd trimester while severity of fetal damage is decreased, i.e. infant is usually asymptomatic if infection transmit in 3rd trimester.
- It causes:
  - hydrocephalous
  - diffuse cerebral calcification
  - hepatosplenomegaly
  - mental retardation
  - myocarditis
  - lymphadenitis
  - microencephaly
  - myocarditis
  - chorioretinitis
  - multiorgan failure
  - pneumonitis

Summary
- **Asexual** (schizogony) forms of parasite — Trophozoite and tissue cyst
- **Sexual** form (gametogony or sporogony) — Oocyst
- **Definitive** host — Domestic cat and other felines.
  - *All three forms present.*
- *Intermediate host* – Man, mammals and birds; only asexual forms present.
- *Infective stage* for man – Oocyst with sporozoites and tissue cyst with bradyzoites.
- Freshly passed oocyst is not infectious (needs development in soil).
- Mature Oocyst containing 8 sporozoites is the infective form.
- Human infection is dead end for the parasite.

18. **Ans. (d) Arthralgia, sore throat and abdominal pain are the most common manifestation**

Ref. Paniker 7/e, p 87 - 89; Harrison 20/e p 1611-1613

Already explained see answer 17

19. **Ans. (a) Plasmodium falciparum** *Ref. Paniken 7/e, p 80*

Multiple ring form suggest diagnosis of P. Falciparum

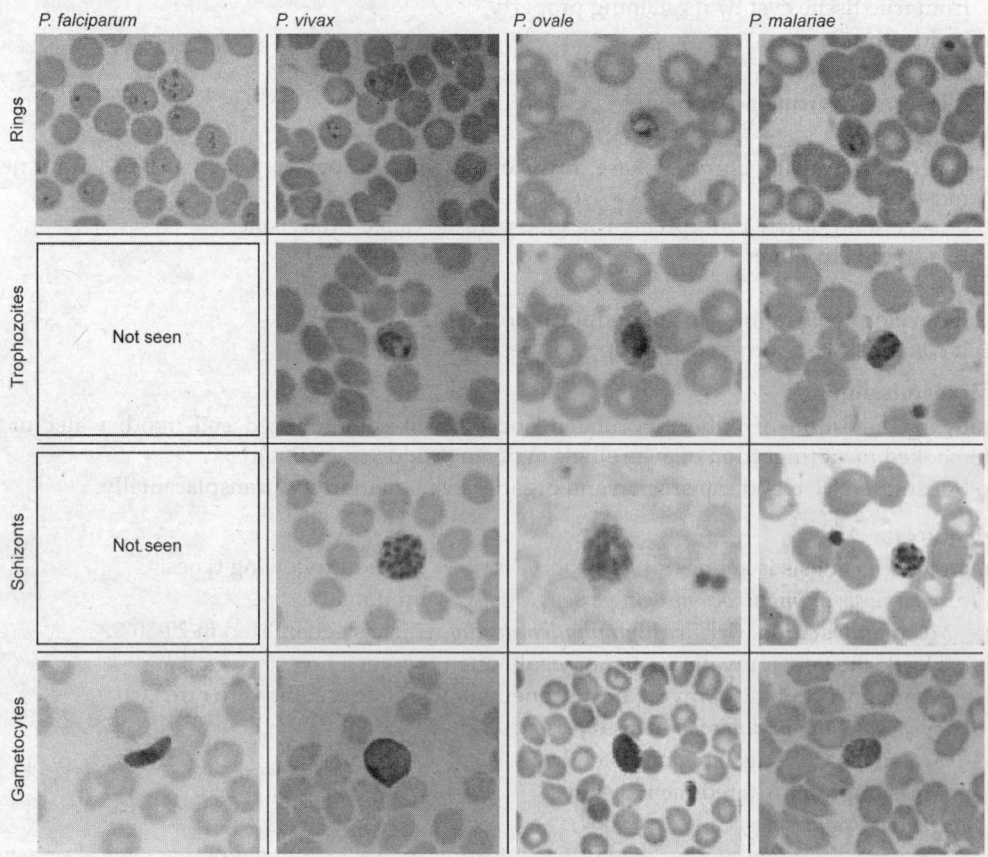

Blood picture in different species of plasmodium

Important features of Falciparum malaria
- Most virulent
- Sporozoites are sickle shaped. Tissue phase consist of only a single cycle of pre-erythrocytic schizogony. No hypnozoites occur
- Ring forms are often seen attached to the margin of red cell forming applique. There can be multiple rings in single RBC
- Late trophozoites and mature schizonts are not ordinarily seen in peripheral blood. The presence of P. falciparum schizonts in peripheral smear indicates a grave prognosis.
- Infected erythrocyte are of normal size and exhibit Maurer's cleft.
- Cause black water fever, pernicious malaria, malignant malaria and septicemic malaria

> **Why trophozoites and mature schizonts are not seen?**
>
> The erythrocytes infected with trophozoites extrudes a strain specific erythrocytes membrane adhesive protein, (PMPI) that mediate erythrocytic attachment to receptors on venular capillary endothelium (RA M-1 in brain, chondroitin sulfate B in placenta).
>
> The infected erythrocyte stick inside and block capillaries and venules. At the same time infected RBC adhere to uninfected RBC to form rosette. This result in sequestration of infected RBC containing mature form of parasite in vital organs like brain, kidney, spleen, etc.

Blood Smears of Plasmodium

Features	P. falciparum	P. vivax	P. malariae	P. ovale
Features of red cells				
Size	All sizes/normal	Large (young), pale	Small (Old) / Normal	Large (Young)
Shape	Round may be crenated	Round or oval	Round	Round or pear-shaped, fimbriated
Stippling	Maurer's clefts; Large; red up to 20 Basophilic stippling ±	Schuffner's dots: numerous, small, red	None Occasionally, Zieman's stippling	Schuffner's dots, James dot
Features of Parasite				
Ring (early torphozoite)	Theardlike, multiple infections, double chromatin dots, form accole or appluque	Thicker	Compact	Compact
Mature / Late trophozoites (amoeboid form)	Absent/occasionally seen	Ameboid, may fill cell	More regular, smaller; Band form	Less ameboid and smaller than those of P. vivax;
Schizonts	Absent/occasionally 8-24 merozoites in grape like pattern	12 to 24 merozoites grape like pattern	8 to 12 merozoites, often rosetted around pigment	8 to 12 merozoites irregularly arranged
Gametocytes	Sausage or crescentic/banana shaped central chromatin (female) or diffuse (male)	Round, fills cell, pigment often central	Round, large coarse pigment	Smaller and oval, but similar to those of P. vivax
Diagnostic keys				
	Gametocyte; multiple rings; double chromatin dots; accole forms, heavy infection	Schizont; large RBCs; ameboid forms	Schizont; small RBCs; band forms	Schizont and large pear-shaped fimbriated RBCs

Characteristics of Plasmodium Species infecting Humans

Characteristic	P. falciparum	P. vivax	P. ovale	P. malariae
Incubation period	12 days (shortest)	14 days	14 days	30 days (Longest)
Number of merozoites released per infected hepatocyte	30,000	10,000	15,000	15,000

Contd...

Contd...

Characteristics of Plasmodium Species infecting Humans				
Characteristic	P. falciparum	P. vivax	P. ovale	P. malariae
Duration of erythrocytic cycle (hours)	48 (Malignant tertian malaria)	48 (Benign tertian malaria)	50 (Ovale tertian malaria)	72 (Quartan malaria)
Red cell preference	Younger cells (but can invade cells of all ages), > 2% of RBC	Red cells up to 14 days old, < 1% of RBC infect	Reticulocytes	Older cells
Morphology	Usually only ring forms; banana shaped gametocytes	Irregularly shaped large rings and trophozoites; enlarged erythrocytes; Schuffner's dots	Infected erythrocytes enlarged and oval with tufted ends; Schuffner's dots	Band or rectangular forms of trophozoites common
Pigment color	Black	Yellow-brown	Dark brown	Brown-black
Ability to cause relapses = Hypnozoites or exo-erythrocytic schizogony	No	Yes	Yes	No

20. **Ans. (b) i.e Due to adherence** Ref. Paniker 7/e, p 71
    Already explained

21. **Ans. (d) Histidine rich protein II (HRP II)** Ref. Harrison 20/e, p 1575; Park 22/e, p 238
    Diagnosis of Malaria
    a. *Demonstration of parasite (= Asexual forms)*
       - **Thin film** is fixed and stained
         - Giemsa (Romanowsky stains) at p H 7.2 is preferred.
         - RBC is examined in tail region for identification of species/type of malaria.
       - **Thick blood film** is stained without fixing for searching of *parasites. It is more sensitive.*
    b. Rapid, simple, sensitive and specific antibody based diagnostic dip stick (antigen capture assay) or card test that detect *P. falciparum* specific (pf HRP-2) histidine rich protein 2 or lactate dehydrogenase antigen in finger prick blood sample is done.
       • Pf HRP-2 is antibody based test remains positive for several weeks after acute infection so it has disadvantage in high transmission areas.
    c. Malarial fluorescent antibody test is usually becomes positive 2 weeks or more after primary infection so positive test is not necessarily an indication of current infection. It is of greatest value in epidemiological studies and in determining whether a person has had malaria in the past.

    > **Remember:** In severe malaria, poor prognosis is indicated by predominance of more mature P. falciparum parasites (>20% of parasites with visible pigment) in peripheral blood film or presence of phagocytosed malarial pigment in >5% of neutrophils.

22. **Ans. (b) i.e. P. vivax and P. ovale** Ref. Paniker 7/e p 66
    Plasmodium vivax and P. ovale have hypnozoite stage which persist in the liver and causes relapse after clearance of the acute blood stage infection. Period of dormancy may range form weeks to over one year after which replication resumes and relapse.

23. **Ans. (b) IgM antibodies against *Toxoplasma* in the foetus** Ref. Harrison 20/e, p 1613-1614
    Diagnosis of Toxoplasmosis
    Diagnosis can be made by appropriate culture, serologic testing and PCR.
    i. **Tissue and body fluids:** Although difficult and available only at specialized labs isolation of *T gondii*. T gondi from blood or other body fluids can be accomplished after subinoculation of sample. Demonstration of tachyzoites in lymph nodes establishes the diagnosis of acute toxoplasmosis.

ii. **Serology**
   - Commonest method of laboratory diagnosis.
   - Diagnosis of acute infection can be established by detection of simultaneous presence of IgG (by Sabin Feldman dye test, indirect fluorescent antibody test and ELISA) and IgM (by double sandwich IgM ELISA and IgM immunosorbent assay).
   - Presence of IgA also favours diagnosis of acute infection. IgA ELISA is more sensitive than IgM ELISA for detecting congenital infection.

iii. **Molecular diagnosis**
   - Real time PCR for either the B_1 gene or the 529-bp sequence.

Patient type

a. *Immunocompetent adult or child*
   - Patient with lymphadenopathy only, a positive IgM titre is an indication of acute infection and indication of therapy.

b. *Immunocompromised host*
   i. Person should be tested for IgG antibody to *T. gondii* soon after diagnosis of HIV infection.
   ii. IgM serum antibody is usually not detectable.

c. *Congenital infection*
   i. Antibodies in neonate may be either due to congenital infection (IgG, IgM) or due to passive transfer of antibodies from mother (IgG only).
      So detection of IgM specific antibody in fetus is helpful in diagnosing congenital toxoplasmosis since it does not cross placenta.
      Harrison writes: *"Persistence of IgG antibody or positive IgM titer after first week of life – diagnosis of congenital Toxoplasmosis."*
   ii. PCR of amniotic fluid to detect B1 gene of the parasite has replaced fetal blood sampling.

d. *Ocular toxoplasmosis*
   i. Positive IgG titer with typical eye lesions.
   ii. Antibody production is expressed in terms of Goldmann-Witmer coefficient.

Treatment of Toxoplasmosis
- *Congenital infection:*
   - Pyrimethamine and sulfadiazine
   - Spiramycin + prednisone
- *Infection in immunocompetent:*
   - If only lymphadenopathy : No treatment unless have severe persistent symptoms.
   - If ocular toxoplasmosis : Pyrimethamine + sulfadiazine or clindamycin.
- *Infection in pregnancy* : Spiramycin (rovamycine) is **DOC**.
- *Infection in Immunocompromised:*
   - Prophylaxis for AIDS who are seropositive for *T. gondii* and have CD4 T cell <100/µl : Trimethoprim + sulfamethoxazole/Dapsone + Pyrimethamine.
   - Pyrimethamine + Sulfadiazine (preferred but not widely available).

24. **Ans. (b) *Plasmodium vivax*** *Ref. Harrison 19/e, p 1369, 18/e, p 1688*

Catch clue of answer from question. In this question clue is 'colour of pigment' which are:

–	Black pigment	: *P. falciparum*
–	Brown black	: *P. malariae*
–	Dark brown	: *P. ovale*
–	Yellow brown	: *P. vivax*

Mnemonic: Learn dark shade to light shade (black to yellow), so species arranged alphabetically.

25. **Ans. (d, e) Laboratory test are useful for making diagnosis, Infection is severe and progressive in immunocompromised host** *Ref. Harrison 20/e p 1609*

- Principal source of human Toxoplasma infection remains uncertain but infection is though to occur by oral route and can be attributables to ingestion of either sporulated oocysts from contaminated soil, food or water or bradyzoites from under cooked meat.
- Most common site of brain involvement is brain stem.
- Isolation of *T. gondii* from blood or other body fluids is difficult and available only at specialized laboratories.
- Diagnosis of Toxoplasmosis is based on detection of simultaneous presence of IgG and IgM antibodies to Toxoplasma in serum.
- In immunocompetent individuals toxoplasmosis is usually asymptomatic and self-limited, in contrast immunocompromised individuals experience severe and progressive disease.

26. **Ans. (b, c) and (d) Gametocytes, Accole trophozoite and Ring form** *Ref. Harrison 19/e p 1579*
    Already explained

27. **Ans. (a, b, c) and (d) Thrombocytopenia, DIC, Hemolysis, and Hematemesis** *Ref. Harrison 19/e, p 1372, 18/e, p 1692*

    Manifestation of severe *falciparum* malaria:
    i. *Cerebral malaria/unarousable coma:*
       - Coma is characteristic and omnious feature of *falciparum* malaria.
       - Manifest as diffuse symmetric encephalopathy, focal neurologic signs are unusual.
    ii. *Hypoglycemia* – associated with poor prognosis.
    iii. *Lactic acidosis* – Plasma conc of HCO_3^- and lactate are *best* biochemical prognosticators in severe malaria.
    iv. *Noncardiogenic pulmonary edema.*
    v. *Renal impairment.*
    vi. *Hematologic abnormalities:*
       - Anemia due to ↑ RBC destruction, removal by spleen and ineffective erythropoiesis.
       - Mild thrombocytopenia
       - Bleeding with DIC
       - Hematemesis due to stress ulceration or acute gastric erosion.
    vii. *Liver dysfunction* – Associated with poor prognosis.
    viii. *Convulsion, chest infection, catheter induced UTI, septicemia, Salmonella bacteremia.*

28. **Ans. (a) Caused by Babesia microti** *Ref. Harrison 20/e, p 1592-1593*
    Babesia
    - Intraerythrocytic (blood) parasite causing piroplasmosis/Texas fever/Acute hemolytic disease/Babesiosis.
    - *Most* human infection are caused by *B. microti* and *B. divergens*.
    - *Vector* Ixodid ticks (*I. dammini* or *I. scapularis, I. ricinus*).
    - *Mode of transmission* – Tick bite and blood transfusion.
    - **Clinical features**
      - Mostly asymptomatic.
      - Characterized by malaise, fever, sweat, depression, myalgia, arthralgia which resembles malaria and rickettsiosis.
      - Severe illness is seen in immunosuppressed; splenectomized (usually infected by *B. divergens* – may develop jaundice, renal insufficiency) and elderly persons.
      - Rash is absent.
    - **Diagnosis**
      - Giemsa stained thick and thin film shows small intraerythrocytic parasites resembling malaria but *it does not form pigment, schizonts, or gametocytes* and seen as tetrad forms infrequently.
      - *'Maltese cross'* form in RBC *without pigment or gametocyte is diagnostic.*

- **Treatment**

Organisms	Adult/child
B. microti (mild)	Atovaquone + azithromycin
B. divergens and Others	Quinine + Clindamycin + exchange transfusion

29. **Ans. (b) It is one of the common opportunistic infection in AIDS** *Ref. Harrison 20/e, p 1617*

   Cryptosporidium
   - *Cryposporidium* is a Acid fast coccidian intracellular but extracytoplasmic parasite.
   - Completes its life cycle in one host (monoxenous).
   - **Most human** infection is caused by *C. parvum*.
   - **Infective stage:** Oocyst (contain 4 sporozoites) in feces which is *infective immediately* without further development so person to person transmission can occur.
   - **Mode of infection:** Acquired from infected animal or human feces or from feces contaminated food or water.
   - **Principal site of infection:** Surface of villi of lower small bowel.
   - **Clinical features**

In immunocompetent	In immunosuppressed AIDS patient
• Self limited watery non-bloody diarrhoea	• Chronic, persistent and profuse diarrhoea
• Traveller's diarrhoea can occur	• Due to involvement of biliary tract papillary stenosis, sclerosing cholangitis or cholecystitis can occur

   - **Diagnosis**
     - Fecal examination for small oocyst of 4-5 µm in diameter.
     - Modified acid fast staining for oocyst
     - Fluorescent staining with auramine phenol is advantageous
     - Direct immunofluorescent stains and enzyme immunoassay (for fecal antigen).
     - Biopsy may show *Cryptosporidium* at apical surfaces of intestinal epithelium.
   - **Treatment:**
     - No chemotherapy is effective
     - Paromomycin — partially effective in HIV patient
     - Nitrazoxanide — in children
     - Spiramycin or combination therapy with azithromycin is also effective.

30. **Ans (a) *Cryptosporidium*** *Ref. Harrison 20/e, p 1617-1618; Paniker 7/e, p 96*

Parasite causing diarrhea on AIDS patient			
Parasite	**Site**	**Mode of infection**	**Oocyst**
Cryptosporidia	Enterocyte in small intestine	Ingestion of oocyst	Blue spherical (≈ 5 mm) bodies in acid fast stain
Microsporidia	Intestine, Muscle, CNS	Spore ingestion	Spores are 2-4 µm in size with polar filaments or tubules
Isospora belli	Epithelial cells of small intestine	Ingestion of mature oocyst	Oval or flask shaped, 25 µm × 15 µm with two sporocyst and four sporozoites. Also acid fast

   Remember: Coccidian parasites are *Isospora*, *Toxoplasma* and *Cryptosporidia*
   Blastocytis hominis is round cell of 6-40 µm containing large membrane bound central body with nuclei in cytoplasm peripherally.

31. **Ans. (a) Gametocyte** *Ref: Paniker Parasitology 7/e, p 66, 67*
   - Infective forms for human is sporozoites in saliva of mosquito
   - Infective forms for mosquito is gametocytes in human blood. At least 12 gametocytes per cubic mm of blood must be present to infect mosquito.
     - Gametocytes are maximum in number during the early stages of infections (may exceed 1000 per cubic mm of blood).
     - Nonmotile zygote converted into motile ookinete in about 18 - 24 hours.
   - Human reservoir is one who harbours the sexual forms (gametocytes) of the parasite which is infective for mosquito.

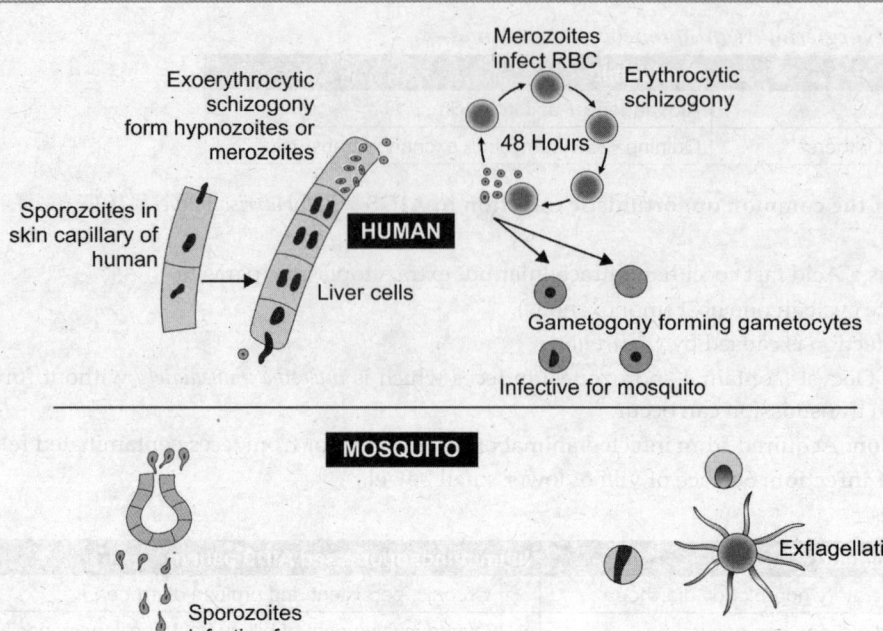
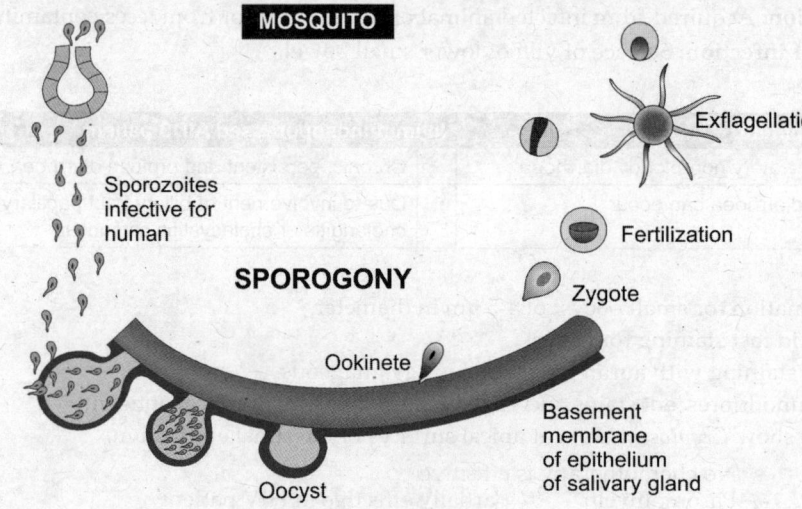

Life cycle of Plasmodium vivax

32. **Ans. (d) Detects histidine rich protein 1** Ref. Harrison 19/e, p 1376
    Antigen capture assay detects histidine rich protein II not HRP-I

33. **Ans. (c) IgG is diagnostic** Ref. Harrison 20/e, p 1614
    Already explained

34. **Ans. (c) Isospora** Ref: Harrision 20/e, p 1618; Paniker 7/e 93

    Isospora belli (Cytoisosporiasis)
    - Coccidian parasite
    - *Site of infection* – Epithelial cells of small intestine where schizogony (sickle shaped merozoites are formed) as well as sporogony occur.
    - *Infective stage* – Mature oocyst. (forms outside the human body) containing two sporocyst with four sporozoites each.
    - *Mode of transmission* – Ingestion of mature oocyst in food or drink.

    Clinical features
    - Usually asymptomatic or abdominal discomfort, mild fever and diarrhea in self-limited manner
    - Protracted diarrhea can occur in immunocompromised person especially in HIV patient.
      – Diagnosis – demonstration of acid fast oocyst in fecal smears.

    Treatment
    - Cotrimoxazole is effective
    - It is easy to treat but relapses are common in comparison to diarrhea of cryptosporidium

    > **Remember:** Oocyst of cryptosporidium is small, hard and is fully mature on release while that of isospora oocyst is large, transparent, thin walled, flask shaped and mature outside the human body.

35. **Ans. (b, c) and (d) Naegleria, Acanthamoeba and Balamuthia** *Ref. Harrison 17/e, p 2632*

Encephalitis (Infection of brain parenchyma)			
Viral	**Bacterial**	**Fungal**	**Parasitic**
– HSV1 *(MC)* – VZV – Enterovirus	– Listeria – Mycoplasma – Leptospira	– Cryptococcus – Mucor	– Naegleria – Acanthamoeba – Balamuthia – Baylisascaris procyonis – Toxoplasma

36. **Ans. (b) and (e) It is a protozoa and It is associated with diarrhoea in HIV patients** *Ref. Harrison 19/e, p 1408, 18/e, p 1732*
    - **Microsporidia** are gram-positive, obligate intracellular, spore forming protozoa that cause disease in humans especially as opportunistic pathogens in **AIDS**. It reside in cytoplasm of enteric cells.
    - Main species causing infection in humans is Enterocytozoon bieneusi.
    - Also seen in extraintestinal locations like muscles, eye (conjunctivitis) and liver (hepatitis) in comparison of isospora or cryptosporidium.
    - In **AIDS** patient microsporidium cause diarrhoea.
    - **Diagnosis** is made by demonstration of spore in smear of faeces or duodenal aspirate by modified trichome or chromotrope 2R based staining or Uveitx 2B or calcofluor fluorescent staining.

37. **Ans. (b) Opisthorchis viverni** *Ref. Internet reference*

Organism	Size	
	Cyst	**Trophozoite**
E. histolytica	12-15 µm	15-30 µm
E. Coli	10-35 µm	20-50 µm
Giardia	9-12 µm	12-15 µm
B. coli	30-200 µm	30-50 µm
C. Cryptosporidium parvum	4-5 µm	3-5 µm
Isospora belli	25-30 µm	

Opisthorchis: Trematode fluke resembling C. sinesis.

38. **Ans. (a) Amphotericin B** *Ref. Paniker 7/e, p 58*

    RK 39, is a rapid dip stick method for detecting antileishmanial antibodies has been developed using a recombinant leishmanial antigen rk 39 consisting of 39 amino acids conserved in kinesin region of L. infantum. The sensitivity of test is 98% and specificity is 90%. Thus, a positive rk39 test indicates Lishmenial infection

    Treatment of Leishmaniasis
    - Kala-azar responds better to treatment than visceral leishmaniasis
    - Pentavalent antimonial compound is the drug of choice in most of the endemic region except Bihar, where there is resistance to pentavalent compound
    - Amphotericin B is the first line drug to be used in Bihar
    - Liposomal Amphotericin B: It is the only drug approved by FDA for treatment if visceral leishmaniasis

    Note: Other important Rapid dipstick test:
    - RDT dipsticks for HRP-2 and pLDH: Plasmodium
    - Optimal rapid dipstick test: Plasmodium falciparum > Plasmodium vivax
    - RDT for F1 antigen: Yersinia pestis
    - RDT for O1 and O139: Rapid detection of *Vibrio cholerae* serotypes
    - Strep A Rapid Test Dipstick (GIMA): Streptococcus pyogenes is throat swab

NEET Pattern Questions

1. **The most common cause of malaria in India:**
   a. P. vivax
   b. P. falciparum
   c. P. malariae
   d. P. ovale
   [Ref. Park 22/e, p 234]

   In India, 50% of infections are reported to be due to P. falciparum; 4-8% due to mixed infection and rest due to P. vivax

2. **True about P. falciparum includes, all except:**
   a. Duration of erythrocytic cycle is 48 hrs
   b. Exo-erythrocytic phase is absent
   c. Parasitic burden can be estimated by peripheral parasitemia
   d. Cause rosette promotion [Ref. Harrison 20/e, p 1579]

   RBC infected with P. falciparum adhere to venous wall and other RBC's (to form rosette). This results in sequestration of infected RBC's in vital organs. As a consiquence the level of peripheral parasitemia under estimates the true number of parasites.

3. **Which type of malaria is associated with renal failure?**
   a. Falciparum
   b. Vivax
   c. Malariae
   d. Ovale
   [Ref. Paniker 7/e, p 77]

   Renal failure occurs in malignant tertian malaria (particularly in black water fever) which is caused by P. falciparum.

4. **Causative agent of malaria:**
   a. Protozoa
   b. Mosquito
   c. Bacteria
   d. Virus
   [Ref. Paniker 7/e, p 64]

   Mosquito is the vector where as plasmodium is the causative agent which is a protozoa.

5. **Malaria causing nephrotic syndrome:**
   [Ref. Harrison 20/e, p 1580]
   a. P. vivax
   b. P falciparum
   c. P. malariae
   d. P. ovale

   Acute kidney injury is common is severe falciparum malaria

6. **In malaria, sexual cycle is:**
   a. Sporozoite to gametocytes
   b. Gametocytes to sporozoite
   c. Occurs in human
   d. Responsible for relapse [Ref. Paniker 7/e, p 65]

Sexual cycle of plasmodium occurs in mosquitos and is called as sporogony.

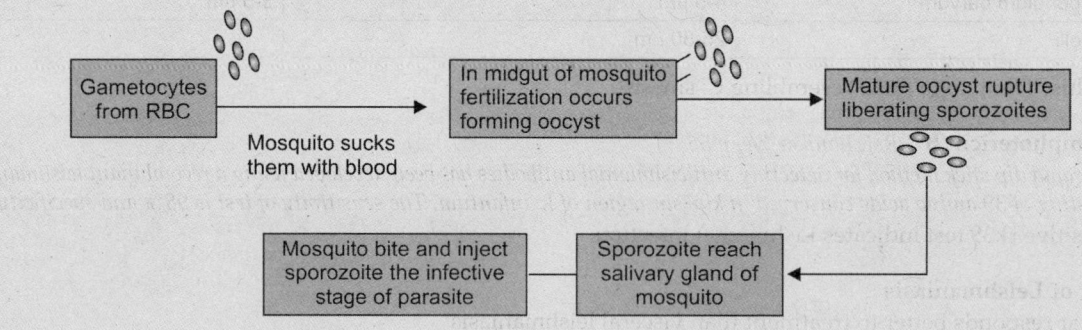

7. **Malaria parasite was discovered by:**
   a. Ronald Ross
   b. Paul Muller
   c. Laveran
   d. Pampania
   [Ref. Paniker 7/e, p 64]

   Laveran discovered the malarial parasite in RBC of a patient in Algeria. Whereas Ronald Ross established its mode of transmission in Secundrabad.

8. **Malaria carriers contain:**
   a. Trophozoite
   b. Gametocytes
   c. Merozoites
   d. Trophozoites
   [Ref. Park 22/e, p 233]

   Note: Gametocyte appear in circulation 4-5 days after the appearance of asexual form in case of P. vivax and 10-12 days in P. falciparum. Gametocyte concentration >12/cubic mm is necessary for the infection of mosquitoes.

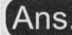 **Ans.**
1. b. P. falciparum
2. c. Parasitic burden can...
3. a. Falciparum
4. a. Protozoa
5. b. P. falciparum
6. b. Gametocytes to sporozoite
7. c. Laveran
8. b. Gametocytes

9. The scientist who discovered the transmission of malaria by anopheline mosquito:
   a. Laveran
   b. Paul Muller
   c. Ronald Ross
   d. Pampana [Ref. Paniker 7/e p 64]

10. Protozoa associated with megaesophagus:
    a. Trypanosome
    b. Ameba
    c. Giardia
    d. Gnathostoma [Ref. Paniker 7/e, p 47]

In chronic phase T. cruzi produces inflammatory response, cellular destruction and fibrosis of muscles and nerves that control tone of hollow organs like heart, oesophagus, colon etc. Thus it can lead to cardiac myopathy and mega-oesophagus and megacolon

11. Largest intestinal protozoa is:
    a. E. coli
    b. Balantidium coli
    c. Giardia
    d. T. gondii [Ref. Paniker 7/e, p 107]

Balantidium coli is the largest protozoan parasite. It resides in large intestine. It is the only ciliate protozoan parasite of human.

12. Definite host of toxoplasma:
    a. Man
    b. Dog
    c. Cat
    d. Rat [Ref. Harrison 20/e, p 1609]

Giardia lives in small intestine.

13. Toxoplasma in children causes:
    a. Chorioretinitis
    b. Conjunctivities
    c. Keratitis
    d. Papillitis [Ref. Harrison 20/e, p 1611]

In the eye infiltrates of monocytes, lymphocytes and plasma cells may produce uni or multifocal lesion. Granulomatous lesions and chorioretinitis may be observed in posterior chamber after acute necrotizing retinitis

14. True about Giardiasis:
    a. Only cyst is infective
    b. Reside in caecum
    c. Only man to man transmission
    d. Exist in one phase [Ref. Paniker 7/e, p 31]

15. Most common clinical feature of toxoplasmosis in an immunocompetent adult:
    a. Encephalitis
    b. Lymphadenopathy
    c. Chorioretinitis
    d. Glaucoma [Ref. Paniker 7/e, p 91]

Commonest manifestation of toxoplasmosis:
Acquired: Lymphadenopathy
Congenital: Chorioretinitis, cerebral calcifications
In immunocompromised: Encephalitis, altered mental state.

16. Band form of P malariae is:
    a. Schizont stage
    b. Trophozoite stage
    c. Merozoite stage
    d. Gametocyte stage [Ref. Paniker 7/e, p 73]

The old trophozoites are seen stretched across the erythrocyte as a broad band. These band forms are unique feature of P.malariae.

17. Which of the following is true about P. falciparum?
    a. James dots are seen
    b. Accole forms are seen
    c. Relapses are frequent
    d. Longest incubation period [Ref. Paniker 7/e, p 71]

18. Schizonts are not seen in peripheral blood of which malarial parasites?
    a. P vivax
    b. P falciparum
    c. P ovale
    d. P malariae [Ref. Paniker 7/e, p 67]

In P.falciparum, erythrocytic schizogony takes place inside the capillaries and vascular led of internal organs. So, in P.falciparum infections schizonts and merozoites are usually not seen in peripheral blood.

19. Mucocutaneous leishmaniasis is caused by:
    a. L-braziliensis
    b. L. tropica
    c. L. donovani
    d. L. orientalis [Ref. Paniker 7/e, p 50]

Muco-cutoneous leishmania is caused by L.braziliensis and L. mexicana complex.

20. Invasive amoebiasis can be best diagnosed by:
    a. ELISA
    b. Countercurrent immunoelectrophoresis
    c. Indirect hemaglutination test.
    d. Complement fixation text [Ref. Paniker 7/e, p 22]

Ans.
9. c. Ronald Ross
10. a. Trypanosome
11. b. Balantidium coli
12. c. Cat
13. a. Chorioretinitis
14. a. Only cyst...
15. a. Encephalitis
16. b. Trophozoite...
17. b. Accole forms...
18. b. P falciparum
19. a. L-braziliensis
20. c. Indirect...

21. Trophozoite of Entamoeba histolytica:
    a. Has eccentric Karyosome
    b. Shows erythrocyte in cytosol
    c. Central nucleus
    d. Non motile [Ref. Paniker 7/e, p 15]

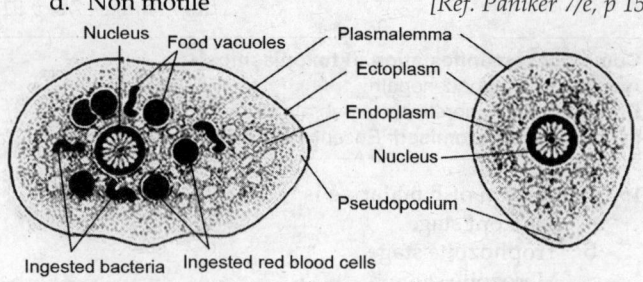

A-Trophozoite form   B-Minuta form

22. A patient presents with fever. Peripheral smear shows band across the erythrocytes. Diagnosis is:
    a. P Falciparum
    b. P vivax
    c. P ovale
    d. P malariae [Ref. Paniker 7/e, p 73]

23. The cystic form of all are seen in man except:
    a. E. histolytica
    b. Giardia
    c. Trichomonas
    d. Toxoplasma [Ref. Paniker 7/e, p 91]

24. For which parasite modified ZN stain is used:
    a. Isospora
    b. Microsporidia
    c. Plasmodium
    d. Echinococcus [Ref. Paniker 7/e, p 231]

Modified Ziehn-Neelsen stain
- Oocyst of cryptosporidium and isospora in fecal specimens may be difficult to detect without special staining. Application of heat to the carbol fuchsin assists in staining.

25. Giardiasis true is all except:
    a. Diarrhea with steatosis
    b. Bloody diarrhea
    c. Metronidazole is the drug of choice
    d. Absent fever [Ref. Paniker 7/e, p 33]

26. A patient presents with headache, high fever and meningismus. Within 3 days he becomes unconscious. Most probable causative agent:
    a. Naegleria fowleri
    b. Acanthamoeba castellani
    c. Entamoeba histolytica
    d. Trypanosoma cruzi [Ref. Paniker 7/e, p 29]

27. The normal habitat of giardia is:
    a. Duodenum and jejunum
    b. Stomach
    c. Caecum
    d. Ileum [Ref. Paniker 7/e, p 30]

28. Kala azar is:
    a. Mucocutaneous leishmaniasis
    b. Cutaneous leishmaniasis
    c. Oriental sore
    d. Visceral leishmaniasis [Ref. Paniker 7/e, p 54]

29. Amoebiasis is not transmitted by:
    a. Feco-oral route
    b. Sexual transmission
    c. Blood and blood products
    d. Vector transmission [Ref. Harrison, 19/e, p 1362]

30. Trypanosoma cruzi is transmitted by:
    a. Tse tse fly   b. Reduviid bug
    c. Culex mosquito   d. Sand fly
    [Ref. Paniker 8/e, p 42]

31. Amastigote form of which parasite is found in human?
    a. Trypanosoma cruzi
    b. Trypanosoma brucei
    c. Trypanosoma gambiense
    d. Trypanosoma rhodesiense [Ref. Paniker 7/e, p 39]

Amastigote form is found in humans in Trypanosoma cruzi and leishmania

32. Which of the following is true about mature cysts of E. histolytica?
    a. Endoplasm and ectoplasm are clearly defined
    b. Eight chromatid bodies
    c. Shows chromatid bodies and glycogen mass
    d. Nuclear structure retains characteristics of trophozoite

33. The pathogencity of Entamoeba histolytica is indicated by:
    a. Isoenzyme pattern   b. Size
    c. Nuclear pattern   d. ELISA test
    [Ref. Paniker 7/e, p 18]

34. Duodenal aspirate is used in diagnosis of:
    a. E histolytica   b. Giardia lamblia
    c. Taenia solium   d. Leishmania
    [Ref. Paniker 7/e, p 33]

35. Recrudescences are commonly seen in which malaria?
    a. P vivax   b. P ovale
    c. P malariae   d. P falciparum
    [Ref. Paniker 7/e, p 78]

Recrudescence is commonest in falciparum malaria

Ans.
21. b. Shows erythrocyte 22. d. P malariae 23. c. Trichomonas 24. a. Isospora 25. b. Bloody diarrhea
26. a. Naegleria fowleri 27. a. Duodenum... 28. d. Visceral leishm... 29. d. Vector trans... 30. a. Tse tse fly
31. a. Trypanosoma cruzi 32. d. Nuclear... 33. a. Isoenzyme... 34. b. Giardia lamblia 35. d. P falciparum

36. Cerebral amoebiasis is not caused by:
    a. Naegleria   b. Acanthamoeba
    c. Dientamoeba   d. Balamuthia
    [Ref. Paniker 7/e, p 24]

Cerebral amoebiasis
- Acanthamoeba
- Naegleria Fowleri
- Balamuthia mandrillaris

37. The cystic form of all are seen in man except:
    a. *E. histolytica*   b. *Giardia*
    c. *Trichomonas*   d. *Toxoplasma*
    [Ref. Paniker 7/e, p 35]

T. vaginalis does not form cyst and the trophozoite itself is the infective form.

38. Which is true of trophozoites of *E. histolytica*?
    a. Has eccentric karyosome
    b. Nuclear membrane without chromatin
    c. Shows erythrophagocytosis
    d. Presence of bacteria inside cell [Ref. Paniker 7/e, p 15]

39. Largest intestinal protozoa is:
    a. *Entamoeba coli*   b. *Balantidium coli*
    c. *Giardia lamblia*   d. *Toxoplasma gondii*
    [Ref. Panikar 7/e, p 107]

B. coli is the only ciliate protozoan parasite of human. It is the largest protozoan parasite of human.

40. Amoebae not found in human intestine:
    a. *E. histolytica*   b. *E. coli*
    c. *E. nana*   d. *E. gingivalis*
    [Ref. Paniker 7/e, p 24]

- Entamoeba gingivalis is present in the mouth, being found in large numbers when oral hygiene is poor.
- It has no cystic stage and is transmit by kissing, airborne droplet and by fomites.

41. Tachyzoites are seen in:
    a. *Toxoplasma*   b. *Toxocara*
    c. Pulm eosinophilia d. *Ascaris* [Ref. Paniker 7/e 88]

Rapidly proliferating trophozoites of toxoplasma in acute infections are called tachyzoites.

42. Charcot Leyden crystal in stool is seen in:
    a. Amoebic dysentery b. bacillary dysentery
    c. Shigella   d. bacillus cereus
    [Ref. Paniker 7/e, p 20]

43. Compound used for fixation of protozoa found in stool is:
    a. Phenol   b. Hypochlorite
    c. Formalin   d. Alcohol
    [Ref. Paniker 6/e, p 233]

44. MC anopheles vector for transmission of malaria in urban area is:
    a. An stephensi
    b. A. gambiae
    c. Both
    d. None   [Ref. Park 22/e p 236]

In India An. culicifacies acts as malaria vector in rural areas and An. steptosis in urban areas

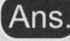
Ans. 36. c. Dientamoeba   37. c. Trichomonas   38. c. Shows ...   39. b. Balantidium   40. d. E. gingi...
         41. a. Toxoplasma   42. a. Amoebic dysentery   43. d. Alcohol   44. a. An stephensi

Helminths

CHAPTER 35

Bilaterally symmetrical metazoa belonging to phylum-scolecida. They have 3 germ layers (triploblastic metazoa).

Classification

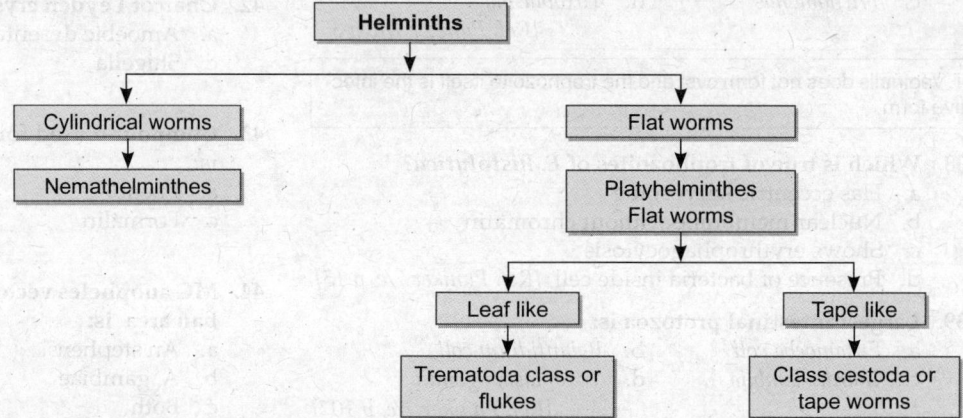

Trematode: Fasciola, Clonorchis.

TREMATODES

- Flat, fleshy, unsegmented worms
- Alimentary canal present, but incomplete without an anus
- Possess suckers, but hooks are lacking
- Sexes may be separate (as in schistosomes) or hermaphroditic.

S. hematoblum: Endemic humaturia
S. japonium: Katayama fever

Classification according to habitat		
Category	**Trematode**	**Habitat**
Blood fluke	Schistosoma haematobium Schistosoma mansoni Schistosoma japonicum	Vesical and pelvic venous plexus Inferior mesenteric vein Superior mesenteric vein
Liver fluke	Clonorchis sinensis	Biliary tract and pancreatic duct
	Fasciola hepatica, opisthorchis	Liver and biliary passages
Intestinal fluke	Fasciolopsis buski, heterophyes heterophyes (**smallest trematode**)	Small intestine
	Gastrodiscoides nominis	Large intestine
Lung fluke	Paragonimus westermani	Lung

Cestodes: Taenia, Echinococcus

CLONORCHIS SINENSIS

- Chinese liver fluke, oriental liver fluke
- Adult worm lives in biliary tract and sometimes in the pancreatic duct
- Definitive host: Humans
- Intermediate host: 1st: Snail
  2nd: Fish
- *Infective form:* Metacercaria larva
- *Mode of infection:* Eating under cooked fresh water fish carrying metacercariae larvae

Longest Cestode infecting man: Diphyllobothrium latum
Smallest cestode infecting man: hymenolepsis nana

- *Pathogenesis*: Metacerceriat excyst in the duodenum. The adolescent that came out enter the common bile duct through the ampulla of Vater and proceed to distal bile capillaries:
  - In distal bile capillaries it can cause cholangitis and calculus formation.
  - Biliary cirrhosis, portal hypertension and cholangio carcinoma are other manifestaion
- **Treatment:** Praziquantel is the drug of choice.

CESTODES

- Segmented tape like worms with variable size (few mm to several meters)
- Lacks alimentary canal
- Possess suckers and in some members hooks too
- Sexually hermaphrodites *(see Table 1 for important features)*

NEMATODES

- Resemble common earthworms
- Elongated cylindrical unsegmented worms with tapering ends
- Body is covered with tough cuticle
- Possess alimentary canal
- Sexes are separate *(see Table 2 for important features)*

FILARIAL WORMS

- Nematodes belonging to the super family Filarioidea
- Worms resides in:
  - Subcutaneous tissue (subcutaneous filariasis) : Loa loa, Onchocerca volvulus, Mansonella streptocerea
  - Lymphatic filariasis: Wuchereria boncrofti, Brugia malayi, Brugia timorii.
  - Serous cavity (serous cavity filariasis): Monsonella
  - Female worms are viviparous and give birth to larvae known as microfilariae.

> **Nematodes:**
> **Ascaris:** Largest
> **Parthenogenetic:** Strongyloides.
> **Lives in appendix:** Trichuris.

> Monsonella ozzardi is virtually nonpathogenic filariasis.

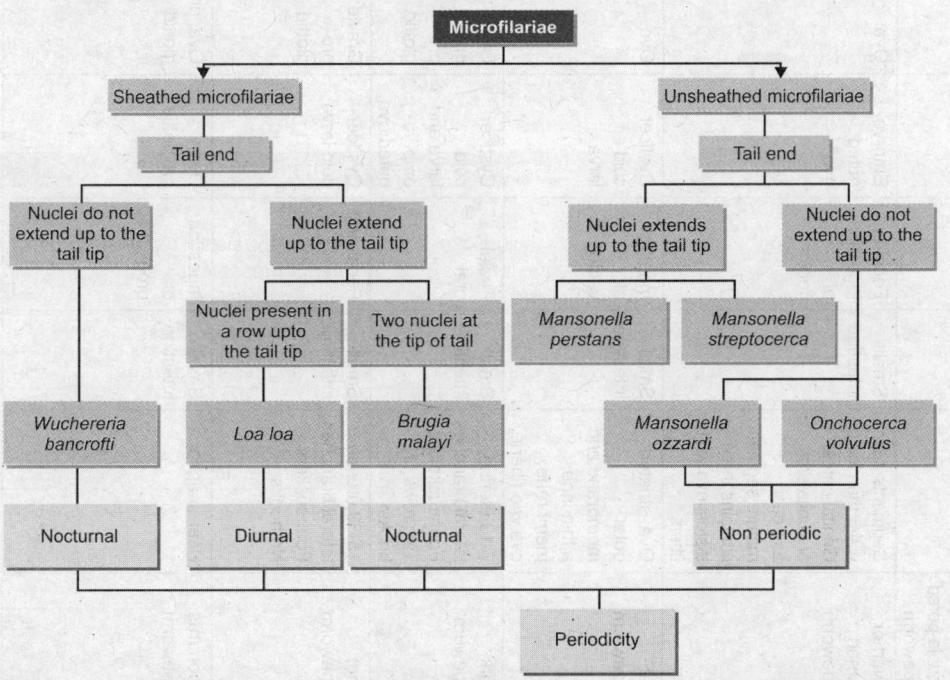

Note:

Filarial worm	Disease
• Onchocerca volvulus	River blindness or onchocericiasis
• Loa loa	Fugitive swellings or calabar swellings
• Wuchereria bancrofti	Filariasis

TABLE 1: IMPORTANT FEATRUES OF CESTODES

Organism	Common name	Distinct characteristics	Habitat	Mode of Transmission	Infective stage	Diagnostic stage	Host	Vector	Diagnosis	Pathogenicity	Treatment	Clinical manifestations
Dihyllobothrium latum	Fish tapeworm broad tapeworm	Longest tapeworm; operculated ova at one end and a knob at the other end	Small intestine	Ingestion of infected raw/undercooked fish	Plerocercoid larva	Ova	DH: human IH: crustacean, small fish		Endoscopy	Diphyllobothriasis	Praziquantel	Megaloblastic anemia
Dipylidium caninum	Dog tapeworm Cucumber tapeworm Double-pored tapeworm	2 reproductive system; 8 egg packet	Small intestine	Fecal-oral ingestion of vector	Cysticercoid larva	Proglottid	DH: dog and cat OH: human	Fleas; dog lice	Direct fecal smear	Dypilidiasis, dog dog tapeworm infection	Niclosamide, Prazinquantel	Abdominal pain; Diarrhea; itchy anus; Urticaria
Hymenolepis nana	Dwarf or human tapeworm	Segments are wider than long; Genital pores are unilateral, and each mature segment contains three testes; ova with fibers	Small intestine	Fecal-oral ingestion of vector	Embryonated ova	Ova	DH: human, mice IH: grain beetle		Fecal smear	Hymenolepiasis	Prazinquantel niclosamide	Induce enteritis with nausea and vomiting, diarrhea, abdominal pain, and dizziness
Hymenolepis diminuta	Rat tapeworm	Ova: striated outer membrane and a thin inner membrane; ova w/o fibers	Small intestine	Ingestion of vector	Cysticercoid larva	Ova	DH: human, rat IH: beetle, caprophilic arthropods	Beetle, caprophilic arthropods	Direct fecal smear	Hymenolepiasis	Prazinquantel	Induce enteritis with nausea and vomiting, diarrhea, abdominal pain, and dizziness
Taenia solium	Pork tapeworm	7-13 uterine lateral branches Four suckers Two rows of hooks	Small intestine	Fecial-oral	Cysticercoid larva and embryonated ova	Ova, gravid proglottid	DH: human IH: pig		Fecal smear	Cysticercosis	Prazinquantel, niclosamide	Seizure, abdominal pain, blurry vision, eosinophilia
Taenia saginata	Beef tapeworm	15-30 uterine lateral branches Four suckers No hooks	Small intestine	Fecal-oral	Cysticercoid larva	Gravid proglottid	DH: human IH: beef		Scotch tape swab, ELISA	TAENIASIS SAGINATA	Niclosamide, Quinacrine hydrochloride Bithionol, Mebendazole, Prazinquantel	Proglottids may also crawl out of the anus
Multiceps multiceps	Coenurus tapeworm	Pear-shaped	Small intestine	Ingestion of proglottid	Ova, proglottid	Ova, proglottid	DH: dogs, fox IH: sheep PH: human		Gross examination of proglottid, fecal floatation method, necroscopy	Coenurosis	Prazinquantel, Epsiprantel, Febendazole	Presence of painless nodules

(DH: Definitive host; IH: Intermediate host)

TABLE 2: IMPORTANT FEATURES OF NEMATODES (ROUNDWORMS)

Organism	Common name	Distinct characteristics	Habitat	Mode of Transmission	Infective stage	Diagnostic stage	Host	Vector	Diagnosis	Pathogenicity	Treatment	Clinical manifestations
Ascaris lumbricoides	Human roundworm	Largest nematode; presence of albuminoid coat in fertilized egg	Small intestine	Ingestion of fertilized egg (oral-fecal)	Fertilized ova	Unfertilized and fertilized ova	DH: human		Kato technique	Ascariasis (P)	Albendazole	
Enterobius vermicularis	Human pinworm	Colorless, D-shaped ova	Colon	Inhalation of ova; oral-fecal	Ova	Ova	DH: human		Scotch tape swab	Enterobiasis	Mebendazole	Pruritus ani
Ancylostoma duodenale	Old world hookworm	2 pairs of ventral teeth; c-shaped	Small intestine	Skin penetration	Filariform larvae	Ova	DH: human		Ancylostomiasis (Wakana disease) (P)	Culture of larvae	Albendazole	Ground itch
Necator americanus	New world hookworm	1 pair of cutting plated; s-shaped	Small intestine	Skin penetration	Filariform larvae	Ova	DH: human		Direct fecal smear/culture	Necatoriasis (Uncinariasis) (P)	Albendazole	Ground itch
Strongyloides stercoralis	Human threadworm		Small intestine	Skin penetration	Filariform larvae	Rhabditiform larvae	DH: human (may be dogs and cats)		Direct fecal smear/culture	Strongyloidiasis	Albendazole, Ivermectin, Thiabendazole	Larva currens
Trichostrongylus spp.			Small intestine	Ingestion of filariform larvae; skin penetration	Filariform larvae	Ova	DH: cattle, sheep, etc. IN: human		Fecal smear	Trichostrongyliasis	Thiabendazole Fenbendazole, Ivermectin, Mebendazole	
Trichuris trichiura	Human whipworm	Barrel/football-shaped ova; 2 prominent polar plugs	Colon	Oral-fecal	Embryonated ova	Embryonated and unembryonated ova	DH: human		Zinc sulfate floatation	Trichuriasis	Albendazole	Prolapse of the rectum
		Nematode	Tissue	Undercooked meat			Human					Damage, pneumonia, meningitis, pleurisy, etc.

Contd...

Section - B

442 Self-Assessment and Review of Microbiology and Immunology

Contd...

Organism	Common name	Distinct characteristics	Habitat	Mode of Transmission	Infective stage	Diagnostic stage	Host	Vector	Diagnosis	Pathogenicity	Treatment	Clinical manifestations
Toxocara canis	Dog roundworm		Small intestine	**Dogs:** transmammary, transplacental **Human:** Ingestion of embryonated ova	Embryonated ova	Larvae	DH: Dogs PH: Human		ELISA/EIA Western-Blot analysis	Toxocariasis	**Dogs:** Antihelminthics **Humans:** Albendazole	Visceral larva migrans, Ocular larva migrans
Dracunculus medinensis	Guinea worm	Triangular mouth with sclerotized plate	Abdominal tissue; lower limbs	Drinking of contaminated water (with infected copepods)	Larvae	Adult female worm	DH: Human IH: Water fleas or copepods	Water fleas or copepods	Direct observation	Dracunculiasis	Stick; no antihelminthic treatment	Blister formation
Angiostrongylus cantonensis	Rat lungworm	Lacks buccal capsule; adult female show red digestive organ	Brain CSF, eyes	Ingestion of undercooked infected snails and fish and infected vegetables; ingestion of rat feces	L3	L3	DH: Rat IH: Snails IncH: Human PH: Prawn, crab	Snails	CT or MRI scan Immuno-PCR	Angiostrongyliasis	Surgical operation	Eosinophilic meningitis

Helminths 443

Multiple Choice Questions

1. **Adult form of echinococcus granulosus lies in:**
   [NEET Pattern 2019]
   a. Man
   b. Sheep
   c. Dog
   d. Pig

2. **Megaloblastic anemia is caused by:** [AIIMS 15]
   a. *Diphyllobothrium latum*
   b. *Schistosoma hematobium*
   c. *Echinococcus granulosus*
   d. *Taenia solium*

3. **Skin ectoparasite as shown in figure:** [NEET Pattern 2019]

   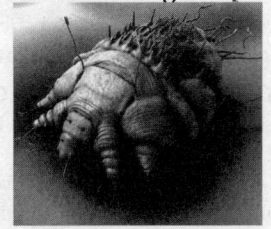

   Figure for Q. No. 3

   a. Leptospiridium
   b. Ioxodes
   c. Sarcoptes scabei
   d. Pediculus humanus capitis

4. **Which of the following parasite's life cycle is shown below?**
   [AIIMS May 17]

   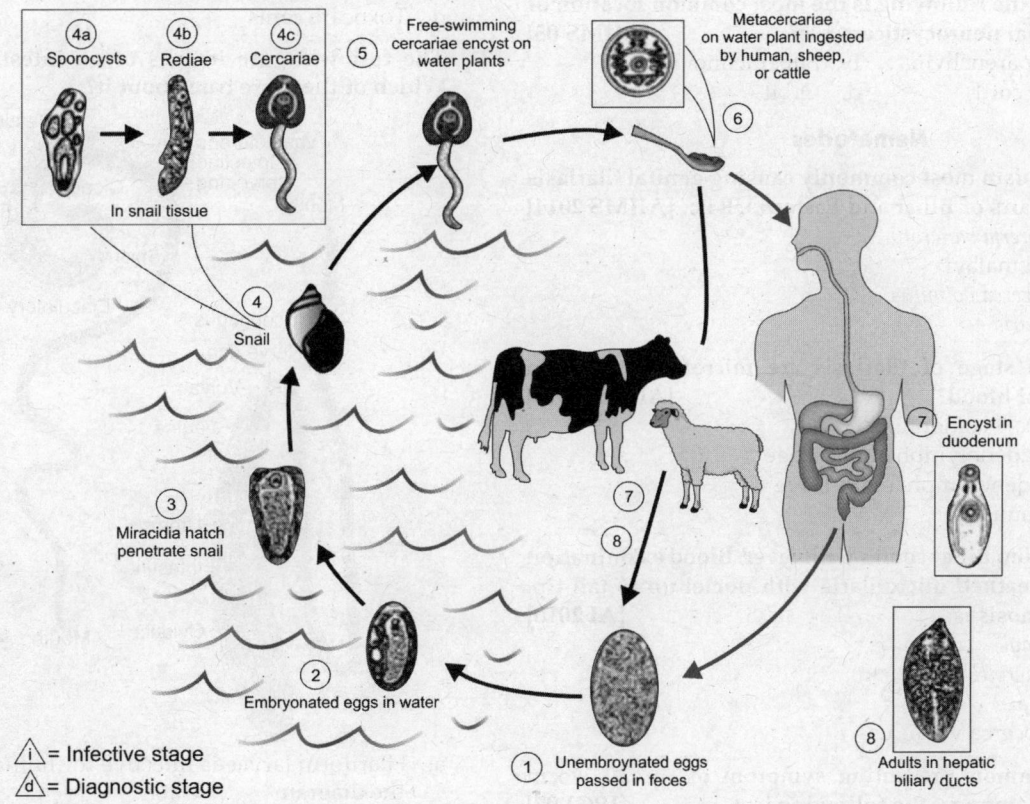

   a. Fasciola abuski
   b. Fasciola hepatica
   c. Paragonimus westermani
   d. Clonorchissinensis

5. **Organism causing biliary tract obstruction:**
   [AIIMS Nov 10]
   a. *Clonorchis sinensis*
   b. *Ankylostoma duodenale*
   c. *Strongyloides stericoralis*
   d. *Enterobius vermicularis*

6. **Ingestion of raw fish leads to gallbladder cancer due to:**
   [AIIMS Nov 10]
   a. *Clonorchis sinensis*
   b. *Hymenolepis diminuta*
   c. *Angiostrongylus*
   d. *D. latum*

Tapeworms

7. **Contact isolation is indicated for:** [NEET Pattern 2019]
   a. Scabies
   b. Diphtheria
   c. Pertussis
   d. Typhoid

UNIT-IV: Parasitology

8. Consumption of uncooked pork is likely to cause which of the following helminthic disease? [AI 11]
   a. *Taenia saginata*   b. *Taenia solium*
   c. Hydatid cyst   d. *Trichuris trichiura*

9. Commonest parasite of CNS in India is: [NEET Pattern 2018]
   a. Schistosomiasis   b. Cysticercosis
   c. *Trichinella spiralis*   d. Hydatid cyst

10. An IT professional visit medicine OPD with productive rusty cough night sweat, AFB was found to be negative. Most likely casuse is: [NEET Pattern 2019]
    a. *Fasciola hepatica*   b. *Fasciola*
    c. *Paragominus*   d. *Opisthotorchus*

11. Organism responsible for neurocysticercosis: [NEET Pattern 2019]
    a. *Cysticercus cellulosae*
    b. *Fasciola hepatica*
    c. *Ancylostoma*
    d. *Enterobius vermicularis*

12. Which of the following is the most common location of intracranial neurocysticercosis? [AIIMS 05]
    a. Brain parenchyma   b. Subarachnoid space
    c. Spinal cord   d. Orbit

Nematodes

13. The organism most commonly causing genital filariasis in most parts of Bihar and Eastern UP is: [AIIMS 2014]
    a. *Wuchereria bancrofti*
    b. *Brugia malayi*
    c. *Onchocerca volvulus*
    d. *Dirofilaria*

14. In which stage of filariasis are microfilaria seen in peripheral blood? [AIIMS 2015]
    a. Tropical eosinophilia
    b. Early adenolymphangitis stage
    c. Late adenolymphangitis stage
    d. Elephantiasis

15. A child from Bihar comes with fever. Blood examination shows sheathed microfilaria with nuclei up to tail tip. The diagnosis is: [AI 2010]
    a. *B. malayi*
    b. *W. bancrofti*
    c. *Loa loa*
    d. *Onchocerca volvulus*

16. Most common presenting symptom of thread worm infection amongst the following is: [PGI 07]
    a. Abdominal pain
    b. Rectal prolapse
    c. Urticaria
    d. Vaginitis

17. Kalu, 30-year-old man, presented with subcutaneous itchy nodules over left iliac crest. On examination they are firm, nontender, and mobile skin scrappings contain microfilaria and adult worms of: [NEET Pattern 2018]
    a. *Loa loa*
    b. *Onchocerca volvulus*
    c. *Brugia malayi*
    d. *Mansonella persetans*

18. Larva found in muscle is: [AIIMS 18]
    a. *Trichinella spiralis*
    b. *Ancylostoma duodenale*
    c. *Trichuris trichiura*
    d. *Enterobius vermicularis*

19. Nematodes are differentiated from other worms by:
    a. Absent fragmentation   [PGI 05]
    b. Flat or fleshy leaf-like worms
    c. Separate sexes
    d. Cylindrical body
    e. GIT is formed completely

20. Cutaneous larva migrans is caused most commonly by:
    a. *Ancylostoma duodenale*   [NEET Pattern 2019]
    b. *Ancylostoma braziliense*
    c. *Nectar americans*
    d. *Toxocara canis*

21. The following are images of an intestinal nematode. Which of these are true about it? [AIIMS 16]

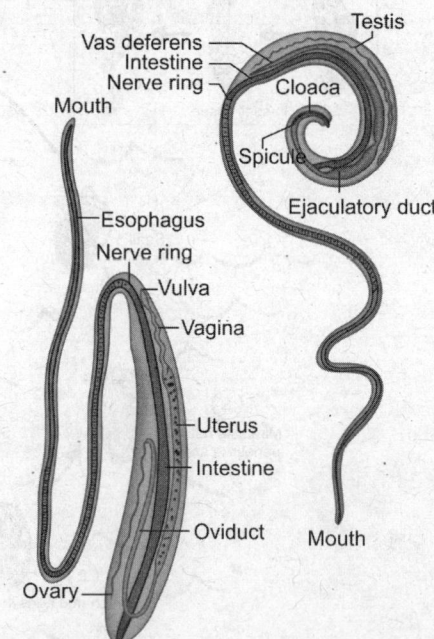

    a. Filariform larvae is infective for humans as shown in the diagram
    b. Transmitted through contaminated food and water usually
    c. Females of these species show parthenogenesis
    d. Triclabendazole is the drug of choice

22. Which of the following has barrel shaped eggs? [PGI 17]
    a. *E. vermicularis*   b. *Ascaris lumbricoides*
    c. *A. duodenale*   d. *N. americanus*
    e. *Trichuris trichiura*

Miscellaneous

23. All of the following causes biliary obstruction except:
    a. Clonorchis
    b. Ascaris [AI 08]
    c. Ancylostoma duodenale
    d. Fasciola

24. Which of the following is not a neuroparasite? [AI 05; PGI 05]
    a. Taenia solium
    b. Acanthamoeba
    c. Naegleria
    d. Trichinella spiralis

25. Autoinfection is seen with: [AIIMS May 09]
    a. Cryptosporodium
    b. Strongyloides
    c. Giardia
    d. Gnathostoma

26. Pigs are resevoir for: [AIIMS 06]
    a. T. solium
    b. T. saginata
    c. Trichinella spiralis
    d. Ancyclostoma

27. Sputum examination is not useful in diagnosis of: [PGI 08]
    a. Trichuriasis trichiura
    b. Ancylostoma duodenale
    c. Paragonimus
    d. Strongyloides

28. Which of the following disease is transmitted by egg ingestion? [AI 06]
    a. Taeniasis
    b. Trichinosis
    c. Hydatidosis
    d. Strongyloidosis

29. Liver is the target organ for: [PGI 08]
    a. Fasciola buski
    b. Paragonimus westermani
    c. Clonorchis sinenses
    d. Schistosoma Hematobium

30. Fish acts as intermediate host in: [PGI 13]
    a. D. latum
    b. Clonorchis sinensis
    c. H. diminuta
    d. H. nana

31. Parasites causing lung infestation are: [PGI 03]
    a. H. nana
    b. Paragonimus westermani
    c. Taenia saginata
    d. E. granulosus
    e. E. multiocularis

32. Visceral larva migrans caused by: [AI 2011]
    a. Strongyloides
    b. Toxocara canis
    c. Ankylostoma
    d. Dirofilaria

33. Small intestine helminth are: [PGI-11]
    a. Ascaris
    b. Necator
    c. Trichuris
    d. Enterobius
    e. Ancyclostoma

34. Identify the organism from its egg in the picture: [AIIMS 2017]

    a. Enterobius vermicularis
    b. Trichuris trichura
    c. Ascaris lumbricoides
    d. Necator Americanus

35. Filarial stage of adult worms responsible for diseases in all of the following except: [AIIMS 18]
    a. Onchocerca volvulus
    b. Brugia
    c. Wuchereria
    d. Mansonella ozzardi

Explanations and References with Illustrative Answers

1. **Ans. (c) Dog** *Ref. Paniker 7/e, 129*

   Echinococcus granulosus = Dog or Hydatid tape worm
   - Causative agent of **cystic or unilocular hydatid disease.**
   - *Definitive host* — Dog and other canine carnivora.
     Infective stage — Fertile hydatid containing fully developed scolex.
   - *Intermediate host* — Sheep and man (**Dead end** in man).
     Infective stage — Egg during grazing or ingestion of Eggs passed by infected dogs.

   Remember: Alveolar or multilocular hydatid disease is caused by *E.multilocularis*.

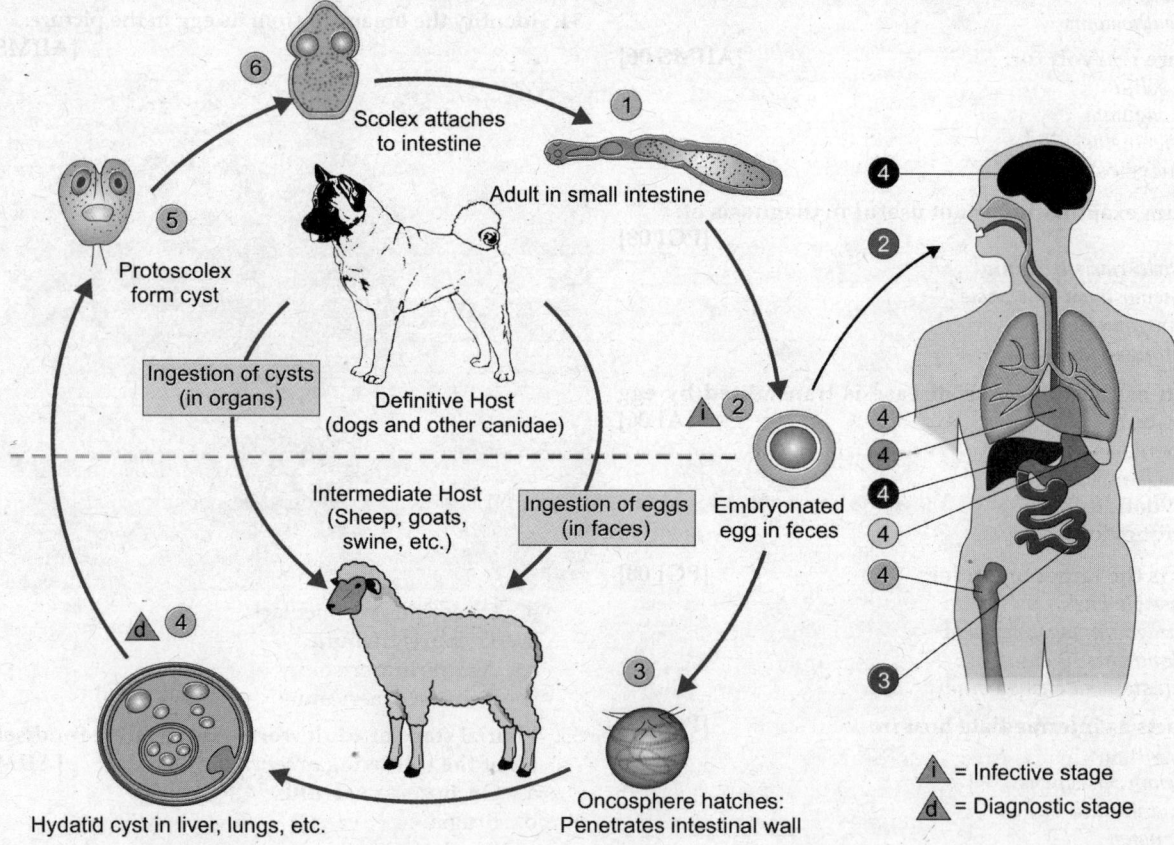

2. **Ans. (a)** *Diphyllobothrium latum* *Ref. Paniker 7/e, p 115; Harrison 19/e, p 1434, 18/e, 1765*

   Diphyllobothrium (Fish Tapeworm = Broad Tapeworm)

   - *Definitive host* – Adult worm lives in small intestine *(usually in the ileum)* of man, cat, dog and other fish eating mammals.
     Infective stage for man – Third stage larva/Plerocercoid larva/sparganum.
   - *Intermediate host*
     First – Cyclops infected by coracidium larva.
     Second – Freshwater fish infected by procercoid larvae.

- **Eggs** – Operculated, shed in feces but are not infective to man.
- **Mode of infection** – Ingestion of imperfectly cooked infected fish containing plerocercoid larva.
- **Clinical features:**
  - Mechanical obstruction
  - Abdominal discomfort
  - Diarrhoea
  - Nausea
  - Anaemia (pernicious type called as ***Bothriocephalus Anaemia***) which is due to vitamin B_{12} deficiency.
- **Diagnosis:** Demonstration of eggs in feces.
- **Treatment:** Praziquantel/Niclosamide.

3. **Ans. is (c) Sarcoptes scabei**

    Ref. Laboratory Identification of Arthropod Ectoparasites Review article by Blaine A. Mathison, Bobbi S. Pritt

   The figure shows sarcoptes scabei, causative agent of Scabies

   ### Sarcoptes scabiei (Scabies)
   - Human itch mite and the causative agent of scabies.
   - Scabies is a highly contagious condition that results in the formation of open sores and linear tracks as the mites burrow in the skin.
   - In severe cases, patients may present with thick layers of crust on the skin, a condition referred to as Norwegian, or crusted, scabies.
   - The infection is highly contagious and requires barrier precautions, including gloves and gowns, for individuals coming into contact with the patients.
   - If any person touches the infected individual without barrier he needs to be isolate till the precautionary treatment has been completed.
   - Sarcoptes mites reside in the epidermis, generally in the stratum corneum. Identification is usually made by the examination of mites, their eggs, or their feces in skin scrapings. Skin scrapings are occasionally submitted to a clinical parasitology laboratory for diagnosis of scabies.
   - Skin scrapings are best performed at the end of the burrows in nonexcoriated and noninflamed areas by using a sterile scalpel blade containing a drop of mineral oil.

   ### Treatment
   a. General Guidelines

   Recently infected person usually have no symptoms. (Symptoms typically take 4-8 weeks to develop); however they can still spread scabies during this time. Therefore in addition to the infested person, treatment also is recommended for household members and sexual contacts, particularly those who have had prolonged direct skin-to-skin contact with the infested person.

   All persons should be treated at the same time to prevent reinfestation. Scabies may sometimes be sexually-acquired in adults, but is rarely sexually-acquired in children.

   Bedding, clothing, and towels used by infested persons or their household, sexual, and close contacts (as defined above) anytime during the three days before treatment should be decontaminated by washing in hot water and drying in a hot dryer, by dry-cleaning, or by sealing in a plastic bag for at least 72 hours. (Scabies mites generally do not survive more than 2 to 3 days away from human skin.)

   b. Medications Used to Treat Scabies

   Scabicide lotion or cream should be applied to all areas of the body from the neck down to the feet and toes.

   Permethrin 5% cream, Lindane (gamma benzene hexachloride) 1% lotion or cream, Benzyl benzoate 10% and 25% lotion or emulsion, Malathion 0.5% lotion are commonly used scabicidal agents in adults.

   Only permethrin or sulfur ointment may be used in infants. The lotion or cream should be applied to a clean body and left on for the recommended time before washing it off. Clean clothing should be worn after treatment.

   Both sexual and close personal contacts who have had direct prolonged skin-to-skin contact with an infested person within the preceding month should be examined and treated. All persons should be treated at the same time to prevent reinfestation.

   > **Note:** The symptoms of scabies are due to a hypersensitivity reaction (allergy) to mites and their faeces (scybala), itching still may continue for several weeks after treatment even if all the mites and eggs are killed. If itching still is present more than 2 to 4 weeks after treatment or if new burrows or pimple-like rash lesions continue to appear, re-treatment may be necessary

4. **Ans. (b) Fasciola hepatica** *Ref. Paniker 7/e, p 150*

Snail as intermediate host suggest f. hepatica.

Fasciola hepatica
- Sheep lines fluke, its a large leaf shaped feshy hermaphrodite fluke.
- Parasite resides in liver and biliary passages of the definitive host
- Life cycle:
    1. Definitive host: Man, Sheep
    2. Intermediate host: Snail of genus lymnaea
       Aquatic plants

Life cycle from page 152 Pankier 7/e, p 149
- Mode of infection: Ingestion of metacercariae
- Pathogenesis: In comparison to clonorchis fasciola produce more hepatic damage, cause parenchymal injury and patient present with fever tender hepatomegaly.
  In chronic phase biliary obstruction and cirrhosis develops.
- Treatment: Triclabendazole is the treatment of choice.

5. **Ans. (a) *Clonorchis* sinensis** *Ref. Paniker 7/e, p 148*

Clonorchis Sinensis
- Also called as **Chinese liver fluke**
- Human clonorchiasis occurs in Japan, Korea, Taiwan etc.
- *Host* –   Definitive: Human
   - *Reservoir:* Dogs and other fish eating canines
   - *Intermediate:* First is snail and second is fresh water fish.
- *Life cycle* – Adult worm lay eggs in biliary tract (brown shell, operculum at one pole and small hook like spine at other pole) which passed in feces

  ↓

  Eggs containing ciliated miracida are ingested by snail

  ↓

  Miracida converts into cercaria and escape from snail

  ↓

  Cercaria attached to 2nd intermediate host and encyst to become metacercariae (infective stage for humans)

- *Mode of infection:*
  - Ingestion of raw or inadequately processed fish or contaminated fingers/utensils used for cooking for fish.
  - Metacercariae excyst in duodenum of human and enter CBD through ampulla of Vater.
- *Pathogenicity:*
  - Cystic dilatation/obstruction of CBD causing cholangitis/Jaundice/calculus formation/fever/epigastric pain/diarrhea/tender hepatomegaly
  - Biliary cirrhosis and portal hypertension
  - Cholangiocarcinoma/increased tendency to become biliary carriers of typhoid bacilli.
- *Diagnosis:*
  - Demonstration of eggs in feces or aspirated bile
  - Liver imaging can show eggs/dilated biliary tract.

> **Remember:** Infection of **fasciolopsis buski/giant intestinal fluke (largest trematode)** present with partial obstruction of bowel, diarrhea, abdominal pain, oedema, ascites, anemia, prostration and persistent diarrhea.
> **Gnathostoma spinigerum/G.hispidium** cause indurated nodules or abscess or creeping eruption (larva migrans) or wandering larvae may damage brain/eyes. Humans are infected by ingestion of fish containing third stage of larvae but worm does not develop further. So humans are paratenic host.

6. **Ans. (a) Clonorchis sinensis**   *Ref. Paniker 7/e, p 149, 225*

   Already explained

   Other option

   Angiostrongylus cantonensis

   Also called as rat lungworm

   - Natural host — Rat, crabs, fresh water prawns and frogs
   - Intermediate host — Molluscs, slugs, and snails
   - Mode of transmission — Eating infected molluscs etc. containing third stage larva
   - Pathogenicity — Meningoencephalitis by died larvae, so antihelminthic is not recommended
   - Diagnosis — Peripheral and CSF eosinophilia
     — Demonstration of larvae/adult worm in CSF
   - Angiostrongylos costaricensis causes inflammation of lower bowel as abdominal angiostrongyliasis

   > **Remember:** H. diminuta (rat tapeworm) is common parasite of rat and mice. Similar to H. nana in its life cycle but is larger (10-60 cm) than H. nana. Human infection is rare, asymptomatic, occur by accidental ingestion of infected rat fleas.
   > A. Cantonensis is the commnest cause of cosinopholic miningitis.

7. **Ans. (a) i.e. Scabies**

   Contact isolation means isolating the patient to avoid any physical contact with any individual without barrier. It is indicated for scabies, *Clostridium difficile*, Methicillin resistant *Staph aureus*.
   For details see answer 3.

8. **Ans. (b) Taenia solium**   *Ref. Paniker 6/e, p 144 - 145, 7/e, p 120 - 121*

   Taenia Solium (Pork Tape Worm)
   - Causative agent of *cysticercosis*.
   - **Definitive host** = Adult worm lives in jejunum of man.
     Infective stage for man:
     – Pork's flesh containing cysticercus cellulosae larvae or bladder worm.
     – Also by eggs either by ingestion in water/vegetables; Autoinfection by fingers contaminated with eggs from perianal skin or feces and retrograde peristalsis.
   - **Intermediate host** = Pig
     Infected stage for pig = Eggs containing hexacanth larvae, so eggs are infective for both man and pig.

   > **Remember:**
   > • Larvae is found in both man and pig.
   > • But in man it is dead end Infection.
   > • Infection occur in both vegetarian and non vegetarian.

   Taenia saginata
   - Causative agent of *Cysticercosis bovis*.
   - **Definitive host** = Adult worm lives in jejunum of man.
     Infected stage for man – Undercooked beef containing *Cysticercus bovis* larvae in striated muscle.
   - **Intermediate host** = Cow/bufflao = harbors larval stage.
     Infective stage of intermediate host = Eggs containing oncosphere during grazing.

   > **Remember:**
   > • Larva is absent in man.
   > • Eggs does not infect man.
   > • Infection does not occur in vegetarians.
   > • MC site involved in man is striated muscles particularly muscles of tongue, neck, shoulder, and myocardium.

Trichuris trichiura = **Whipworm**
- Life cycle in *one host only* (monoxenous).
- Adult worm lives in cecum and appendix *(Large intestine)*.
- *Mode of infection:* Feco-oral when mature embryonated eggs containing infective rhabditiform larva are swallowed in food or water.

Remember: All nematodes are monoxenous (one host) except *T. spiralis*, Filaria, Guinea worm.

9. **Ans. (b) Cysticercosis** *Ref. Harrison 19/e, p 902; Paniker 7/e, p 125*

   "Neurocysticercosis is the most common parasitic disease of CNS worldwide."

   Neurocysticercosis = Cysticercosis of CNS

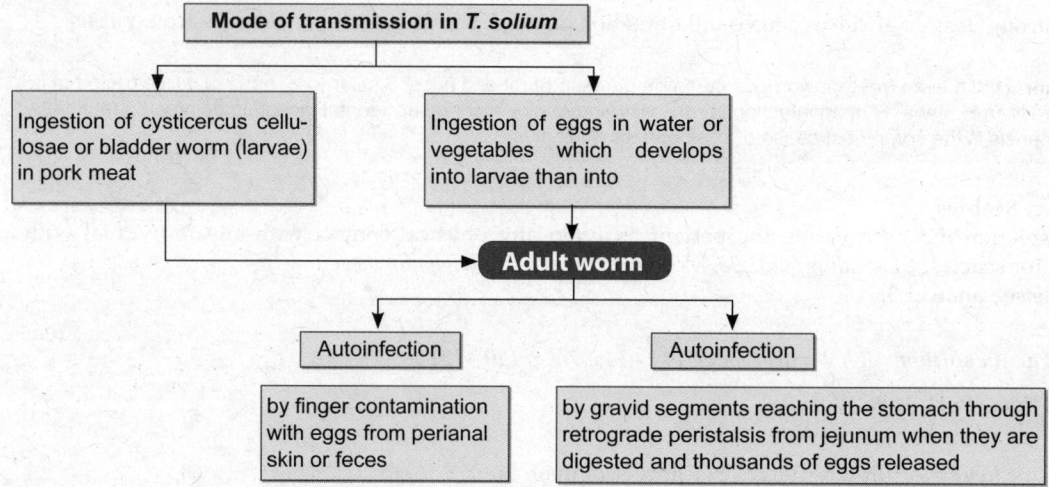

- So man is *both* definitive and intermediate host for *T. solium* but in man it is Dead end infection.
- Adult tape worm lives in the human intestine usually in the jejunum

Clinical features:
- MC manifestation is new-onset partial seizures with or without secondary generalization.

Site	Symptoms
Brain parenchyma **(MC)**	Seizures or focal neurological defects
Subarachnoid or ventricular space	Increased intra-cranial tension
Spinal cyst	Mimic intraspinal tumour

Diagnosis: – By non-contrast CT.
– MC finding on neuroimaging is parenchymal brain calcification.
Treatment: Antiepileptic therapy + Albendazole or praziquantel.

Remember: Site of cysticercosis – CNS > Subcutaneous tissue > globe of eye.

10. **Ans. (c) Paragominus**

    Paragonimiasis casued by *Paragonimus westermani* (lung flukes) mimics tuberculosis and present with chronic cough, fever, malaise
    Paragonimus westermani
    - Trematode of genus Paragonimus, usually ingested through food.
    - Paragonimus has a quite complex life-cycle that involves two intermediate hosts as well as humans.
    - First intermediate host is fresh water snail, second intermediate host is crab or cray fish
    - Human acquire infection after eating ras fish or crab.

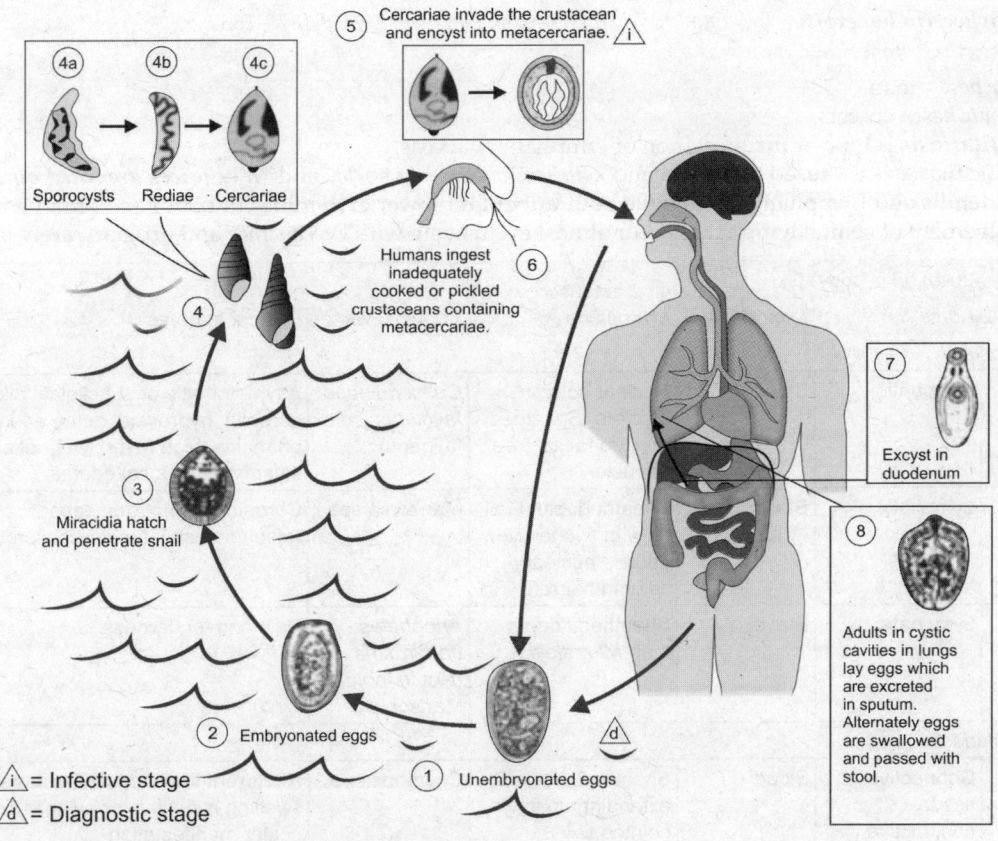

1. In the external environment, the eggs become embryonated
2. And miracidia hatch and seek the first intermediate host, a snail, and penetrate its soft tissues
3. Miracidia go through several developmental stages inside the snail
4. Sporocysts
4a. Rediae
4b. With the latter giving rise to many cercariae
4c. Which emerge from the snail. The cercariae invade the second intermediate host, a crustacean such as a crab or crayfish, where they encyst and become **metacercariae**. *This is the infective stage for the mammalian host*
5. Human infection with P. westermani occurs by eating inadequately cooked or pickled crab or crayfish that harbor metacercariae of the parasite
6. The metacercariae excyst in the duodenum
7. Penetrate through the intestinal wall into the peritoneal cavity, then through the abdominal wall and diaphragm into the lungs, where they become encapsulated and develop into adults
8. (7.5 to 12 mm by 4 to 6 mm). The worms can also reach other organs and tissues, such as the brain and striated muscles, respectively.

Treatment: Praziquental is the drug of choice. Recommended dose is 75 mg/kg/day

11. Ans. (a) Cysticercus cellulosae   *Ref. Paniker 7/e p 123*

Infective larval form of T. solium is called cysticercus cellulosae, the organism responsible for cysticercosis

> **Note:** Cysticercus cellulosae can develop into adult worm in various organs of pig as well as man.

12. Ans. (a) Brain parenchyma   *Ref. Harrison 20/e, p 1015*
Already explained

> **Note:**
> - Most common manifestation of neurocysticercosis is new onset seizure
> - Spinal cysticercosis mimics intraspinal tumors
> - MRI is the modality of choice for diagnosis of neurocysticercosis

13. Ans. (a) Wuchereria bancrofti *Ref. Paniker 7/e, p 205 - 206; Harrison 20/e, p 1629-1630*

Filariasis
- *Definitive host* – man.
- *Intermediate host* – insects
- **Genital filariasis** is type or manifestation of lymphatic filariasis.
- Lymphatic filariasis is caused by Brugia and *Wuchereria bancrofti* so "c" and "d" choices are ruled out.
- Lymphadenitis and Lymphangiitis involve both upper and lower extremities in both bancroftian and *brugian filariasis* but involvement of genital lymphatics occur almost exclusively with *W. bancrofti* and brugian rarely involved genitalia.

Parasite	Location in body		Characteristics of Microfilaria	Principal vector	Clinical features	DOC
	Adult	Microfilaria				
I. Lymphatic Filariasis						
Wuchereria bancrofti	Lymphatic	Blood	Nuclear column discrete, Sheathed, pointed tail tip free of nuclei	*Culex quinque fasciatus* (culex fatigans)	Asymptomatic or subclinical microflaremia; hydrocele; acute adenolymphangitis (high fever, lymphatic inflammation, local edema.	Dec
Burgia malayi	Lymphatic	Blood	Sheathed, blunt tail tip with two terminal nuclei, nuclear column blurred	Mansonia spp	Chronic lymphatic disease (elephantiasis); funiculitis; scrotal	
Burgia timori	Lymphatic	Blood	Sheathed, longer than *Mf malayi*	Anopheles barbirostris (Not in India) Mansonia	Pain and tenderness	
II. Subcutaneous filariasis						
Loa loa	Connective tissue, conjunctiva	Blood	Sheathed, nuclei extending up to pointed tail	Chyrsops spp	Recurrent transients subcutaneous swelling is fugitive or calabar swellings, ocular manifestation	Dec
Onchocerca volvulus= Convulated = binding filaria	Subcutaneous nodules	Skin, eyes	Unsheathed, blunt tail tip free of nuclei	Simulium spp.	Pruritus, and rash (MC; Iverm palpable subcutaneous ectin nodules; lymphadenopathy; visual impairment (River blindness)	Ivermectin
Mansonella streptocerca	Subcutaneous	Skin	Unsheathed; blunt tail tip with nuclei	Culicoides	Pruritus, papular rash, Ivermpigmentation; inguinal ectin, adenopathy	Dec, Ivermectin
III. Serous cavity filariasis						
Mansonella ozzardi	Peritoneum and pleura	Blood	Unsheathed pointed tail tip without nuclei	Culicoides	Headache articular Iverm pain, fever, pulmonary ectin symptoms, adenopathy, hepatomegaly, pruritus, eosinophilia	Ivermectin
Mansonella perstans	Peritoneum; and pleura, mesentery, perirenal tissue	Blood	Unsheathed, pointed tail tip with nuclei	Culicoides	Asymptomatic mostly; transient angioedema; pruritus of arm, face; fever; headache; arthralgia; right upper quadrant pain	Dec

DEC: Diethylcarbomazine

14. Ans. (b) Early adenolymphangiitis stage *Ref. Park 21/e, p 246; Paniker 7/e, p 205; Chatterjee 12/e, p 195 - 197*

Clinical manifestations		
Lymphatic filariasis		
i.	*Asymptomatic amicrofilaremia*	– No microfilarae and no clinical manifestation.
ii.	Asymptomatic microfilaremia	– Positive for Mf without any symptoms.
iii.	Stage of acute manifestation	– Recurrent episodes of acute inflammation in lymph glands and vessels characterized by lymphadenitis, lymphangitis, filarial fever, lymphangiovarix and lymphorrhagia. It is caused by adult worm but blood **may reveal microfilarae in early phase.**

Contd...

Contd...

Clinical manifestations		
Lymphatic filariasis		
iv. Stage of chronic obstructive lesions	–	Caused by adult worm blocking lymph nodes and vessels either mechanically or are commonly due to allergic inflammatory reactions to worm antigens and secretions. Granuloma may form. Main features are hydrocele, elephantiasis (*MC* site is leg), Lymphedema *(non pitting or brawny edema)*.
	–	Microfilaria in blood are absent either due to death or their failure to reach the systemic circulation due to lymphatic obstruction.
Occult filariasis		
Meyers Kouwenaar syndrome	–	It is due to hypersensitivity reactions to filarial antigens. It *includes Tropical pulmonary eosinophilia* characterized by nocturnal paroxysmal cough, wheeze and blood eosinophil count is above 3000 per cmm.
	–	*Microfilariae* are *not usually* detectable in blood but lung biopsies may show microfilariae
	–	Antifilarial antibody titres are characteristically elevated

15. **Ans. (a) B. malayi** *Ref. Paniker 7/e, p 214; Park 21/e, 244*
    - Heavily infected areas of lymphatic filariasis are found in Uttar Pradesh, Bihar, Jharkand, Andhra Pradesh, Orissa, Tamil Nadu, Kerala and Gujarat. So, it is case of lymphatic filariasis.

    Sheathed microfilaria are:
    - Loa-loa ⎫ Tail tip has nuclei but loa-loa cause subcutaneous filariasis
    - *Burgia malayi* ⎬ found in Africa (not in Bihar.)
    - *W. bancrofti* ⎭ Tail tip free of nuclei.

    Mnemonic: **L**ow (L); **B**irth (B); **W**eight (W)

Features	Mf bancrofti	Mf. malayi
Length	250-300 µm (longer)	175-300 µm
Appearance	Graceful sweeping curves	Kinky, with secondary curves
Cephalic space	Length and breadth equal	Almost twice as long as broad
Stylet at anterior end	Single	Double
Excretory pore	Not prominent	Prominent
Nuclear column	Discrete nuclei	Blurred/smudged
Tail tip	Pointed, free of nuclei	Kinkled and 2 distinct nuclei one at tip, the other subterminal
Sheath	Faintly stained	Well stained

    Microfilaria tail free of nuclei
    - *W. Bancrofti*
    - *O. Volvulus*
    - *M. Ozzardi*

    Mnemonic: **BOO**

16. **Ans. (a) Abdominal pain** *Ref. Paniker 7/e, p 190 - 192; Harrison 19/e, p 1416; 18/e, p 1743*

    Enterobius vermicularis = Pinworm = thread worm = seat worm
    - Life cycle in *one host only (man)*.
    - *No* intermediate host.
    - Adult worm live in caecum, appendix and adjacent part of ascending colon (i.e. in large intestine).
    - *Mode of infection* – By ingestion of egg containing infective larvae (=autoinfection) and retroinfection.
    - **Clinical features:**
      - Mostly asymptomatic.
      - *Cardinal symptoms:* Perianal pruritus (It is nocturnal and cause excoriation + bacterial superinfection).
      - Abdominal pain and weight loss.
      - Vulvovaginitis and pelvic or peritoneal granuloma.
    - **Diagnosis:**
      - Fecal examination is not useful.
      - Apply clear cellulose acetate tape to perianal region in the morning and see characteristic *planoconvex, non-bile stained* pin worm *eggs* (containing tadpole shaped coiled embryo) on microscopy.
      - Sampling can also be done by NIH swab, scotch tape, glass pestle swab.
    - **Treatment:**
      - Mebendazole/Albendazole/Pyrantel pamoate.

17. **Ans. (b) Onchocerca volvulus** *Ref. Paniker 7/e, p 216 - 217*

    - *It is a case of subcutaneous filariasis* so causes of lymphatic filariasis (Brugia) and serous cavity filariasis (M.perstans) are ruled out. Thus, we left with only 2 options:
      Loa Loa = Eye Worm: Cause Loiasis/Fugitive Swellings Or Calabar Swellings
      - *Definitive host* = Man (in subcutaneous tissue)
      - *Intermediate host* = Vector – day biting flies (Chyrysops)
      - *Mode of trnsmission*: Bite of infected Chyrysops
      - *Microfilariae*: Are sheathed and show diurnal periodicity and appear in blood only during day and taken by chyrysops in which Mf develop into infective third stage larvae.
      - Clinical features: Is due to migration of adult worms causing fugitive swellings (which disappear in few days only to reappear elsewhere); Ocular manifestations.
      - Diagnosis   :   Demonstration of adult worm from scraping of skin or conjunctiva.
      - Treatment   :   Surgery to remove worms; DEC; corticosteroids
      Onchocerca Volvulus:
      - Convulated or blinding filaria causing *onchocerciasis or river blindness.*
      - It is 2nd major cause of blindness in the world.
      - **Vector:** Day biting female black flies (are pool feeders) Simulium, which breed in fast flowing rivers.
      - *Microfilariae:* Unsheathed; non-periodic; found in skin, subcutaneous lymphatics, conjunctiva and rarely in blood.
      - **Clinical features**: Subcutaneous nodule or onchocercoma which is circumscribed, firm, non-tender tumor tend to occur over anatomical sites where bones are superficial such as scalp, scapula, ribs, elbow, iliac crest, sacrum, knees.
      - Lesions in skin (pruritus, pigmentation, atrophy, fibrosis) and eyes (photophobia to blindness, glaucoma, punctate or sclerosing keratitis, iridocyclitis, glaucoma) also seen.
    - **Diagnosis:** Demonstrating microfilariae by slicing off a silver of skin; aspirating subcutaneous nodules, conjunctival biopsies.
      - **Treatment:** *Ivermectin; Enucleation of nodules; DEC (cause Mazotti reaction) and Suramin.*

18. **Ans. (a) Trichinella spiralis** *Ref. Paniker 7/e, p 168*

    Classification of Nematodes on the basis of Mode of infection.

Ingestion	Penetration of skin	By blood sucking insect	Inhalation of dust containing eggs

• Eggs
  – Ascaris
  – Enterobius
  – Trichuris
	• **A**ncylostoma
	• **N**ecator
	• **S**trongyloides
		• Filariae	• Ascaris
			• Enterobius

• *Larvae within Intermediate host* or drinking water containing cyclops – Dracunculus	Mnemonic: **ANS**		
• *Encysted larvae in muscle*: Trichinella			

19. **Ans. (a, c, d) and (e) Absent fragmentation, Separate sexes, Cylindrical body and GIT is formed completely**

    Ref. Paniker 6/e, p 113-114

Features	Nematodes	Trematodes	Cestodes
Shape	Cylindrical/thread	Flat or fleshy leaf-like or flukes	Tape like
Segmentation	Unsegmented	Unsegmented	Segmented
GIT	Complete	Incomplete	Absent
Suckers	Absent	Present	Present
Hooks	Absent	Absent	May present
Sex	Separate (Dioecious)	Monoecious except Schistosomes	Monoecious
Number of host	Monoxenous except *Trichinella*, filarial, *Dracunculus medinensis*	Digenetic	Digenetic except *H.nana*
Body cavity	Present	Absent	Absent

    Remember: Nematodes may be viviparous or oviparous or Ovo-viviparous but other worms are oviparous

20. **Ans. (b) Ancylostome braziliense** *Ref. Harrison 20/e p 1623*

    Cutaneous Larva Migrans
    - Serpengenous skin eruptions caused by burrowing larvae of animal hook worms usually the dog and cat hook worm Ancytostoma braziliense
    - More prevalent in children and travelers to endemic
    - Larvae hatch from eggs passed in dog and cat and mature in soil
    - Human become infected after skin contact with soil
    - As Larvae penetrates the skin erythematous lesion form along the tortous tract of their migration through the dermal epidermal junction.

21. **Ans. (b) Transmitted** *Ref. Paniker 7/e, p 173*

    This is the figure denoting longitudinal section of trichuris trichiura as characterized by coiled posterior end of male. Now let us consider each option
    Option "a"
    Infective form is rhabditiform larvae.
    Option "b"
    Mode of transmission: Infection occurs in human when mature embryonated eggs containing the infective larvae are swallowed in contaminated food or water.
    Option "c"
    Pathogenicity: Usually asymptomatic, however when worm load is heavy, disease may result either due to mechanical effects or allergic reactions.
    The whip like anterior portion of worm (both male and female) usually attaches it self to the mucosa of caecum and upper colon. One worm is believed to suck about 0.005 mL of blood.

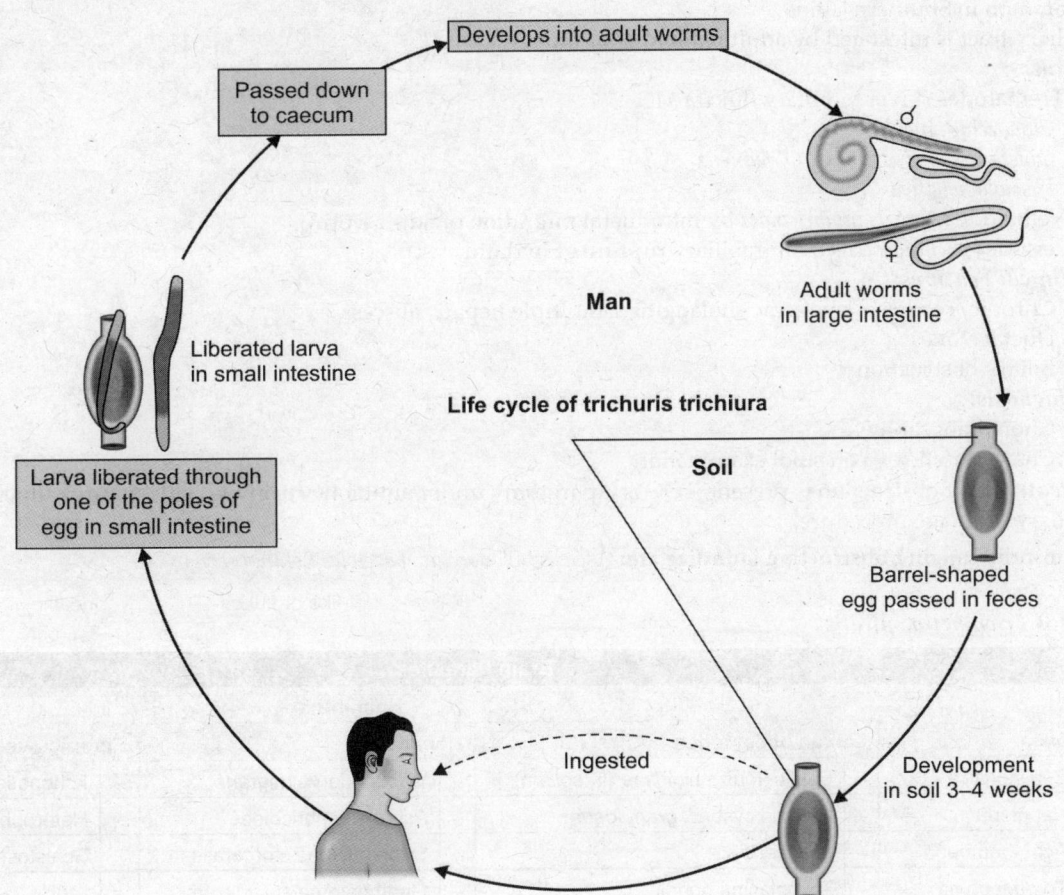

Life cycle of trichuris trichiura

Option "d"

Mebendazole or albendazole are drug of choice: Important points about trichuris:

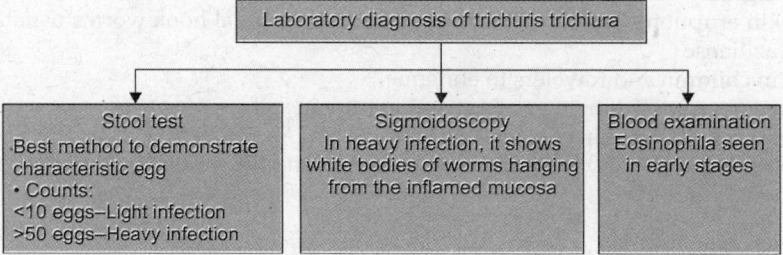

22. **Ans. (e) Trichuris trichiura** Ref. Paniker 7/e p 173
    "Barrel-shaped eggs are characteristic of trichuris trichiura".
    Important points about trichuris trichiura:
    - First described by Linnaeus
    - Lives in large intestine, adult worms are attached to the wall of caecum.
    - Adult worm resemble whip
    - Egg are characteristically barrel-shaped and possess triple shell. Eggs flot in saturated salt solution. They hatch in small intestine.
    - Mebendazole or albendazole is the treatment.

23. **Ans. (c) Ankylostoma duodenale** Ref. Harrison 17/e p 1334, 1335, 2000
    Hepatobiliary Parasitism
    - Common in Southern China
    - Biliary tract is infestated by adult helminths or their ova
    - *Causes:*
      (a) Trematodes (Liver or biliary flukes) MC
        – Clonorchis sinensis
        – Opisthorchis viverrini or O. felineus
        – Fasciola hepatica
      (b) Nematode (Ascaris lumbricoides by intraductal migration of adult worm)
      (c) Cestodes (Echinococcus by intrabiliary rupture of hydatid cyst)
    - *Clinical Features:*
      – Chronic/recurrent pyogenic cholangitis ± multiple hepatic abscess
      – Ductal stones
      – Biliary obstruction
    - *Diagnosis:*
      – Cholangiography
      – Characteristic ova on stool examination
    - *Treatment:* If obstruction is present, TOC is laparotomy under antibiotic coverage with common duct exploration and biliary drainage procedure.

    Helminths causing obstructive jaundice are: *Ascaris, Clonorchis, Fasciola, Echinococcus.*

24. **Ans. (d) Trichinella spiralis**

Brain Parasites							
		Helminths					
Protozoa		**Larvae of cestodes**		**Nematodes**		**Ectopic ova**	
–	E. histolytica	–	Cysticercus cellulosae (T. solium)	–	Visceral larva migrans	–	F. hepatica
–	Naegleria	–	Hydatid cyst (E. granulosus)	–	Ascaris lumbricoides	–	Heterophyes hyterophyes
–	Acanthamoeba	–	Multiceps sp	–	Strongyloides stercoralis		Schistosoma hematobium
–	Trypanosoma	–	Toxoplasma gondii	–	Gnathostoma spinigerum		
–	P. falciparum						

25. **Ans. (b) Strongyloides** *Ref. Paniker 7/e, p 4*

    > **Autoinfection is seen in:**
    > C = *Capillaria philippinensis*
    > H = *Hymenolepis nana*
    > E = *Enterobius vermicularis*
    > S = *Strongyloides stercoralis*
    > T = *Taenia solium* (cysticercosis)
    > C = *Cryptosporidium Parvum*
    >
    > **Mnemonic:** CHEST congestion

    - Autoinfection in cysticercosis occurs by finger contamination with the eggs from the perianal skin or feces and by gravid segments reaching the stomach by retrograde peristalsis from jejunum.

26. **Ans. (a) and (c) *T. solium*; and *Trichinella spiralis*** *Ref. Paniker 7/e, p 123, 167*

    Taenia solium
    - Also known as *pork tapeworm.*
    - Intermediate host is pig.

    Trichinella spiralis
    - *Primary host* = Man – Mucosal epithelium of small intestine.
    - *Infective form* is the encysted larvae found in the muscles of pig and other animals (larvae is tissue parasite).
    - *Intermediate host* = Pig
    - *Mode of Infection* – Uncooked pork meat containing encysted larvae.
    - Female worm is viviparous (eggs are absent).
    - Human infection is dead end infection.

27. **Ans. (a) *Trichuris trichiura*** *Ref. Paniker 7/e, p 172, 238*
    - Sputum examination can be useful for any parasite which pass through lungs at some or other stage during their life cycle.
    - **These parasites are:**
      - Rhabditiform larva of Ascaris
      - Golden brown eggs of *Paragonimus westermani* (Lung fluke)
      - Migrating larvae of *Strongyloides, Ancylostoma, Ancylostoma ducdenale, nector americanus*
      - *Entamoeba histolytica* - Chocolate brown sputum due to hepatobronchial fistula.

28. **Ans. (c) Hydatidosis** *Ref. Paniker 6/e, p 159*

    Following parasitic infection occur by ingestion of eggs:
    - *Echinococcus granulosus*
    - *Hymenolepis nana*
    - *Ascaris*   **Mnemonic:** Esha HATE Tushar
    - *Trichuris*
    - *Enterobius*
    - *Taenia solium* (but mainly transmit by ingestion of undercooked pork meat containing cysticercus cellulose).

29. **Ans. (c) *Clonorchis sinensis*** *Ref. Paniker 7/e, p 148*
    - All are trematodes (also known as *flukes*).
    - Man is definitive and snails are intermediate host usually.
    - They are classified as:

	Flukes	Habitat	Intermediate host	Mode of transmission
a. Blood Flukes				
i.	*Schistosoma* (Bilharzia) *hematobium*	Vesical and pelvic vein plexuses	Snail which is infected by miracidium	– Water borne disease – Man is infected by bathing in contaminated water when cercaria penetrates unbroken skin
ii.	*S. mansoni*	Inferior mesentric vein (Intestinal bilharziasis) or Schistosomal dysentry		
iii.	*S. japonicum* or oriental schistosomiasis	Superior mesenteric vein (katayama disease)		
b. Liver Flukes				
i.	Clonorchis sinensis (=Chinese liver flukes)	Biliary tract (associated with Cholangiocarcinoma)	1st intermediate host: snail 2nd intermediate host: fish	Fish containing metacercariae are eaten raw or inadequately processed
ii.	*Fasciola hepatica* (=sheep liver fluke)	Biliary tract	Primary host: man/sheep Intermediate host: snails	Ingestion of watercress or other water vegetation containing metacercaria
c. Intestinal Flukes				
i.	*Fasciolopsis buski* (Giant intestinal fluke)	Duodenum or jejunum	Molluscum Snails	Ingestion of roots of lotus, bulb of water chestnut and other acquatic vegetations
ii.	Heterophyes	Small intestine	Molluscum Snails	Ingestion of fishes since cercariae encyst on fishes
iii.	Metagonimus Yokogawai	Small intestine	1st intermediate host: fresh water snail; 2nd intermediate host: fish	Ingestion of raw fish
v.	*Gastrodiscoides hominis* (only fluke inhabiting human large intestine)	Large intestine	Molluscum	Ingestion of water plants
d. Lung Fluke				
	Paragonimus Westermani = Oriental lung fluke	Cystic space of lung	1st intermediate host: snail 2nd intermediate host: fresh water cray fish or crab fish	Inadequately cooked crabs, cray fish

30. **Ans. (a) and (b)** *D. latum* and *Clonorchis sinensis*   *Ref. See below*
    Two intermediate host with fish as one of them are seen in:

	Parasite	Ist intermediate host	IInd intermediate host
i.	*Paragonimus westermani* (Trematode)	Snail	Fresh water cray fish or crab
ii.	*Clonorchis sinensis* (Trematode)	Snail	Fish
iii.	*Metagonimus yokogawai* (Trematode)	Fresh water snail	Fish
iv.	*Diphyllobothrium latum* (Cestode)	Cyclops	Fresh water fish

Remember:
- All cestodes are digenetic (require 2 host) except *H. nana*.
- Intermediate host for *H. diminuta* is Rat flea.

31. **Ans. (b, d and e)** *Paragonimus westermani, E. granulosus* and *E. multiocularis*   *Ref. Paniker 6/e, 150 - 1555*
    - *Taenia saginata* and *H. nana* are intestinal cestodes.
    - Paragonimus is lung fluke, so there is no doubt about this.

    Clinical manifestations of hydatid cyst
    - **MC** site of Hydatid cyst (*E. granulosus* typically develops unilocular cyst): **Liver**; mostly in right lobe presenting as Hepatomegaly, pain, obstructive jaundice.
    - **Next common** site is **lung** usually in the lower lobe of right lung – cough, hemoptysis, chest pain, dyspnea.

- Hypersensitivity, fatal anaphylaxis if cyst ruptures.
- Kidney - pain, hematuria.
- Osseus hydatid.

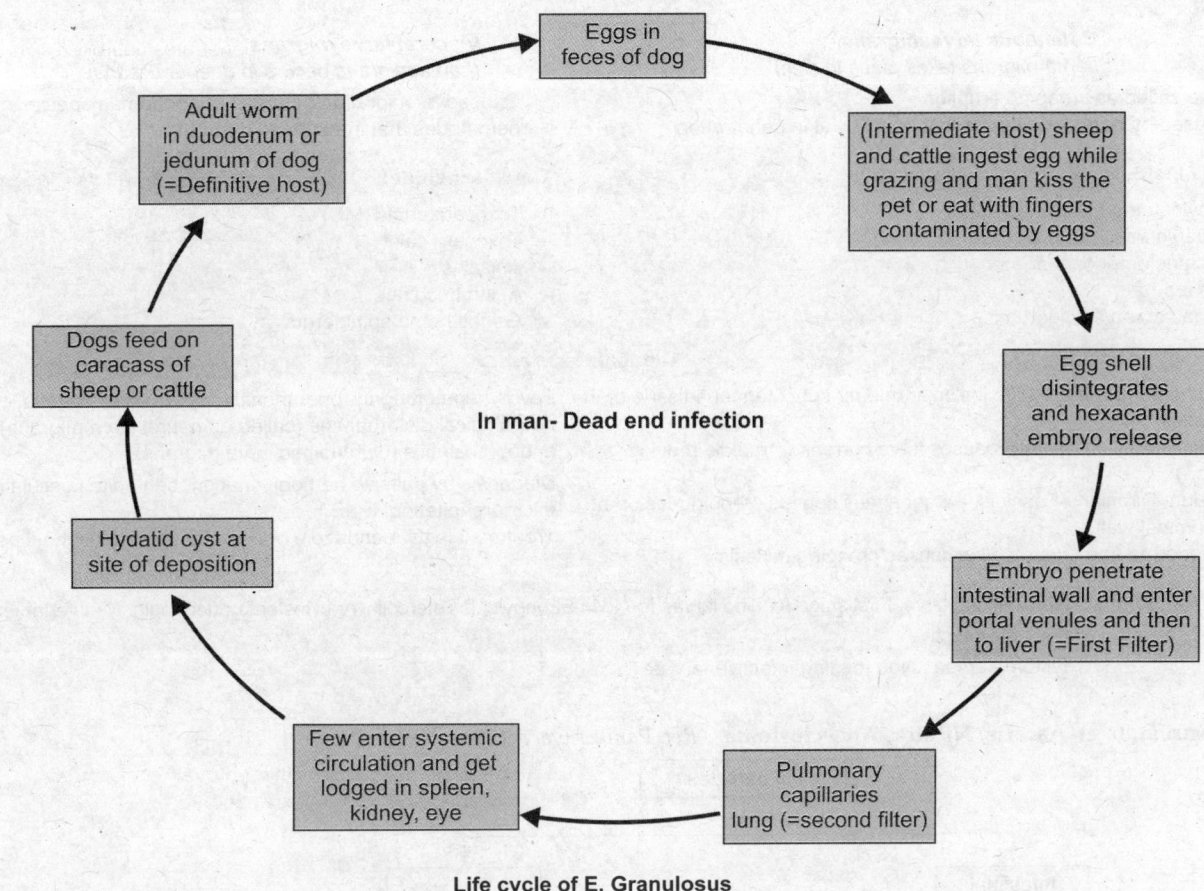

Life cycle of E. Granulosus

E. Multilocularies:
- *Cause alveolar or multilocular hydatid disease in man.*
- *Definitive host:* Foxes, dogs, cats
- *Intermediate host:* Rodents (main), man
- Man infected by eating fruits or vegetables contaminated with feces.
- *Clinical features:*
  - *MC* site liver: Multilocular infiltrating lesion mistaken for malignant tumor.
  - Also metastasize to lungs and brain.
- *Treatment:* Resection is *TOC*.

> **Remember:** Malignant hydatid disease:
> - Caused by Echinococcus multilocularis. Present with multiple small cysts in both lobe of liver
> - Mimics malignancy and most patient die of liver failure

32. **Ans (b) Toxocara canis** *Ref. Paniker 7/e, p 162 - 166*

Larva migrans occur when larvae lose their normal pathway and wander around aimlessly

It is generally seen when human infection occurs with non-human species of nematodes so larvae is unable to complete its normal development. It can also occur when parasitic nematodes infect immune person, so that its immunity does not allow normal progression of infection.

It can be of two types:

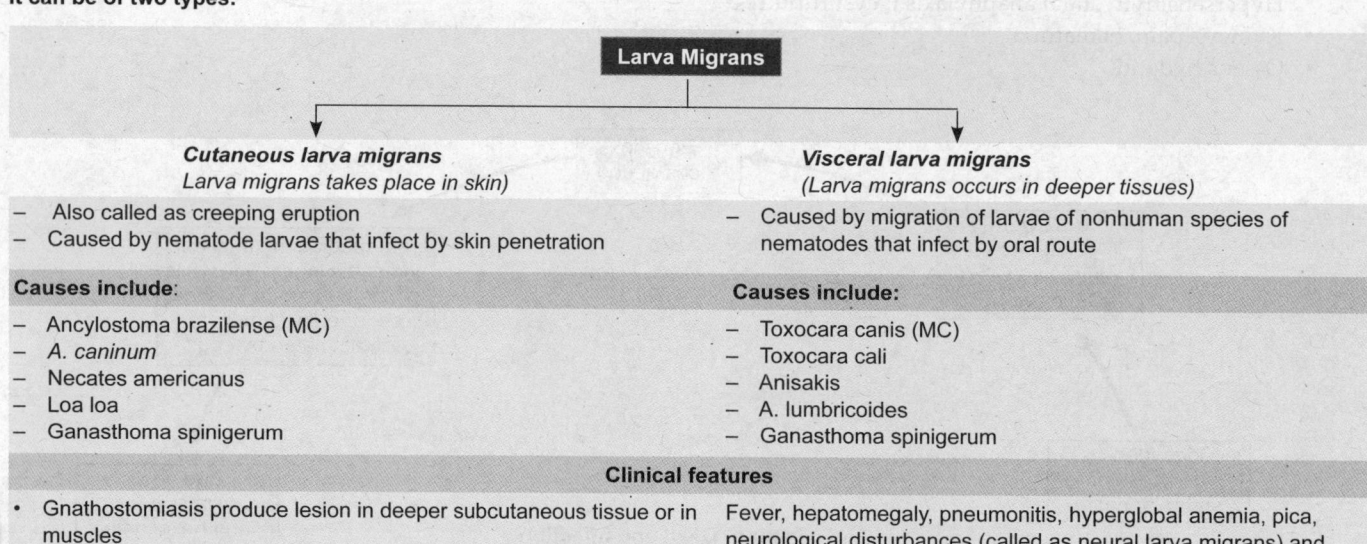

- Gnathostomiasis produce lesion in deeper subcutaneous tissue or in muscles
- Strongyloides stercoralis causes larva currens (= rapidly moving lesion)
- Loa loa, Dirofilaria Fasciola, paragonimus causes creeping lesion of abdominal wall
- Hypoderma and Gastrophilus causes creeping myiasis

Fever, hepatomegaly, pneumonitis, hyperglobal anemia, pica, neurological disturbances (called as neural larva migrans) and endophthalmitis (Ophthalmic larva migrans)

Diagnosis by passive hemoglutination, bentonite flocculation, micropreapitation, ELISA

Treatment is thiabendazole or deworming of household pets

Remember: Rhabditiform larva: First stage feeding larvae found in Strongyloides stercolis, Ancylostoma duodenale, Necater americanus.
It is non-infective
Filiform larvae : Non feeding infective larvae

33. **Ans. (a, b, e) Ascaris, Nicator, Ancyclostoma** *Ref. Paniker 6/e, p 159*

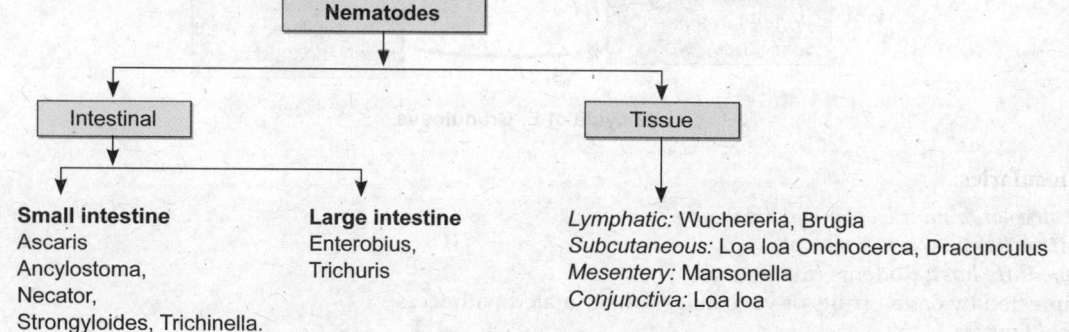

34. **Ans. (d) Necator Americanus** *Ref. Paniker 7/e p 183, 186*

The figure represents egg of ancylostoma duodenale and Necator americanus.
As guided by clear space between hyaline shell and blastomere.

35. **Ans. (d) Mansonella ozzardi** *Ref. Paniker 7/e p 219*

Mansonella Ozzardi

M. ozzardi is a new world filaria seen only in central and south America and the West Indies.
- The adult worms live in the **body cavities** of humans, mainly in **peritoneum**, less often in **pleura**, and rarely in **pericardium**.
- The microfilariae are unsheathed and nonperiodic.
- Vectors are *Culicoides* species.
- Infection does not cause any illness.

NEET Pattern Questions

1. **Katayama fever is caused by:**
   a. F. hepatica
   b. C. sinensis
   c. S. haematobium
   d. A. lumbricoide
   [Ref. Paniker 7/e, p 147]

   > Katayama fever on oriental schistosomiasis is caused by schistosoma japonicum.
   > • Katayama fever is characterized by eosinophilia, enlarged tender liver, and a palpable spleen. In the chronic stages several manifestations associated with portal hypertension are seen. Pathologically it is characterized by periportal fibrosis (clay pipe stem fibrosis)

2. **Schistosomiasis is transmitted by:**
   a. Cyclops
   b. Fish
   c. Snails
   d. Cattle
   [Ref. Paniker 7/e, p 143]

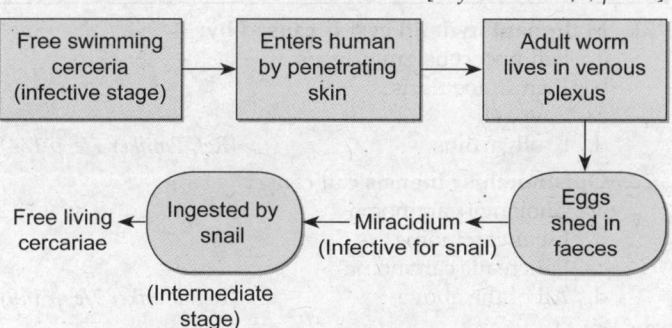

3. **Schistosomiasis is an example of:**
   a. Meta-zoonoses
   b. Cyclo-zoonoses
   c. Direct-zoonoses
   d. Sporo-zoonoses

   > **Metazoonosis:** Disease transmitted by invertebrate host.

4. **Cercariae are infective form of:**
   a. S. hematobium
   b. P. westermanii
   c. F. hepatica
   d. T. solium
   [Ref. Paniker 7/e, p 143]

5. **Water host required for schistosomiasis:**
   a. Fish
   b. Cyclops
   c. Snails
   d. Crabs
   [Ref. Paniker 7/e, p 143]

6. **Hydatid disease is caused by:**
   a. Echinococcus
   b. Tapeworm
   c. Ascaris
   d. Clonorchis
   [Ref. Paniker 7/e, p 127]

7. **Wucheria bancrofti, true is:**
   a. Unsheathed
   b. Tail tip free from nuclei
   c. Non-periodic
   d. All
   [Ref. Paniker 7/e, p 205]

8. **Which is non lymphatic filariasis?**
   a. Loa loa
   b. Wucheria bancrofti
   c. Brugia malai
   d. Brugia timori
   [Ref. Paniker 7/e, p 205]

   > Loa Loa cause subcutaneous filariasis affecting subcutaneous tissue (calabor swelling) and conjunctivitis.

Lymphatic filariasis	Subcutaneous filariasis	Serous cavity filariasis
• Wuchereria bancrofti • Brugia malayi • Brugia timori	• Loa loa • Onchocerca vovulus • Mansonella streptocerca	• Mansonella perstans • Mansonella ozzard

9. **True about diphyllobothrium:**
   a. Man is single host
   b. Iron deficiency anemia is seen
   c. Operculated egg is diagnostic
   d. Fish is the definitive host
   [Ref. Paniker 7/e, p 115-118]

   > Anaemia of Diphyllobothrium latum is due to vit B_{12} deficiency.

10. **Unsegmented eggs are in which parasite?**
    a. Trichuris trichiura
    b. Ancylostoma
    c. Necator americanus
    d. Dracunculus
    [Ref. Paniker 7/e, p 161]

    > Ascaris and Trichuris lay unsegmented eggs

11. **Flame cells are seen in:**
    a. Protozoa
    b. Cestode
    c. Nematodes
    d. None

    > Flame cells (solenocyte) are the excretory cell in cestodes and trematodes Arrangement and number of flame cell forms the basis for identification.

12. **Rhabditiform larvae is seen in:**
    a. Tenia solium
    b. Strongyloides
    c. D. latum
    d. Trichenella
    [Ref. Paniker 7/e, p 179]

Ans.
1. c. S. haematobium
2. c. Snails
3. a. Meta-zoonoses
4. a. S. hematobium
5. c. Snails
6. a. Echinococcus
7. b. Tail tip free from nuclei
8. a. Loa loa
9. c. Operculated egg is diagnostic
10. a. Trichuris trichiura
11. b. Cestode
12. b. Strongyloides

UNIT-IV: Parasitology

13. Which organism can be isolated from stool and sputum?
    a. Paragnomus   b. Fasciola
    c. Chlornchis   d. P. carinii
    [Ref. Paniker 7/e, p 157]

Helminth present in lung		
Trematode	Cestode	Nematodes
– Paragonimus westermani	– Echinoccocus granulosis	– Capillaria aerophila – Dicrofilaria imnitus

14. Ankylostoma duodenale commonly lives in:
    a. Upper 1/3rd of duodenum
    b. Lower 1/3rd of duodenum
    c. Jejunum
    d. Ileum   [Ref. Paniker 7/e p 182]

15. Ovoviviparous parasite which is associated with auto-infection:
    a. Ancylostoma duodenale
    b. Strongyloides stercoralis
    c. Enterobius vermicularis
    d. Ascaris   [Ref. Paniker 7/e, p 179]

Autoinfection is seen in both Enterobius vermicularies and S. stercoralis. Enterobius is **oviparous** whereas strongyloides is ovoviviparous.

16. Chlonorchis sinensis infection is due to ingestion of:
    a. Fish   b. Pork
    c. Snail   d. Beef   [Ref. Paniker 7/e, p 148]

17. Chlonorchis sinenensis is:
    a. Tapeworm   b. Roundworm
    c. Threadworm d. Fluke   [Ref. Paniker 7/e, p 148]

Clonorchis sinopsis is called Chinese liver fluke.

18. The following infection resembles malignancy:
    a. Echinococcus granulosus
    b. E.multilocularis
    c. E.vogeli
    d. E.oligarthus   [Ref. Paniker 7/e, p 134]

Echinococcus multilocularis cause malignant hydatid disease, a benign condition that resembles clinically and prognosis wise to malignancy. Clinically it presents with multiple small cysts in both lobes of liver.
Most patients die of liver failure.

19. Skin penetration not seen in:
    a. Taenia saginata
    b. Nectator americanus
    c. Ankylostoma duodenale
    d. Strongyloides stercoralis   [Ref. Paniker 7/e, p 122]

20. Larvae of Ascaris lumbricoides most commonly causes:
    a. Cardiac symptoms
    b. Respiratory symptoms
    c. Genitourinary symptoms
    d. Cerebral symptoms   [Ref. Paniker 7/e, p 198]

Clinical presentation of ascaris lumbricoides:
• Symptom due to larvae
  – Usually asymptomatic
  – Pathogenic effect of larval migration are due to allergic reaction and occur only when larval load is very heavy.
  – Pneumonitis is the commonest manifestation
• Symptom due to adult worm
  – Protein-energy malnutrition
  – Colicky abdominal pain
  – Intestinal obstruction
  – Acute biliary obstruction
  – Pancreatitis
  – Obstructive appendicitis
  – Liver abscess

21. Malignant hydatid cyst is caused by:
    a. Echinococcus granulosus
    b. E. multilocularis
    c. E. vogeli
    d. E. oligarthus   [Ref. Paniker 7/e, p 134]

22. Opisthorchis sinensis can cause:
    a. Cholangiocarcinoma
    b. Liver carcinoma
    c. Pancreatic carcinoma
    d. All of the above   [Ref. Paniker 7/e, p 149]

23. Cholangiocarcinoma is caused by:
    a. Giardia lamblia
    b. Clonorchis infestation
    c. Paragonimus infestation
    d. Ascaris infestation   [Ref. Paniker 7/e, p 149]

24. Infective stage of hook worm is:
    a. Trophozoite form   b. Filiform larva
    c. Cyst   d. None
    [Ref. Paniker 7/e p 104]

25. River blindness is caused by:
    a. Onchocerca
    b. Loa loa
    c. Ascaris
    d. B. malayi   [Ref. Paniker 7/e, p 217]

Ans.					
13. a. Paragnomus	14. c. Jejunum	15. b. Strongyloides...	16. a. Fish	17. d. Fluke
18. b. E.multilocularis	19. a. Taenia saginata	20. b. Respiratory symptoms	21. b. E. multilocularis
22. a. Cholangiocarcinoma	23. b. Clonorchis...	24. b. Filiform larva	25. a. Onchocerca

SECTION B

UNIT V

Immunology

- Basics of Immune System
- Antigen and Antibody
- Hypersensitivity

CHAPTER 36

Basics of Immune System

CLASSIFICATION

Immunity

- **Innate Immunity / I I**
  (Natural immunity
  = native immunity)
  - Include defense mechanism that are present even before infection i.e. since birth
  - It is the first line of defense

- **Adaptive Immunity / A I**
  (Acquired immunity)
  - Include mechanism that are stimulated by microbes and are capable of recognizing microbial and non-microbial substances

Includes

- **Humoral Component of I I**
  - Acute phase reactants
  - Interferons
  - Complements
  - Lysozyme

- **Cell mediators of I I**
  - Natural killer cells
  - Phagocytes

- **Humoral Component of A I**
  - Antibody

- **Cell mediators of A I**
  - T lymphocytes

Characteristics

- **Innate immunity**
  - Broad specificity
  - No change with repeat exposure
  - Mechanical barrier
  - Natural flora

- **Acquired immunity**
  - Specific to microbe
  - Generates memory
  - Repeat exposure shows rapid and enhanced response

Innate immunity is the first line of defense and most potential pathogen are checked before they establish an overt infection. If these defenses are breached, the acquired immune system is called into play.

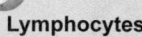

Lymphocytes
- B lymphocytes: Constitute 10-20% of peripheral lymphocyte. Provides humoral immunity.
- T lymphocyte: 60-70% of peripheral lymphocyte.

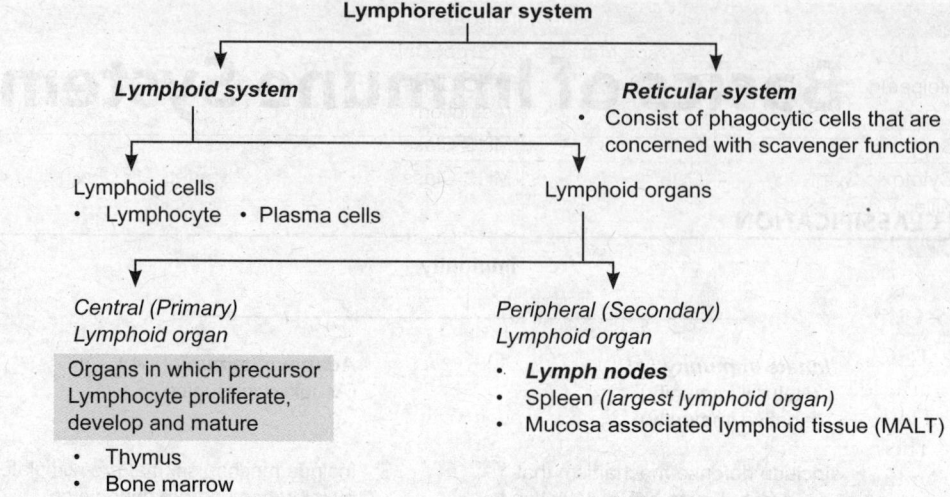

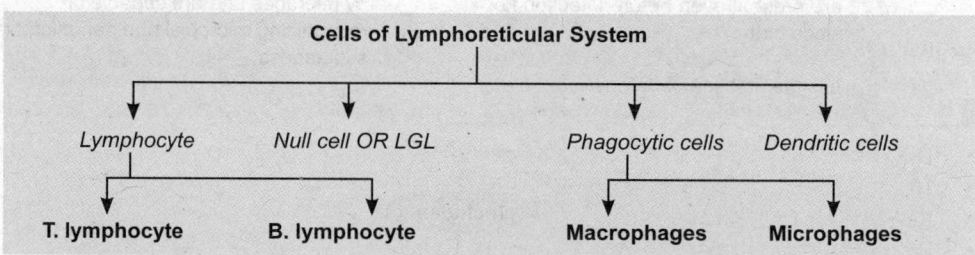

Lymphocyte - Human body contain 10^{12} lymphocyte out of which 10^9 are renewed daily. Mature B and T cells before they encounter antigen are called **naive cells**.

T. LYMPHOCYTE

- Thymus derived lymphocyte, constitute 60-70% of peripheral lymphocyte.
- Found in *paracortical* area of lymph nodes and periarteriolar sheaths of **spleen**.
- Antigen binds to TCR [T cell receptor] which is responsible for signal 1.
- Demonstration of TCR gene by southern blot analysis is a molecular *marker of T lineage cell*.
- All T-lymphocyte contain **CD-3 molecule** which are involved in transduction of signal 1.
- Other surface molecules or co-receptors include CD 2, CD 4 or CD 8, CD 11a, ***CD 28 (Binds to B 7-1 and B 7-2 of antigen presenting cells and provide signal 2)***, CD 40.
- CD 4 is expressed on 60% of T cells, while *30% expressed CD 8*.

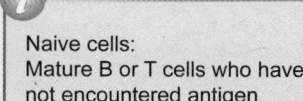

Naive cells:
Mature B or T cells who have not encountered antigen

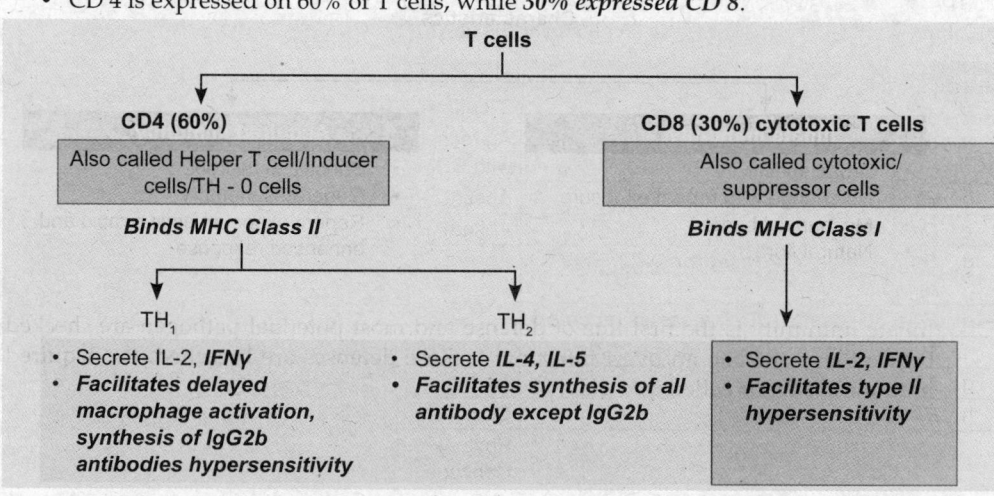

Classification of T Cells

Type of Cells	Surface Markers	Target Cells	Functions
Helper/inducer cell (TH)	CD4	MHC Class II restriction	Growth of T cells and Macrophages
Suppressor T cell (Ts)	CD8	MHC Class I	Down regulate the immune response
Cytotoxic/Cytolytic/Killer T Cell (Tc)	CD8	MHC Class I	Kill and lyse target cells carrying foreign antigen
Memory cells (Tm)	CD4 and CD8	MHC Class I	Provide memory and anamnestic responses

Post-thymectomy Changes

- T. lymphocytes are seeded into certain sites in peripheral lymphatic tissue around central arterioles, white pulp of spleen, paracortical area of lymph nodes.
- However these regions also become grossly depleted after neonatal thymectomy.
- Though thymectomy primarily affects the cell mediated immunity, it also diminishes antibody response to many types of antigens (thymus dependent antigens) such as sheep erythrocytes and bovine serum albumin. Humoral response to other antigens remains unaffected.

B. LYMPHOCYTE

- Develop from precursors in bone marrow.
- 10 - 20% of peripheral lymphocyte.
- Responsible for *humoral immunity*.
- Present in bone marrow, peripheral lymphoid tissue, e.g. lymph node (superficial cortex), spleen (white pulp), tonsils and extra lymphatic organs, e.g. GIT.
- In spleen and lymph node it *form lymphoid follicles*.
- Unlike T cell, it responds to *free Ag*.
- B cell act as *Antigen presenting* cells.
- Other molecules are complement receptor, Fc receptors, *CD 21 (receptor of EBV)*, CD 40 (essential for interaction of T and B cell which cause B cell *maturation* so mutation in **CD 40** ligand cause immunodeficiency called *X-linked hyper - IgM syndrome*).
- Membrane bound antibodies called IgM and IgD present on the surface of all nature naive B-cells and represent antigen-binding component of the B-cell receptor complex.
- RAG mediated rearrangement of Ig genes imparts B-cell receptor an unique antigen specificity.
- After stimulation by an antigen, B-cell develop into plasma cells that secrete antibodies.
- In addition to membrane Ig, the B-cell antigen receptor complex contains a heterodimer of two invariant protein called Igα and Igβ.
- First Ig class to appear on the B cell surface is Ig M. subsequently other classes may appear.

B. Lymphocytes:
- Act as APC
- Secrete Ig
- Responsible for humoral antibody

Differentiation of T and B cells

		T cells	B cells
a.	*Ag binding site*	Ag receptor (= TCR with CD. 3)	Surface Ig
b.	*Fc receptor*	Absent	Present
c.	*Complement receptor*	Absent	Present
d.	*EAC rosette (C 3 receptor CR 2; EBV receptor)*	Absent	Present
e.	*E/SRBC rosette (CD 2; measles receptor)*	+	−
f.	*Microvilli on surface*	−	+
g.	*Thymus specific Ag*	+	−
h.	*Blast transformation*	Occurs by anti CD-3, Phytohemagglutinin Concanavalin	Occurs by anti-Ig Endotoxin *S. aureus* (cowan I strain) EBV

Surface markers	T cells	B cells
CD-3 receptor	+	–
Surface Ig	–	+
Thymus specific Ag	+	–
Ag receptor	+	–
Fc receptor	–	+
Complement receptor	–	+
Rosettes	SRBC or E. rosette (CD-2; measles receptor)	EAC rosette (C3 receptor; CR-2; EBV receptor)
Numerous microvilli	–	+

NULL CELL/LARGE GRANULAR LYMPHOCYTE (LGL)

- Constitute approximately 10–15% of peripheral blood lymphocyte.
- Differentiate and mature in bone marrow, lymph node, thymus, spleen.
- Morphologically NK cells are some what larger than small lymphocyte and contain abundant azurophilic granules.
- Functional activity is regulated by a balance between signals from activating and inhibitory receptors. NKG2D is the main activating receptor. CD–94 and killer cell Ig, like receptor are inhibitory receptor.
- *Do not bear* TCR or surface Ig and are non adherent, non-phagocytic.
- They together with macrophage *form innate immunity* in comparison *of adaptive* immunity *by lymphocytes.*
- **LGL express:**
  - Receptor for Fc portion of IgG (CD-16) which is used for ADCC (**antibody dependent cell mediated cytotoxicity**).
  - Receptor for NCAM-I (CD 56).
- Many LGL express some T lineage markers particularly CD-8, CD-2.
- Usually CD-3 negative but subset of NK cell are *CD-3 positive* called NK/T cell.
- Some NK proliferate in the presence of *IL-2* called as LAK cells.
- **Target cell killing by NK cell is:**
  - Inversely related to target cell expression of MHC class I molecule.
  - So, it kills the cell that express little or no HLA class I molecule (provide immunosurveillance) such as *virus infected cells, certain tumor cells and allogenic cells.*
  - Non-immune i.e. without previous sensitization, MHC unrestricted and non-antibody mediated.
  - It kill host cell infected with intracellular bacteria eg. Mycobacteria, TB, listeria monocytogens.
  - Not kill cells which express class I MHC (all normal nucleated cell express it).
- **Receptors**
  - *NK has two receptors:*
    a. Killer cell inhibitory receptors (KIRs) which recognized classic MHC-I and
    b. CD 94/NKG- 2 receptor which recognized MHCIb or HLA - E.
- **NK cell secrete**
  - TNF α, GMCSF, IFN - γ, Cytolytic factors (perforin).
  - Also secrete IL-4 to recruit TH.2 T cell; IgG1, IgE.

> **Remember:**
> - IFNγ favors differentiation of T_H 1 cell so NK cell can influence CD4 and B cell.
> - NK cell is abnormal in HIV disease and hyporesponsive in Chediak-Higashi syndrome.

Recently two subsets of NK cell are identified CD56^{bright} and CD56^{dim} NK cell. These subsets exhibit differential receptor profiles and innate immune functions.

a. **CD56^{bright} CD16$^{dim/neg}$ NK cells** produce abundant immunoregulatory cytokines and exhibit potent LAK activity but are less effective mediators of ADCC and natural cytotoxicity. They have a less granular morphology.

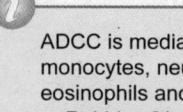

ADCC is mediated by monocytes, neutrophils, eosinophils and NK-cells
...Robbins 8/e, p 202

b. **CD56^{dim} CD16^{bright} NK cells** produce low levels of NK-derived cytokines and are potent mediators of ADCC, LAK activity, and natural cytotoxicity.

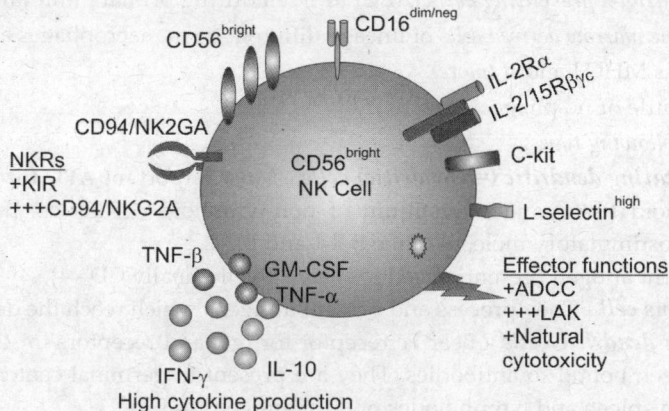

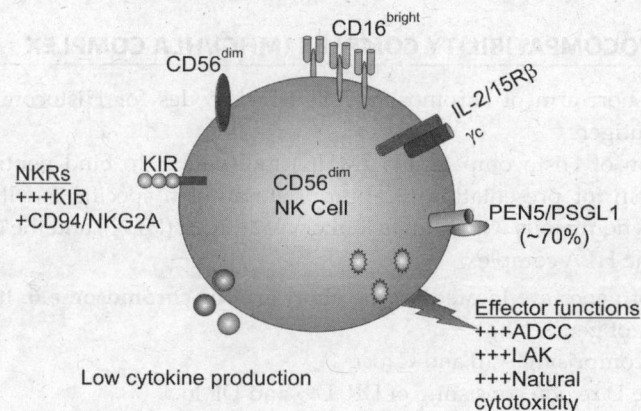

>
> **Phagocytic cells include**
> - Macrophages
> - Microglia in CNS
> - Kupffer cells of liver
> - Osteoclast
> - Sinus histiocytes.

>
> **Dendritic cells**
> - Main antigen presenting cells
> - Include: Interdigitating dendritic cells
>   – Langerhans cell
>   – Follicular dendritic cells

PHAGOCYTIC CELLS

It is of two types:

i. **Mononuclear macrophages of blood and tissues :**
   - Blood macrophages (monocytes) are *largest* of lymphoid cells.
   - Tissue macrophages (histiocytes) are:
     – Microglia in CNS
     – Kupffer in liver
     – Alveolar macrophage in lung
     – Osteoclast in bone
     – Sinus histiocyte—spleen, lymph node.
   - Half-life of *blood monocyte* is about *1 day* while life span of *tissue macrophage* is *several months.*
   - Most important cell in chronic inflammation in the form of activated macrophages, fusion giant cell and epithelioid cell of granulomatous lesion.
   - When a monocyte reaches extravascular tissue, it undergoes transformation in to a larger phagocytic cell, macrophage. This macrophage activated by IFN - γ and other variety of stimuli secrete number of nflammatory mediators like IL-1, IL-6, INF - α.
   - They are obligatory for induction of cell mediated immunity since they are required *to process and present antigen* to immuno competent T cell.
   - Like other Ag presenting/processing cell, it has both class of MHC I and *II (more).*
   - Also important for effector phase of humoral immunity.

ii. **Microphages** which are polymorphonuclear leucocytes of blood-neutrophil, eosinophil and basophil.

>
> **MHC**
> - Located on short arm of 6th chromosome
> - MHC gene products:
> a. Class I: Glycoprotein
> b. Class II: Glycoprotein of antigen presenting cells
> c. Class III: Soluble protein of complement.

DENDRITIC CELLS

- These are *Antigen presenting cells (APC)* to T cell during primary immune response.
- They are *bone marrow derived cells* of lineage different from macrophages and T or B cell.
- They possess MHC I and *II (more)*.
- They have little or no phagocytic activity.
- *They are of following types:*
  a. *Interdigitating dendritic (= Dendritic) cells* - **Most important APC for T-cells.** Found in lymphoid tissue and interstitium of non-lymphoid organs eg. heart and lung. Possess costimulatory molecules like B 7-1 and B 7-2.
  Most potent antigen presenting cell for naive T cell (ideally CD - 4).
  b. *Langerhans cell* - They process and present antigens which reach the dermis.
  c. *Follicular dendritic cells* - Bear Fc receptor for IgG and receptors for C3b. Hence can trap antigen bound to antibodies. They are present in germinal centers of lymphoid follicles in spleen and lymph nodes present antigens to B-cell.

MAJOR HISTOCOMPATIBILITY COMPLEX (MHC)/HLA COMPLEX

- Located on short arm of chromosome six which codes for Histocompatibility (transplantation) antigen.
- Main function of Histocompatibility (MHC) molecule is to bind peptide fragments of foreign protein for presentation to appropriate antigen specific T cells. Human MHC antigen are synonymous with human leukocyte antigen (HLA), and the MHC complex of genes with the HLA complex.

HLA complex of genes are located on the **short arm of chromosome 6**. It consist of three separates cluster of genes:
1. HLA class 1 comprising A, B and C loci
2. Class II or the D region consisting of DR, DQ and DP loci.
3. Class III or the complement region containing genes for complement components C_2 and C_4.

HLA Molecules

HLA antigens are two-chain glycoprotein molecules anchored on the surface membrane of cells.

Class I molecules

- Consists of a heavy peptide chain (α chain) noncovalently linked to a much smaller peptide called β 2-microglobulin (β chain)
- The beta chain has a constant sequence which is coded by chromosomes 15.
- Alpha chain has got three domains (alpha 1, alpha 2 and alpha 3). The distal domain (alpha 1 and alpha 2) have highly variable amino acid sequences and are folded to form a groove.
- Protein antigen processed by macrophages or dendritic cells to form small peptides, are bound to this groove for presentation to CD8 T cells.
- HLA class 1 antigen are found on the surface of all nucleated cells.

Class II molecules

- HLA class II antigen are found only on cells of the immune system—macrophages, dendritic cells, activated T cells, and particularly on B cells.
- Class II antigen are heterodimers, consisting of an alpha and a beta chain.
- Each chain has two domains, the proximal domain being the constant region and the distal the variable.
- The two distal domains (alpha 1, beta 1) constitute the antigen-binding site, for recognition by CD4 lymphocytes.
- Responsible for graft versus host response and mixed leucocyte reaction (MLR).

- Classic C3 convertase: **C4b2b**
- Classic C5 convertase: **C4b2b3b**

C5a is the most effective chemotaxis substance

Class III molecules
- HLA class III molecules are heterogeneous. They include complement components linked to the formation of C3 convertases, heat shock proteins and tumor necrosis factors. They also display polymorphism.
- Soluble protein of complement system; (C_2 and C_4 of classical pathway; properdin factor B of alternative pathway); heat shock protein; TNF alpha and beta.

Note: As you see above, human MHC complex of genes is synonymous with HLA.

> **Complement function**
> Inflammation: C3a, C5a, C4a act as anaphylatoxin
> C5a: Chemotaxin
> Phagocytosis: C3b and C3bi,
> Cell lysis: C5b–9

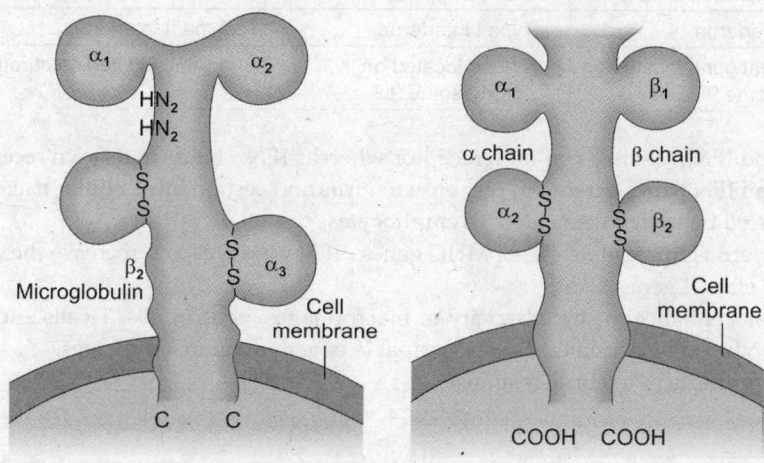

HLA Class I and HLA Class II molecules

COMPLEMENT SYSTEM

Consist of at least 30 chemically and immunologically distinct serum proteins.
Fixation of complement is not influenced by nature of antigens but only by class of Ig.
- $IgM > IgG_3 > IgG_1 > IgG_2$ – Classic pathway activators
- IgA_1, IgA_2, IgD, IgG_4 – Alternative pathway activators

Fractions: Complement is a complex of 9 different fractions
- *Classic C3 convertase*
  – C4b2b
- *Classic C5 convertase*
  – C4b2b3b
- *Alternate C3 convertase*
  – C3bBb
- *Alternate C5 convertase*
  – C3bBb3b
- Role of complement derived factors in inflammation:
  i. C3b and C3bi - act as opsonin so cause phagocytosis.
  ii. C3a + C5a [= Anaphylatoxin] - ↑ vascular permeability, vasodilation.
  iii. C5a - activate lipoxygenase pathway, chemotaxis, activation and adhesion.
  iv. C5b-9 (= Membrane attack complex) - Lysis of cell.
- Biosynthesis of complements:
  a. Intestinal epithelium: C1
  b. Macrophages: C2, C4
  c. Liver: C3, C6, C9
  d. Spleen: C5, C8

| Clinical problems associated with genetic deficiencies of complement components ||
Deficiency	Syndrome
CL inhibitor	Hereditary angioneurotic edema
Early components of classical pathway C1, C2, C4	SLE and other collagen vascular diseases
C3 and its regulatory protein C3b in activator	Severe recurrent pyogenic infections
C5 to C8	Bacteremia, mainly with Gram-negative diplococci, toxoplasmosis
C9	No particular diseases

INTERFERONS

- Originally discovered as factors produced by cells in response to viral infections.
- There are three main interferons:

α Interferon	β Interferon	γ Interferon
Part of Innate immunity	Part of innate immunity	Part of acquired immunity
Produced by peripheral blood mononuclear cells	Produced predominanty by fibroblasts	A lymphokine produce in response to a specific antigenic signal
Type I interferon	Type I interferon	Type II interferon
18 different gene located on chromosome 9	1 gene located on chromosome 9	1 gene located on chromosome 9

- IFN α and IFN β share a common receptor whereas IFN γ binds to its own receptor.
- IFN α and IFN β are secreted in response to virus and certain intracellular bacteria. IFN γ is produced by antigen activated T-lymphocytes.
- All interferons upregulate class I MHC genes. IFN γ induces and increase the expression of MHC class II genes also.
- Interferons enhance the cytotoxcicity of macrophages, neutrophils, T-cells and NK cells. IFN γ produced by activated T-cells is capable of activating macrophages.
- Interferons induces a febrile response.

Multiple Choice Questions

1. Adenosine deaminase deficiency is seen in the following: [AI 05, 01]
   a. Common variable immunodeficiency
   b. Severe combined immunodeficiency
   c. Chronic granulomatous disease
   d. Nezelof syndrome

2. A woman with infertility receives an ovary transplant from her sister who is an identical twin. What type of graft is it? [AI 05]
   a. Xenograft
   b. Autograft
   c. Allograft
   d. Isograft

3. Which of the following statements is true about hapten? [AIIMS 09]
   a. It induces brisk immune response
   b. It needs carrier to induce immune response
   c. It is a T-independent antigen
   d. It has no association with MHC

4. Neonatal thymectomy leads to: [AIIMS 08]
   a. Decreased size of germinal center
   b. Decreased size of paracortical areas
   c. Increased antibody marrow production by B cells
   d. Increased bone marrow production of lymphocytes

5. IL-I produces: [NEET Pattern 2018]
   a. T-lymphocyte activation
   b. Delayed wound healing
   c. Increased pain perception
   d. Decreased PMN release from bone marrow

6. NK cells kill the viral infected cells due to: [AIIMS 06]
   a. Increased expression of MHC class I molecules
   b. Decreased expression of MHC class I molecules
   c. Increased expression of MHC class II molecules
   d. Decreased expression of MHC class II molecules

7. Which of the following best denotes classical complement pathway activation in immuno- inflammatory condition? [AIIMS 05]
   a. C2, C4 and C3 decreased
   b. C2 and C4 normal, C3 is decreased
   c. C3 normal and C2 C4 decreased
   d. C2, C4, C3 all are elevated

8. Which of the following cell types are the most potent activator of T-cell? [AI 2012]
   a. Bell
   b. Follicular Dendritic Cells
   c. Mature dendritic cells
   d. Macrophages

9. Which of the following is an opsonin? [NEET Pattern 2018]
   a. C5a   b. C3b
   c. C3a   d. C5b

10. True about class II MHC molecules:
    a. Polypeptide in nature [NEET Pattern 2019]
    b. Present in antigen presenting cells only
    c. No role in graft rejection
    d. Contains two alpha chain

11. Nude mouse is used in immunological studies as it lacks: [NEET Pattern 2018]
    a. B cells
    b. T cells
    c. NK cells
    d. Both B and T cells

12. What enhances multiplication of T cells in culture?
    a. Phytohemagglutinin b. Chemotactic factor
    c. Leukotrienes   d. Prostaglandins [AIIMS 16]

13. All of the following are part of innate immunity except:
    a. Complement   b. NK cells   [AIIMS 05]
    c. Macrophages   d. T cells

14. Common between B and T cells: [PGI June 07]
    a. Origin from same cell lineage
    b. Site differentiation
    c. Antigenic marker
    d. Both humoral and cellular immunity
    e. Further differentiation seen

15. All of these are antigens presenting cells except:
    a. T cells   [PGI 12]
    b. B cells
    c. Fibroblasts
    d. Dendritic cells
    e. Langerhans cells

16. Which complement component is involved in both classical and alternate pathway? [AI 2011]
    a. C_1
    b. C_2
    c. C_3
    d. All

17. Which of the following features is not shared between T cells and B cells? [AIIMS Nov 2012]
    a. Positive selection during development
    b. Class I MHC expression
    c. Antigen specific receptors
    d. All of the above

18. **First chemical barrier encountered by microorganism for common exposed sites:** [AIIMS Nov 2011]
    a. Lysozyme
    b. Acidic pH
    c. Skin
    d. Lactose

19. **Active immunity can be induced by:** [PGI May 2013]
    a. Toxoids
    b. Subclinical infection
    c. Antitoxin
    d. Immunoglobulins
    e. Antigen exposure

20. **True about passive immunity:** [PGI May 2013]
    a. Can not be given with active immunity
    b. Last for 4-5 days only
    c. It can be given before disease occurrence
    d. Can be transferred by antibodies from another host
    e. Takes long time to develop

21. **The role played by Major Histocompatibility Complex-1 and 2 is to:** [AIIMS 2013, 2014]
    a. Transduce the signal to T cells following antigen recognition
    b. Mediate immunogenic class switching
    c. Present antigens for recognition by T cell antigen receptors
    d. Enhance the secretion of cytokines

Explanations and References with Illustrative Answers

1. **Ans. (b) Severe combined immunodeficiency** *Ref. Ananthanarayan 10/e, p 176; Harrison 19/e, p 2108*

   Immunodeficiency
   - Primary immunodeficiency syndrome - genetically determined
   - Secondary immunodeficiency syndrome, e.g. AIDS.

Classification of important Immunodeficiency syndrome	
Name of syndrome	Defect
i. Humoral immunodeficiency (B cell defects)	
a. X linked agammaglobulinemia:	Mutation in bruton tyrosine kinase
	Pre/pro B cell →✗→ B cell
b. Common variable immunodeficiency:	B cell →✗→ Plasma cells
c. Immunodeficiency with hyper IgM:	Mutation in CD40 ligand gene
ii. Cellular immunodeficiency (T cell defect)	
a. Thymic hypoplasia **(Di George's syndrome):**	Failure of development of 3rd and 4th pharyngeal pouch (hypoplasia of thyroid and parathyroid also).
b. Chronic mucocutaneous candidiasis	
c. Purine nucleoside phosphorylase (PNP) deficiency	
iii. Combined immunodeficiencies (B and T cell defect)	
a. Cellular immunodeficiency with abnormal: Ig synthesis **(Nezlof syndrome)**	Abnormal T cell maturation in thymus with normal, ↓ or ↑ Ig
b. Ataxia telangiectasia:	DNA repair defect
c. **Wiskott-Aldrich syndrome:**	WASP gene mutation (secondary ↓ of T lymphocytes)
d. Severe combined immunodeficiency:	Variable defect

   Severe Combined Immunodeficiency
   - Includes syndromes with severe combined deficiency of both humoral and cell mediated immunity, inherited in **autosomal recessive mode**.
   - Defects are at the level of early precursors of immunocompetent cells in the fetal liver and bone marrow.
   - Some important types include:
     - **Swiss type agammaglobulinemia:** Basic defect is at the level of *lymphoid stem cell*.
     - **Reticular dysgenesis of de Waal:** Defect is at the level of *multipotent hemopoietic stem cell,* as a result of which there is total failure of myelopoiesis leading to leukopenia, thrombocytopenia and
     - **Adenosine deaminase deficiency:** Range of immunodeficiency varies from complete absence to mild abnormalities of B and T cell functions.

2. **Ans. (d) Isograft** *Ref. Ananthanarayan 10/e, p 186*

Terminology of grafts		
Donor	**Term**	**Synonyms**
Self	Autograft	Autogenous or autogenic graft
Different individual, genetically identical with recipient. Identical twin or member of same inbred strain	Isograft	Isologous or syngeneic graft or syngraft
Genetically unrelated member of same species	Allograft	Allogeneic graft. Formerly called homograft
Different species	Xenograft	Xenogeneic. Formerly called heterograft

Type of graft
- *Orthotopic graft:* Graft applied in anatomically normal site, e.g. skin graft.
- *Heterotopic graft:* Graft applied in anatomicaly abnormal site, e.g. thyroid tissues transplanted in subcutaneous pocket.

3. **Ans. (b) It needs carrier to induce immune response** *Ref. Ananthanarayan 10/e, p 89*
   Haptens
   - Substances that are incapable of inducing antibody formation by themselves but can react specifically with antibodies.
   - Haptens become immunogenic on combining with a larger molecule or carrier.
   - They are of two types:
     - Complex hapten: Precipitate with specific antibody
     - Simple hapten: Non precipitating.

4. **Ans. (b) Decreased size of paracortical areas** *Ref. Ananthanarayan 10/e, p 132*
   - Neonatal thymectomy leads to depletion of thymus dependent areas.
   - *Peripheral lymphoid tissue is of two types:*

Features	Thymus dependent (contain T lymphocytes)	Bone marrow dependent (contain B lymphocytes)
Spleen	Lymphatic sheath surrounding the central arteriole known as Malpighian corpuscles in white pulp.	Perifollicular region, Germinal center, Mantle layer
Lymph node	Between cortical follicles and medullary cords there is ill-defined paracortical area.	The Corticle follicles and Medullary cords

- B cells also found in tonsils, extralymphoid organs such as GIT.

5. **Ans. (a) T lymphocyte activation** *Ref. Ananthanarayan 10/e, p 156; Robbin's 7/e, p 82*
   IL-1
   - Formerly called as the leucocyte activating factor (LAF) and as the B-cell activating factor (BAF)
   - Stable polypeptide; secreted by macrophages and monocytes but can be produced by most other nucleated cells also.
   - Presence of antigens, toxins, injury and inflammation, stimulates its production, while cyclosporin A, corticosteroids and prostaglandins inhibits it.

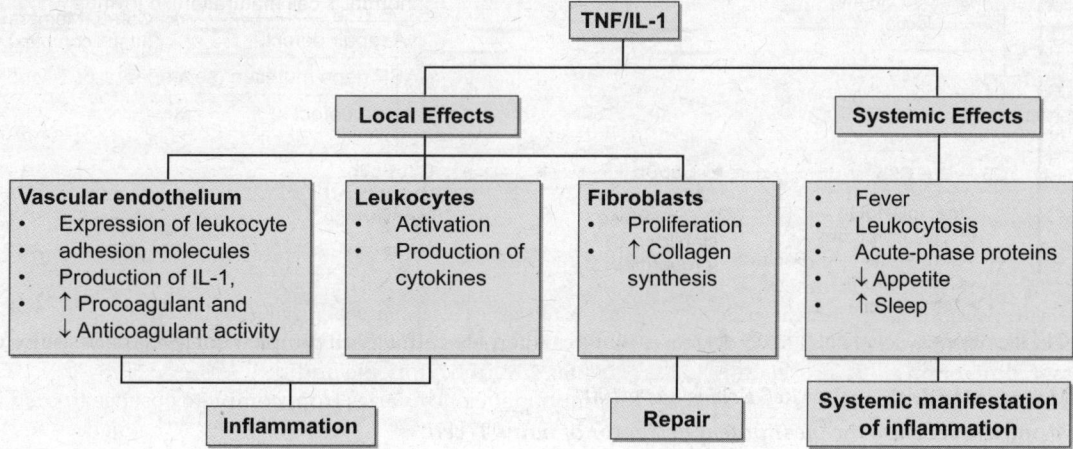

Interleukins	Main source	Major function
IL-1 (α + β)	Macrophage	Proliferation and differentiation of T,B cells; pyrogenic; ↑ acute phase reactants; BM cell proliferation.
IL-2	TH1 cells	Growth and differentiation of T and B cells; cytotoxicity of T and NK cells.
IL-3	T cells	Stimulation of hematopoietic progenitors.
IL-4	TH2 cells	Proliferation of B and cytotoxic T cells; ↑ IgG1 and IgE production; ↑ MHC class II and IgE receptor.
IL-5	TH2 cells	Proliferation of eosinophil; ↑ IgA and IgM production.
IL-6	TH1, macrophages,	Promote B cell differentiation, IgA production, Acute phase proteins.
IL-7	Spleen, BM stromal cells	B and T cell growth factor.

6. **Ans. (a) Increased expression of MHC class I molecules** *Ref. Harrison 20/e p 2450*
   NK cell activity is non-immune; MHC unrestricted; non-antibody mediated killer of target cells which are usually malignant cells types, transplanted foreign cells or virus infected cells.
   Thus NK cells play an important role in immune surveillance and destruction of malignant and virally infected host cells.

   NK cells
   - Accounts for 5-10% of peripheral blood lymphocytes. They are non adherent, non phagocytic cells with large azurophilic cytoplasmic granules.
   - NK cells express surface receptors for the F_c portion of IgG (CD-16) and for CD-56. Many NK cells express CD8, where as some NK cells (called as NK/T cells) express CD-3.
   - NK cells proliferate in response to IL-2. NK cells arise in both bone marrow and thymic microenvironment.
   - Three molecules of NK cells; NKp46; NK p30 and NKp44 are collectively referred as *natural cytotoxicity receptors* (NCRs) and mediate NK cell activation against target cells.

   Features of target cell killing by NK cell:
   - Inversely related to target cell expression of MHC class I molecule.
     - So, it kills the cell that expresses little or no HLA class I molecule (provide immunosurveillance) such as *virus infected cells, certain tumor cells and allogenic cells.*
   - It kills host cell infected with intracellular bacteria, e.g. Mycobacteria, *TB. Listeria, monocytogens.*
   - Do not kill cells which express class I MHC (all normal nucleated cells express it).

7. **Ans. (a) C2, C4, C3 decreased** *Ref. Jawetz 27/e, p 141; Harrison 20/e, p 2464; Robbins 7/e, p 66*
   Complements are activated by 3 pathways.

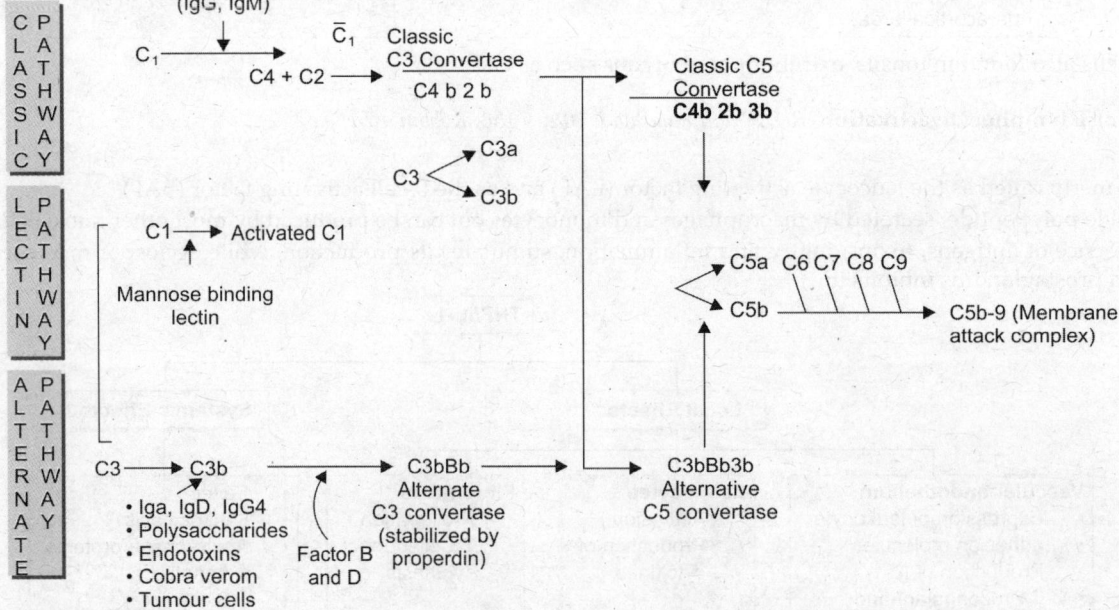

   - So, in Classic pathway level of C1 to C9 decreases while in Alternate pathway all complement levels decrease except C1, C2, C4.

8. **Ans. (c) Mature Dendritic cells** *Ref. Robins 8/e, p 190*
   "Mature dendritic cells are the most potent activator of naive T-cell"

Dendritic Cells:
- Bone marrow derived cells
- There are two types of cells with dendritic morphology:
  - Interdigitating dendritic cells
  - Follicular dendritic cells
- *Interdigitating dendritic cells* or just dendritic cells are the most important antigen presenting cells for initiating primary immune response against protein antigens. This is due to following reasons:
  - These cells are located at the right place to capture antigens, i.e. under epithelia, in the interstitial of all tissue.
  - They express variety of receptors (including TLR, mannose) for capturing microbes.
  - In response to microbes dendritic cells express the same chemokine receptors as to naive T-cells.
  - They express high levels of MHC class II molecules as well as co-stimulatory molecules B.7-1 and B.7-2. Or in other words they possess all the machinery needed for presenting antigens to and activating CD4 + T cells.
- On the other hand *follicular dendritic cells* (*does not arise from bone marrow*) are present in the germinal centres of lymphoid follicles where they trap antigens bound to antibodies or complement. Follicular dendritic cells plays a role in ongoing immune response by presenting antigens to B-cells and selecting the B-cells that have the highest affinity for the antigen.

Naïve Cells:
- Mature T and B cells before they encounter antigens are called naïve cells
- In the lymph node, a naïve T cell may encounter the antigen that is specifically recognizes on the surface of activated APC most likely dendritic cells
- Naïve lymphocyte that have exited the thymus migrate to lymph node and enter the T cell zones through specialized venules called high endothelial venules.
- Naïve T cells recognize MHC associated peptide antigens displayed on dendritic cells
- The naïve T cells are then activated to proliferate and to differentiate into cells of T_{H-1} subset.

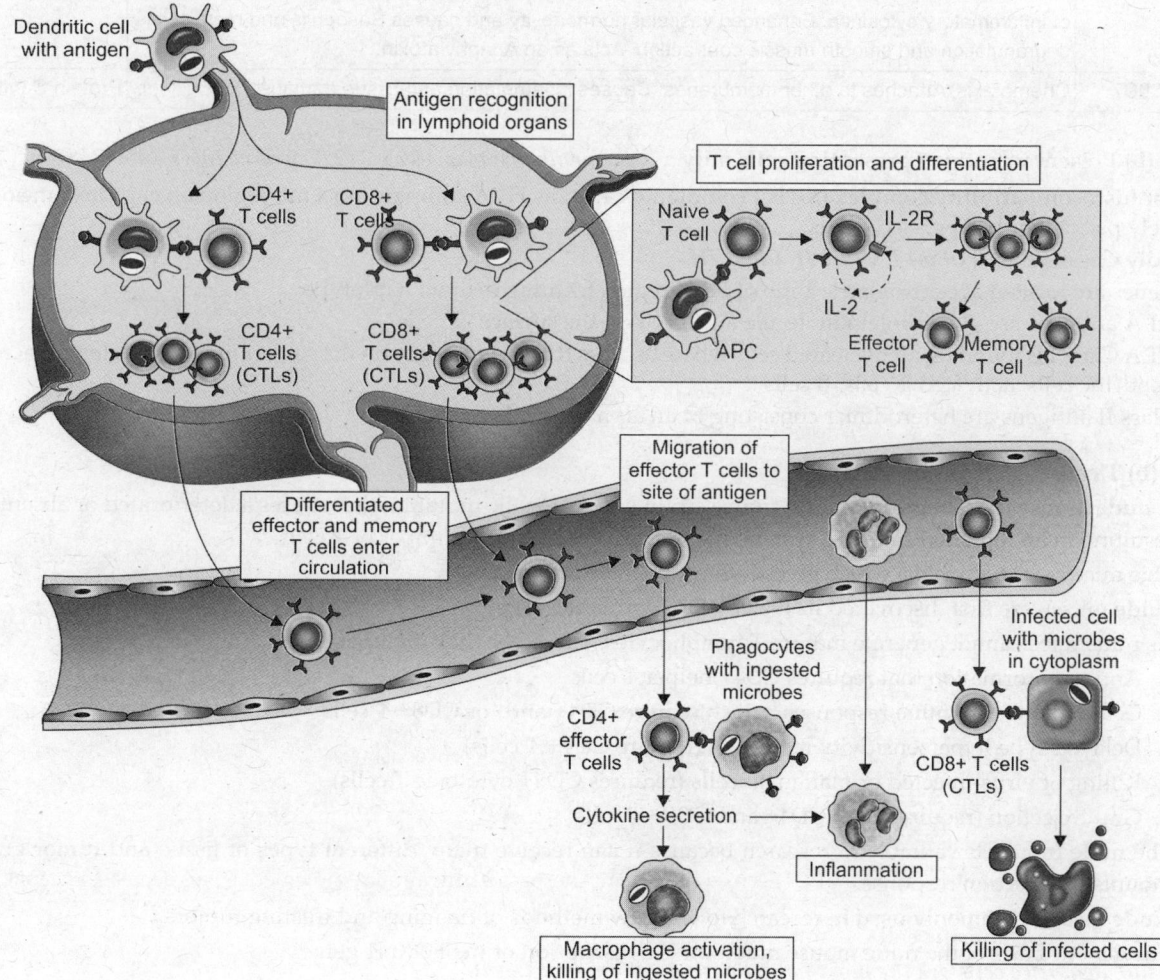

Cell-mediated immunity. Naïve T cells recognize MHC-associated peptide antigens displayed on dendritic cells in lymph nodes. The T cells are activated to proliferate (under the influence of the cytokine IL-2) and to differentiate into effector and memory cells, which migrate to sites of infection and serve various functions in cell-mediated immunity. Effector CD4+ T cells of the T_H1 subset recognize the antigens of microbes ingested by phagocytes and activate the phagocytes to kill the microbes; T_H17 effector cells enhance leukocyte recruitment and stimulate inflammation; T_H2 cells activate eosinophils. CD8+CTLs kill infected cells harbouring microbes in the cytoplasm. Some activated T cells differentiate into long-lived memory cells. APC, antigen-presenting cell; CTLs, cytotoxic T lymphocytes.

9. **Ans. (b) C3b**   *Ref. Robbins 9/e, p 78*

Components of complement system, their actions and their controls		
Component	Action	Control
C2a	Proinflammatory, accumulation of fluids causes edema	C1-INH
C3a	Basophils and mast cells degranulation; enhanced vascular permeability, smooth muscle contraction. Anaphylatoxin	C3a-INA
C3b	Opsonin, phagocyte activation	Factors H and I
C4a	Enhanced vascular permeability causes Basophils and mast cells degranulation and smooth muscle contraction. Acts as an Anaphylatoxin	C3a-INA
C4b	Opsonin causes Phagocytosis	C4-BP and Factor I
C5a	It leads to chemotaxis, stimulation of respiratory burst, activation of phagocytes and stimulation of inflammatory cytokines. Enhanced vascular permeability and causes Basophils and mast cells degranulation and smooth muscle contraction. Acts as an Anaphylatoxin.	C3a-INA
C5bC6C7	Chemotaxis, Attaches to other membranes. Causes inflammation and tissue damage.	Protein S (vitronectin)

10. **Ans. (b) Present in antigen presenting cells only**   *Ref.. Ananthanarayan 10/e p 142; Harrison 20/e p 2480-2481*

    Major histocompatibility complex (MHC) commonly called as HLA complex is a 4 mb region on chromosome 6 which is densely packed with expressed genes.
    Broadly classified into **Class I, Class II, Class III**
    - Genes are located at centromatric 1 mb of HLA region forming distinct haplotype
    - HLA antigens are glycoprotein molecule anchored on the surface of cells
    - HLA Class I is found on all nucleated cells where as class II are found only on the cells of immune system: macrophages, dendritic cells, activated T cells, B cells
    - Class II antigens are heterodimer consisting of an alpha and a beta chain

11. **Ans (b) T cells**   *Ref. Journals*
    - A **nude mouse** is a laboratory mouse from a strain with a genetic mutation that causes a deteriorated or absent thymus, resulting in an inhibited immune system due to a greatly reduced number of T cells.
    - This mice lacks body hair, which gives it the "nude" nickname.
    - Nude mice were first discovered in 1962 by Dr. Norman R. Grist
    - As nude mice cannot generate mature T lymphocytes. Therefore they are unable to exhibit:
        1. Antibody formation that requires CD4+ helper T cells
        2. Cell-mediated immune responses, which require CD4+ and/or CD8+ T cells
        3. Delayed-type hypersensitivity responses (require CD4+ T cells)
        4. Killing of virus-infected or malignant cells (requires CD8+ cytotoxic T cells)
        5. Graft rejection (requires both CD4+ and CD8+ T cells)
    - The nude mouse is valuable to research because it can receive many different types of tissue and tumor grafts, as it mounts no rejection response.
    - Nude mice is commonly used in research to test new methods of imaging and treating tumors.
    - The genetic basis of the nude mouse mutation is a disruption of the FOXN1 gene

12. Ans. (a) Phytohemagglutinin *Ref. Ananthanarayan 10/e, p 135*

Blast transformation or proliferation stimuli are:

Stimulus	T cell	B cell
Anti CD-3	+	–
Anti Ig.	–	+
PHA (Phytohemagglutinin)	+	–
Concanavalin A	+	–
Endotoxins	–	+
S-aureus (Cowan strain)	–	+
EB virus	–	+

Note: (+) means proliferation occurs and (–) means no proliferation

13. Ans. (d) T cells *Ref. Harrison 20/e, p 2452, 2466*

Components of the Adaptive Immune System	
Cellular	Thymus-derived (T) lymphocytes - T cell precursors in the thymus; naive mature T lymphocytes before antigen exposure; memory T lymphocytes after antigen contact; helper T lymphocytes for B and T cell responses; cytotoxic T lymphocytes that kill pathogen- infected target cells.
Humoral	Bone-marrow-derived (B) lymphocytes - B cell precursors in bone marrow; naive B cells prior to antigen recognition; memory B cells after antigen contact; plasma cells that secrete specific antibody.
Cytokines	Soluble proteins that direct focus and regulate specific T versus B lymphocyte immune responses.

Major Components of the Innate Immune System	
Pattern recognition receptors (PRR)	C type lectins, leucine-rich proteins, scavenger receptors, pentraxins, lipid transferases; integrins.
Antimicrobial peptides	α-Defensins, β-defensins, cathelin, protegrin, granulysin, histatin, secretory leukoprotease inhibitor, and probiotics.
Cells	Macrophages, dendritic cells, NK cells, NK-T cells, neutrophils, eosinophils, mast cells, basophils, and epithelial cells.
Complement components	Classic and alternative complement pathway, and proteins that bind complement components.
Cytokines	Autocrine, paracrine, endocrine cytokines that mediate host defence and inflammation, as well as recruit, direct, and regulate adaptive immune responses.

14. Ans. (a) and (e) Origin from same cell lineage; Further differentiation seen *Ref. Ganong 22/e, p 525*

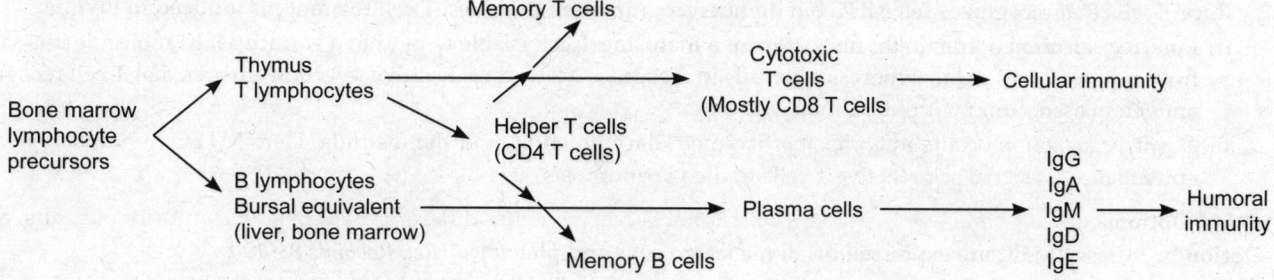

15. **Ans. (a) and (c) T cells and Fibroblast** Ref. Robbin's 8/e, p 192
    Antigen presenting cells are:
    - Macrophages
    - B cells
    - Dendritic cells (*most potent*)
    - Activated T cells.

    Antigen Presenting Cell
    - An antigen presenting cell (APC) can be defined as any cell that expresses MHC or related molecule (eg CD1) that can bind antigenic components such as peptide, and can be recognized by one or another class of T-cell. T-cell can not recognize and therefore can't react to free antigen. T-cell can only see antigen which has been processed or presented by antigen presenting cells. Broadly on the basis of MHC class II expression APC can be divided into:
        a. **Professional APC's :** APC's that express MHC II molecules, they are very efficient cells and include:
           - Macrophages
           - Dendritic cells
           - Certain activated epithelial cells
           - Few B-cells
        b. **Non professional APC:** They do not express MHC II molecule constitutively but only upon stimulation by certain cytokines. They include:
           - Fibroblast
           - Thymic epithelial cells
           - Thyroid epithelial cells
           - Glial cells
           - Pancreatic beta cells
           - Vascular endothelial cells

    For examination purpose, only professional APC's are considered as APC.

16. **Ans. (c) C_3** Ref. Jawetz 27/e, p 142
    Already explained

    > **Remember:** Biosynthesis of complement
    > - C_1 is synthesized in intestinal epithelium
    > - C_2, C_4 by macrophages
    > - C_5, C_8 in spleen
    > - C_3, C_6, C_9 in liver

17. **Ans. (a) Positive selection** Ref. Internet references
    B cell undergoes negative selection, whereas T cells undergoes both positive and negative selection.

    Mechanism of central tolerance:
    B cell:
    - The recognition of antigens by the immature B-cells in the bone marrow is critical to the development of immunological tolerance to self. For proper immunological function it is essential B cell do not recognize self antigen and should recognize antigen derived from pathogens.
    - In the bone marrow the immature B cells bearing surface IgM, if recognizes self molecule undergo negative selection. This self antigen induce loss of cells from the B cell repertoire is called as ***clonal deletion.*** Thus only those B cells that do not recognizes self molecules as antigen comes out of bone marrow.

    T cells tolerance:
    - T cells are selected for survival more rigorously than B cells. They undergo both positive and negative selection to produce T cells that recognizes self MHC but do not recognizes self peptides. T cell tolerance is induced in thymus.
        (i) ***Positive selection*** occurs in thymic cortex, if a maturing T cell is able to bind to a surface MHC molecule it is saved from program cells death; whereas cells fails to recognize MHC dies. Positive selection ensures that T cell recognize antigen in association with MHC molecule only.
        (ii) ***Negative selection*** occurs in cortex, cortico-medullary junction, and the medulla. Here MTEC (modullary thymic epithelial cells) signal self reactive T cells to die via apoptosis.

    Other Options
    Option b: Class I MHC are expressed by all nucleated cells and platelets. Ref. Robbin's 8/e 190
    Option c: Both B cells and T cell possess antigen receptors. On B cells surface Ig acts as antigenic receptor whereas on T cell, TCR along with CD_3 acts as antigenic receptors. Ref. AA 8/e 128, 9/e, p 133

18. **Ans. (b) Acidic pH** *Ref. Jawetz 27/e 126*
    Physiological barriers at the portal of entry:
    a. Skin:
       - Skin provide the very efficient barrier against all sort of microbes, and only few bacteria can penetrate the skin.
       - Sweat and sebaceous secretions by virtue of their acidic pH and certain chemical substances (fatty acids) have antimicrobial including antifungal properties.
       - Lysozymes present on skin and other secretions also provide additional protection by lysing the microbes.
    b. Mucous membrane:
       - In the respiratory tract a film of mucous covers the surface. Bacteria tend to stick to this film. In addition there are lysozyme, and other antimicrobial substance.
       - Saliva contains many enzyme.
       - Gastric acidity kills almost all bacteria, ingested.

    > **Remember:** Innate immune system use pattern recognition receptor (like lipo-polysaccharide of Gr (−)ve bacteria, to sense the presence of pathogens.
    > **Innate immune mechanism involves:**
    > - Phagocytosis
    > - Inflammatory responses
    > - Interferons
    > - Alternate pathway of complement activation
    > - Fever
    > - Natural killer cells.

19. **Ans. a, b and e. Toxoids, Subclinical infection, Antigen exposure** *Ref. Harrison 20/e, p 2466*

    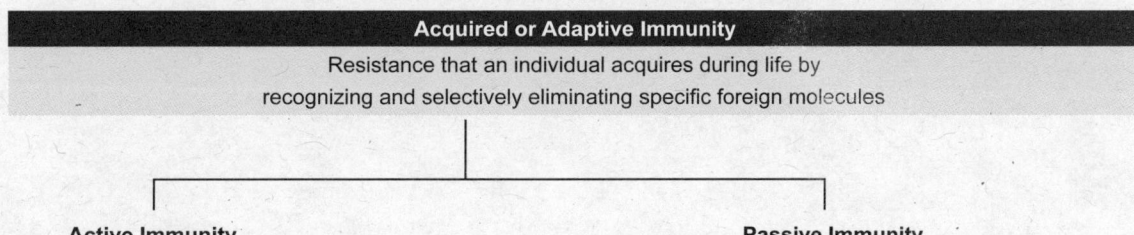

    Active Immunity
    - Induced by infections or by immunogens (Antigens, toxoid)
    - Provide effective protection for long period
    - Immunity effective only after lag period
    - Immunological memory present
    - Booster effect is there on subsequent exposure
    - Negative phase may occur
    - Not applicable in the immunodeficients
    - Live attenuated vaccines provide active immunity

    Passive Immunity
    - Received passively, e.g. injection of readymade antibodies
    - Effect is transient only immediate immunity
    - No memory
    - Subsequent dose is less effective
    - No negative phase
    - Applicable in the immunodeficient
    - Anti rabies immunoglobulins are the example of passive immunity

20. **Ans. c and d. It can be given before disease occurrence, Can be transferred by antibodies from another host**
    Ref. Ananthanarayan 10/e, p 84

    The duration of passive immunity is approximately equal to the half life of the immunoglobulin injected, which varies from disease to disease.
    Example: 7 days in case of antitetanus serum.
    For full details See Previous Answer.

21. **Ans. (c) Present antigen for recognition by T cell antigen** *Ref. Jawetz 27/e, p 132*

    Both Class I and Class II antigen are involved in presentation of processed antigen on microphage and other accessary cells to T-cell.
    - Cytotoxic T-cell recognize Class I MHC antigen on target cells
    - Helper T cell can accept antigens presented by macrophages/dendritic cells only when they bear some Class II MHC molecules

- **MHC Class I molecules** consist of two non covalently associated polypeptide chains A, B, C. Present on all human nucleated cells except neurons
- **MHC Class II Molecules:** are composed of two chains DP, DQ and DR. Found on immune cells (dendritis cells, macrophages, monocytes and activated T lymphocytes
- **MHC Class III genes:** They are grouped together in a region between D and B.

Important features of human MHC Classes I and II Gene products		
	Class I	Class II
Genetic loci (partial list)	HLA-A, -B, and -C	HLA-DP, -DQ and -DR
Polypeptide composition	MW 45,000 + β_2M (MW 12,000)	α chain (MW 33,000) β (MW 30,000), Ii chain (MW 30,000)
Cell distribution	Most nucleated somatic cells, except cells of the brain and retina	Antigen-presenting cells (macrophages, dendritic cells, B cells, etc.), and IFN-γ-activated cells
Present peptide antigens to	CD8 T cells	CD4 T cells
Size of peptide bound	8–10 residues	10–30 or more residues

NEET Pattern Questions

1. **Complement formed in liver:**
   a. C2, C4
   b. C3, C6, C9
   c. C5, C8
   d. C1

Sites of complement protein synthesis			
	Classical pathway proteins	Alternative pathway proteins	Effector proteins
Liver (hepatocyte)	C1r, s, C4, C2, C1-inh	C3, B, H, I	C3, C5, C6, C7, C8, C9
Mononuclear phagocytes	C1q, r, s, C4, C2, C1-inh	C3, B, P, D, H, I	C3, C5
Fibroblasts*	C1q, r, s, C4, C2, C1-inh	C3, B, H	C3
Epithelial cells	C1q, r, s	C3, B	C3
Endothelial cells	C1-inh	C3, B, H, I	C3
Alveolar type II epithelial cells	C4, C2	C3, B	C3, C5

*Studies with primary human fibroblast cultures indicated that I, P, C4, and C5 are not synthesized in these cells. Rodent fibroblasts synthesize C4[8]. Studies in a transformed fibroblast line demonstrated synthesis of C5[105].

2. **C-3 convertase in alternate complement pathway:**
   a. C4b2a
   b. C3b
   c. C3bBb
   d. C3a
   [Ref. Ananthanarayan, 10/e, p 175]

3. **Activation of classical complement pathway:**
   a. IgA
   b. IgG
   c. IgM
   d. IgD
   [Ref. Ananthanarayan, 10/e, p 123]

   First step of activation of complement pathway is binding of C1 to the antigen-antibody complex. One molecule of IgM or two molecules, IgG can initiate this process

4. **Fever is caused by:**
   a. IL 3
   b. **IL 6**
   c. IL 5
   d. IL 9
   [Ref. Robbin's, 8/e, p 55]

5. **Center of complement pathway:**
   a. C3
   b. C1
   c. C5
   d. C2
   [Ref. Ananthanarayan, 10/e, p 124]

   Once C3 activation occurs, the subsequent steps are common in classic, alternate and lectin pathways

6. **Gene components of HLA class I includes:**
   a. A, B, C
   b. DR
   c. DQ
   d. DP
   [Ref. Ananthanarayan, 10/e, p 142]

HLA class	Product
Class I	A, B, C loci
Class II	DR, DQ, DP
Class III	C2, C4, TNF α and β, properdin factor B

7. **HLA complex is on chromosome:**
   a. 6
   b. 7
   c. 8
   d. 9
   [Ref. Ananthanarayan, 10/e, p 141]

8. **Chediak Higashi syndrome, defect is:**
   a. Fusion of lysosome
   b. T-cells
   c. B-cells
   d. Complement
   [Ref. Ananthanarayan, 10/e, p 177]

   In chediak-Higashi syndrome (Autosomal recessive) there is reduced chemotaxis and phagolysosome fusion. Blood picture show giant primary granules in neutrophils and other granule bearing cells. Clinically these patients present with decreased pigmentation of eye, skin and hair.

9. **Hereditary angioneurotic edema is due to:**
   a. Deficiency of C1 inhibitor
   b. Deficiency of NADPH oxidase
   c. Deficiency of MPO
   d. Deficiency of properdin
   [Ref. Ananthanarayan, 10/e, p 126]

Ans.
1. b. C3, C6, C9
2. c. C3bBb
3. b, c. IgG, IgM
4. b. IL 6
5. a. C3
6. a. A, B, C
7. a. 6
8. a. Fusion of...
9. a. Deficiency of...

10. **SCID which is true:**
    a. Adenosine deaminase deficiency
    b. Decreased circulating lymphocytes
    c. NADPH oxidase deficiency
    d. C1 esterase deficiency
    [Ref. Ananthanarayan, 10/e, p 176]

> **Severe combined immunodeficiency:**
> - Deficiency of both humoral and cell mediated immune response.
> - Include:
>   a. Swiss type agammaglobulinemia: Defect at the level of lymphoid stem cell
>   b. Reticular dysgenesis of deVaal: Defect at the level of multi-potent stem cell which result in total failure of myelopoiesis
>   c. Adenosine deaminase deficiency: ADA catalyzes the conversion of adenosine to inosine. The range of immunodeficiency varies from complete absence to mild abnormalities in B and T cell junction.

11. **Nucleotidase deficiency:**
    a. Humoral immunity deficiency
    b. Acquired immunity deficiency
    c. SCIDs
    d. Cell mediated immunity deficiency
    [Ref. Ananthanarayan, 9/e, p 124]

> Ecto-5 nucleotidase deficiency is associated by B cell defect

12. **All are true about innate immunity except:**
    a. Non-specific
    b. First line of defence
    c. Not affected by genetic make up
    d. Includes complement
    [Ref. Ananthanarayan, 10/e, p 81]

13. **Which of the following acts as a chemoattractant?**
    a. C3a
    b. C3b
    c. C5a
    d. LTB4
    [Ref. Robbin's 8/e, 50]

> **CHEMOATTRACTANTS**
>
> | Endogenous | Exogenous |
> |---|---|
> | – Cytokines (IL-8) | – Bacterial products that possess N-formyl methionine terminal amino acid and some lipids |
> | – Components of complement system (C5a) | |
> | – Arachidonic acid metabolites (leukotriene B4) | |

14. **Not true about innate immunity:**
    a. Not influenced by hormones
    b. Dependent on genetic constitution
    c. Identical twins have same degree of resistance
    d. Not influenced by exposure to antigen
    [Ref. Ananthanarayan, 10/e, p 81]

> Endocrine disorders such as diabetes mellitus, hypothyroidism and adrenal dysfunction are associated with increased susceptibility to infection

15. **When transfer factor is given as treatment results in:**
    a. Natural active immunity
    b. Artificial active immunity
    c. Artificial passive immunity
    d. Adoptive immunity
    [Ref. Ananthanarayan, 10/e, p 86]

> **Adoptive Immunity:** Special type of immunisation by infection of immunologically competent lymphocytes. Instead of whole lymphocyte an extract of immunologically competent lymphocyte known as transfer factor. Not much application – attempted in leptomatous leprosy.

16. **Most potent chemoattractant is:**
    a. Leukotriene B4
    b. Leukotriene C4
    c. Leukotriene D4
    d. Leukotriene E4
    [Ref. Robbins, 8/e, p 57]

17. **T cells in lymph node are present in:**
    a. Paracortical area
    b. Mantle layer
    c. Medullary cords
    d. Cortical follicles
    [Ref. Ananthanarayan, 10/e, p 133]

18. **Which cells cause rosette formation with sheep RBCs:**
    a. T-Cells
    b. NK cells
    c. Monocytes
    d. B cells

> - T cells bind to sheep erythrocytes, forming rosettes (SRBC or E rosette) by the CD2 antigen. B. cells do not.
> - B cells bind to sheep erythrocytes coated with antibody and complement, forming EAC rosettes, due to the presence of a C3 receptor (CR2) on the B cell surface. CR2 also acts as a receptor for the Epstein-Barr virus. T cells do not possess this.

19. **Cellular immunity is induced by:**
    a. NK-Cells
    b. Dendritic-cells
    c. TH1-cells
    d. TH2-cells
    [Ref. Ananthanarayan, 10/e, p 134]

> TH1 cells promote cell mediate immunity by producing IL-2, which activate macrophages and T-cells. TH-2 cells produce cytokines IL4, 5 and 6 which stimulate B cells to form antibodies. TH1t cells produce cytokine IL17 and promote inflammation.

Ans.
10. a. Adenosine...
11. a. Humoral...
12. c. Not affected by...
13. d. LTB4
14. a. Not influenced...
15. d. Adoptive...
16. a. Leukotriene B4
17. a. Paracortical area
18. a. T-Cells
19. c. TH1-cells

20. In cell lysis by compliments:
    a. They activate cyclaise
    b. Inhibits elongation factor p
    c. Destruction of cell wall
    d. Increased permeability of cell membrane
    [Ref. Ananthanarayan, 10/e, p 124]

> The mechanism of complement mediated cytolysis is the production of holes, approx. 100 Å diameter on cell membrane, which disrupts the osmotic integrity of membrane and lysis.

21. True about interferon is:
    a. Host protein
    b. Viral protein
    c. Inactivated by nucleases
    d. Virus specific
    [Ref. Ananthanarayan, 10/e, p 157]

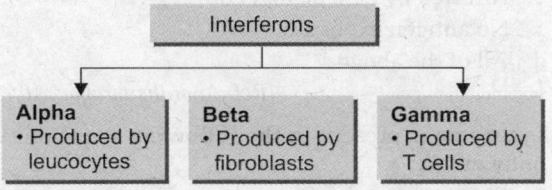

22. Chronic granulomatous disorder is due to defect in:
    a. B-cell
    b. NADPH oxidase
    c. IgA
    d. T-cell
    [Ref. Ananthanarayan, 10/e, p 177]

23. Anaphylatoxin in complement system:
    a. C_{3b} b. C_{5-9}
    c. C_{5a} d. C_{1-3}
    [Ref. Jawetz, 27/e, p 141]

24. Most chemotactic property is with:
    a. C3a   b. C5a
    c. C5-9   d. C3b
    [Ref. Jawetz, 27/e, p 141]

25. Membrane attack complex (MAC) in complement system is:
    a. C_{3b} b. C_{1-3}
    c. C_{5-9} d. C_{2-4}
    [Ref. Jawetz, 27/e, p 142]

26. Complement components are:
    a. Lipids   b. Proteins
    c. Lipoproteins   d. Polysaccharide
    [Ref. Ananthanarayan, 10/e, p 123]

> Complement system consist of atleast 30 chemically and immunologically distinct serum proteins.

27. Which is not true about macrophages:
    a. Activation by IFN-γ
    b. Major cells in chronic inflammation
    c. M_2 type involved in inflammation
    d. Phagocytic cells
    [Ref. Robbins, 8/e, p 70, Greenwood, 18/e, p 121]

28. Natural killer cell is:
    a. MHC restricted
    b. Antibody dependent
    c. Null cells
    d. B-lymphocytes
    [Ref. Robbins, 8/e, p 188]

29. Which does not stimulate active immunity:
    a. Subclinical infection
    b. Clinical infection
    c. Vaccination
    d. Transplacental antibody in newborn
    [Ref. Ananthanarayan, 10/e, p 84]

30. Complement deficiency has not been associated with:
    a. SLE
    b. PNH
    c. Hereditary angioedema
    d. Membranous nephritis
    [Ref. Ananthanarayan, 10/e, p 128]

Clinical syndromes associated with genetic deficiencies of complement components		
Group	Deficiency	Syndrome
I	Cl inhibitor	Hereditary angioneurotic edema
II	Early components of classical pathway C1, C2, C4	SLE and other collagen vascular diseases
III	C3 and its regulatory protein C3b inactivator	Severe recurrent pyogenic infections
IV	C5 to C8	Bacteremia, mainly with Gram-negative diplococci, toxoplasmosis
V	C9	No particular disease

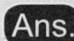 **Ans.**
20. d. Increased permeability of cell membrane   21. a. Host protein   22. b. NADPH oxidase   23. c. C_{5a}
24. b. C5a   25. c. C_{5-9} 26. b. Proteins   27. c. M_2 type...   28. c. Null cells
29. d. Transplacental antibody in newborn   30. d. Membranous nephritis

31. **Primary T-cell deficiency is:**
    a. Ecto-5 nucleotidase deficiency
    b. Common variable immunodeficiency
    c. DiGeorge syndrome
    d. Wiskott-Aldrich syndrome
    [Ref. Ananthanarayan, 10/e, p 175]

32. **DiGeorge syndrome is characterized by all *except*:**
    a. Congenital thymic hypoplasia
    b. Abnormal developmental of third and fourth pouches
    c. Hypothyroidism
    d. Hypocalcemic tetany
    [Ref. Ananthanarayan 10/e, p 175]

- **Thymic hypoplasia (DiGeorge syndrome)**
    - It is a developmental defect involving the endodermal derivatives of the third and fourth pharyngeal pouches, leading to aplasia on hypoplasia of the thymus and parathyroid gland.
    - It is nonhereditary and is supposed to be due to intrauterine infection
    - It is associated with tetralogy of Fallot.
    - Neonatal tetany is present
    - There is defect in cell mediated immunity and humoral immunity is largely unaffected.

33. **Antibody dependent cytotoxicity is seen with:**
    a. Cytotoxic T-cells
    b. Natural killer cells
    c. ADCC
    d. All of the above
    [Ref. Robbins, 8/e, p 203]

34. **Functions of complement include all *except*:**
    a. Chemotaxis   b. Opsonization
    c. Cell lysis   d. Antigen presentation
    [Ref. Robbins, 8/e, p 64]

35. **T-cell multiplication is stimulated by:**
    a. Macrolin   b. Heat
    c. Bovine serum   d. Phytohemagglutin
    [Ref. Ananthanarayan 10/e, p 135]

- T-cells undergo blast transformation on treatment with mitogens such as phytohemagglutinin, concanavalin A, while B-cells undergo similar transformation with bacterial endotoxins on E-B virus.

36. **Which is specific for acquired immunity?**
    a. Immunological memory
    b. Affected by genetic makeup
    c. No antigen exposure
    d. All of the above
    [Ref. Ananthanarayan, 10/e, p 83]

37. **Lysozyme is present in the following secretions of the body *except*:**
    a. Lacrimal secretions
    b. CSF
    c. Saliva
    d. Respiratory tract secretions
    [Ref. Ananthanarayan 10/e, p 82]

- Lysozyme is a thermolabile, low molecular weight basic protein which acts as neuraminidase. It is present in tissue fluids, and in nearly all secretions except CSF, sweat and urine. It acts by splitting certain polysaccharide components of the cell walls of susceptible bacteria.

Ans.
31. **c.** DiGeorge syndrome   32. **c.** Hypothy ...   33. **b.** Natural killer...
34. **d.** Antigen presentation   35. **d.** Phytohe ...   36. **a.** Immunological memory
37. **c.** Saliva

Antigen and Antibody

CHAPTER 37

ANTIGENS

Substance that can provoke the production of antibody.

Determinants of Antigenicity
- Molecular size (< 5000 are non-antigenic)
- Chemical nature (usually protein and polysaccharide are more antigenic than lipid and nucleic acid)
- Susceptibility to tissue enzymes
- Foreignness
- Antigen specificity
- Species specificity
- Isospecificity
- Autospecificity (except lens protein and sperm)
- Organ specificity
- Heterogenetic/heterophile specificity (Forssman antigen; Weil-Felix reaction in typhus fever, Paul-Bunnel test in infectious mononucleosis; Cold agglutinin test in primary atypical pneumonia).

Haptens – Non-immunogenic but has immunological reactivity, i.e. incapable of inducing antibody formation but can react with antibodies.

They become immunogenic on combining with larger molecule carrier.

Hapten is of two types:
i. Simple haptens are non-precipitating.
ii. Complex haptens are precipitating, since they have two or more antibody combining sites.

> - **Haptens:** Nonimmune, but react with antibody
> - **Epitope:** Smallest unit of antigenicity
> - **Paratope:** Area on antibody that bind epitope.
> - **Idiotopes:** Specific antigen determinant on paratope.

Epitope or antigenic determinant
- It is *smallest unit of antigenicity* (small area on the antigen) which is capable of sensitising an immunocyte and of reacting with its complementary site on specific antibody or T cell receptor.
- *T cell identify linear or sequential* epitope, whereas *B cell identify conformational* epitope.

Paratope
- It is combining area of the antibody molecule, corresponding to the epitope.
- Epitope and paratope determine **specificity** which is hallmark of immunological reaction.
- Bacteria/virus may contain antigen mosaic (different epitopes) while same epitope on different antigen may present causing antigenic cross-reaction.
- Specific antigen determinants on paratope are called *IDIOTOPES*.

Human immune system

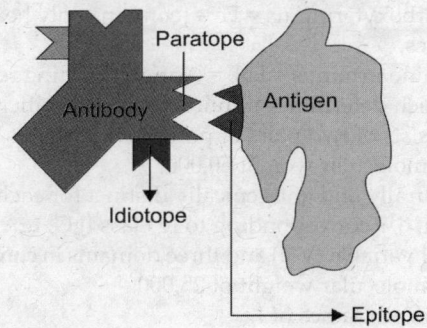

Antibody and Antigen with paratope, epitope and idiotope

ANTIBODIES

Plasma		
Fractionation of serum proteins by NH_4SO_4		
Soluble albumins	Insoluble globulin	
	Water soluble (pseudoglobulins)	Insoluble (Euglobulin)

Antibodies:
- Globulin in nature
- Contains 2 heavy chain and 2 light chain
- Heavy chain has 4 highly variable region.
- Light chain has 3 highly variable region.

- *Most* of the human antibody is euglobulin and are usually gammaglobulin (but equine antitoxin is beta or alpha globulins).
- All antibodies are Ig but all Ig may not be antibodies because Ig not only includes antibody globulins but also includes abnormal proteins of myeloma macroglobulinemia, cryoglobulinemia and naturally occurring subunits of Ig.
- Ig constitutes 20-25% of total serum proteins.

Structure of Ig

- **VL** = Variable domain of light chain.
- **CL** = Constant domain of light chain.
- **VH** = Variable domain of heavy chain.
- **CH** = Constant domain of heavy chain.
- **S-S** = Disulphide bond.

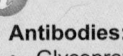

Antibodies:
- Glycoproteins
- Present in serum and body fluids.

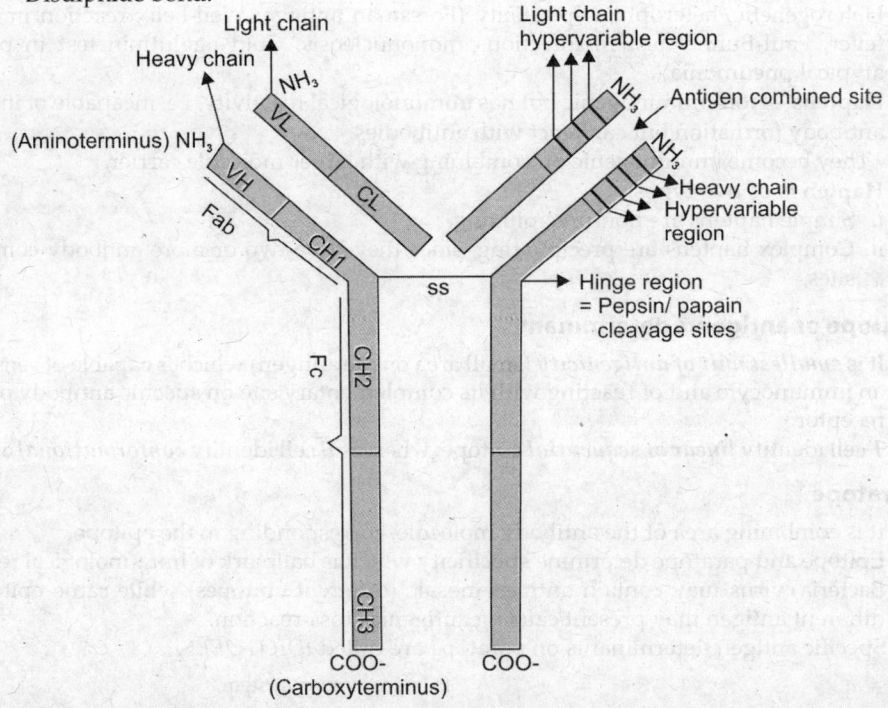

- *Constant region* = Carboxyterminus = Fc = [contains only heavy chain] which determines Ig biological properties.
- *Variable region* = Aminoterminus = Fab = Antigen binding region [= contains both Heavy and Light chains] which determines immunological specificity of antibody molecule.
- Ig (glycoprotein) consists of two pairs of polypeptide chains **(2H and 2L)**.
- H = heavy chain has molecular weight 50,000.
  - H chain are structurally and antigenically distinct for each class and are designated by Greek letter γ, α, μ, δ, ε corresponding to Ig class IgG, IgA, IgM, IgD, IgE. respectively.
  - H chain consist of 1 variable (VH) and three domains in constant region (CH_1, CH_2, CH_3).
- L = Light chain with molecular weight of 25,000.
  - L chain is similar in all classes of Ig.

- 2 types of L chain are kappa (κ) and lambda (λ).
- 1 molecule of Ig may have either kappa or lambda chains but never both.
- Kappa and Lambda occur in ratio of about κ : λ = 2 : 1.
- L chain consists of 1 variable (V_L) and 1 constant domain (C_L).
- Highly variable zones (3 in L and 4 in H chain) are known as *Hypervariable regions* or *Hot spots*. They are involved in the formation of antigen-binding sites. Sites on the hypervariable regions which make actual contact with the epitope are called *complementarity determining regions* or *CDRs*.
- Fd piece - is portion of H chain present in Fab fragment.
- Immunoglobin isotype (G, M, A, D, E) is determined on the basis of Ig heavy chain present.

Digestion of Antibody

- Papain cleaves antibody to produce two fab fragment and 1 fc fragement.
- Enzyme pepsin produce a f(ab)$_2$ and fragment of antibody.

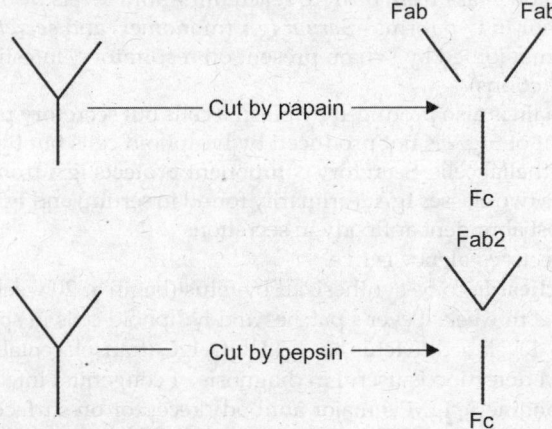

IMMUNOGLOBULIN CLASSES

It has following properties:
- *Sedimentation coefficient* - **max** IgM
- *Molecular weight* - **max** IgM **min** - IgG
- *Serum concentration, Half life in days, Daily production (mg/kg)* – G > A > M > D > E
- *Intravascular distribution (%)* - **max** IgM, **min** IgA
- *Carbohydrate (%)* **max** IgE
- *Complement fixation:* Classical - IgM > IgG
  Alternative - IgA, IgD, IgG
- *Placental transport* - only IgG
- *Present in milk* - IgG and IgA
- *Selective secretion by seromucinous gland* - IgA
- *Heat labile* - **only** IgE
- J chain - IgA and IgM

Heaviest Ig	:	IgM
Lightest Ig	:	IgA
Heat labile	:	IgE
Most abundant	:	IgG in serum, IgM in plasma

Properties of various immunoglobulin classes					
	IgG	IgA	IgM	IgD	IgE
1. Molecular weight in kDa	150	160,385*	900	180	190
2. Sedimentation coefficient	7	7,11	19	7	8
3. Carbohydrate content (%)	3	8	12	13	12
4. Heavy chain	$\gamma_1, \gamma_2, \gamma_3, \gamma_4$	α_1, α_2	μ	δ	ε
5. Light chain	κ, or λ	κ, or λ	κ, or λ	κ, or λ	κ, or λ
6. Serum concentration (mg/ml)	12	2	1.2	0.03	0.00004
7. Half-life (days)	21	6	5	3	2

Contd...

Contd...

	Properties of various immunoglobulin classes				
	IgG	IgA	IgM	IgD	IgE
8. Complement binding	Classical pathway	Alternative pathway	Classical pathway	None	None
9. Binding to tissue	Heterologous	None	None	None	Homologous
10. Secretion from serous membranes	No	Yes*	No	No	Yes
11. Placental Passage	Yes	No	No	No	No
12. Heat stability (56°C)	Yes	Yes	Yes	Yes	No

Immunoglobulin classes

i. **IgG**
   - Most abundant immunoglobulin of serum, making up 75% of total
   - General purpose antibody, enhances phagocytosis by opsonization.
   - It has four subclasses G_1 (65%), > G_2 (23%), > G_3 (8%) > G_4 (4%)
   - IgG decrease from birth to reach minimum levels by 3rd month.

ii. **IgA**
   - Occur in two forms - *Serum IgA* (monomer) and *secretory IgA*, i.e. SIgA (dimer joined by J chain present on respiratory/intestinal mucosa and in secretions).
   - J chain is also produced by plasma cells but secretory piece/secretory component of SIgA is not produced by lymphoid cells but by mucosal or glandular epithelial cells. Secretory component protects IgA from denaturation.
   - Has two classes IgA_1 (primarily found in serum) and IgA_2 (found in secretions)
   - Most abundant antibody in secretions

iii. **IgM**
   - Effective valency is five.
   - **Earliest Ig** to be synthesized by fetus (begin at 20 week of age) is IgM.
   - At 20th weeks Peyer's patches and lymphoid cells in spleen, and lymph nodes are developed so fetus has IgM, IgD, IgG (transplacentally) but not IgA and IgE.
   - IgM detection is useful in diagnosis of congenital infection.
   - Monomeric IgM is major antibody receptor on surface of B lymphocytes for antigen recognition.
   - IgM synthesis is five times more costly for a cell in comparison to IgG, this is the reason for IgM to IgG switch.

iv. **IgD** — Resemble IgG structurally and also serve as recognition receptor for antigen.

v. **IgE**
   - Mostly extravascular and exhibits Homocytotrophism.
   - Chiefly produced in the lining of intestinal and respiratory tract.
   - It mediates Reaginic hypersensitivity and Prausnitz-Küstner (PK) reaction.

> **Remember:** *IgG protect body fluids, IgA body surfaces and IgM the blood stream. IgE is not secreted by eosinophils, rather eosinophils get activated with IgE.*

Types of Antibody in various conditions:

IgM
- Biological false positive Ab in syphilis
- Rheumatoid factor
- Ab against ABO
- Ab to typhoid O Ag (endotoxin).

IgG
- Ab against Rh factor (Anti Rh D)
- (LATS) long acting thyroid stimulator Ab in Graves'
- AutoAb in SLE, GB Syndrome
- Reagin Ab in syphilis (Lupus anticoagulant, anticardiolipin).

Abnormal Ig

i. *Bence Jones Protein (BJP)*
   - Monoclonal Ig consists of light chain found typically in multiple myeloma.
   - Identified in urine by its characteristic property of coagulation when heated to 50°C but redissolving at 70°C.

ii. *Myeloma (M) protein*
   - Monoclonal Ab seen in multiple myeloma (IgG, IgA, IgD, IgE) and Waldenstrom's macroglobulinemia (IgM).

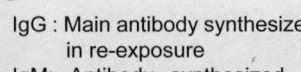

IgG : Main antibody synthesized in re-exposure
IgM: Antibody synthesized in first exposure
IgA: Antibody found in secretions
IgE: Antibody involved in activating mast cells and basophills

IgM Vs IgG

IgM is 500-1000 times more effective than IgG in opsonisation.
100 times more effective in bactericidal action
20 times more effective in bacterial agglutination

iii. *F_c parts of Ig heavy chain*
   - ↑ in Heavy chain disease.
iv. *Cryoglobulinemia*
   - Formation of gel or precipitate on cooling the serum, which redissolves on warming.
   - Most cryoglobulin consist of either IgG, IgM or mixed precipitates.

IMMUNOGLOBULIN SPECIFICITIES

- It is of great importance in immumology. The antigenic determinants on immuglobulin molecule fall in to three main category.
- **Isotype:** Isotype variations refers to genetic variations and differences in the constant region of the heavy chain of the Ig class or subclass within a species. Within a species each normal individuals will express all isotypes in the serum whereas different species inherit different constant region and therefore express differet isotypes.
- **Allotype:** It refers to multiple allele that exists for some of the genes and which lead to subtle amino acid difference in some but not all members of species, e.g. Allotype have been characterized for all IgG subclass. Each of these allotypic determinants represent differences in one to four amino acid that are encoded by different alleles.
- **Idiotype:** These determinants arise from the sequence of the heavy and light chain variables region. The sum of all idiotopes on an Ig molecule constitute idiotype. This results due to the variability in amino acid sequence in variable region. Antibodies against the idiotypic portion of an antibody molecule are called anti-idiotype antibodies.

> IgG protects body fluid
> IgA protects body surface
> IgM protects blood stream
> IgE produce hypersensitivity
> IgD is the recognition molecule on the surface of B lymphocyte

ANTIGEN – ANTIBODY REACTIONS

Ag-Ab reaction is reversible, occur *at surface* and there is no denaturation of Ag or Ab during reaction. Reactions occur in three stages:

i. *Primary stage:*
   Ag-Ab combined by weaker intermolecular forces such as van der Waals, ionic bond and H_2 binding rather than by firmer covalent bonding; without any visible effects.
   Firmness is influenced by affinity and avidity. Affinity is intensity of attraction, avidity is strength of bond after formation of antigen antibody complex.

ii. *Secondary stage:*
   Usually present but not always. It leads to demonstrable events such as precipitation, agglutination, lysis of cells etc.

iii. *Tertiary stage (reaction):*
   Leads to tissue damage e.g. allergy and other immunological diseases.

> **Serological Reactions:**
> - **Precipitation:** Soluble Antigen + Antibody in presence of electrolyte
> - **Agglutination:** Particulate antigen + antibody in presence of electrolyte. More sensitive include, tube and slide agglutination

SEROLOGICAL REACTIONS

Comparative efficiency of Ig in different serological reactions:

Reaction	IgG	IgM	IgA
• *Neutralization (N)*	More effective	Less effective	Variable
• *Precipitation (P)*	Strong	Weak	Variable
• *Classical complement fixation (C)*	Strong	Strongest	Negative
• *Immunohemolysis (I)* and *Bactericidal (opsonization) (O)*	Less effective	More effective	Moderate
• *Agglutination (A)*	Weak	Strong	Moderate
• *Lysis (L)*	Weak	Strong	Negative

Mnemonic for strong reaction in IgG = *G*-N-P (Neutralization, Precipitation).
Mnemonic for strong reaction in IgM = CO-*M*-ALI (Classical Complement fixation, Opsonization, Agglutination, lysis, Immunohemolysis).

Precipitation Reaction

When **soluble antigen** combines with its antibody in presence of electrolytes, it forms *insoluble precipitates/floccules*.
- This reaction show "zone phenomenon" *(also in agglutination)* either in the form of prozone (*antibody* excess) or postzone (*antigen* excess).

> Prozone phenomenon is clinically seen in secondary syphillis

Precipitation literally means formation of insoluble product

- It occurs in zone of equivalence due to lattice formation *(also in agglutination)*.
- It is very *sensitive* in antigen detection (but relatively less sensitive for antibody detection).
- It is of following types:
    a. *Ring test* – Simplest type, e.g. Ascoli's thermoprecipitin test and streptococcal lancefield grouping.
    b. *Slide test* – VDRL test of syphilis
    c. *Tube test* – Kahn test of syphilis
    d. *Immunodiffusion (ppt in gel)* – e.g. Elek test for toxigenicity in diphtheria (double diffusion).
    e. *Electroimmunodiffusion* – e.g. rocket electrophoresis for quantitative estimation of antigen.

Immunodiffusion
- Possess advantage of visible and stable reaction. It includes:
    - – Single diffusion in one dimension (Oudin procedure)
    - – Double diffusion in one dimension (Oakle-Fulthorpe procedure)
    - – Single diffusion in two dimension (Radial immunodiffusion)
    - – Double diffusion in two dimension (Ouchter lony procedure)

Agglutination Reaction
- When *particulate antigen* combines with its antibody in the presence of electrolyte at suitable pH and temperature. The particles gets clumped or agglutinated.
- It is more sensitive than precipitation for antibody detection. Occur in presence of electrolytes.
- Incomplete or monovalent antibodies (usually Ab are bivalent) do not cause agglutination, though they combine with the antigen. They also act as blocking Ab since they inhibit agglutination by complete Ab.
- Agglutination is of following types:

- Complement fixation test: **Wassermann reaction**
- Neutralization test: **Schick test**

    a. *Slide agglutination* – used for blood grouping and cross matching.
    b. *Tube agglutination* – e.g. Widal test, Brucellosis, Weil-Felix reaction, Paul Bunnel test, cold agglutination and *Streptococcus* MG test.
    c. *Antiglobulin (Coombs) test* – used for detecting incomplete Ab of brucellosis; anti-Rh Ab.
    d. *Passive agglutination test* – used to detect Ab by adsorbing soluble Ag on carrier particles so precipitation reaction converts into agglutination test which are *more convenient* and *more sensitive*. e.g. Rose Waller test, a hemagglutination test detecting RA factor by using amboceptor.
    e. *Latex agglutination test (latex fixation test)* – for detection of ASO, CRP, RA factor, HCG; Streptozyme test.
    f. *Reversed passive agglutination* – Estimation of antigen by adsorbing antibody to carrier particles.

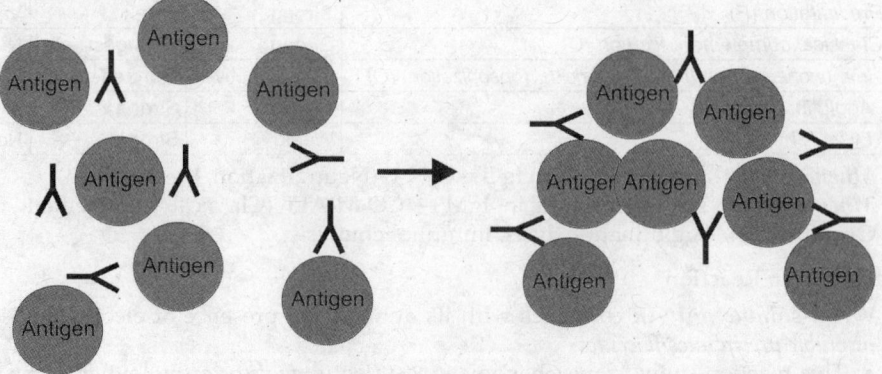

Agglutination reaction

Complement Fixation Test (CFT)
- Antigen may be soluble or particulate.
- Source of complement is guinea pig serum, e.g. Wassermann reaction; coagglutinating complement adsorption test using horse complement; immuno adherence of *V. cholera* and *T. pallidum*; Immobilization test of *T. pallidum*; Cytolytic or cytocidal test.

Neutralisation Tests
- Includes virus neutralization test *(plaque inhibition test)*, Toxin neutralization *(Schick, antistreptolysin O)* test; Nagler's reaction

Radio-Immunoassay (RIA)
- MC labels used are radio-isotopes and enzymes.
- It measures analytes upto picogram (10^{-12}g) quantities.
- Used for quantitation of hormones, drugs, tumour markers, IgE and viral antigen.

Enzyme Immunoassay (EIA)
- Measures enzyme labelled antigen, hapten or antibody.
- It may be homogenous or heterogenous.
- Major type of heterogenous EIA is ELISA which involves the use of immunosorbent - an absorbing material specific for one of components of reaction, the antigen or antibody, e.g. ELISA for detection of *Rotavirus in feces or HIV antibody in serum.*

Lattice Hypothesis
- Explains precipitation and agglutination.
- Multivalent antigen combines with bivalent antibodies in varying proportion
- Precipitation and agglutination occurs at zone of equivalence.
- In zone of antibody excess (prozone phenomenon) or antigen excess (post zone) lattice do not form.

Immunofluorescence
- Detect antigen by using fluorescent dye labelled antibodies
- Two types
  (a) Direct immunofluorescence
   - Used for identification of bacteria, virus or other antigen using the specific antiserum labelled with fluorescent dye. Main limitation is requirement for separate fluorescent conjugates for each antigen.
  (b) Indirect immunofluorescence
   - Here labelled antibody against antiserum is used. This overcomes the difficulties of direct immunofluorescence.

Multiple Choice Questions

1. The following methods of diagnosis utilize labelled antibodies *except*: [NEET Pattern 2019, AIIMS 05]
   a. ELISA
   b. Hemagglutination inhibition test
   c. Radioimmunoassay
   d. Immunofluorescence

2. A child has recurrent infection with encapsulated bacteria. Which IgG subclass is deficient? [NEET Pattern 2019]
   a. IgG1
   b. IgG2
   c. IgG3
   d. IgG4

3. Which of the following immunological disorder is associated with recurrent Staphylococcal abscess:
   a. Hyper IgE [NEET Pattern 2019]
   b. Hyper IgN
   c. Transient hypogammaglobulinemia of infancy
   d. X-linked agammaglobulinemia

4. The serum concentration of which of the following human IgG subclasses is maximum? [AI 05]
   a. IgG1
   b. IgG2
   c. IgG3
   d. IgG4

5. The earliest immunoglobulin to be synthesized by the fetus is: [AIIMS 09]
   a. IgA
   b. IgG
   c. IgE
   d. IgM

6. Which precipitates at 50°C-60°C but disappears on heating? [AI 06]
   a. Heavy chain
   b. Light chain
   c. Both
   d. None of the above

7. Prozone phenomenon is due to: [AIIMS 18]
   a. Antigen excess
   b. Antibody excess
   c. False +ve reaction
   d. False -ve reaction

8. In a 5-year-old boy who has history of recurrent pyogenic infections by bacteria with polysaccharide-rich capsules, which of the following investigations should be done? [AI 2012, AIIMS May 2012]
   a. IgA deficiency
   b. IgG_1 deficiency
   c. IgG_2 deficiency
   d. IgA and IgG_2 deficiency

9. The most avidly complement fixing antibody is:
   a. IgA
   b. IgG [AIIMS 15]
   c. IgM
   d. IgE

10. All of the following statements about carbohydrate antigens are true *except*: [AI 2011]
    a. Good memory response
    b. Poor immunogenicity
    c. T-cell independent immunity
    d. Polyclonal response

11. Vaccination is based on the principle of: [AI 2012]
    a. Agglutination
    b. Phagocytosis
    c. Immunological memory
    d. Clonal detection

12. The reaction between antibody and soluble antigen is demonstrated by: [AIIMS 16]
    a. Agglutination
    b. Precipitation
    c. Complement fixation
    d. Hemagglutination test

13. Antibody diversity is due to: [PGI Dec 07]
    a. Gene rearrangement
    b. Gene translocation
    c. Antigenic variation
    d. CD40 molecules
    e. Mutation

14. MHC class III genes encode: [PGI 06]
    a. Complement component C3
    b. Tumor necrosis factor - alpha
    c. Tumor necrosis factor - beta
    d. Interleukin 2
    e. Beta 2 microglobulin

15. Acute phase reactants (APR) in acute inflammation are: [PGI 07]
    a. Albumin
    b. Fibrinogen
    c. Haptoglobulin
    d. Gammaglobulin

16. Antigen binding site on antibody is: [AMIS 14]
    a. Hinge region
    b. Constant region
    c. Variable region
    d. Hypervariable region

17. True regarding clonal selection: [PGI 2008]
    a. Specific
    b. Secondary response is rapid
    c. Variable region of Ig is involved in Ab production

18. Which of the following is true about isotypic variation? [AIIMS 09]
    a. Subtle amino acid changes due to allelic difference
    b. Changes in a heavy and light chain in variable region
    c. Changes in heavy and light chain in constant region responsible for class and subtype
    d. These are areas in antigen that bind specifically to antibody

19. Superantigens true statement is: [AIIMS May 10]
    a. They bind to the cleft of the MHC
    b. Needs to be processed before presentation
    c. They are presented by APCs to T-cells
    d. Directly attached to lateral aspect of TCR β chain

20. Antigen antibody precipitation is maximally seen in which of the following? [AIIMS May 10]
    a. Excess of antibody
    b. Excess of antigen
    c. Equivalent of antibody and antigen
    d. Antigen-Hapten interaction

21. **Antigen-antibody complexes are detected by:** [PGI 09]
    a. Western blot
    b. Southern blot
    c. Northern blot
    d. ELISA

22. **Which portion of MHC 1 complex forms the component of antigen presenting part:** [AIIMS 2011]
    a. Between alpha1-beta 2 microglobulin
    b. Distal part of alpha chain
    c. Proximal part of alpha chain
    d. Between a_s and b_2 microglobulin

23. **C in C-reactive protein stands for:** [AI 2011]
    a. Capsular polysaccharide of S. pneumoniae
    b. Concanavalin-A
    c. Calretinin
    d. Cellular

24. **Ova albumin antigen was injected into a rabbit. What antibody will it produce initially?** [AI 2011]
    a. IgG
    b. IgM
    c. IgE
    d. IgD

25. **Role of adjuvant in vaccine is/are:** [PGI Nov 2011]
    a. Stimulation of Toll-like receptors
    b. Activate B-lymphocyte only
    c. Increase both adaptive and innate immune response
    d. Activate both B and T lymphocyte
    e. Ensure prolonged delivery of antigen

26. **Synthesis of an immunoglobulin in membrane bound or secretory form is determined by:** [AIIMS: May 2012]
    a. One turn to two turn joining rule
    b. Class switching
    c. Differential RNA processing
    d. Alletic exclusion

27. **Immunoglobulin bound on the surface of bacteria mediates phagocytosis by:** [AIIMS: Nov 2011]
    a. C3b and Fc
    b. Receptor mediated endocytosis
    c. Oxidase action
    d. Lysosomal burst

28. **Heterophile agglutination is/are used in all test *except*:** [PGI May 2013]
    a. Widal test
    b. Weil-Felix reaction
    c. Paul-Bunnell test
    d. ELISA
    e. Cold agglutination test

29. **True about antibody:** [PGI May 2013]
    a. IgM is produced in primary response
    b. IgD protects mucosa
    c. IgE is main antibody in secondary response
    d. IgG is main antibody in secondary response
    e. IgA protects body surface

30. **Antibodies present in person with O blood group:** [PGI May 2013]
    a. Anti-A antibody only
    b. Anti-B antibody only
    c. Both Anti-A and Anti-B antibody
    d. No antibody
    e. Anti-O antibody

31. **Regarding IgE which of the following is false:** [AIIMS 2014]
    a. Cause anaphylaxis
    b. Immediate reaction
    c. Fix complement
    d. Cross placenta

32. **Papain cleaves the immunoglobin molecule into:** [AIIMS 2017]
    a. 1 Fc and 1 Fab
    b. 1 Fc and 2 Fab
    c. 2 Fc and 1 Fab
    d. 2 Fc and 2 Fab

Explanations and References with Illustrative Answers

1. **Ans. (b) Hemagglutination inhibition test** *Ref. Ananthanarayan 10/e, p 107-111*

    Following serological test, use labeled antibodies:

    A. Immunofluorescence (IF) = Fluorescent Antibody Technique
    - **Principle:** Labels (fluorescent dyes) conjugated with Antibodies of serum = labelled antibodies which is used to locate and identify *antigens* in tissues.
    - Fluorescent dyes commonly used are *fluorescein Isothiocynate and lissamine - rhodamine*

Immunofluorescence may be	
Direct IF test	Indirect IF test
• Antigen + labeled antibodies ↓ Antigen - Antibody complex is fluorescent e.g. detection of *rabies virus* antigen in brain smears	• Antigen + Antibody ↓ • Antigen - Antibody complex + fluorescent conjugated antiglobulin serum ↓ • Final product is fluorescent e.g. fluorescent *treponemal antibody* test for syphilis
• Disadvantage - Separate fluorescent conjugates have to be prepared against each antigen to be tested	• Advantage - A single antihuman globulin fluorescent conjugate can be used for detecting human antibody to any antigen

- Fluorescent dyes can also be conjugated with *complement*.
- Labelled complement can be used for detection of antigen or antibody.
- Antibody is detected by Sandwich technique.
- **Major disadvantage** of immunofluorescence is frequent occurence of nonspecific fluorescence in tissues and other materials.

B. **Radioimmunoassay (RIA) = Binder Ligand Assays**
   - *Principle:* Radiolabelled ***Radioisotopes (MC) and enzyme*** conjugated to antigen / antibody = labelled reactants which *measure* antigen *and* antibodies.
   - The substance (antigen) whose concentration is to be determined is termed the analyte or ligand.
   - Binding protein (usually antibody) which binds to ligand is called the binder.
   - RIA measure analytes up to picogram 10^{-12}g quantities.
   - RIA has application in quantitation of hormones, drugs, tumor markers, IgE and viral antigens.
   - Fixed amount of antibody reacts with radiolabelled antigen as well as varying known amount of unlabelled (test) antigen competitively.
   - Concentration of test antigen is calculated from standard dose response or calibrating curve.

C. **Enzyme Immunoassays (EIA)**
   - It is the most widely used procedure in clinical serology.
   - It uses enzyme labelled antigen and antibodies as serological reagents, for the assay of antibodies and antigens.
   - It is of two types:
     i. **Homogenous EIA (one step test) -**
        - Used only for assay of haptens such as drugs (opiates, cocaine, etc.)
     ii. **Heterogenous EIA (multistep test) -**
        - Major type of heterogenous EIA is **ELISA** which involves the use of immunosorbent specific for one of the components of reaction, the antigen or antibody.
        - Immunosorbent may be particulate or solid phase
          e.g. - *Noncompetitive sandwich ELISA*
             - ***Detection of rotavirus antigen in feces.***
             - *Anti-HIV antibody test.*
             - *Competitive ELISA*
             - *IgM specific ELISA*
             - *Capture ELISA*
             - *Immunometric ELISA*
             - *Card and dipstick methods*
             - *Cylinder or* Casette *ELISA* for the detection of HIV type 1 and 2 antibodies. It is rapid.

D. **Chemiluminescence Immunoassay (CLIA)**
   - Uses chemiluminescent compounds (such as luminol or acridinium esters) as the label to provide signal during antigen-antibody reaction.

E. **Immunoelectroblot Techniques**
   - e.g. western blot test.

F. **Immunochromatographic Tests**
   - Test system is a small cassette containing membrane impregnated with anti-HbsAg antibody - colloidal gold dye conjugate, *e.g. HBsAg detection.*

G. **Immunoferritin Test**
   - Antibody conjugate with ferritin.

H. **Immunoenzyme Test**
   - Stable enzyme like peroxidase conjugated with antibodies.

> **Remember:** *Hemagglutination inhibition test* - convenient method for detection and quantitation of antibody to the virus.

2. **Ans. (b) IgG2 class** ...*Ref. Journals*
   Selective IgG class Deficiency
   - Patients with persistently low levels of one or two IgG subclasses and a normal total IgG level have a selective IgG subclass deficiency.

- IgG1 and IgG3 subclasses are rich in antibodies against proteins such as the toxins produced by the diphtheria and tetanus bacteria, as well as antibodies against viral proteins. Whereas, IgG2 antibodies are predominantly against the polysaccharide (complex sugar) coating (capsule) of certain disease-producing bacteria (such as, *Streptococcus pneumoniae* and *Haemophilus influenzae*).
- IgG subclass deficiencies affect only IgG subclasses, with normal total IgG and IgM immunoglobulins and other components of the immune system being at normal levels. IgG2 or IgG3 deficiencies are the most common IgG subclass deficiencies.
- **Treatment:**
  - Recurrent or chronic infections of the ears, sinuses and lungs need comprehensive treatment to prevent permanent damage that might result in hearing loss or chronic lung disease. It is also important to encourage patients to continue normal activities of daily living, such as school or work.
  - The mainstay of treatment includes appropriate use of antibiotics to treat and to prevent infections.
  - Additional immunization with pneumococcal vaccines may also be used to enhance immunity.
  - Ig therapy is an option for selected symptomatic patients that have persistent IgG subclass deficiencies, documented poor responses to polysaccharide vaccines and who fail prophylactic antibiotic therapy

Note: The IgG in the bloodstream is 60-70% IgG1, 20-30% IgG2, 5-8% IgG3 and 1-3% IgG4. IgG1 and IgG3 reach normal adult levels by 5-7 years of age while IgG2 and IgG4 levels rise more slowly, reaching adult levels at about 10 years of age.

Association of abnormal serum IgG	
Infections	**Change in IgG subclass**
Recurrent infections with capsulated bacteria	↓IgG2/IgG4
Recurrent sinopulmonary infections, Bronchiectasis	↓IgG2/IgG3/IgG4
Otitis media in children	↓IgG2 antibodies to pneumococcus
Cystic fibrosis with chronic *P. aeruginosa* infection	↑IgG2
Mothers of children with group B streptococcal sepsis	↓IgG1,2,3
AIDS	Variable IgG subclass deficiencies
Gastro-intestinal symptoms	
Diarrhoea, failure to thrive, food intolerance	Variable subclass deficiencies
Allergic disease	
Bronchial asthma	↓IgG2,3,4
Atopic eczema, dermatitis	↑IgG4
Vasculitis, including Henoch-Schönlein purpura	Variable subclass deficiencies
Autoimmune diseases	↓IgG2
(diabetes mellitus type I)	↓IgG3
Neurological disorders	
Treatment refractory epilepsy	↓IgG2
Friedreich's ataxia	↓IgG3
Ataxia telangiectasia	↓IgG2/IgG4
Miscellaneous immunodeficiencies	
Inherited deficiency of classical complement. Pathway components	↓IgG4
C3 deficiency	↓IgG2
IgA deficiency	↓IgG2/IgG4/IgG3
Post bone marrow transplantation	Variable IgG subclass deficiencies
Adenosine deaminase deficiency	↓IgG2

3. **Ans. (a) Hyper IgE** *Ref. Ananthanarayan 10/e p 178*
   Hyper IgE syndrome
   - Characterized by unusually high serum IgE level (usually 10 times)
   - Patient present with early onset eczema and recurrent bacterial infection such as abscess, pneumonia
   - Organism responsible include *Staph aureus, Strep pyogenes*
   - Cellular and humoral immune system mechanism are normal.

   Other options
   X-linked agammaglobulinemia
   - First immunodeficiency disease to be recognised
   - Seen only in male infant

- Present with recurrent serious infection with pyogenic bacteria like pneumococci, streptococci, meningococci, pseudomones and *H. influenzae*
- Response to viral infection is normal
- All classes of immunoglobulins are grossly depleted in the serum
- **Management:** Initial administration of 300 mg of gammaglobulin per kg of body weight in three doses followed by monthly injection of 100 mg per kg.

Transient hypogammaglobulinemia of infancy:
- Abnormal delay in initiation of IgG synthesis in some infants
- Recurrent otitis media and respiratory infection are common disease.
- Spontaneous recovery occurs between 18 and 30 months of age
- Seen in both sexes

Hyper IgM

Include some X-linked and autosomal recessive disorders

Patients show increased susceptibility to infections and autoimmune processus such as thrombocytopenia neutropenia, haemolytic anemia and renal lesions.

4. **Ans. (a) IgG1** *Ref. Jawetz 27/e, p 137; Ananthanarayan 10/e, p 98*

   IgG
   - Most abundant serum immunoglobulin (80%) with molecular weight of 1,50,000 and half-life of 21 days.
   - Distributed equally between extravascular and intravascular compartment.
   - Carbohydrate content is less if compared to other Ig.
   - *IgG is divalent.*
   - They are distributed as G1 (65%) > G2 (23%) > G3 (8%) > G4 (4%).
   - The subclasses of IgG differ from one another in the size of hinge region and number and position of the interchain disulphide bond between the heavy chains.
   - *IgG2 is directed against polysaccharide antigen, so it is important in defence against encapsulated bacteria.*
   - IgG is produced in secondary response of immunity.

   > **Remember:**
   > - Most abundant Ig in newborns–IgG.
   > - Only immunoglobulin which crosses placenta – IgG
   > - Basic structure of all Ig is 2 pairs of polypeptide chains (2H and 2L).

5. **Ans. (d) IgM** *Ref. Ananthanarayan 10/e, p 100; Jawetz 27/e, p 137*
   - Main immunoglobulin produced early in the primary response.
   - **IgM**, composed of five H_2L_2 and 1 J chain and is heaviest immunoglobulin with molecular weight of 1000,000 (hence called millionaire molecule)
   - It has valency of 10 (effective valency - 5, due to steritic hindrance)
   - Its presence in the serum indicates recent infection (primary response).
   - IgM is present on the surface of virtually all uncommitent B-cells.
   - It is the most efficient immunoglobin for agglutinations, complement fixation.
   - It has *highest avidity* among all Ig.
   - *By 20th week, fetus produce IgM, IgD and receives maternal IgG so IgA and IgE are not present.*
   - Phylogenetically it is the oldest immunoglobulin class.
   - Treatment of serum with 0.12mM2 mercaptoethanol selectively destroys IgM. This is a simple method for differential estimation of IgG and IgM.

6. **Ans. (b) Light chain** *Ref. Ananthanarayan 10/e, p 101*
   - BJP are identified in urine by its characteristic property of coagulation when heated at 50°C and dissolved at 70°C.
   - BJP (abnormal Ig) are light chain of Ig (so may occur as kappa or lambda form) found typically in multiple myeloma.
   - But in one patient, chain is either kappa or lambda, never both.

7. **Ans. (b) and (d) Antibody excess and False-negative reaction** *Ref. Ananthanarayan 10/e, p 107*

   Zone phenomenon (seen in agglutination and precipitation) consists of 3 parts:
   i. **Prozone** = Ab excess = weak or absent precipitation reaction = False –ve
   ii. **Zone of equivalence** = peak amount of precipitation.
   iii. **Post zone** = Ag excess = weak or absent precipitation reaction.

8. **Ans. (d) IgA and IgG$_2$ deficiency** *Ref. Harrison 20/e p 2496*

    "IgG subclass deficiency may be suspected in children and adults who have a history of recurrent infections of the ears, sinuses, bronchi and/or lungs."
    - Antibodies against the polysaccharide, coating (capsule) of certain disease-producing bacteria (e.g. the pneumococcus and Haemophilus influenzae) are predominantly of the IgG$_2$ type.
    - These patients are unable to produce protective levels of antibody when immunized with unconjugated polysaccharide vaccines against Streptococcus pneumoniae (the pneumococcus) or Haemophilus influenzae bacteria and are prone for infections by capsulated bacteria.
    - IgG$_2$ deficiency is frequently associated with deficiency of IgA.

    Note: Overall IgA deficiency is the most common primary immunodeficiency.

    See Ans 2 for details

9. **Ans. (c) IgM** *Ref. Ananthanarayan 10/e, p 100*

    IgM in comparison to IgG:
    - 500-1000 times more effective in opsonization
    - 100 times more effective in bactericidal action
    - 20 times more effective in bactericidal agglutination

    Note: A single molecule of IgM can bring immune hemolysis whereas 1000 molecule of IgG molecules are required for some effect

10. **Ans. (a) Good memory response** *Ref. Understand the immune system Elgert (wiley/Black well)*

    "Polysaccharide antigens are ineffective in producing immunogenic memory and this is the reason behind the protein conjugation of polysaccharide vacines."

    Carbohydrate Polysaccharide antigens:
    - T-cell independent antigens, hence they do not evoke T-cell response which is essential for memory response.
    - Usually present in bacterial cell wall and capsule
    - Stimulates B-cell directly without involving antigen presenting cells, or else produce polyclonal activation of B-cells.
    - Considerably less immunogenic in comparison to peptide antigen
    - Don't exhibit delayed type hypersensitivity
    - In large doses induce tolerance.

11. **Ans. (c) Immunological memory** *See below*
    - During the development of a primary immune respone to a pathogen, **memory cells are produced**.
    - These lie dormant in the lymphatic system for many years.
    - If they detect the same pathogen later on, they can clone rapidly and secrete antibodies.
    - So, secondary exposure to a pathogen produces a much enhanced and rapid secondary response which kills the bacteria before clinical symptom appear.
    - Vaccine takes advantage of this secondary response effect.
    - Vaccine contains antigen from pathogens, which induces the production of memory cells–giving protection from the same pathogen, if encountered later on in life.

12. **Ans. (b) Precipitation** *Ref. Ananthanarayan 10/e, p 107*

Serological reactions type		
	Precipitation	**Agglutination**
Pre-requisite	Soluble antigen, antibody, electrolytes, at suitable temperature and pH	Particulate antigen, antibody, electrolytes at suitable temperature and pH
Optimal proportion	Precipitation is abundant and rapid if antigen and antibody are present in optimal or equivalent proportion	Occurs optimally when antigens and antibodies react in equivalent proportion
Application	Sensitive test for detection of antigen (can detect as tittle as 1 µg protein). Therefore used in forensic applications for identification of blood and seminal stains, testing for food adultrants	Slide agglutination for blood grouping and cross matching. Tube agglutination is standard method for quantitative assessment of antibodies
Limitation	Relatively less sensitive for detection of antibody	More sensitive than precipitation for detection of antibodies

- Hemagglutination is a type of agglutination
- *Agglutination* (e.g. indirect HA) is *more sensitive* than precipitation (e.g. gel diffusion test) *for antibody* detection.

Remember:
Flocculation: – When instead of sedimenting, precipitate remains suspended as floccules, the reaction is known as flocculation.
Zone phenomen: – In agglutination reactions when either an antibody or antigen is in excess, agglutination does'ntoccur.
Passive agglutination: – The only difference between requirement for precipitation and agglutination reaction is the physical nature of antigen. By attaching soluble antigen to the surface of carrier particle, it is possible to convert precipitation test into agglutination test which are more sensitive for detection of antibodies. Such tests are known as passive agglutination tests.

13. **Ans. (c) Antigenic variation** *Ref. Harrison 17/e, p 2035*
    Learn it

14. **Ans. (b) and (c) Tumor necrosis factor - alpha and Tumor necrosis factor - beta**
    "MHC class genes is classified as Class I, Class II, Class III."

Products of Class III genes includes:	• C_2 and C_4 of classical pathway • Heat shock protein • Soluble protein of complement system • Properdin factor B of alternative pathway • TNF alpha and beta.

15. **Ans. (b) and (c) Fibrinogen and Haptoglobin**
    Ref. Ananthanarayan 10/e, p 83; Infectious disease by Jonathan 2/e, p 856; Greenwood 18/e, p 114

    Acute phase reactants (APR)
    - APR is the generic name given to a approx. 30 biochemically different and functionally unrelated proteins which are synthesized and secreted by hepatocytes. Their level in the serum are either increased (positive APR) or reduced (negative APR), approx. 90 minutes after the onset of systemic inflammatory reaction. Some important APR includes:
      i. C-reactive protein (B1 globulin)
      ii. α 1 Antitrypsin
      iii. Haptoglobin (α2 glycoprotein)   ↑ **with inflammation** (Positive APR)
      iv. Mannose binding protein
      v. Serum anyloid
      vi. α1 acid glycoprotein (orosomucoid)
      vii. Fibrinogen
      viii. Pre-albumin
      ix. Albumin   **Decreased with inflammation** (Negative APR)
      x. Transferrin

    These acute phase reactants enhance host resistance, prevent tissues injury, promotes repair of inflammatory lesions

16. **Ans. (d) Hypervariable region** *Ref. Harper 24/e, p 746; Ananthanarayan 10/e, p 96*
    - Each H and L chain of Ig consists of variable (V) region/domain and constant (C) region/domain.
    - H has 1 V_H and 3(CH1, CH2, CH3) constant region.
    - L has 1 V_L and $1C_L$ region.
    - V_H and V_L domain (formed by amino terminal portion) is specific antigen binding region (=Fab) (not antibody binding region as given in *Harrison, p 1922*)
    - V_L and V_H region have hypervariable regions (hot-spots=extreme sequence variability) that constitute Ag binding 'Site' (not region) unique to each Ig molecule (at tip).
    - L chain has 3 (in V_L) and H chain has 4 (in VH) Hypervariable regions. Also called as complementarity determinig regions (CDRs).
    - Idiotype is specific region of Fab portion to which antigen binds.
    - CH2 of IgG binds C1q in classical component, CH3 domain mediates adherence to monocyte surface.
    - The area of H chain in C region between CH1 and CH2 is hinge region which cleaves by papain to form 1Fc and 2 Fab fragments.

17. **Ans (a), (b) (c) Specific, secondary response is rapid, variable region of Ig is involved in Ab production**
    Ref. Ananthanarayan 10/e, p 161; Greenwood 18/e, p 122

    Clonal selection theory of immune response
    - During development B and T cells acquire specific cell surface receptor that commit them to a single antigen specificity. The lymphocytes are activated when they bind to their specific antigen.
    - The lymphocyte reactives to any particular antigen, are only a small proportion of the total pool.
    - When an antigen is encountered, the cell specific for that antigen gets activated, and trigger proliferation of cells with an identical genetic makeup (clones). This phenomenon is called as *clonal selection.*
    - *During embryonic life the lymphocyte clones acting against self-receptor are eliminated,* such clones are called *forbidden clones.*
    - For the mechanism of regulation of antibody response *network hypothesis* was postulated, according to which variable region of Ig carrying the antigen binding site is different in different antibodies. The distinct AA sequence at the Ag combining sites and the adjacent part of variable region are termed iditype. The idiotype in turn acts as antigenic determinent and can induce antidiotypic antibodies. These, in turn can induce antibodies against them and so on forming an idiotype network.
    - Immunological memory is another consequence of clonal selection, due to which secondary response is rapid and heightened.
    - Genetic basis of all this can be explained by *split genes.*

18. **Ans (c) Changes in heavy and light chain in constant region responsible for class and subtype** *Ref. Ananthanarayan 10/e p 91*

    Isotopic specificities
    - The antigenic specificities which distinguish between the different classes and subclasses of immunoglobulin present in all individual of a species,. e.g. Antigen specificity of IgA and IgG.
    - They are located on (Constant) domains of Ig chains in all individual.

    Other immunoglobulin Specificity
    - *Idiotypic specificity*
        – Specificity of greatest biological importance is idiotypic specificity, pertaining to the nature of antigen binding site. These are located on V region.
    - *Allotypic-specificity*
        – Antigenic specificity which distinguishes immunoglobulins of the same class, between different groups of individual in the same species.

19. **Ans (d) Directly attached to lateral aspect of TCR β chain** *Ref. Ananthanarayan 10/e, p 92; Jawetz 27/e p 134*

    Superantigen
    - Superantigens are certain antigens that can interact with antigen presenting cells and T-cells in non-specific manner.
    - Conventional antigens binds to the α β heterodimer groove of the MHC molecule through the V regions of TCR α and β chains, super antigens bind directly to the lateral aspect of the TCR β chain. Moreover, this activity does not involve the endocytic processing required for typical antigen presentation.
    - This interaction activates a larger number of T-cells (10%) than conventional antigen (about 1%) resulting in massive cytokine expression and immuno-modulation.
    - Various superantigens include: Staphylococcal enterotoxin, toxic shock syndrome toxin, etc.

    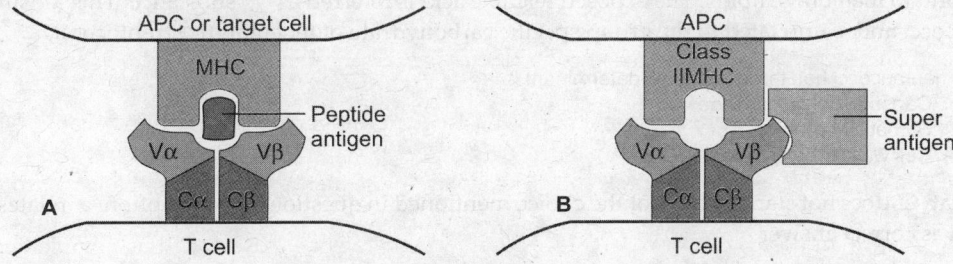

    Fig. A. Interaction between peptide antigen. MHC, and ther T cell eceptor.
    Fig. B. Interaction between a superantigen, MHC, and the T cell receptor

20. **Ans. (c) Equivalent of antigen and antibody** *Ref. Ananthanarayan 10/e, p 107*

    "Amount of precipitate formed is greately influenced by the relative proportions of antigen and antibodies, Precipitation reaction is rapid and abundant when antien and antibody are *present* in optimal or equivalent proportion."

Prozone : Zone of antibody excess
Peak : Zone of equivalence
Post zone: Zone of antigen excess

21. **Ans (a; d) Western blot; ELISA** *Ref. Ananthanarayan 10/e, p 107*
    Precipitation reactions are seen in:
    - Agglutination
    - Precipitation
    - Complement fixation
    - ELISA
    - Immunofluorescene (Director/indirect)
    - Radioimmunoassay
    - Chemiluminescence immunoassay (CLIA)
    - Immunoblot techniques e.g. western blot
    - Immunochromatographic test
    - Immune electron microscopy tests

22. **Ans. (b) Distal part of alpha chain** *Ref. Ananthanarayan 10/e p 142*
    MHC I/HLA I
    - Class 1 molecule consists of a three domains of heavy alpha peptide chain (a1; a2; a3) which are non-covalently linked to smaller β_2 microglobulin peptide.
    - The *distal domain* (alpha 1 and alpha 2) of MHC 1 have highly variable amino acid sequences and are folded to form a cavity or groove. Protein antigens are bound to this groove for presentation to CD8 T cells.

    MHC II/HLA II
    - MHC II antigens are heterodimer consisting of an alpha and beta chain. Each chain has two domain proximal one is constant and distal one is variable.
    - The two *distal domain* (alpha 1 , beta 1) *constitute the antigen binding site*, for recognition by CD4 T cells.
    - Both class 1 and class 2 are members of immunoglobulin gene super family.

    MHC III/HLA III
    - MHC III are heterogenous they include complement components involved in the formation of C3 convertase, heat shock protein and tumor necrosis factor.

23. **Ans. (a) Capsular polysaccharide of S. pneumoniae** *Ref. Ananthanarayan 10/e p 226*
    'C' Reactive protein
    An abnormal protein (beta 1 globulin) that precipitates with the somatic 'C' antigen of pneumococci, appears in the acute phase of pneumonia and disappears during convalescence. This protein found in other conditions also is called as C-reactive protein, where C stands for the C substance of pneumococci. This C-RP is not an antibody, rather a acute phase reactant synthesised in liver in response to bacterial infection, inflammation.

    What is C substance?
    Cell wall of pneumococci contains two types of teichoic acid; one exposed on the cell surface and the other similar form covolently bound to membrane lipids. The exposed teichoic acid is referred as 'C' substance. This 'C' substance is common to all pneumococci and is unrelated to the group specific carbohydrate of β hemolytic streptococci.

    > **Remember:** Pneumococci has three antigenic determinants:
    > - Capsular polysaccharide
    > - Somatic M protein
    > - Cell wall carbohydrate

    So it is clear that 'C' does not stand for any of the choice mentioned in question, as only option 'a' relates it to pneumococci it can be taken as correct answer.

24. **Ans. (b) IgM** *Ref. Jawetz 27/e p 98*
    IgM is the first antibody to be produced, after exposure to both antigen or allergin
    "IgM is the first antibody formed in every response"   ...Medical Microbiology by BS Napoba
    Thogh ovaalbumin is an allergin, its initial injection would produce IgM first, then IgE. If it is injected again IgE production would be first response.

25. **Ans. (a, c, d and e) Stimulation of Toll-like receptors, Increase both adaptive and innate immune response, Activate both B and T lymphocyte, Ensure prolonged delivery of antigen**

[Ref: Ananthanarayan 10/e p 152: Medical microbiology by Greenwood 16/e110, 671]

Role of Adjuvants
- Adjuvants are substances that stimulate the immune response, They enhance the immunogenicity of a vaccines for example, by facilitating uptake into antigen-presenting cells.
- Adjuvants are essential for enhancing and directing the adaptavie immune response to vaccine antigens, which is mediated by both B and T cells
- Due to the variety of mechanism and links between the innate and adaptive immune response, an adjuvant-enhanced innate immune response results in an enhanced adaptive immune response.
- **Adjuvants exert their immune-enhancing effects by following immune-functional activities:**
  1. Adjuvants help in the translocation of antigens to the lymph nodes where they can be recognized by T cells. Thereby producing greater T cell activity
  2. Adjuvants provide physical protection to antigens which grants the antigen a prolonged delivery. This means that the cell will be exposed to the antigen for a longer duration.
  3. They increase the capacity to cause local reactions at the injection site (during vaccination), inducing greater release of danger signals like chemokines.
  4. They induce the release of inflammatory cytokines which helps to not only recruit B and T cells at sites of infection but also to increase transcriptional events leading to a net increase of immune cells as a whole.
  5. Finally they are believed to increase the innate immune response to antigen by interacting with pattern recognition receptors (PRRs), specifically Toll-like receptors (TLRs), on accessory cells.

26. **Ans. (c) Differential RNA processing** *Ref. Internet*

Membrane bound versus secreted immunoglobulin
- A primitive B-cell (virgin B cell) bears IgM (and possibly IgD) in its membrane; however after stimulation, it begins to secrete IgM into its surrounding environment.
  These two form of IgM are different:
- The secreted form of IgM has a different C-terminal sequence which, lacks a membrane anchoring region.
- Membrane bound IgM is not capable of associating with J Chain and forming its normal pentameric structure. So, membrane bound IgM remains exclusively in monomeric form.
  These two forms differs basically in their *mu*-chain which is synthesized to via an alternative splicing scheme.

Other options
- *Allelic Exclusion:* Though diploid cells have two copies of every immunoglobulin gene, only one of the two is expressed in a given B cell. This allelic exclusion ensures the symmetry of antibody.
- *Class switching:* A particular antibody forming cell can switch from production of IgM to IgG from IgD to IgA, etc. In this switch only CH (heavy chain) changes, so that the original combining site remains same, however gets associated with a molecule of a different class or subclass.

Note: Such switching is undirectional, i.e. once IgM cell begin to secrete IgG, it can't go back to secrete IgM.

27. **Ans. (a) C3b and Fc** *Ref. Robbin's 8/e 202*
- Cells coated by antibodies are cleared through phagocytosis. These bacterial cells are recognized by phagocytic Fc receptors.
- In addition when IgM on IgG antibodies are deposited on the surfaces of cells they may activate the complement system by the classical pathway and generates C3b and C4b.
- C3b and C4b gets deposited over the surface of bacterial cell and are recognized by the phagocytes. The net result is phagocytosis.

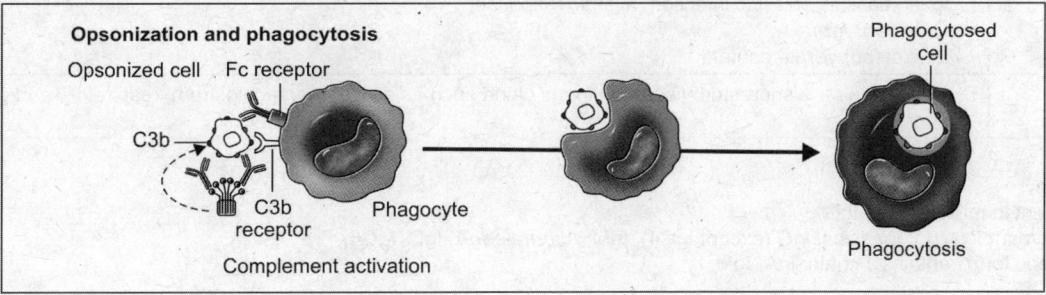

Remember: Antibody mediated destruction of cells may occur by antibody dependent cellular cytotoxicity (ADCC) also, where cells are lysed with out phagocytosis. ADCC is mediated by monocytes, neutrophills, eosinophils and NK cells.

28. **Ans. a and d, i.e. Widal test, ELISA** *Ref. Ananthanarayan 10/e 110*

    Heterophile Antigen: Similar antigen present on dissimilar organisms are heterophile antigens.
    Heterophile Antibodies: Antibodies reacting with heterophile antigens are called heterophile agglutinations.
    Heterophile Agglutination: Antibodies derived from one species reacting with heterophile antigen of another species causing agglutination.
    Example: Agglutination of horse RBCs by the heterophile antibodies present in infectious mononucleosis patient serum.

Heterophile Agglutination Tests		Application
Weil-Felix reaction	– Typhus rickettsiae, some strains of proteus bacilli	– Serodiagnosis of Typhus fever
Paul-Bunnell test	– Sheep horse red cell agglutinins in the serum of infectious mononucleosis patient	– Infectious mononucleosis
Cold Agglutination test	– Test is positive in mycoplasma pneumoniae. The patients sera agglutinate human O group erythrocytes at 4°C, the agglutination is reversible at 37°C	– Mycoplasma
Streptococcus Mg agglutination test	– For diagnosis of primarily atypical pneumonia	

Serological test	Type	Used to diagnose
i. Ascolis Thermoprecipitin test	Ring precipitation	Anthrax
ii. Lancefield test	Ring precipitation	Grouping of streptococci
iii. Kahn flocculation test	Tube precipitation	Syphilis
iv. VDRL test	Slide precipitation	Syphilis
v. Paul-Bunnell test	Tube agglutination	Infectious mononucleosis
vi. Rose-Waaler test	Passive hemagglutination	Rheumatoid arthritis
vii. Widal test	Tube agglutination	Typhoid
viii. Weil-Felix test	Heterophile tube agglutination	Rickettsiae
ix. Wassermann reaction	Complement fixation test	Syphilis

29. **Ans. (a, d and e) IgM is produced..., IgG is main..., IgA protects...** *Ref. Ananthanarayan 10/e 99*

IgM	• Antigen receptor on B cells • Useful for diagnosing congenital infections • **Earliest Ig** to be synthesized by fetus • Increased in **primary** response • **Max** sedementation coefficient, max molecular weight and max intravascular distribution. • Exhibits strong classical complement fixation, opsonization, agglutination, lysis, immunohemolysis.
IgG	• Max serum conc. and half-life • Ig increase in **secondary** immune response and is opsonizing antibody. • Only Ig which **crosses placenta** so its presence in fetus indicates immunity not infection. • Exhibits strong precipitation and neutralization reaction.
IgE	• Ig increase in parasitic infection, allergic response • Only **heat labile** Ig • Max carbohydrate content
IgA	• Only Ig which is secreted by seromucinous gland such as saliva, tears, colostrum, respiratory and gastrointestinal secretions.

Remember:
- Ig present in milk: IgA and IgG
- Complement fixation: *Classical IgG* (except IgG4), IgM; *Alternate IgA*, IgD, IgG4.
- Polymeric form contains J chain: IgA, IgM.

30. Ans. (c) Both Anti-A and Anti-B antibody *Ref. Ananthanarayan 10/e 193*

	Distribution of ABO antigen and antibodies in red cells and serum				
	Red cells			**Serum**	
Group	**Antigen present**	**Agglutinated by serum of group**		**Antibody present**	**Agglutinates cells of group**
A	A	B, O		Anti-B	B, AB
B	B	A, O		Anti-A	A, AB
AB	A and B	A, B, O		None	None
O	None	None		Anti-A and Anti-B	A, B, AB

31. Ans. (d) Cross placenta *Ref. Ananthanarayan 10/e 100*

IgE
- 8S molecule immunoglobulin with a half-life of two days and molecular weight of about 190,000
- Structurally resemble IgG
- Heat labile and affinity for the surface of tissue cells
- Susceptible to mercaptoethanol.
- Does not cross the placental barrier or fix complement.
- Mostly extravascular in distribution.
- Mainly produced by linings of respiratory and intestinal tracts.
- IgE is responsible for type I hypersensitivity.
- Protect against pathogens by mast cell degranulation. Believed to have a special role in defence against helminth infections.

32. Ans. (b) 1 Fc and 2 Fab
(see below)

Antibody Fragmentation
The performances of certain immunoassay procedures are enhanced by using antibody fragments, such as Fab and $F(ab')_2$. Antibody fragmentation is accomplished using reducing agents and proteases that digest or cleave certain portions of the immunoglobulin protein structure.

Antibody fragments of primary interest are:
a. Antigen-binding fragments such as Fab and
b. Class-defining fragments such as Fc that do not bind antigen.

Technique of antibody fragmentation
a. **Papain digestion:**
   A nonspecific, thiol-endopeptidase defragment IgG molecules into three fragments of similar size: two Fab fragment and one Fc fragment.
b. **Pepsin digestion:**
   A nonspecific endopeptidase produces one $F(ab')_2$ fragment and numerous small peptides of the Fc portion. The resulting $F(ab')_2$ fragment is composed of two disulfide-connected Fab units.
c. **Ficin digestion**
   A thiol protease that can digest mouse monoclonal IgG1 into either $F(ab')2$ or Fab fragments, depending on the concentration of cysteine included.

Types of antibody fragments
- **$F(ab')_2$ fragments:** $F(ab')_2$ (110,000 daltons) fragments contain two antigen-binding regions joined at the hinge through disulfides. This fragment is void of most, but not all, of the Fc region.
- **Fab' fragments:** Fab' (55,000 daltons) fragments can be formed by the reduction of $F(ab')_2$ fragments. The Fab' fragment contains a free sulfhydryl group that may be alkylated or utilized in conjugation with an enzyme, toxin or other protein of interest. Fab' is derived from $F(ab')_2$.
- **Fab fragments:** Fab (50,000 daltons) is a monovalent fragment that is produced from IgG and IgM, consisting of the VH, CH1 and VL, CL regions, linked by an intramolecular disulfide bond.
- **Fv fragments:** Fv (25,000 daltons) is the smallest fragment produced from IgG and IgM that contains a complete antigen-binding site. Fv fragments have the same binding properties and similar three-dimensional binding characteristics as Fab.
- **Fc fragments:** Fc (50,000 daltons) fragments contain the CH_2 and CH_3 region and part of the hinge region held together by one or more disulfides and noncovalent interactions. Fc and Fc5μ fragments are produced from fragmentation of IgG and IgM, respectively. The term Fc is derived from the ability of these antibody fragments to crystallize. The Fc fragment cannot bind antigen, but it is responsible for the effector functions of antibodies, such as complement fixation.

NEET Pattern Questions

1. Most abundant immunoglobulin in human body:
   a. IgM
   b. IgG1
   c. IgG2
   d. IgG3
   [Ref. Ananthanarayan, 10/e, p 98]

   IgG contribute 80% of the total serum immunoglobulins. There are four subclasses IgG1, IgG2, IgG3, IgG4 which are disbributed in human serum in the approximate proportions of 65%, 23%, 8% and 4% respectively.

2. When a particulate antigen combines with an antibody in approximate proportion, the resulting reaction is:
   a. Agglutination
   b. Prozone phenomenon
   c. Precipitation
   d. Flocculation
   [Ref. Ananthanarayan, 10/e, p 109]

3. Immunoglobulin changes in variable region:
   a. Idiotype
   b. Isotope
   c. Allotype
   d. Epitope
   [Ref. Ananthanarayan, 10/e, p 102]

   Variability of amino acid sequence in the variable region from the sepcific antigen binding site idiotype

4. Maximum half life:
   a. IgG
   b. IgA
   c. IgM
   d. IgE
   [Ref. Ananthanarayan, 10/e, p98]

5. Pentameric structure:
   a. IgM
   b. IgG
   c. IgA
   d. IgD
   [Ref. Ananthanarayan, 10/e, p100]

   IgM are polymers of five four peptide subunits, each bearing on C_H domain

6. Which of the following immunoglobulin is responsible for opsonisation:
   a. IgA
   b. IgG
   c. IgM
   d. IgE
   [Ref. Ananthanarayan, 10/e, p 100]

   IgM is 500–100 times more effective in opsonization.

7. Immunoglobulin isotype class switching is determined by:
   a. Constant region of light chain
   b. Constant region of heavy chain
   c. Variable region of light chain
   d. Variable region of heavy chain
   [Ref. Ananthanarayan, 10/e, p 101]

8. Antigen idiotype is related to:
   a. Fc fragment
   b. Hinge region
   c. C-terminal
   d. N-terminal
   [Ref. Ananthanarayan, 10/e, p 97]

   Amino terminal variable region of light and heavy chains participates in antigen recognition. Carboxyl terminal constant region of heavy chain mediates the effector functions.

9. Haptens are immunogenic when they covalently bind to: **[NEET Pattern 2016]**
   a. Lipid carrier
   b. Polysaccharide carrier
   c. Protein carrier
   d. Any of the above carrier
   [Ref. Ananthanarayan 10/e, p 89]

10. Nagler reaction is type of:
    a. Neutralization reaction
    b. CFT
    c. Precipitation
    d. Agglutination
    [Ref. Ananthanarayan, 10/e, p 114]

11. Coombs test is:
    a. Precipitation test
    b. Agglutination test
    c. CFT
    d. Neutrilization test
    [Ref. Ananthanarayan, 10/e, p 111]

12. Most sensitive test for antigen detection is:
    a. RIA **[NEET Pattern 2016]**
    b. ELISA
    c. Immunofluorescence
    d. Passive hemagglutination
    [Ref. Ananthanarayan 10/e, p 115]

    RIA permits the measurement of analytes (antigen) up to picogram quantities.

13. Monoclonal antibody binds to:
    a. Epitope
    b. Paratope
    c. Both epitope and paratope
    d. None of the above *[Ref. Ananthanarayan, 10/e, p 90]*

    Paratope is on antibody.

Ans.
1. b. IgG1
2. a. Agglutination
3. a. Idiotype
4. a. IgG
5. a. IgM
6. c. IgM
7. b. Constant region...
8. d. N-terminal
9. d. Any of the above...
10. a. Neutralization
11. b. Agglutination test
12. a. RIA
13. a. Epitope

14. Which of the following is agglutination test:
    a. Widal test   b. VDRL
    c. Ascoli test   d. Kahn test
    [Ref. Ananthanarayan, 10/e, p 109]

15. Prozone phenomenon is seen with:
    a. Same concentration of antibody and antigen
    b. In antigen excess to antibody
    c. Antibody excess to antigen
    d. Hyperimmune reaction
    [Ref. Ananthanarayan, 10/e, p 107]

16. Quantitative estimation of antibody is done by:
    a. Ziehl-Neelsen procedure
    b. Ouchterlony procedure
    c. Halden procedure
    d. Spaulding procedure

> **Ouchterlony procedure:**
> - Diffusion of both antigen and antibody in two dimensions.
> - It is used to detect identity, cross reaction, and non-identity between different antigen in a reacting mixture.
> - It is one of the simplest technique to determine the presence of an antibody in serum.

17. Gammaglobulins are synthesized in:
    a. Liver   b. Lung
    c. Plasma cells   d. Spleen
    [Ref. Jawetz, 27/e, p 138]

18. Antigen-antibody binding occurs at:
    a. Surface   b. Center
    c. Inside molecule d. Anywhere in structure
    [Ref. Ananthanarayan, 10/e, p 104]

19. IgE binds to which cell:
    a. T cells   b. B cells
    c. Mast cells   d. NK cells
    [Ref. Jawetz, 27/e, p 137]

> Fc region of IgE binds to the high affinity receptor or the surface of mast cells.

20. Neutralization test is:
    a. Widal test   b. Weil-Felix test
    c. Paul Bunnell test d. Nagler reaction
    [Ref. Ananthanarayan, 10/e, p 114]

> Nagler reaction is a neutralization test for identification of alpha toxin of Cl. perfringens
> Note: Schick test is another neutralization test.

21. Which of the following is a superantigen:
    a. Exfoliative toxin of Staphylococcus
    b. Lipopolysaccharide of gram negative bacteria
    c. Enterotoxin of V cholerae
    d. Shiga toxin of EHEC   [Ref. Ananthanarayan, 10/e, p 93]

22. Rose-Waaler test is:
    a. Complement fixation test
    b. Pricipitation in gel
    c. Ring precipitation   [Ref. Ananthanarayan, 10/e, p 112]
    d. Passive hemagglutination test

> Rose-Waaler test is passive hemogglutination test for detection of RA factor.

23. Example of agglutination test:
    a. Widal test   b. Schick test
    c. VDRL test   d. Ascoli test
    [Ref. Ananthanarayan, 10/e, p 110]

24. Example of precipitation test is:
    a. Rose-Waaler test
    b. Widal test
    c. Latex agglutination
    d. Kahn test   [Ref. Ananthanarayan, 10/e, p 107]

25. Immunoglobulin variation does not depend on:
    a. Light chain
    b. Heavy chain
    c. Amino acid sequence
    d. Constant region [Ref. Ananthanarayan, 10/e, p 96]

26. Molecular mass of IgG (in K Da):
    a. 150   b. 400
    c. 1000   d. 1500
    [Ref. Ananthanarayan, 10/e, p 98]

27. Weil-Felix reaction is:
    a. Heterophile agglutination
    b. Tube precipitation test
    c. Slide agglutination test
    d. Tube agglutination test
    [Ref. Ananthanarayan, 10/e, p 111]

> Can be done as either a slide or tube method.

28. Lattice phenomenon is seen in:
    a. Neutralization reaction
    b. Complement fixation test
    c. Precipitation test
    d. All of the above   [Ref. Ananthanarayan, 10/e, p 105]

29. Which is an example of antigen-antibody reaction:
    a. Flocculation reaction
    b. Precipitation
    c. Agglutination
    d. All of the above   [Ref. Ananthanarayan, 10/e, p 104]

30. Which of the following is a complement fixation test:
    a. Wassermann test for syphilis
    b. VDRL test for syphilis
    c. Kahn test for syphilis
    d. Rose-Waaler test for RA
    [Ref. Ananthanarayan, 10/e, p 113]

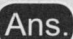

Ans.
14. **a.** Widal test	15. **c.** Antibody excess...	16. **b.** Ouchterlony...	17. **c.** Plasma cells	18. **a.** Surface
19. **c.** Mast cells	20. **d.** Nagler reaction	21. **a.** Exfoliative toxin...	22. **d.** Passive hemag...	23. **a.** Widal test
24. **d.** Kahn test	25. **d.** Constant region	26. **a.** 150	27. **a.** Heterophile...	28. **c.** Precipitation...
29. **d.** All of the above	30. **a.** Wassermann...			

CHAPTER 38

Hypersensitivity

Hypersensitivity is defined as immunologic tissue injury in response of subsequent exposure with the allergen (shocking or challenge dose). It is of following types:

Types	Mechanism and Effects	Examples
1. Type I (Immediate or reaginic HSN) Systemic acute anaphylaxis — Local anaphylaxis = atopy	• **Ab** - IgE (cytotropic) • **Cells** - IgE B cell, mast cells, basophils, eosinophil • **Pivotal role** - by $T_H 2$ cell • Most important **vasoactive amine**: Histamine • Slow reacting substance of anaphylaxis **(SRS-A)** = Leukotrienes **(LT B_4, C_4, D_4, E_4)**	• Urticaria; angioedema; hay fever and some forms of asthma; eczema • Anaphylactic shock • Casoni's test, • Theobald Smith phenomenon • Schultz Dale phenomenon • Prausnitz Kustner (PK) reaction
2. Type II [cytotoxic or cytolytic] HSN a. Complement dependent	• **Ab:** IgG or IgM • Lysis or phagocytosis by opsonization • Most commonly involves blood cells (**Mnemonic:** II HSN involves blood: b is second alphabet)	• Transfusion reactions • Erythroblastosis fetalis (Hemolytic disease of neonates) • AI hemolytic anemia or agranulocytosis or thrombocytopenia; • Pemphigus syndrome • Bullous pemphigoid • Pernicious anemia • Thrombotic phenomenon • Acute rheumatic fever • Some forms of vasculitides and certain drug reactions.
b. Type VI HSN = Antibody dependent cell mediated cytotoxicity (ADCC)	• **Ab** - usually IgG sometimes IgE • Cell lysis without phagocytosis by monocytes, neutrophil, eosinophils and NK cells	• Phagocytosis of tumor cells or parasite • Some role in graft rejection
c. Type V HSN = Antibody mediated cellular dysfunction.	**Antireceptor Antibody** • Stimulation • Inhibition	• Thyrotoxicosis/Graves' diseases • Myasthenia gravis
3. Type III [Immune complex] HSN Local immune complex disease [= Arthus reaction] Systemic immune complex [Serum sickness]	• **Ab** - IgG or IgM • Ag-Ab complex activate complement → attack neutrophil → release of lysosomal enzymes	• SLE • Certain forms of acute glomerulonephritis • Rheumatoid arthritis • Hyperacute graft rejection • Hypersensitivity pneumonitis • Infective endocarditis • PAN • Henoch-Schonlein purpura • Schick test • Type 2 lepra reaction (ENL)
4. Type IV [Cell mediated] HSN a. Delayed type by CD4 $T_H 1$ - Induration is its characteristic	• Ab - No antibody • Initiated by specifically sensitized T lymphocytes	• Tuberculin test • Lepromin test • Fairleys (Schistosomiasis) test • Frie's (LGV) test • Granulomatous inflammation • Contact dermatitis • Defense against intracellular pathogen • Type I lepra reaction
b. Cell mediated cytotoxicity by CD - 8 T cells		• Graft rejection • Resistance to virus infection • Tumor immunity

* HSN: Hypersensitivity

Multiple Choice Questions

1. Which of the following is false? [AI 95]
   a. Theobald-Smith phenomenon is a type I hyper-sensitivity reaction
   b. Serum sickness is a type II hypersensitivity reaction
   c. Allograft rejection is a type IV hypersensitivity reaction
   d. Transfusion reaction is a type II hypersensitivity reaction

2. Hemolytic disease of newborn is which type of hypersensitivity reaction? [PGI June 07]
   a. Type - I   b. Type - II
   c. Type - III   d. Type - IV
   e. Type - V

3. Skin test is used for which hypersensitivity reaction? [PGI June 07]
   a. I   b. II
   c. III d. IV

4. Skin test based on neutralization reaction is/are:
   a. Casoni test   b. Lepromin test
   c. Tuberculin test d. Schick test
   [NEET 18 pattern]

5. Disorders of phagocytosis are all, except:
   a. Job's syndrome [PGI May 2013]
   b. Chediak-Higashi syndrome
   c. Myeloperoxidase deficiency
   d. Wiskott-Aldrich syndrome
   e. Tuftsin deficiency

6. Anaphylaxis is mediated by: [PGI May 2013]
   a. 5-hydroxytryptamine b. Heparin
   c. Prostaglandin   d. Platelet activating factor

Explanations and References with Illustrative Answers

1. **Ans. (b) Serum sickness is type II HSN** *Ref. Taylor 3/e, p 119*

Type of Rejection	Type of HSN	Target Sites in Transplantation
Hyperacute rejection (preformed Ab against donor transplantation Ag)	Type II cytotoxic Type III HSN	Small blood vessels in donor tissues
Acute rejection	Type II cytotoxic	Parenchymal cells
	Type III HSN	Small blood vessels
Chronic rejection	Type III HSN	Small blood vessels
	Type IV HSN	

2. **Ans. (b) Type - II** *Ref. Taylor 3/e, p 107*

Type I HSN (IgE mediated)	Type II HSN (IgG and IgM mediated)
• Eczema • Hay fever • **Asthma** (atopy) • Urticaria • Anaphylactic shock • Acute dermatitis • **Theobald Smith phenomenon** • PK (**Prausnitz Kustner**) reaction • Casoni's skin test • **Schultz** Dale phenomenon	• **Blood transfusion reactions** • Erythroblastosis fetalis • **AI Hemolytic anemia** or agranulocytosis or thrombocytopenia • Pemphigus vulgaris • **Good Pasture** syndrome • Bullous pemphigoid • Pernicious anemia • **Acute rheumatic** fever • Diabetes mellitus • **Graves disease** • Myasthenia gravis

Contd...

Contd...

Type III HSN (IgM or IgG mediated)	Type IV HSN (cell mediated)
• Local - **Arthus** reaction	• Tuberculin skin test
• **Systemic-serum sickness**	• Lepromin skin test
• Lepromin skin test	• Contact dermatitis
• Schick skin test	• Jones Mote reaction (**cutaneous basophilic HSN**)
• PAN	• **TB**
• **Rheumatoid** arthritis	• Sarcoidosis
• SLE	• Temporal arteritis
• Acute viral hepatitis	• Patch test
• Penicillamine toxicity	• **Granulomatous inflammation**
• **Hyperacute graft rejection**	• Type I lepra reaction
• Type 2 lepra reaction (ENL)	
• Hypersensitivity pneumonitis	

Type V hypersensitivity: Stimulatory hypersensitive. Here the antibody activates receptor sites and enhance the activity of the cell.
Example: Long acting thyroid stimulation which stimulates excessive secretion of thyroid hormone.

3. **Ans. (a), (c) and (d) I, III and IV** *Ref. Taylor 3/e, p 107; Jawetz 24/e, p 142-43*
   Already explained

4. **Ans. (d) Schick test** *Ref. Ananthanarayan 7/e, p 103, 8/e, p 111*

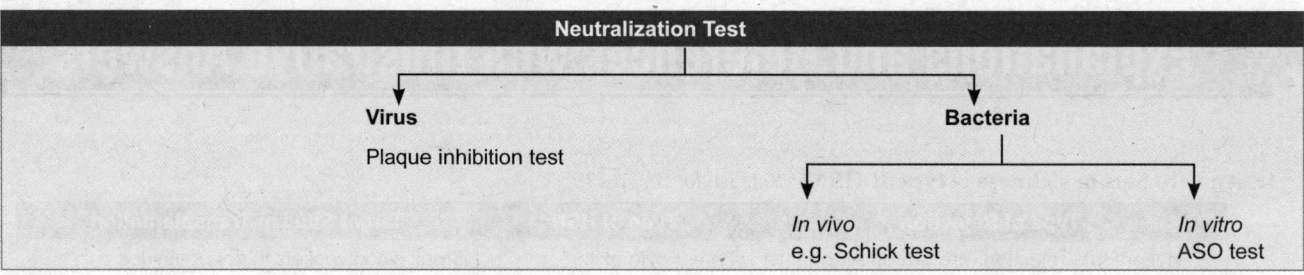

- Bacterial exotoxin can be neutralized (e.g. diphtheria, tetanus) while endotoxins can't be neutralized by antitoxin.

5. **Ans. (d) Wiskott-Aldrich syndrome** *Ref. Ananthanarayan 10/e, p 177*
   Disorders of phagocytosis:
   - Chronic granulomatous disease
   - Myeloperoxidase deficiency
   - Chediak-Higashi syndrome
   - Leukocyte G6PD deficiency
   - Job's syndrome
   - Tuftsin deficiency
   - Lazy leukocyte syndrome
   - Hyper-IgE syndrome
   - Actin binding protein deficiency
   - Shwachman's disease

6. **Ans. (a, b, c, d), All options** *Ref. Ananthanarayan 9/e, p 164; Robbins 7/e, p 209*
   Mediators of Anaphylactic Reaction
   a. **Primary mediators** (These are present in mast cell granules) Includes:
      - Biogenic Amines   : Histamine, 5 Hydroxytryptamine
      - Enzymes   : Neutral protease (Chymase, tryptase) and several acid hydrolases
      - Proteoglycans   : Heparin

b. **Secondary mediators:**
   - Leukotrienes : LTC4, D4, B4
   - Prostaglandin D_2
   - Platelet activating factor
   - Cytokines : IL1, IL3, IL-4, IL-5, IL-6 TNF and GMCSF

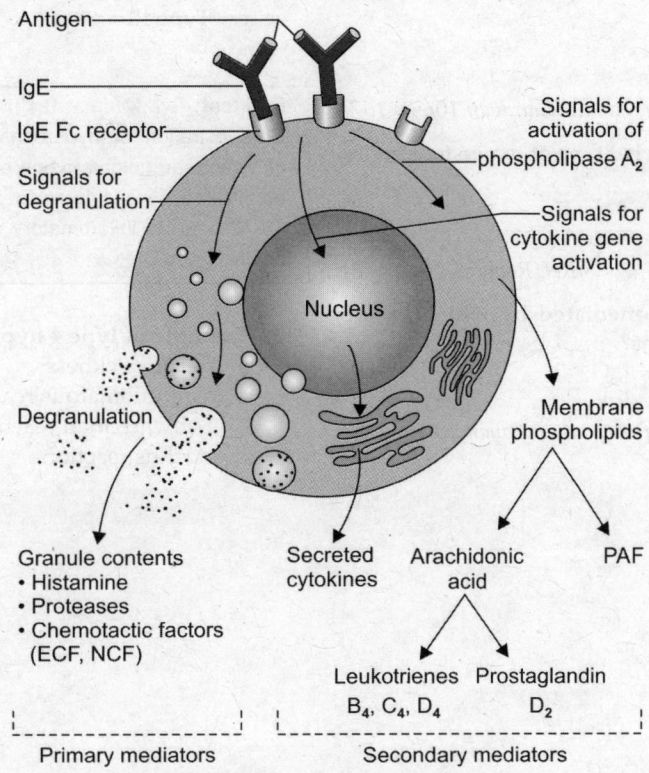

Mediators of Anaphylactic Reaction

NEET Pattern Questions

1. Type IV hypersensitivity includes all, except:
   a. Paul Bunnell test
   b. Lepromin test
   c. Tuberculin test
   d. Granulomatous reactions
   [Ref. Ananthanarayan 10/e, p 167]

2. Wheal and flare reaction is what type of hyperstensitivity reaction?
   a. Type I
   b. Type II
   c. Type III
   d. Type IV
   [Ref. Robbins 8/e, p 128]

3. Type I hypersensitivity is mediated by which of the following immunoglobulins?
   a. IgA
   b. IgG
   c. IgM
   d. IgE
   [Ref. Ananthanarayan 10/e, p 165]

4. Frei test which type of hypersensitivity?
   a. Type I
   b. Type II
   c. Type III
   d. Type IV
   [Ref. Ananthanarayan 10/e, p 426]

Frei test:
Demonstration of hypersensitivity by skin testing in a patient of lymphogranuloma venereum. In this test a heat inactivated LGV 0.1 ml is infected intradermally on the forearm. After 48-72 hour an inflammatory nodule > 60 mm diameter suggests positive result.

5. Example of type 4 hypersensitivity is:
   a. Serum sickness
   b. Granulomatous reaction
   c. Schwartzman reaction
   d. Arthus reaction
   [Ref. Ananthanarayan 10/e, p 169]

Ans.
1. a. Paul Bunnell test
2. a. Type I
3. d. IgE
4. d. Type IV
5. b. Granulomatous...

SECTION B

UNIT VI

Miscellaneous

- Miscellaneous

CHAPTER 39

Miscellaneous

Multiple Choice Questions

1. Which of the following is not transmitted by soil?
   a. Coccidiodomycosis   b. Tetanus   [AI 08]
   c. Brucella   d. Anthrax

2. Isolation is not useful for all *except*:   [AI 08]
   a. Mumps   b. Measles
   c. Hepatitis A   d. Pneumonic plague

3. Congenital infection affecting fetus with minimal teratogenic risk is: [AI 08]
   a. HIV   b. Rubella
   c. Varicella   d. CMV

4. Which of the following congenital infection leads to maximum CNS damage in the fetus: [AI 08]
   a. Rubella and CMV
   b. Rubella and toxoplasmosis
   c. CMV and toxoplasmosis
   d. HIV and CMV

5. With reference to *Bacteroides fragilis* the following statements are true *except*:
   [AI 07; AIIMS 06, AIIMS 2011, 2012]
   a. *B. fragilis* is the most frequent anaerobe isolated from clinical samples
   b. *B. fragilis* is not uniformly sensitive to metroni-dazole
   c. The lipopolysaccharide formed by *B. fragilis* is structurally and functionally different from the conventional endotoxin
   d. Shock and disseminated intravascular coagulation are common in *Bacteroides* bacteremia

6. Which of the following is least likely to cause infective endocarditis: [AI 06]
   a. *Staphylococcus albus*
   b. *Streptococcus faecalis*
   c. *Salmonella typhi*
   d. *Pseudomonas aeruginosa*

7. A 40-year-old woman presented to the gynecologist with complaint of profuse vaginal discharge. There was no discharge from the cervical os on the speculum examination. The diagnosis of bacterial vaginosis was made based upon all of the following findings on microscopy *except*:   [AI 06]
   a. Abundance of gram variable coccobacilli
   b. Absence of Lactobacilli
   c. Abundance of polymorphs
   d. Presence of clue cells

8. Apart from *Escherichia coli*, the other most common organism implicated in acute suppurative bacterial peritonitis is: [AI 06]
   a. *Bacteroides*
   b. *Klebsiella*
   c. *Peptostreptococcus*
   d. *Pseudomonas*

9. All cause malabsorption syndrome *except*:
   [AIIMS May 09, May 10]
   a. Giardiasis   b. *Ascaris*
   c. *Strongyloides*   d. *Capillaria phillipinesis*

10. All of the following organisms are known to survive intracellularly *except*:   [AI 05]
    a. *Neisseria meningitides*
    b. *Salmonella typhi*
    c. *Streptococcus pyogenes*
    d. *Legionella pneumophilia*

11. Virus can be isolated from clinical samples by cultivation in the following *except*:   [AI 05]
    a. Tissue culture
    b. Embryonated eggs
    c. Animals
    d. Chemically defined media

12. It is true regarding the normal microbial flora present on the skin and mucous membranes that: [AI 05]
    a. It cannot be eradicated by antimicrobial agents
    b. It is absent in the stomach due to acidic pH
    c. It establishes in the body only after the neonatal period
    d. The flora in the small bronchi is similar to that of the trachea

13. The most common pathogens responsible for nosocomial pneumonia in the ICU: [AI 05]
    a. Gram +ve organism
    b. Gram −ve organism
    c. Mycoplasma
    d. Virus infections

14. Which of the following is the common cause of acute prostatitis: [NEET Pattern 2018]
    a. Peptostreptococci
    b. S. agalactiae
    c. Neisseria gonorrhoea
    d. S. agitans

15. All vaccines developed from embryonated eggs *except*:
    a. Influenza   b. Hepatitis A   [AIIMS 2018]
    c. Yellow fever   d. Rabies
    e. CMV

16. Plaque formation in virus is done for:
    a. Isolation and typing of viurses   [NEET Pattern 2018]
    b. Cloning separation of specific viruses
    c. Determining infectivity of virus
    d. Assessing multiplication of virus

17. Which of the following are bacteria?   [PGI June 09]
    a. Bacteriophage   b. Chlamydia
    c. Mycoplasma   d. Spirochete

18. The following diagnostic tests are useful for corresponding purpose *except*:   [NEET Pattern 2018]
    a. Ziehl-Neelsen staining - Detection of mycobacteria
    b. Immunofluorescence - Detection of Influenza virus
    c. Specific IgM antibodies - Immunity against Rubella
    d. Specific IgM antibodies - Detection of acute infection

19. All of the following are sexually transmitted *except*:
    a. *Candida albicans*   [AI 12]
    b. *Echinococcus granulosus*
    c. *Molluscum contagiosum*
    d. Group B *Streptococcus*

20. All of the following infections may be transmitted via blood transfusion *except*:   [AIIMS 09]
    a. Parvo B-19   b. Dengue virus
    c. CMV   d. Hepatitis G virus

21. Normal commensal of skin: [PGI June 08]
    a. *Staph. aureus*   b. *Candida albicans*
    c. *Bacteroides fragilis*   d. *Propiobacterium*
    e. *Corynebacterium*

22. Most common agents responsible, for human, bite infections are: [PGI 07]
    a. Gram –ve bacilli   b. Gram +ve bacilli
    c. Spirochaete   d. Anaerobic streptococci

23. Prokaryotes differs from eukaryotes in being: [PGI 12]
    a. Absence of nuclear membrane
    b. Presence of microvilli on its surface
    c. Presence of smooth endoplasmic reticulum
    d. All of the above

24. HACEK group includes all of the following *except*:
    a. *Hemophilus arophilus*   [AIIMS 08]
    b. *Acinetobacter baumanni*
    c. *Eikenella corrodens*
    d. *Cardiobacterium hominis*

25. Cy Bromide green dye is used for: [AIIMS 06]
    a. HLPR   b. PCR
    c. ELISA   d. Immunofluorescence

26. The single most common cause of pyrexia of unknown origin is: [AIIMS 06, 03]
    a. *Mycobacterium tuberculosis*
    b. *Salmonella typhi*
    c. *Brucella* sp.
    d. *Salmonella paratyphi A*

27. In the gut, anaerobic bacteria outnumber the aerobes by a ratio of: [AIIMS 06]
    a. 10: 1   b. 100: 1
    c. 1000: 1   d. 10,000: 1

28. In all of the following diseases chronic carriers are found *except*:   [AIIMS 06]
    a. Measles   b. Typhoid
    c. Hepatitis B   d. Gonorrhea

29. Humoral immunodeficiency is suspected in patient and he is under investigation. Which of the following infections would be consistent with the diagnosis: [AIIMS 15]
    a. Giardiasis
    b. Pneumocystis carinii pneumonia
    c. Recurrent sinusitis
    d. Recurrent subcutaneous abscess

30. All the following are common nosocomial infection *except*:   [AIIMS 03]
    a. Staph. aureus   b. P. aeroginosa
    c. Enterobacteriaceae   d. Mycobacterium

31. Latent infection is seen in viral infections *except*:   [PGI Dec 08]
    a. HSV-2   b. CMV
    c. EBV   d. HIV
    e. Rotavirus

32. The term "viable not cultivable" (VNC) is used for:
    a. *M. leprae*   b. *M. tuberculosis*
    c. *Trepenoma pallidum*   d. *Salmonella*   [PGI Dec 07]
    e. *Staph.*

33. Microorganisms invading the GIT causing gastro-enteritis: [PGI Dec 07]
    a. EHEC
    b. *Shigella*
    c. *Vibrio parahemolyticus*
    d. *Campylobacter*
    e. *Salmonella*

34. Which of the following can cause rhabdomyolysis?
    a. *Clostridium perfringens*   [PGI June 07]
    b. *Streptococcus*
    c. *Clostridium difficle*
    d. *Cl. tetani*

35. Genital elephantiasis is seen in: [PGI 06]
    a. Donovanosis
    b. Lymphogranuloma venereum
    c. Congenital syphilis
    d. Herpes simplex

36. Rhinosporidiosis is caused by: [PGI 06]
    a. Fungus
    b. Bacteria
    c. Virus
    d. Protozoan
    e. Parasite

37. Which human infection spreads through urine:
    a. *Leptospira*
    b. *Legionella* [PGI 06]
    c. Plague
    d. Diphtheria

38. Urease test is positive in: [PGI 05]
    a. *H. pylori*
    b. *S. aureus*
    c. *Klebsiella*
    d. *Bacillus cereus*
    e. *Pseudomonas*

39. Resolution provided by light microscope is: [PGI 11]
    a. 200 nm
    b. 20 nm
    c. 0.2 nm
    d. 2.0 nm
    e. 120 nm

40. Pus cell in diarrhea seen in: [PGI 09]
    a. Vibrio cholera
    b. EPEC
    c. Rotavirus
    d. Shigella
    e. *Campylobacter*

41. Man is intermediate host in: [PGI 14]
    a. *Taenia saginata*
    b. *Trichenella spiralis*
    c. *Strongyloidis*
    d. *P. falciparum*

42. Capsulated organism: [PGI 15]
    a. *Candida*
    b. *Klebsiella*
    c. *Proteus*
    d. *Cryptococcus*
    e. *Histoplasma*

43. One virus particles prevents multiplication of 2nd virus. This phenomena is: [PGI 12]
    a. Viral interference
    b. Mutation
    c. Supervision
    d. Permutation

44. DNA covering material in a virus is called as: [NEET Pattern 2018]
    a. Capsomere
    b. Capsid
    c. Nucleocapsid
    d. Envelope

45. The virus causing gastroenteritis are: [PGI Dec 08]
    a. Rotavirus
    b. Norwalk virus
    c. Adenovirus
    d. Hepatadenovirus
    e. Enterovirus

46. A male patient presented with granulomatous penile ulcer. On Wright Giemsa stain tiny organisms of 2 microns within macrophages seen. What is the causative organism?
    a. LGV [AIIMS May 10]
    b. Calymmatobacterium granulomatis
    c. Neisseria
    d. Staph aureus

47. Which ones can be easily cultured from CSF? [PGI 09]
    a. Polio
    b. Coxsackie
    c. Echo
    d. Mumps
    e. Rubella

48. Which of the following does not have non human reservoirs: [PGI 09]
    a. Polio
    b. Pertussis
    c. Salmonella Typhi
    d. Neisseria
    e. Cl. tetani

49. Which of the following is best stain for fungus: [AIIMS Nov 09]
    a. Muciramine
    b. Methenamine silver
    c. Alcian blue
    d. Hematoxylin and eosin

50. A patient with history of discharge from right ear for past 1 year presented with severe earache. The discharge was cultured and the organism was found to be gram positive cocci. The least likely cause is? [AI 2011]
    a. Pseudomonas
    b. Streptococcus pneumoniae
    c. Staphylococcus
    d. Haemophilus influenzae

51. Most common cause of meningo-encephalitis in children is: [AI 2011]
    a. Arbo virus
    b. Entero virus
    c. HSV
    d. Polio virus

52. Correct combination of incubation period is:
    a. Sypillis : 9-90 days [PGI 2011]
    b. Herpes genitalis : 4-5 weeks
    c. LGV : 3 day-6 weeks
    d. Donovanosis : 1-4 weeks
    e. Chancroid : 2-3 weeks

53. With reference to antibiotic resistance all of following statements are true *except*: [AI 12, AIIMS 11, May 12]
    a. The most common mechanism is production of neutralizing enzymes by bacteria
    b. Plasmid mediated resistance is exclusively transferred vertically
    c. Complete elimination of target is the mechanism by which enterococci develop resistance to vancomycin
    d. Alteration of target leisons leads to development of resistance in pneumococci

54. Which organism cannot be cultured in cell free media:
    a. Klebsiella rhinoscleromatis [PGI 2011]
    b. Klebsiella ozaenae
    c. Treponema pallidum
    d. Pneumocystis jiroveci
    e. Rhinosporidium seeberi

55. The endotoxin of the following gram negative bacteria does not play any part in the pathogenesis of the natural disease. [AIIMS Nov 2012]
    a. E. coli
    b. Klebsiella
    c. Vibrio cholerae
    d. Pseudomonas

518 Self-Assessment and Review of Microbiology and Immunology

56. Which of the following is not a common case of neonatal sepsis in India: [AIIMS 2013]
    a. Staphylococci   b. Klebsiella
    c. E.coli   d. Group B Streptococci

57. Common stain for fungal hyphae: [AIIMS 2013]
    a. Methylene blue
    b. Gomori Methenamine silver
    c. Congo red
    d. Oil red O

58. Real Time PCR is used for: [AIIMS 2013]
    a. Multiplication of RNA
    b. Multiplication of specific segments of DNA
    c. Multiplication of Proteins
    d. To know how much amplification of DNA has occurred

59. True about mechanism of bacterial toxins:
    a. Cholera toxin acts by inhibition of guanyl cyclase
    b. Botulinum toxin inhibits Ach release
    c. Shiga toxin of shigella dysenteriae act by inhibiting protein synthesis [PGI 2013]
    d. Diphtheria toxin act by inhibiting protein synthesis

60. Duration of isolation for bacterial meningitis?
    a. Until culture is negative [AIIMS 2018]
    b. 24 hrs of antibiotic treatment
    c. 7 days of subside of fever
    d. 3 days of neck rigidity

61. Incubation period of LGV: [AIIMS 2018]
    a. 3-12 days   b. 15-45 days
    c. 1 month   d. 6 months

Explanations and References with Illustrative Answers

Section - B

1. **Ans. (c) Brucella**   *Ref. Park 22/e, p 265*

   Modes of transmission of Brucella:
   - *Contact infection (MC)*: Through direct contact with infected tissue, blood, urine, vaginal discharge. Mostly occupational.
   - *Food borne infection*: Through ingestion of raw milk, dairy products.
   - *Air borne infection*: In the environment of slaughter house.

   Infection transmitted through soil:
   - Man-soil-man–All the disease transmitted fecorally, e.g. typhoid, hepatitis A, etc.
   - Soil as storehouse of spores–tetanus, mycosis, botulism.

2. **Ans. (d) Pneumonic plague**   *Ref. Park 22/e, p 112*

Periods of isolation recommended	
Disease	**Duration of isolation**
Chickenpox	Until all lesions crusted; usually about 6 days after onset of rash
Measles	From the onset of catarrhal stage through 3rd day of rash
German measles	None, except that women in the first trimester or sexually active, non-immune women in child-bearing years not using contraceptive measures should not be exposed
Cholera, Diphtheria	3 days after tetracyclines started, until 48 hours of antibiotics (or negative cultures after treatment)
Shigellosis Salmonellosis	Until 3 consecutive negative stool cultures
Hepatitis A	3 weeks
Influenza	3 days after onset
Polio	2 weeks adult, 6 weeks pediatric
Tuberculosis (sputum +)	Until 3 weeks of effective chemotherapy
Herpes zoster	6 days after onset of rash
Mumps	Until swelling subsides
Pertussis	4 weeks or until paroxysms cease
Meningococcal meningitis / Streptococcal pharyngitis	Until the first 6 hours of effective antibiotic therapy completed

3. **Ans. (a) HIV**   *Ref. Dutta 6/e, p 301*

   HIV has got no teratogenic effect on fetus.

Viral infection in pregnancy:

Infection	Fetal effect
Rubella	Sensoneural deafness
Varicella	Septal defect, PDA, cataract, retinopathy
CMV	Hypoplasia of limbs, limb deformity, choroidoretinal scarring, cataract, microcephaly
Parvo virus	IUGR, microcephaly, Intracranial calcification, Mental retardation, choriodoretinitis, deafness
Mumps	Aplastric crisic, CHF, hydrops
HIV	No ill effect on fetus

4. **Ans. (b) Rubella and toxoplasmosis** *Ref. Dutta 6/e, p 296, 299*
   - Among Rubella and CMV, rubella is mainly associated with cardiac anomalies while CMV is associated with CNS anomalies.
   - Toxoplasmosis leads to hydrocephalus, choriodoretinitis, cerebral calicfication, microcephaly and mental retardation.

5. **Ans. (d) Shock and disseminated intravascular coagulation are common in Bacteroides bacteremia**
   Ref. Ananthanarayan 10/e, p 274

   Anaerobic Gram negative bacilli. includes Bacteroides, Fusobacterium, Leptotrichia, Prophyromonas, Prevatella.

   Bacteroides
   MC anaerobe isolated from clinical specimen.
   - They are Non-sporing, Non-motile, strict anaerobes and capsulated (Virulence factor).
   - They are classified on *the basis of colonial, biochemical features (Sacchrolytic effects) and on characteristics of short chain fatty acid patterns in gas liquid chromatography.*
   - MC isolate of *Bacteroides* is *B. fragilis.*
   - They grows well on media such as brain heart infusion agar in an anaerobic atmosphere containing 10% Co_2.
   - *B. fragilis* (also *Prevotella melaninogenic*) possess **lipopolysaccharides (endotoxin)** that are **less biologically potent than endotoxins associated with aerobic gram negative bacteria.** Due to this relative biologic inactivity, infection caused by *Bacteroides* less frequently *produce the clinical signs of sepsis.*
   - *First line therapy* for anaerobes includes Metronidazole, Ticarcillin/Clavulanic acid, Piperacillin/tazobactan, Imipenem.
   - Resistance to metronidazole is seen in <2% cases, i.e. not uniformly sensitive.   ... *Harrison 18/e, p 1338, 19/e, p 1101*

6. **Ans. (c) *Salmonella typhi*** *Ref. Harrison 20/e, p 922*

   Though both salmonella and pseudomonas cause endocarditis, pseudomonas is a more common etiologic agent than salmonella.

Organism causing endocarditis		
• Streptococci **(MC)** (60-80%):	– S. viridans (30-40%) – Other streptococci (15-25%)	– Enterococci (5-18%)
• Staphylococci (20-35%):	– Coagulase positive (10-27%)	– CoNS (1-3%)
• Gram negative bacilli (1.5-13%):	– Enterobacteriaceae	– Pseudomonas
• HACEK Group of Organisms		
• Fungi	– Candida	– Cryptococcus

   Remember:
   - Among streptococci **MC** cause are S. sanguis, S. bovis, S. mutans, S. mitior.
   - Among enterobacteriaeeae **MC** cause – Salmonella.
   - P. aeroginosa is **MC** gram negative bacilli causing endocarditis.

7. **Ans. (c) Abundance of polymorphs** *Ref. Shaw's 13/e, p 129; COGDT 10/e, p 670*

   Bacterial Vaginosis
   - Defined as alteration in normal vaginal flora rather than true infection
   - Causative organism:
     – *G. vaginalis*
     – *H. vaginalis*
     – *Mobiluncus*
   - **Microscopy of vaginal secretions** in *bacterial vaginosis* shows:
     – Characteristic **clue cells**
     – Decreased or absent lactobacillus
     – Decreased leucocytes.

- **Clinical criteria for diagnosis:**
  - Homogenous white non inflammatory discharge with fishy odour.
  - Microscopic presence of >20% clue cells.
  - Vaginal discharge with pH > 4.5
  - Fishy odor with or without addition of 10% KOH.
- **Treatment:** Metronidazole for both pregnant and non-pregnant women.

> **Remember:**
> - Clue cells represent epithelial cells adherant to G. vaginalis.
> - Bacterial vaginosis is most prevalent vaginal infection.

8. **Ans. (b) Klebsiella**   [Ref. CSDT 13/e, p 465; Harrison 20/e, p 953]
   Causative organism of acute bacterial peritonitis:

Aerobic (30%)	Anaerobic (10%)
• E. coli **(MC)** • Klebsiella • Enterococci	• Bacteroides • Peptostreptococci • Enterococci

> **Remember:** In 60% of cases mixed anaerobic and aerobic infection is found.

9. **Ans. (b) Ascaris**   Ref. Journal of digestive disease and sciences 53(3) March 2008 672-679

Parasites causing Malabsorption	
Adults	**Children**
• Giardia lamblia (MC) • E. histolytica/dispar • Ankylostoma duodenale • H. nana • Stronglyoids* • Capillaria philipinesis**	• Giardia lamblia (MC) • Cryptosporidium • E. histolytica/dispar • A. duodenale

10. **Ans (c) Streptococcus pyogenes**   See below

Intracellular organisms			
a. Bacteria	**b. Parasites**	**c. Viruses are obligate intracellular parasite**	**d. Fungi**
• **L**isteria monocytogens • **L**egionella • **R**ickettsia • **M**ycobacteria TB and mycobacteria leprae • **C**hlamydia • **N**eisseria meningococci and Gonococci • **Y**ersinia pestis • **B**ordetella • **S**almonella • Calymmatobacterium Gronunomatis (**D**onovania) • **S**higella • **B**rucella • **P**neumococci	• Babesia • Plasmodium • Cryptosporidium parvum • Microsporidia sp. • Toxoplasma		• Histoplasma capsulatum

> **Mnemonic:** LLRM Medical College Ne Yaha Bulakar, SDS ko Bahut Pareshaan kiya.

> **Remember:** Cell Mediated Immunity play vital role against these organisms.

11. **Ans. (d) Chemically defined media**   Ref. Ananthanarayan 10/e, p 457
    Method of isolation consists of:
    "Inoculation into animals, eggs or tissue culture after the processed to remove bacterial contaminants."
    ..... *Ananthanarayan 8/e, p 450, 9/e, p 451*

    As many viruses (adenoviruses, enteroviruses) are frequently found in normal individuals, so only recovery of viral agent from patient doesn't prove that it is the causative agent of the patient illness.

Organism not grown in artificial cultural media are:		
• **C**hlamydia • **P**athogenic **t**reponemes • **V**iruses.	• **R**ickettsia • M. **l**eprae	• **R**hinosporidium • **P**neumocystis

Mnemonic: Rahul Chalo TV Remote Lao Please

12. **Ans. (c). It establishes in the body only after the neonatal period** *Ref. Jawetz 27/e, p 169-170*
    - "Term normal microbial flora" denotes the population of microorganisms that inhabit the skin and mucous membranes of healthy normal persons. They are not essential to life.
    - MC resident organisms of upper respiratory tract is streptococci of viridans group.
    - MC resident bacteria of large intestine is bacteroides species.

    Lines from Jawetz clears all choice to you -

    "Mucus membranes of mouth and pharynx are often sterile at birth, within 4-12 hrs after birth, viridans streptococci become establish as most prominent member of resident flora and remain so for life."

    "In the pharynx and trachea, similar flora establish itself whereas few bacteria are found in normal bronchi. Small bronchi and alveoli are normally sterile."

    "Stomach acidity keep the number of microorganisms at a minimum (10^3-10^5) unless obstruction at the pylorus favours the proliferation of gram positive cocci and bacilli."

    "Antimicrobials drugs taken orally can, in humans, temporilly suppress the drug susceptible components of the fecal flora."

13. **Ans. (b) Gram –ve organisms** *Ref. Harrison, 19/e, p 810; 20/e, 1023*
    Guys, this is a twisted question, understand the choice clearly.
    - MC cause of nosocomial pneumonia in **ICU** now is *S. aureus* (Gram +ve)
    - After this comes enterobacteriaceae followed by *Pseudomonas aeruginosa* (Gram –ve).
        - But if we take Enterobacteriaceae and *P. aeruginosa* (Gram –ve organism) together they can outnumber *S. aureus* (Gram +ve organism).

    So, the answer will be *Gram –ve organism.*

    Note: Now word nosocomial has been replaced by hospital acquired pneumonia.

14. **Ans. (c) Neisseria gonorrhoeae**
    Acute Bacterial Prostatitis
    - Usually a complication of UTI
    - Microbiology resemble that of UTI
    - Commonest cause are:
        - E. coli (most common), Pseudomonas, Proteus sp, Klebsiela sp.
        - In patients with STD Neisseria gonorrheae and Chlamydia are also common
    - Disease usually ascend through infected urine. Prostatic biopsy is an important risk factor.

15. **Ans (b, e) Hepatitis A, CMV** *See below*

Vaccine	Source	Nature
Varicella	Tissue culture	Live attenuated
Polio		
– Salk	Tissue culture	Killed
– Sabin	Tissue culture	Live
Influenza		
Inactivated	Allantoic cavity of egg	Killed
Live	Egg	Live
Mumps	Chick embryo fibroblast culture	Live
Measles	Human diploid cells	Live
Rabies	Duck egg	Killed
	Chick embryo	
	Tissue culture	
Hepatitis A	Human diploid cell	Live
Hepatitis B	Genetically engineered Clone of S-gene	–
Rubella	Tissue culture	Live

16. **Ans. (c) Determining infectivity of virus** *Ref. Ananthanarayan 10/e, p 435*

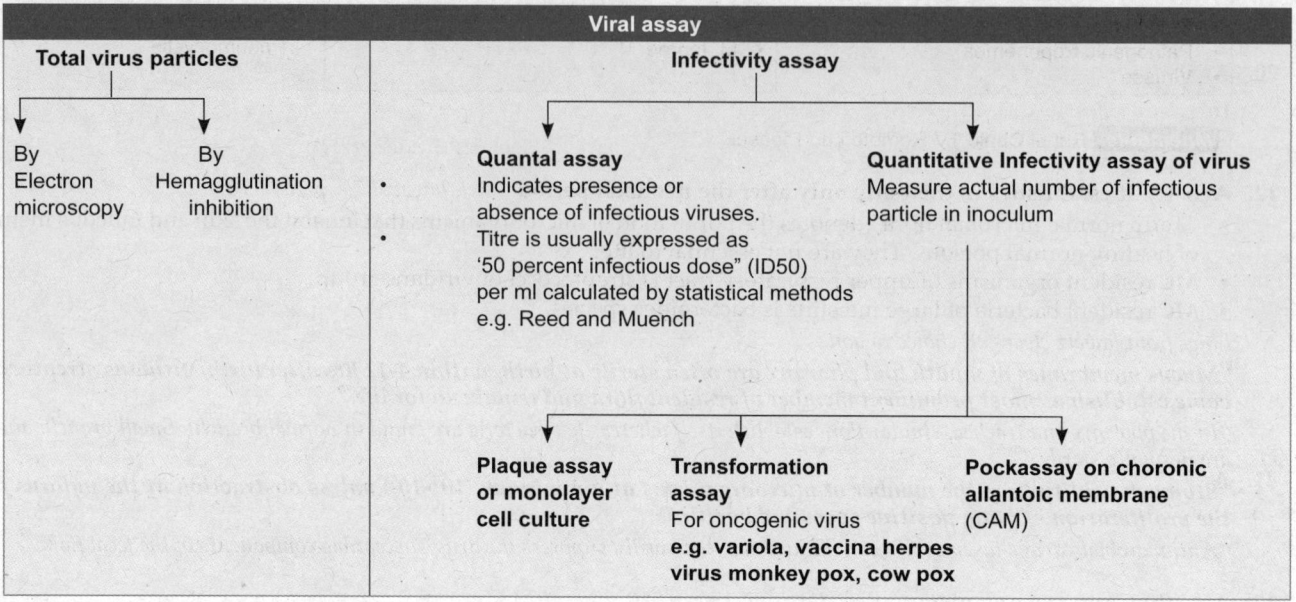

Plaque assay: Each infectious particle give rise to a localized focus of infected cells that can be seen with naked eye. Such foci are knows as plaque and each plaque indicates an infectious virus.

17. **Ans. (b, c) and (d)** *Chlamydia, Mycoplasma* **and Spirochete** *See below*
    Bacteriophage are virus infecting bacteria

18. **Ans. (c) Specific IgM antibodies - Immunity against Rubella** *Ref. Ananthanarayan 8/e, p 498, 9/e, p 555*
    - **Ziehl-Neelsen Staining** (Acid fast staining) is used for Mycobacteria detection.
    - Rapid diagnosis of Influenza is made by demonstration of virus antigen on the surface of nasopharyngeal cells by immunofluorescence.
    - IgM antibodies are antibodies of primary response (IgG is antibody of secondary response). So IgM indicates acute or recent infection. Its production signify that immune response of individual is proper but doesn't mean that person has immunity against that infection (e.g. Rubella).

19. **Ans. (b)** *Echinococcus granulosus* *Ref. Harrison 20/e, p 977*

Bacteria	Viruses	Other
TRANSMITTED IN ADULTS PREDOMINANTLY BY SEXUAL INTERCOURSE		
Neisseria gonorrhoeae	HIV (types 1 and 2)	Trichomonas vaginalis
Chlamydia trachomatis	Human T-cell lymphotropic virus Type I	Phthirus pubis
Treponema pallidum	Molluscum contagiosum virus	
Haemophilus ducreyi	Herpes simplex virus type 2	
Calymmatobacterium granulomatis	Human papillomavirus	
Ureaplasma urealyticum	Hepatitis B virus	
SEXUAL TRANSMISSION REPEATEDLY DESCRIBED BUT NOT WELL-DEFINED OR NOT the PREDOMINAT MODE		
Mycoplasma hominis	*Cytomegalovirus*	Candida albicans
Mycoplasma genitalium	HTLV - II	Sarcoptes scabiei
Gardnerella vaginalis and other	Hepatitis C, D viruses	
Vaginal bacteria	Herpes simplex virus type 1	
Group b Streptococcus	Epstein-Barr virus	
Mobiluncus spp.	Transfusion-transmitted virus	
Helicobacter cinaedi		
Sporothrix fennelliae		

Remember: E. granulosus spread by feco-oral route when eggs in dog's feces are ingested either by direct contact with infected dogs or by taking vegetable contaminated with dog's feces.

20. **Ans. (b) Dengue virus** *Ref. Harrison 20/e, p 815*

Infectious complications of blood transfusion

Viral infection	• Hepatitis C virus • Hepatitis G virus • TTV and SENV virus • Cytomegalovirus • Parovirus B-09 • Variant Creutzfeilt jakob disease	• Hepatitis B virus • Hepatitis A virus (rarely) • HIV • HTLV type I • West nile virus • Hepatitis E virus
Bacterial infection	• Syphilis • Pseudomonas • Lyme disease	• Yersinia • Gram +ve cocci including coagulase negative staphylococci.
Parasites	• Malaria • Trypanosoma cruzi	• Babesia • Toxoplasmosis

.....Harrison 17/e, p 1305

21. **Ans. (a, b, d) and (e) Staph. aureus; Candida albicans; Propiobacterium; Corynebacterium**

Ref. Ananthanarayn 10/e, p 625-626

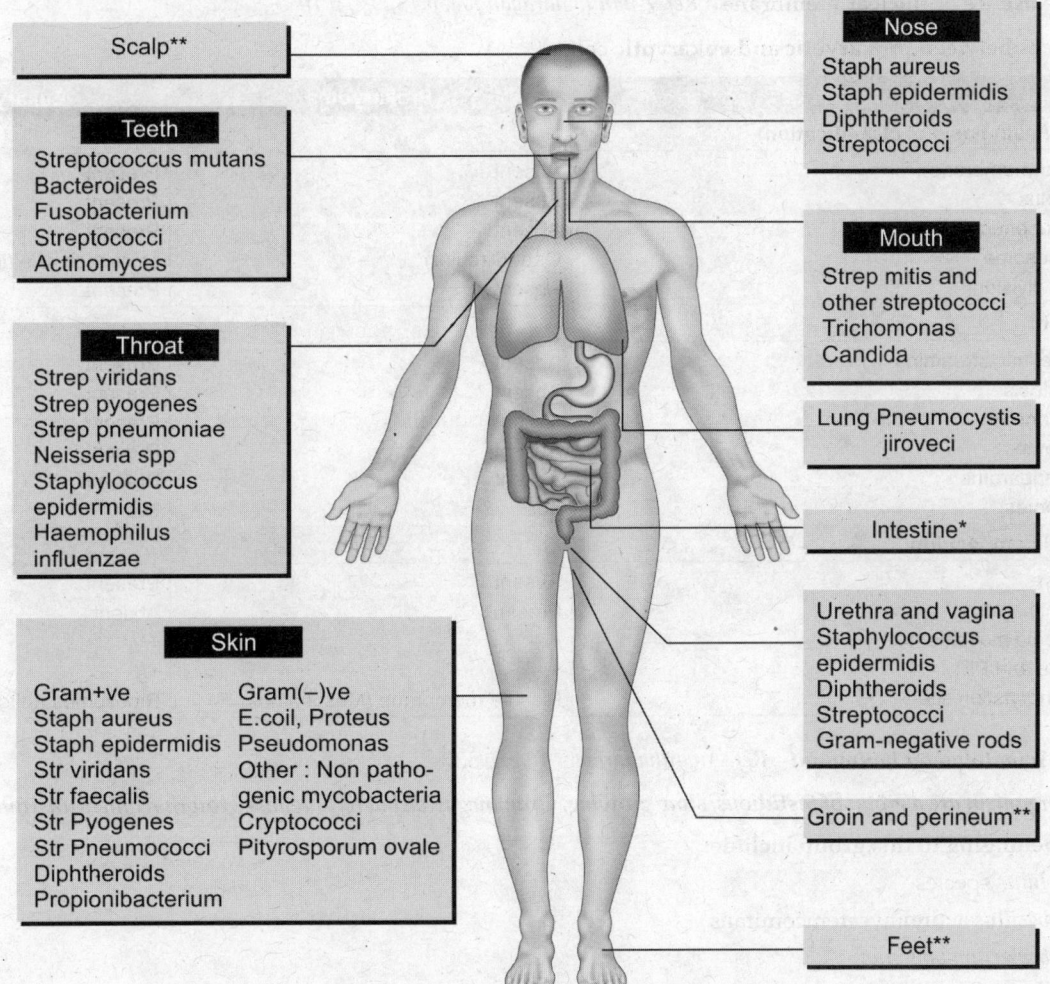

Normal microbial flora according to location.

22. **Ans. (d) Anaerobic streptococci**   *Ref. CMDT 2014, p 1243*

    Human bites
    - Human bites are usually inflicted by children; in adults bites are associated with alcohol use and closed fist injury.
    - Bites inflicted by children rarely get infected and bites by adults become infected in 15-30% of cases.
    - Bacteriology of bite infection:
        - Human bites are mixture of aerobes and anaerobes (54%) or due to aerobes only (44%).
        - *Streptococcus*, *staphylococcus* and *Eikenella corrodens* are most common aerobes.
        - *Prevotella* and *fusobacterium* are the most common anaerobe

    Remember:
    - Cat bites are most likely to become infected (30-50%)
    - Dog bite become infected only in 5% of cases.
    - Pasturella species are the single most common isolate in dog and cat bites.

    About the question
    This question is of 1998, at that time Harrison 15/e was running. In 15/e, Anaerobes (including pepto streptococcus) were given as more common, So, was the answer.

23. **Ans. (a) Absence of nuclear membrane**   *Ref. Ananthanarayan 8/e, p 13, 9/e, p 10*

    Differences between prokaryotic and eukaryotic cells

Character	Prokaryotes	Eukaryotes
Nucleus (Main basis of classification)		
Nuclear membrane	Absent	Present
Nucleolus	Absent	Present
Deoxyribonucleoprotein	Absent	Present
Chromosome	One (Circular)	More than one (linear)
Mitotic division	Absent	Present
Cytoplasm		
Cytoplasmic streaming	Absent	Present
Pinocytosis	Absent	Present
Mitochondria	Absent	Present
Lysosomes	Absent	Present
Golgi apparatus	Absent	Present
Ribosomes	70s	80s
Chemical composition		
Sterols	Absent	Present
Muramic acid	Present	Absent
Amoeboid movement	+/–	+/–
Flagella and Pilli	+/–	+/–
Phosphorylation site	Plasma membrane (Mesosomes)	Ribosomes (Mitochondria)

24. **Ans. (b) *Acinetobacter baumanni***   *Ref. Ananthanarayan 10/e, p 337*

    HACEK organism are a group of fastidious, slow growing, Gram negative bacteria whose growth requires an atmosphere of CO_2.

    Species belonging to this group include:
    - *Hemophilus* species
    - *Actinobacillus* actinomycetemcomitans
    - *Cardiobacterium hominus*
    - *Eikenella corrodens*
    - *Kingella kingae*
    - They are normally resident in mouth. Endocarditis is the *most common* disease caused by them.

25. **Ans. (b) PCR**   *See below*

Cy Bromide green dye is a dye that binds to minor groove of double stranded DNA and generates fluorescence.
Uses:
- To determine presence of amplified DNA product.
- For optimizing PCR reaction.

26. **Ans. (a) *Mycobacterium tuberculosis***   *Ref. Harrison 16/e, p 117, 18/e, p 159, 19/e, p 136*

    Fever of unknown origin
    Defined as:
    - Temperature > 38.3°C (> 101°F) on several occasions
    - Duration of fever > 3 weeks
    - Failure to reach diagnosis despite 1 week of inpatient investigations

Causes				
Infections (13%)	Neoplasm (7%)	Non-infectious inflammatory (22%)	Miscellaneous (7%)	Undiagnosed (51%)
• *Mycobacterium TB* • Abdominal abscess • Endocarditis • UTI • Viral infections: • CMV • EBV • Kala azar • Brucellosis	• Lymphoma • Leukemia • Solid tumours			

Infections such as extrapulmonary TB and in endemic areas: typhoid fever and malaria remain a leading diagnosable-cause of FUO.

27. **Ans. (c) 1000:1**   *Ref. Jawetz 25/e, p 162, 27/e, p 169*

    Anaerobes outnumber facultative organism by 1000 fold.

    Normal flora of intestinal tract
    - At *birth* the intestine is sterile, but organism are soon introduced after birth.
    - In breastfeed children lactic acid streptococci and lactobacilli seen.
    - Microorganism are *minimum* (10^3-10^5g/ of contents) in stomach.
    - In *upper intestine* lactobacilli and enterococci predominate.
    - In *colon Bacteroides fragilis* is the *most common* organism found.
    - Intestinal bacteria are important in synthesis of vitamin K.

28. **Ans. (a) Measles**   *Ref. Park 22/e, p 154*

    In measles and whooping cough only cases are found with no carriers.
    Chronic carriers seen in:
    - Typhoid
    - Dysentery
    - Hepatitis B
    - Cerebrospinal meningitis
    - Malaria
    - Gonorrhea

29. **Ans. (b) *Pneumocystis carinii* pneumonia**   *See below*

    Infection in patients with defects in humoral immunity:
    - Recurrent or chronic sinopulmonary infection otitis media, meningitis and bacteremia; *MC* by pyogenic bacteria such as *H. influenzae*; *Strep pneumoniae*; *Staphylococci*
    - Response to viral infection is good except increased risk of:
        - HBV
        - Polio
        - Echoviruses
        - Adenoviruses

- **Parasitic** – Giardial diarrhea
- Less frequent – Bacterial infection of skin and urinary tract.

Infection in patient with deficient cell mediated immunity:
- Disseminates virus infection of Herpes simplex, Varicella zoster, and CMV
- *Mucocutaneous candidiasis* – Almost invariably
- Pneumonia caused by *P. carinii*
- Severe Enteritis caused by Cryptosporidium
- T cell deficiency is always accompanied by some abnormality of antibody response so patient with T cell defect are also subject to overwhelming bacterial infection.

30. **Ans. (d)** *Mycobacterium* Ref. Harrison 20/e, p 1024
    - **Most important group of hospital pathogens are:**
        i. Enteric gram negative bacilli:
            - E. coli
            - Klebsiella
            - Enterobacter
            - Proteus
            - Serratia
        ii. S. aureus
        iii. *Pseudomonas aeruginosa* and other pseudomonas
        iv. Tetanus spores
        v. Yeast (*Candida albicans*), moulds (*Aspergillus mucor*)
        vi. Protozoa (*E. histolytica, Plasmodia, P. carinii, T. gondii*)

Nosocomial infection	Most common causative organism
Urinary tract infection (**MC Nosocomial infection**)	E. coli; Candida
Early onset pneumonia (within 4 days)	Strept pneumoniae
Late onset pneumonia	S. aureus, P. aeruginosa
Surgical wound infections	**S.aureus**, coagulase negative staphylococcus
Infections related to vascular acess	**Coagulase negative Staph**, S. aureus

Remember:
- ***Candida is now the MC pathogen in nosocomial UTI in ICU patients.***   ..... Harrison 19/e, p 914
- Examples of some emerging and potential, epidemic problems in hospitals are: Chickenpox TB, Group A streptococci, Aspergillus, Legionella

31. **Ans. (e)** Rotavirus   Ref. Ananthanarayan 10/e, p 451
    Latent Infection
    - Infection in which the infectious agents lies dormant within the host without *symptoms* (often without detectable presence in blood, tissue or other secretion) and without release from host.

Virus causing latent infection		
• HSV 1 and 2	• EBV	• CMV
• VZV	• HHV-6	• HHV-7
• HHV-8	• HIV	• Human papilloma virus
• Prions	• Slow virus infection	• Oncogenic virus

32. **Ans. (a) and (c)** *M. Leprae*, *Treponema pallidum*
    Already explained

33. **Ans. (b, c, d) and (e)** Shigella, *Vibrio parahemolyticus, Campylobacter* and *Salmonella*

Invasive Diarrhea		
Minimal inflammation	**Variable inflammation**	**Severe**
• Rotavirus • Norwalk agent	• Salmonella • Campylobacter • Aeromonas • Vibrio parahaemolyticus • Yersinia	• Shigella • EIEC • Entamoeba histolytica

34. **Ans. (a, b, d)** *Clostridium perfringens, Streptococcus* and *Cl. tetani*

Rhabdomyolysis			
Viral causes	**Bacterial causes**		**Fungal causes**
• Influenzae types A and B (most common) • HIV • Ebstein-Barr virus • Echovirus • Cytomegalovirus • Adenovirus • Herpes simplex virus • Parainfluenza virus • Varicella-zoster virus • Coxsackievirus	• *Francisella tularensis* • *Streptococcus pneumoniae* • Group B streptococci • *Streptococcus pyogenes* • *Staphylococcus epidermidis* • *Escherichia coli* • *Borrelia burgdorferi* • *Clostridium tetani* • *Viridans streptococci*	• *Rickettsia* species • *Salmonella* species • *Listeria* species • *Legionella* species • *Mycoplasma* species • *Vibrio* species • *Brucella* species • *Bacillus* species • *Leptospira* species	• Candida • Aspergillus

Infection associated with severe hemolysis are:

• **B**artonella • **C**lostridium welchii	• **M**alaria (*Plasmodium falciparum*) • **B**acteremia with *pneumococci, staphylococi, escherichia coli.*	• **B**abesiosis

35. **Ans. (a) and (b)** Donovanosis and Lymphogranuloma venerum *Ref. Ananthanarayan 8/e, p 396, 9/e, p 397*

Genital elephantiasis is seen in Donovanosis which is caused by Klebsiella granulomatis (Calymmatobacterium granulomatosis or Granuloma inguinale/venerum).

Donovanosis
- Chronic progressive bacterial infection of the genital region that is generally sexually transmitted.
- **Causative organism:**
  - *Klebsiella granulomatis (formerly called Calymmatobacterium granulomatis*: Gram negative, nonmotile, encapsulated bacterium.
  - Morphologically and antigenically related to Klebsiella.
  - Grow on egg yolk or modified levinthal agar.
- I.P. – 1-4 weeks.
- **Clinical features:**
  - Disease begin as one or more subcutaneous nodules that erode through the skin to produce clean ulcers, (sharply defined) which is usually painless lesion.
  - Genitalia are involved in 90% of cases.
  - Genital swelling particularly of labia is common and may progress to pseudoelephantiasis.
  - Complications include phimosis and paraphimosis.
- **Diagnosis:**
  - Diagnosis is made by demonstration of typical intracellular Donovan bodies (safety pin appearance) in Wright Giemsa stain.
- **Treatment:**
  - Azithromycin - *DOC.*
  - Doxycycline - Second *DOC.*

Remember:
- Genital elephantiasis is also seen in lymphatic filariasis.
- Vulval elephantiasis or esthiomene is seen in lymphogranuloma venerum

528 Self-Assessment and Review of Microbiology and Immunology

36. **Ans. (a) Fungus** *Ref. Ananthanarayan 10/e, p 607*
    - Rhinosporidiosis is a chronic granulomatous disease characterized by development of friable polyp usually confined to the nose, mouth or eye.
    - Polyp is highly vascular which bleeds easily on touch. Its surface is studded with white dots which represents the sporangia of fungus.
    - **Causative agent**
        - *Rhinosporidium seeberi*. The fungus has not been cultivated in media.
        - The infection is supposed to originate from stagnant water or aquatic life.
    - **Diagnosis:**
        - Biopsy shows round or oval sporangia filled with spores which may burst through chitinous wall.
    - **Treatment:**
        - Complete excision with diathermy knife and cauterization of its base.
        - Dapsone and Amphotericin B are also effective.

37. **Ans. (a) Leptospira** *Ref. See below*

Disease	Mode of infection
Leptospira	Water contaminated by the urine of carrier animals enter the body through cut or abrasions on the skin or through intact mucosa of mouth, nose or conjunctiva.
Legionella	Inhalation of aerosols produced by AC, cooling towers.
Plague	Bite of rat flea, droplet infection
Diphtheria	Droplet infection

38. **Ans. (a, b, c) *H. pylori*, *S. aureus* and *Klebsiella*** *Ref. See below*

    Urease test is positive in urease producing bacteria which includes:
    i. **P**roteus
    ii. **S**. aureus
    iii. **M**organella
    iv. **K**lebsiella
    v. **Y**ersinia
    vi. **C**ryptococcus
    vii. **D**iptheroids
    viii. **M**ycobacterium except MAC
    ix. **H**. Pylori

    Mnemonic: PSM KY CD Meri Hai

39. **Ans. (a) 200 nm** *Ref. See below*

    Resolving power are:
    Light microscope   –   0.25 µm–0.3 µm   =   200–300 nm
    Electron microscope –   2–10 Å   =   0.2–1 nm

40. **Ans. (d) and (e) *Shigella* and *Campylobacter***

    ### GASTROINTESTINAL PATHOGENS CAUSING ACUTE DIARRHEA

Mechanism	Location	Illness	Stool findings	Examples of pathogens involved
Noninflammatory (enterotoxin)	Proximal small bowel	Watery diarrhea	No fecal leukocytes; mild or no increase in fecal lactoferrin	Vibrio cholerae, enterotoxigenic *Escherichia coli* (LT and /or ST), *Clostridium perfringens*, *Bacillus cereus*, *S. aureus*, shigelloides, rotavirus, Norwalk-like viruses, enteric adenoviruses, *Giardia lamblia*, *Cryptosporidium* spp., microsporidia

    Contd...

Contd...

Mechanism	Location	Illness	Stool findings	Examples of pathogens involved
Inflammatory (invasion or cytotoxin)	Colon or distal small bowel	Dysentery or inflammatory diarrhea	Fecal Polymorphonuclear leukocytes; substantial increase in fecal lactoferrin	Shigella spp., Salmonella spp., Campylobacter jejuni, enterohemorrhagic E. coli, enteroinvasive E. coli, Yersinia enterocolitica, Vibrio parahaemolyticus, Clostridium difficile, Entamoeba histolytica
Penetrating	Distal small bowel	Enteric fever	Fecal mononuclear leukocytes	Salmonella typhi, Y. enterocolitica, Campylobacter fetus

41. **Ans. (d)** *P. falciparum*

   Man is intermediate host (Secondary) in:
   - *Plasmodium*
   - *Toxoplasma gondii*
   - *Echinococcus granulosus* [dog tapeworm/hydatid worm/*Taenia echinococcus*]
   - *Sarcocystis lindemanni*
   - *T. solium* (man also act as definitive host).

42. **Ans. (b) and (d)** *Klebsiella* and *Cryptococcus*

   Capsulated bacterias are:
   - **Pn**eumonococcus
   - **Kl**eibsella
   - **Ye**rsinia
   - N. **Me**ningococci
   - **V**ibrio parahemolyticus
   - Bacillus **an**thrax
   - H. **in**fluenza
   - **Bo**rdetella
   - **Cl**. Perfringe's and butyricum

   Mnemonic: PAKIYB - M.C.V

   Remember : Capsulated fungi is *Cryptococcus neofomans* not *Histoplasma capsulatum*.

43. **Ans. (a) Viral interference**   Ref. Ananthanarayan 10/e, p 442

   Viral interference

   "Interference in which infection of a cell by one virus inhibits simultaneous or subsequent infection by another virus."
   - *Most important* mediator of interference is *interferon*.
   - Interference produced by destruction of cell receptors is seen *with myxoviruses and enterovirus*.

   It is *applied* in the field in *controlling poliomyelitis* outbreaks by introducing into the population, the live attenuated poliovirus vaccine.

   Remember: Interference is *Nongenetic interaction*.

44. **Ans. (b) Capsid**   Ref. Ananthanarayan 10/e, p 434

   "*Capsid is the protein coat which surrounds nucleic acid (RNA or DNA) of virus.*"
   - Capsid + enclosed nucleic acid is known as nucelocapsid.
   - *Function of capsid is:*
     – To *protect the* nucleic acid from inactivation by nucleases and other deleterious agents in the environment.
     – To *introduce viral genome into host cells* by adsorbing readily to cell surfaces.
   - *On the basis of shape capsid can be:*
     – Icosahedral   : Herpes virus, Adenovirus, Poliovirus
     – Helical   : Rabies virus
     – Complex   : Pox virus

45. **Ans. (a, b, c, e) Rotavirus, Norwalk Virus, Adenovirus, Enterovirus** *See below*

Virus causing diarrhea	
• Adenovirus • Rotavirus (MC) • Adenovirus (Specially serotype 40 & 41) • Calcivirus • Corona virus	• Enterovirus • Norwalk virus • Astrovirus • Enterovirus

46. **Ans. (b) Calymmatobacterium granulomatis** *Ref. Ananthanarayan 10/e, p 404*

    "In donovanosis bacteria appear as round coccobacilli of 1-2 µm, with in cystic spaces inside large morphonuclear cells. They show bipolar condensation of chromatin, giving a safety pin appearance in stained smears".
    For details see Answer No. 52.

47. **Ans. (d) Mumps** *Ref. Jawetz 27/e 758*

    Virus can be successfully isolated from the CSF in:
    - Mumps virus
    - Herpers simplex meningitis
    - Enterovirus
    - JC virus

48. **Ans. (a; b; c) Polio; Pertussis; Salmonella typhi** *Ref. Park 22/e, p 154; 185, 213*

Human are the only reservoir for:	
• B. pertusis • V. Cholera • Enterovirus	• Polio • Salmonella typhi

49. **Ans. (b) Methenamine silver** *Ref. Ananthanarayan 10/e 596*

    Stains for fungi
    - Gomori methenamine silver (GMS) (**Better contrast**)
    - Periodic acid Schiff (PAS)
    - Alcian blue
    - Gridley fungus (GF)
    - Giemsa
    - Meyer's mucicarmine

    Out of these **GMS** is the *best stain for fungi*. For studying tissue response secondary to fungal infection, *Haematoxylin and eosin (H&E) is best.*

    > **Remember: Commonly used culture media for fungus are:**
    > - Sabouraud's glucose agar
    > - Corn meal agar
    > - Czapek - Dox medium

50. **Ans. (d) Haemophilus influenzae** *Ref. See below*

    H. influenzae is a gram (–)ve coccobacilli

Otitis media	Etiologic bacteria
Acute otitis media	Pneumococci > H. influenzae > Moraxella > Streptococcus pyogenes
Chronic otitis media	Staph aureus > Pseudomonas

    ... *Infectious disease by Nonathan 2/e, 856*

51. **Ans. (b) Enterovirus** *Ref. Nelson 18/e, p 2521*

    Viral Meningoencephalitis
    An acute inflammatory process involving the meninges and to a variable extent brain tissue.
    Etiology: Enterovirus (MC), Arbovirus, HSV-1, Mumps (in regions where mumps vaccine is not used), EBV, CMV
    Clinical features – Headache (most common), usually frontal or generalized. In adolescent retrobulbar pain is frequent
    – Fever, nausea, vomiting
    Lab finding
    - CSF shows mild mononuclear pleocytosis with absence of bacteremia
    - Detection of viral RNA or DNA by PCR is diagnostic

    Treatment – Symptomatic in all cases except in HSV meningoencephalitis where acyclovur is beneficial

    > **Note:**
    > - Enterovoirus is the MC cause of viral meningitis in mumps immunized population
    > - Enterovirus meningitis is particularly prevalent in infants < 3 months of age. Frequently implicated serotypes include Enterovirus 70 71, coxsackie 4, 6, 7, 9, 11

Miscellaneous

52. Ans. (a, c and d) i.e. Sypillis : 9-90 days, LGV: 3 day-6 weeks, Donovanosis: 1-4 weeks

Incubation period of common Sexually transmitted disease	
Chancroid (Hemophilus ducreyi)	1–14 days
Gonorrhea	2–30 days
Syphilis	10–90 days
Lymphogranuloma venereum (Chlamydia)	3–35 days
HIV	14 days to years
Genital herpes	2–14 days
Scabies	3–60 days
Granuloma inguinale	10–40 days

53. Ans. is (b) Plasmid mediated resistance is exclusively transferred vertically   *Ref: Goodman and Gilman's 12/e, p 1377-78*
- *Drug resistance is more commonly acquired by horizontal transfer.*
- Horizontal transfers occurs through transformation, transduction conjugation. It largely depends on mobile genetic elements like plasmids, bacteriophages. Other mobile elements like transposons, integrin's also participate in acquiring resistance.
- Once acquired resistance in transmitted vertically to its progeny.

Other options
Option 'a'   *...Goodman and Gillman 12/e, p 1541*
- Drug inactivation is a common mechanism of drug resistance. *Example:* Resistance to aminoglycosides and beta lactams are usually secondary to production of aminoglycoside modifying enzymes and beta lactams respectively

Option 'c'   *...Goodman and Gillmann 12/e, p 1541*
- Enterococcal resistance to glycopeptides (vancomycin and teicoplanin) is the result of alteration of the D-alanyl-D-alanine target to D-alanyl-D-lactate which bind glycopeptides poorly due to the lack of a critical site for hydrogen bonding.

Option 'd'   *...Harrison 18/e, p 1157*
- Penicillin resistance in pneumococci is due to alteration in PBP (penicillin binding protein), which is acquired by transformation through horizontal transfer gene from a related streptococci species.

54. Ans. is (c, d, e) Treponema pallidum, Pneumocystis jiroveci, Rhinosporidium seeberi
Ref Ananthanarayan 8/e, p 278, Harrison 18/e, p 1380

Klebsiella can be grown very well on ordinary media
For details see previous answers

55. Ans. is (c) Vibrio Cholerae *Ref Ananthanarayan 10/e, p 316*

Lipopolysaccharide O antigen (endotoxin) of V. Cholera plays no role in the pathogenesis of cholera, but is responsible for the immunity induced by killed vaccine.

Distinguishing features of exotoxins and endotoxins

Exotoxins	Endotoxins
• Proteins	Lipopolysaccharides
• Heat labile	Heat stable
• Actively secreted by cells; diffuse into surrounding medium	Form part of cell wall; do not diffuse into surrounding medium
• Readily separable from cultures by physical means such as filtration	Obtained only by cell lysis
• Action usually enzymic	No enzymic action
• Specific pharmacological effects for each exotoxin	Effect nonspecific; action common to all endotoxins
• Specific tissue affinities	No specific tissue affinity
• Active in very minute doses	Active only in very large doses
• Highly antigenic	Weakly antigenic
• Action specifically neutralized by antibody	Neutralization by antibody ineffective
• Can be toxoided	Can't toxoided
• Generally formed by gram positive including some gram negative *shigella, vibrio cholera,* ETEC, *V. parahemolyticus, Aeromonas Y. enterocolitica, P. aeroginosa*	Generally formed by gram negative bacteria

56. Ans. (d) Group B Streptococci   *Ref. Arch Dis Child Fetal Neonatal Ed2005;90:F220-FF224*

The pathogens most often implicated in neonatal sepsis in developing countries differ from those seen in developed countries:
- Overall, Gram negative organisms are more common and are mainly represented by Klebsiella, Escherichia coli, Pseudomonas, and Salmonella.
- Of the Gram positive organisms, Staphylococcus aureus, coagulase negative staphylococci (CONS), Streptococcus pneumoniae, and Streptococcus pyogenes are most commonly isolated.

Further it is stated that
Group B streptococcus (GBS) is generally rare or not seen at all, although maternal rectovaginal carriage rates of GBS may be similar to those recorded in developed countries.

> **Neonatal Sepsis**
> - **Neonatal sepsis** specifically refers to the presence of a bacteriamic infection (such as meningitis, pneumonia, pyelonephritis, or gastroenteritis) in the setting of fever in a newborn baby.
> - It is divided into two categories:
>   - Early Onset Sepsis (EOS): EOS refers to sepsis presenting in the first 7 days of life
>   - Late Onset Sepsis (LOS). with LOS referring to presentation of sepsis after 7 days
> - *Diagnosis:* Culturing for microorganisms from a sample of CSF, blood or urine, is the gold standard test for definitive diagnosis of neonatal sepsis.

Note: In western countries, Group B streptococci is the most common etiologic organism responsible for neonatal sepsis.

57. Ans. (b) Gomori Methanamine silver   *Ref. Chakraborty 2/e 617*

"Gomori Methenamine Silver (GMS) and Periodic acid-Schiff (PAS) are the two most common stains used to look for fungi in tissues and in cytology specimens."
- The GMS stain is more sensitive than the PAS stain as it stains both viable and non-viable fungal elements (which are refractory to other stains) but it stains inflammatory cells (lysosomes) and tissue reticulin too (in addition to fungi.) PAS staining has the slight advantage that the morphology of the tissue adjacent to the fungi can be better visualized, but this can be addressed using a GMS stain and H and E counterstain (which stains only tissue).

58. Ans. (d) To know how much amplification of DNA has occurred   *Ref. Jawetz 27/e, p 124; Greenwood 18/e 79*

Real Time PCR
- It is the molecular detection technique that discriminates real time amplification from conventional PCR assays.
- The real-time polymerase chain reaction (PCR) uses fluorescent reporter molecules to monitor the production of amplification products during each cycle of the PCR reaction.
- This combines the DNA amplification and detection steps into one homogeneous assay and obviates the requirement for gel electrophoresis to detect amplification products.
- Its simplicity, specificity, and sensitivity, together with its, more reliable instrumentation, and improved protocols, has made realtime PCR the benchmark technology for the detection of DNA.
- Real time PCR is extremely useful in medical microbiology, with greatest impact on virology.

59. Ans. (b, c, d) Botulinum toxin inhibits Ach release, Shiga toxin of shigella dysenteriae act by inhibiting protein synthesis, Diphtheria toxin act by inhibiting protein synthesis   *Ref. Greenwood 18/e p 165, Ananthanarayan 9/e, p 308, 264*

Bacterial Exotoxins
- These are the diffusible protein secreted into the external medium by the pathogen
- According to the mode of action bacterial exotoxin can be classified into:
  a. Type I (Membrane acting): Toxin bind surface receptors and stimulate transmembrane signals and include the super-antigenic toxins
  b. Type II (Membrane damaging): Toxin directly affect membranes, forming pores or disrupting lipid bilayers
  c. Type III (intracellular effector): Toxins translocate an active enzymatic component into the cell and modify an intracellular target molecule.

Mechanism of Action of Important Toxins	
↑ cAMP	Cholera toxin; E. coli heat liable toxin
↓ Acetylcholine release	Bolulinum toxin
↓ Protein synthesis	Diptheria toxin, Shigella toxin, Exotoxin A of pseudomonas
↑ cGMP	Heat stable toxin of E. coli

60. **Ans. (b) 24 hrs of antibiotic treatment** *Ref. Park 22/e 112*
    Patient of meningitis to be isolated until six hours of effective antibiotic therapy

Disease	Duration of isolation
Chickenpox	Until all lesion crusted (usually about 6 days after rash)
Measles	From the onset of catarrhal stage through third day of rash
Hepatitis A	3 weeks
Influenza	Till 3 days of onset
Polio	2 weeks adult; 6 weeks paediatrics
Tuberculosis	Until 3 weeks of effective chemotherapy
Herpes zoster	6 days after onset of rash
Mumps	Until swelling subsides
Pertussis	4 weeks or until paroxysms ceases
Pharyngitis	6 hours of effective antibiotic therapy

61. **Ans. (a) 3-12 days** *Ref. Ananthanarayan 9/2/e 421*
    Incubation period of Lymphogranuloma venereum range from 3 days to 5 weeks.
    For details see Answer 52

NEET Pattern Questions

1. **Eukaryotes are different in causing infection because:**
   a. Divide by binary fission
   b. Highly structured cell with organized cell organelles
   c. Donot have all organelles
   d. Evolutionally ancient *[Ref: Ananthanarayan 10/e p 10]*

2. **Ehrlichia chaffeensis is causative agents of:**
   a. HME
   b. HGE
   c. Glandular fever
   d. None *[Ref: Ananthanarayan 10/e p 416]*

- HME refers to human monocytic ehrlichiosis caused by Ehrlichia chaffeensis. It is transmitted by Amblyomma ticks. Deer and rodents are the reservoir hosts.

Ehrlichia
- Small, Gram negative obligate intracellular bacteria which have an affinities towards blood cells.
- They grow within phagosomes as mulberry like clusters and are transmitted by ticks.

Pathogenicity
- Human Monocytic Ehrlichiosis: Caused by E. chaffeenisis.
- Human granulocytic Ehrlichiosis: Causes by E. equi.
  - In both conditions there is thrombocytopenia and leukopenis.
- Glandular Fever: Caused by Ehrlichia sennetsu
  - There is lymphoid hyperplasia with atypical lymphocytosis.
- Doxycline is the treatments of choice.

3. **Correct order of Gram staining is:**
   [Ref: Ananthanarayan 10/e p 13]
   a. Gention violet → Iodine Carbol → fuchsin
   b. Iodine → Gention violet → Carbol fuchsin
   c. Carbol fuchsin → Iodine → Gention violet
   d. Carbol fuchsin → Gention violet → iodine

Gram staining procedure.
- Primary staining with pararosaniline dye such as crystal violet methyl violet and gentian violet.
- Application of dilute solution of iodine.
- Decolourisation with an organic solvents such as ethanol, acetone or aniline.
- Counter staining with a dye of contrasting colour such as carbol fuchsin safranine or neutral red.

4. **Not a component of Gram stain:**
   [Ref: Ananthanarayan 10/e, p 13]
   a. Methylene blue   b. Ethanol
   c. Iodine   d. Gentian violet

5. **Which part of bacteria is most antigenic:**
   [Ref: Ananthanarayan 10/e, p 89]
   a. Protein coat
   b. Lipopolysaccharide
   c. Nucleic acid
   d. Lipids

6. **Which of the following is a protist:**
   a. Algae
   b. Fungi
   c. Proteus
   d. Bacteria

7. **Non-motile organism:** *[Ref. Ananthanarayan 10/e, p 286]*
   a. E. coli   b. Vibrio cholera
   c. Salmonella   d. Klebsiella

Motile bacteria	
Polar Flagella	**Peri-trichous flagella**
• Vibrio	• E.coli
• Pseudomonas	• Proteus
• H. pylori	• Listeria monocytogenes
• Campylobactor	• All clostridia except Cl. perfringens and and Cl. tetani VI
• Spirochetes	• Bacillus except B. anthrax
• Legionella	• Salmonella except S. gallinarum-pullorum

8. **Flagella not true:** *[Ref. Ananthanarayan 10/e, p 19]*
   a. Locomotion
   b. Attachment
   c. Protein in nature
   d. Antigenic

Flagella is made up of protein called by flagellin, similar to keratin or myosin
- Because of their proteinecious nature they are antigenic.

9. **Which of the following organisms does not enter through abrasions in the skin:** *[See below]*
   a. E. rhusiopathiae
   b. E. corrodens
   c. C. hominis
   d. C. violaceum

Ans.
1. b. Highly....   2. a. HME   3. a. Gention violet...   4. a. Methylene blue
5. a. Protein coat   6. c. Proteus   7. d. Klebsiella   8. b. Attachment
9. c. C. hominis

Organisms entering the body through breaks in the skin or mucous membranes.

Aerobic and facultative microorganisms	Anaerobic bacteria	Aerobic microorganism from unusual, specialized and zonotif infections	Yeast
• Coagulase negative staphylococci • Staphylococcus aureus • Enterococcus spp. • Streptococcus viridans • Coryncbacterium spp. • Bacillus cereus • E.coli • Serratia • Enterobactor • Proteus • Morganella • Pseudomona • Acinetobactor	• Peptostreptococcus spp. • Clostridium spp. • Ebacterium limposum • Bacteriodes fragilis • Prevotella spp. • Prophyromonas • Fusobacterium • Villonella spp.	• Actinobacillus actinomyceteracomitans • Aeromonas spp. • Bacillus anthracis • Bergeyella zoohelcum • Chromobacterium violaceum • Eikenella corrodens • Erysipalothrix rhusiopathial • Francisella tularensis • Haemophillus spp. • Kingella kingae • Pasteurella multocida • Streptobacillus moniliformis • Vibro vulnificus	• Candida albicans • Candida krusei • Candida parapsilosis

10. **True about exotoxin:**
    a. Non-antigenic b. Enzymatic
    c. Non-protein   d. Heat stable
    [Ref. Ananthanarayan 10/e, p 77]

11. **Smallest virus is:**
    a. Herpes virus b. Adenovirus
    c. Parvovirus   d. Poxviurs
    [Ref. Ananthanarayan 10/e, p 558]

12. **KOH wet mount is prepared for:**
    a. Herpes zoster b. Candida
    c. Gonorrhea   d. Trichomonas vaginalis
    [Ref. Ananthanarayan 10/e, p 596]

KOH wet amount digest cell and other tissue material and thus aid in better visualization of fungi

13. **Thermophile bacteria grow at:**
    a. 20°C   b. 20–40°C
    c. 20–60°C   d. 60–80°C
    [Ref. Ananthanarayan 10/e, p 25]

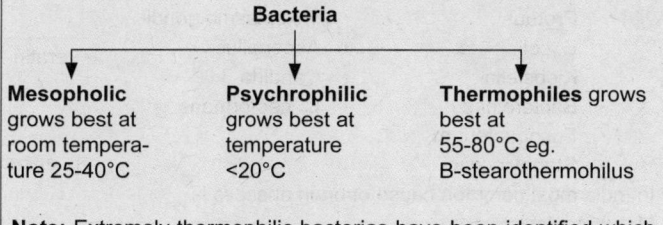

Note: Extremely thermophilic bacterias have been identified which can grow at temperature as high as 250°C

14. **Healthy carriers are seen in all except:**
    a. Polio   b. Meningocpcci
    c. Measles   d. Cholera
    [Ref. Park 22/e, p 92]

15. **Rash is not caused by:** [Ref. Harrison 19/e, p 128]
    a. Salmonella
    b. Shigella
    c. Meningococci
    d. Staphylococcus

16. **Which vaccine can cause adverse effects in persons with allergy to egg:**
    a. Measles   b. Rubella
    c. Rabies   d. Mumps

Vaccines that contain small quantities of egg protein can cause hypersensitivity reactions in some peoples with allergies to egg. Vaccine containing egg component are:
• MMR vaccine
• MMRV vaccine
• Influenzae vaccine
• Yellow fever vaccine
• RabAvert rabies vaccine
• Yellow fever vaccine

17. **Pediculus humanus can transmitt:**
    a. Sleeping sickness
    b. Plague
    c. Chagas disease
    d. Relapsing fever   [Ref. Park 22/e, p 712]

 | 10. **b.** Enzymatic | 11. **c.** Parvovirus | 12. **b.** Candida | 13. **d.** 60–80°C |
| 14. **c.** Measles | 15. **b.** Shigella | 16. **c.** Rabies | 17. **c.** Chagas disease |

18. Southern blotting is used for:
    a. RNA   b. DNA
    c. Protein   d. Antibody

Southern blot: Used for defecting specific DNA sequence in DNA samples.
Western blot: Used to detect specific protein
Northern blot: Used to detect specific RNA
Eastern blot: Used to analyze protein post translational modifications such as lipids.
Southwestern blot: Used to identifying and characterizing DNA binding proteins.

19. Stain use for staining degenerated fungi in tissue is:
    [Ref: Greenwood 18/e 619]
    a. PAS   b. Gomori methamine silver
    c. H and E   d. Muciramine

Gomori-Methenamine silver (GMS) and periodic acid-schiff (PAS) are the two most common stains used to look for fungi in tissues and in cytology specimens

20. Disease transmitted from men to animals:
    a. Antropozoonoses   b. Zooanthroponoses
    c. Amphixenoses   d. Aptozoonoses
    [Ref. Park 22/e, p 19]

Anthropozoonosis: Infection transmitted to man from vertebrate animals eg. rabies.
Zooanthroponoses: Infection transmitted from man to vertebrate animals.
Amphinosis: Infection maintained in both man and lower vertebrate animals that may be transmitted in either direction e.g. T. Cruzi.

21. All are true about chromobacterium violaceum *except*:
    a. Gram negative   [Ref. Ananthanarayan 10/e, p 404]
    b. Produces violet-colored pigment
    c. Normal flora in human
    d. Causes cellulitis

Chromobacterium violaceum
- Gram negative nonsporing bacillus
- Motile with lateral flagella
- Facultative anaerobes growing on ordinary media and produce violet pigment
- Human infections are recorded in tropics and consist of multiple abscess, cellulites, pyemia.

22. Phenol test or Reidel Walker test is done to determine:
    a. Hardness of water   [Ref. Ananthaarayar 10/e 35]
    b. Chlorine demand
    c. Quality of disinfectant
    d. Efficacy of a disinfectants

Reidel Walker test is done to determine the efficacy of a disinfectant in the terms of phenol. The dilution of disinfectant which sterilizes the suspension in a given time, divided by the corresponding dilution of phenol and is stated as phenol coefficient of the said disinfectant.

23. Gram-negative bacteria doesn't take Gram stain because it is made of: [Ref. Greenwood 18/e, p 14; DR Arora 3/e, p 41]
    a. Polysaccharide   b. Lipopolysaccharide
    c. Techoic acid   d. None of the above

- The exact mechanism of Gram reaction is not known. The possible reason are:
  - Gram positive bacteria have a more acidic protoplasm, which account for their retaining the basic primary dye more strongly.
  - Dye iodine complex is retained in gram positive cells by thick peptido glycan mesh and is readily wash through the very thin peptidoglycan layer of gram – ve cells.

24. Which is always present in bacteria?
    [Ref. Ananthanarayan 10/e, p 16]
    a. Cell wall   b. Cytoplasmic membrane
    c. Mitochondria   d. Nucleoli

25. Which of the following does not possess both DNA and RNA? [Ref. Ananthanarayan 10/e, p 18]
    a. Bacteria   b. Fungus
    c. Virus   d. Spirochete

- RNA containing virus are called ribovirus.
- DNA containing virus are called deoxyribovirus.

26. Brain abscess in immunodeficient person is due to:
    [Ref. Harrison 18/e, p 3428]
    a. Cryptococcus   b. Staphylococcus
    c. Pneumococcus   d. E. coli

Etiology of Brain Abscess

Immunocompetent	Immunodeficient
Streptococcus	Nocardia
Proteus	Toxoplasma gondii
E. coli	Aspergillus
Klebsiella	Candida
Bacteroides	C. neoformans
Fusobacterium	
Staphylococci	

In India most common cause of brain abscess is M. tuberculosis

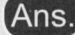

18. b. DNA	19. a, b; PAS, Gomori..	20. b. Zooanthroponoses	21. c. Normal flora...
22. d. Efficacy of a...	23. d. None...	24. b. Cytoplasmic ...	25. c. Virus
26. a. Cryptococcus			

SECTION C

Emerging Diseases

- Swine Flu
- Zika Virus

Swine Flu

CHAPTER 40

Swine influenza (also called **Pig influenza, swine flu, hog flu and pig flu**) is an infection by any one of several types of swine influenza virus. **Swine influenza virus (SIV) or S-OIV (swine-origin influenza virus)** is any strain of the influenza family of viruses that is endemic in pigs. The known SIV strains include influenza C and the subtypes of influenza A known as **H1N1**, H1N2, H3N1, H3N2, and H2N3.

The **2009 flu pandemic** is a global outbreak of a new strain of H1N1 influenza virus. It was first detected in April 2009, contains a **combination of genes** from swine, avian (bird), and human influenza viruses.

The outbreak began in Veracruz, Mexico. The pandemic virus is a type of swine influenza, derived originally from a strain that lived in pigs and this origin gave rise to the common name of "swine flu". However, despite its origin in pigs, this strain is transmitted between people and not from swine to people. The United States Secretary of Agriculture made clear that despite its common name being "swine flu", there is no risk of contracting flu from eating cooked pork products.

TRANSMISSION

Transmission between pigs
- Influenza is common in pigs, about half of breeding pigs have been exposed to influenza.
- The main route of transmission is through direct contact between infected and uninfected animals. Airborne transmission through the aerosols produced by pigs coughing or sneezing are also an important means of infection.
- However, pigs are unusual as they can be infected with influenza strains of different species: pigs, birds and humans. *This makes pigs a host where influenza viruses might exchange genes, producing new and dangerous strains.*

Transmission to humans
- People who work with poultry and swine, especially people with intense exposures, are at increased risk of zoonotic infection with influenza virus
- Other professions at particular risk of infection are veterinarians and meat processing workers, although the risk of infection for both of these groups is lower than that of farm workers.

Transmission in 2009 pandemic
- In human H1N1 virus spread occur in the same way that seasonal flu spreads. Flu viruses are spread mainly from person to person through coughing or sneezing by people with H1N1 infection.
- Sometimes people may become infected by touching something – such as a surface or object – with flu viruses on it and then touching their mouth or nose.
- *The basic reproduction number* (the average number of other individuals that each infected individual will infect, in a population that has no immunity to the disease) for the 2009 novel H1N1 is estimated to be 1.75

Signs and Symptoms

The symptoms of swine flu are similar to other influenzas, and include fever, cough (*typically a "dry cough"*), headache, muscle or joint pain, sore throat, chills, fatigue, and runny nose. Diarrhea, vomiting, and neurological problems have also been reported in some cases.

People at higher risk of serious complications include:
- Age over 65, children younger than 5
- Children with neurodevelopmental conditions
- Pregnant women (especially during the third trimester)
- Underlying medical conditions, such as asthma, diabetes, obesity, heart disease, or a weakened immune system.

Symptoms in severe cases
The World Health Organization reports that the clinical picture in severe cases is strikingly different from the disease pattern. In severe cases, patients generally begin to deteriorate around 3 to 5 days after symptom onset. Deterioration is rapid, with many patients progressing to respiratory failure within 24 hours.

A November 2009 CDC recommendation stated that the following constitute "emergency warning signs" which demands urgent hospitalization include:

In adults:
- Difficulty breathing or shortness of breath
- Pain or pressure in the chest or abdomen
- Sudden dizziness
- Confusion
- Severe or persistent vomiting
- Low temperature

In children:
- Fast breathing or working hard to breathe
- Bluish skin color
- Not drinking enough fluids
- Not waking up or not interacting
- Being so irritable that the child does not want to be held
- Flu-like symptoms that improve but then return with fever and worse cough
- Fever with a rash
- Being unable to eat
- Having no tears when crying

Diagnosis

Confirmed diagnosis of pandemic H1N1/09 flu requires testing of a nasopharyngeal, nasal, or oropharyngeal tissue swab from the patient. Real-time RT-PCR is the recommended test as others are unable to differentiate between pandemic H1N1/09 and regular seasonal flu.

Treatment

- A number of methods have been recommended to help ease symptoms, including adequate liquid intake and rest.
- Over-the-counters pain medications such as acetaminophen and ibuprofen do not kill the virus, but reduce symptoms. Aspirin and other salicylate products should not be used with any flu-type symptoms because of the risk of developing Reye's Syndrome.
- If the fever is mild and there are no other complications, fever medication is not recommended.
- People in at-risk groups should be treated with antivirals (oseltamivir or zanamivir) as soon as possible when they first experience flu symptoms. Antivirals are most useful if given within 48 hours of the start of symptoms and may improve outcomes in hospitalized patients
- Normal individuals who have persistent or rapidly worsening symptoms should also be treated with antivirals.
- If oseltamivir (Tamiflu) is unavailable or cannot be used zanamivir (Relenza) is recommended as a substitute. Peramivir is another antiviral drug approved for hospitalized patients in cases where the other drugs are ineffective or unavailable.

PREVENTION

Vaccine

Two types of influenza vaccines are available:
- TIV [Flu shot (injection) of trivalent (three strains; usually A/H1N1, A/H3N2, and B) inactivated (killed) vaccine] or
- LAIV [nasal spray (mist) of live attenuated influenza vaccine.]
  - LAIV is not recommended for individuals under age 2 or over age 50, but might be comparatively more effective among children over age 2.
  - Children through 9 years of age should get two doses of vaccine, about a month apart. Older children and adults need only one dose.

Zika Virus

CHAPTER 41

INTRODUCTION

Zika virus is an emerging mosquito-borne virus that was first identified in Uganda in 1947 in rhesus monkeys through a monitoring network of sylvatic yellow fever. It was subsequently identified in humans in 1952 in Uganda and the United Republic of Tanzania. Outbreaks of Zika virus disease have been recorded in Africa, the Americas, Asia and the Pacific.

Etiology
- Zika virus is single stranded RNA virus belongs to family flavii virus.
- **Vector**: Aedes mosquitoes (which usually bite during the morning and late afternoon/evening hours)
- **Reservoir:** Unknown

Signs and Symptoms
- The incubation period (not known exactly), but is likely to be a few days.
- The symptoms are similar to other arbovirus infections such as dengue, and include fever, skin rashes, conjunctivitis, muscle and joint pain, malaise, and headache. These symptoms are usually mild and last for 2-7 days.
- Enhances the risk of Guillain-Barré syndrome
- There are evidences that Zika virus enhances the chances of microcephaly if infection is acquired in pregnancy

Transmission
- Zika virus is transmitted to people through the bite of an infected mosquito from the Aedes genus, mainly Aedes aegypti in tropical regions.
- Sexual transmission of Zika virus has also been described.

Diagnosis
- Infection with Zika virus may be suspected based on symptoms and recent history (e.g. residence or travel to an area where Zika virus is known to be present).
- Zika virus diagnosis can only be confirmed by laboratory testing for the presence of Zika virus RNA in the blood or other body fluids, such as urine or saliva.

Treatment
- Zika virus disease is usually relatively mild and requires no specific treatment.
- People sick with Zika virus should get plenty of rest, drink enough fluids, and treat pain and fever with common medicines.
- If symptoms worsen, they should seek medical care and advice. There is currently no vaccine available.

Prevention
- As disease is transmitted through mosquito bite, prevention and control relies on reducing mosquitoes.
- This can be done by using insect repellent regularly; wearing clothes (preferably light-coloured) that cover as much of the body as possible; using physical barriers such as window screens, closed doors and windows;
- People (particularly pregnant females) should avoid travelling in areas with out break or if at all necessary travellers should take the basic precautions described above to protect themselves from mosquito bites.